T0275549

Textbook of Traditional Chinese Medicine

Yong Huang • Lifang Zhu

Editors

Textbook of Traditional Chinese Medicine

Volume 2: Chinese Materia Medica,
Prescription, Acupuncture and Moxibustion,
Other Therapies and Common Diseases

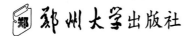 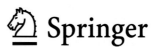 Springer

Editors
Yong Huang
School of Traditional Chinese Medicine
Southern Medical University
Guangzhou, China

Lifang Zhu
College of International Education
Jining Medical University
Jining, China

ISBN 978-981-99-5298-4   ISBN 978-981-99-5299-1   (eBook)
https://doi.org/10.1007/978-981-99-5299-1

Jointly published with Zhengzhou University Press
The print edition is not for sale in China (Mainland). Customers from China (Mainland) please order the print book from: Zhengzhou University Press.

This Springer imprint is published by the registered company Springer Nature Singapore Pte Ltd.
The registered company address is: 152 Beach Road, #21-01/04 Gateway East, Singapore 189721, Singapore

Paper in this product is recyclable

Editorial Committee

Preface

This is a textbook on traditional Chinese medicine (TCM) for international MBBS students studying in universities and colleges in China.

The Belt and Road Development Plan of TCM (2016–2020) was put forward to implement the *Vision and Action on Jointly Building Silk Road Economic Belt and the twenty-first Century Maritime Silk Road (the Belt and Road, BandR)*, issued by the National Development and Reform Commission, Ministry of Foreign Affairs, and Ministry of Commerce of the People's Republic of China, with State Council authorization in March 2015. We aim to enhance communication and strengthen cooperation with foreign countries and create a new pattern of all-facet opening up in the TCM field. Nowadays, TCM has been spread to 183 countries and regions. As an important part of the international medical system, TCM is playing an active role in protecting human health.

In order to introduce TCM with its unique advantages to the world and make contribution to human health cause, Zhengzhou University Press organized the compilation of this English textbook to promote and spread TCM culture.

TCM is a comprehensive discipline, including fundamental theories of TCM, diagnostics of TCM, Chinese materia medica, prescription, acupuncture and moxibustion, traditional Chinese tuina and clinical discipline such as internal medicine, surgery, gynecology, and pediatric of TCM. All these essential parts of TCM are included in this textbook. We cover all the contents from theoretical basis to clinical practice comprehensively, which are under the guideline of classic inheritance and the essence of TCM. The clinical practical parts are also emphasized to enable students to turn knowledge into useful skills. Different topics are designed in detail or briefly under a systematical framework, while practical clinical skills and information are highlighted comparatively.

This is a TCM textbook in English compiled by 36 teachers and experts in universities, colleges, and hospitals with experiences of teaching in English to ensure the accuracy of TCM theory and language expression. During the compilation, drafts were modified, revised, and collated with the help of a great number of professors. Traditional methods and modern pattern of compiling are adopted, including introduction, overview, text segment, summary, reflective problems, references, and so on.

In this textbook, philosophical foundation, physiology and pathology, etiology, differentiation and diagnostics, health preservation of TCM, Chinese materia medica and prescription, acupuncture and moxibustion, characteristic therapies, and common clinical diseases are systematically arranged. From Chaps. 1 to 4, a clear picture of the philosophical foundation of TCM from yin-yang, five-element, qi, blood, body fluids, and zang-fu viscera theory is presented. Chapters 5–7 include etiology, pathogenesis, diagnostic and differentiation of syndromes. Chapter 8 is one of the most popular chapters with a topic of health preservation. Chapters 9, 10 are about Chinese materia medica and prescription, presenting the tropism of natures, flavors and meridians, as well as commonly used prescription. Acupuncture and moxibustion therapy is the topic of Chap. 11; meridians and acupoints and acupuncture techniques are explained systematically and thoroughly. Chapter 12 is about some particular therapies such as massage, dietary therapy, qigong, and Tai Chi. Chapter 13 mainly presents clinical TCM therapies of common diseases. And the last chapter is appendix which provides supplementary materials as references.

Prof. Chunzhi Tang, dean of Clinical Medical College of Acupuncture, Moxibustion and Rehabilitation, Guangzhou University of TCM, is the chief reviser of the compilation board. Prof. Yong Huang, director of Acupuncture and Moxibustion Department, School of TCM, Southern Medical University, and Prof. Lifang Zhu, vice director of International Exchanges and Cooperation Department, Jining Medical University, are chief editors in charge of the compilation. All the editorial board members worked hard with clear division and efficient cooperation of work in compiling this textbook.

It is a great challenge to compile an English textbook of TCM. If you find any errors or mistakes that might exist in the textbook, please do not hesitate to let us know. We are always open to suggestions and comments, and strive to improve it for a new edition.

Chief Reviser: Chunzhi Tang

Chief Editors: Yong Huang and Lifang Zhu

Guangzhou, China   Yong Huang
Jining, China   Lifang Zhu

Contents

Chapter 1
Basic Knowledge of Chinese Materia Medica

Min Sun, Fengting Zhai, Guanli Song, Zhinan Zhang, and Yong Huang

Objectives

Master four properties (cold, hot, warm, and cool) and five flavors (sour, bitter, sweet, pungent, and salty), four directions (ascending, descending, floating, and sinking), meridian entry, toxicity, and indications of the common Chinese medicine.

Get familiar with the theory properties and effects, compatibility, and contraindication of Chinese medicine.

Know the purpose and methods of processing.

Guideline

This chapter focuses on the basic theories and clinical applications of Chinese medicine. It is composed of the general and specific introduction to Chinese medicine. In the general introduction, it covers the common theory about the habitat and collection, processing, properties and effects, compatibility, and contraindication of Chinese medicine. In the specific introduction, according to the main effect, the special discussions classify the common Chinese medicine and chose several representatives to introduce in detail in which the source of each Chinese medicines and their properties, flavor, meridian entry, usage, dosage, precautions, and so on are presented. Others will be listed in a table as reference.

M. Sun
Jining Medical University, Jining, China

F. Zhai
Shandong University of Traditional Chinese Medicine, Jinan, Shandong, China

G. Song
Guang'anmen Hospital, Beijing, China

Z. Zhang
Southern Medical University, Guangzhou, China

Y. Huang (✉)
School of Traditional Chinese Medicine, Southern Medical University, Guangzhou, China

© Zhengzhou University Press 2024
Y. Huang, L. Zhu (eds.), *Textbook of Traditional Chinese Medicine*,
https://doi.org/10.1007/978-981-99-5299-1_1

1.1 Introduction

For thousands of years, Chinese materia medica as the main weapon in the prevention and treatment of disease of the human body and mind has made great contributions to the prosperity of Chinese. Chinese materia medica is a major aspect of traditional Chinese medicine, which focuses on restoring a balance of yin-yang and qi-blood to maintain health rather than treating a particular disease or medical condition.

The vast majority of Chinese medicines are originally produced in China, but even a natural medicine coming from China cannot be called Chinese materia medica. The understanding and application of the Chinese materia medica have a unique theoretical system and application form, which must be based on the theory of traditional Chinese medicine.

Chinese medicines mainly come from natural medicine and its processed products, including plants, animals, mineral medicine, and some chemical and biological drugs. Because plants medicines are the most of the Chinese medicines, as a result, Chinese materia medica has often been called "Bencao" from ancient times.

1.2 Habitat and Collection

Most of the Chinese medicines come from plants, so the production areas and acquisition time are important factors influencing the quality and effectiveness. Chinese ancient doctors attached great importance to this crucial aspect and accumulated rich experience in practice. Modern researches indicate that producing areas and acquisition time are closely related to the type and contents of effective components of Chinese medicine.

1.2.1 Habitat

As for the place of production, the ecological environment such as climate, sunlight, humidity, temperature, and soil in different areas varies considerably. Thus, the quality of Chinese medicine is diverse. A lot of Chinese medicines are known for their origins, from which we know the great significance of producing area. The concept of famous-region drug has gradually formed since *Tang* and *Song* dynasties. It refers to the excellent varieties of Chinese medicine with an obvious regional character, growing environment, reasonable cultivation and processing, concentrated production, large amount of output, and a quality superior to those produced in other regions. In a word, it refers to high-quality Chinese medicines with special regions (Table 1.1).

1.2.2 Collection

In terms of collection period, Chinese medicines should be harvested in different periods of growth. Effective and harmful ingredients of medicinal parts are unequal in different phases; consequently, the efficacy and side effects have considerable differences. Therefore, collecting them properly is crucial to guarantee the quality and clinical effect of Chinese medicine (Table 1.2).

Table 1.1 Examples of famous-region drugs

Areas	Famous-region drugs
Sichuan Province	Huanglian (Rhizoma coptidis), Dahuang (radix et Rhizoma rhei), Chuanxiong (Rhizoma Ligustici Chuanxiong), and Fuzi (Radix Aconiti Lateralis Preparata)
Henan Province	Dihuang (Radix Rehmanniae), Shanyao (Rhizoma Dioscoreae), Juhua (Flos Chrysanthemi), and Niuxi (Radix Achyranthis Bidentatae)
Northeast of China	Renshen (Radix Ginseng), Xixin (Herba Asari), and Wuweizi (Fructus Schisandrae Chinensis)
Guangdong Province	Sharen (Fructus Amomi Villosi), Chenpi (Pericarpium Citri Reticulatae), Huoxiang (Herba Pogostemonis), and Dilong (Lumbricus)
Yunnan Province	Fuling (Poria) and Sanqi (Radix Notoginseng)
Shandong Province	Ejiao (Colla Corii Asini)
Ningxia Province	Gouqizi (Fructus Lycii)

Table 1.2 Collection period of different Chinese medicine

Category		Time	Example
Plant medicine	Whole plant	The period before the blossom or the early period of blossom when the branches and leaves are thriving	Yimucao (Herba Leonuri), Jingjie (Herba Schizonepetae)
	Leaf	The bud period or the full blooming period	Pipaye (Folium Eriobotryae), Aiye (Folium Artemisiae Argyi)
		Late autumn or early winter after frost hit (exception)	Sangye (Folium Mori)
	Flower	The period when they are flower bud or just blooming	Jinyinhua (Flos Lonicerae), Juhua
	Pollen	The full blooming period	Puhuang (Pollen Typhae)
	Fruit	Period when they are going to be	Chenpi, Shanzha (Fructus Crataegi)
		Period when they are mature	Qingpi (Pericarpium Citri Reticulatae Viride), Zhishi (Fructus Aurantii Immaturus)
	Seed	Period when they are mature	Lianzi (Semen Nelumbinis), Gouqizi
	Roots and rhizome	Early spring or late autumn (February or August)	Gegen (Radix Puerariae), Tianma (Rhizoma Gastrodiae)
		Summer (exception)	Banxia (Rhizoma Pinelliae), Yanhusuo (Rhizoma Corydalis)
	Tree buck, root buck	The exuberant growth period of plants (spring or summer)	Huangbai (Cortex Phellodendri), Du Zhong (Cortex Eucommiae)
		After autumn (exception)	Mudanpi (Cortex Moutan Radicis), Digupi (Cortex Lycii)
Animal medicine		Collecting medicine depends on animals' growth and active period to ensure effect	Quanxie (Scorpio), Dilong (Lumbricus), Lurong (Cornu Cervi Pantotrichum), Muli (Concha Ostreae)
Mineral medicine		Any time appropriate	Cishi (Magnetitum), Daizheshi (Haematitum)

1.3   Processing

Processing refers to the process of preparation and manufacturing for Chinese medicines before utilizing or making into other various forms. It includes common treatment of crude medicine or special process of some medicinal materials. This process is important to guarantee the efficacy, medication safety, and preparation.

1.3.1 Purpose of Processing

According to the characteristics of Chinese medicine and the principle of safety and effectiveness, the purpose of processing mainly includes the following four aspects (Table 1.3).

1.3.2 Methods of Processing

Commonly used methods of processing for Chinese medicine are discussed in Table 1.4.

In addition, other adjuvants are often added during processing. Commonly used adjuvant can be divided into liquid adjuvant and solid adjuvant.

Liquid adjuvant includes wine, vinegar, honey, ginger juice, and sesame oil; solid adjuvant includes alum, salt, rice, and bran.

Table 1.3 Purpose of processing

Purpose	Significance	Example
Improving therapeutic effects	Increasing the effective components of the stripping and content or producing new ingredient and enhancing the efficacy of medicine. It is the most common purpose	Frying Chuanxiong Danggui (Radix Angelicae Sinensis) with wine can promote the function of activating blood circulation (add adjuvant material); frying seed Chinese medicine like Juemingzi (Semen Cassiae) and Laifuzi (Semen Raphani) can break their surface to promote the effective components stripping
Reducing toxicity, drastic properties, and side effects	Changing or reducing the toxicity, drastic properties and side effects of some Chinese medicine to ensure safety	Chuanwu (Radix Aconiti), Caowu (Radix Aconiti Kusnezoffii), and Fuzi contain toxic ingredient aconitine which changes to aconine after processing with largely reduced toxicity
Modifying properties and effects	By changing Chinese medicinal meridian entry, four properties, five flavors, four directions to change or broaden the scope of application	In terms of sweating, prepared Mahuang (Herba Ephedrae) is not as good as Mahuang, so it is applied to the disease not for sweating. Sheng Di Huang (Radix Rehmanniae Recens) has cold property to clear heat and cool blood; it turns into Shudihuang (Radix Rehmanniae Preparata) after steaming processing with warm property to tonify blood
Facilitating decocting, making preparation, and storing	Purifying medicine, taking away the impurity, making Chinese medicine herbal tablets, or preserved by drying, which aids the storage of Chinese medicine and preserves effectiveness	Sangpiaoxiao (Oötheca Mantidis) is processed by steaming to kill the egg and made easier to store

Table 1.4 Methods of processing

Methods of processing	Definitions	Examples
Purifying and cutting	In preparation for further processing, preserving, blending, and pharmaceutical preparation	Discarding, impurity, breaking into fine pieces, and cutting
Processing with water	Processing Chinese medicine with water of low temperature or other methods. The purpose of water processing is to clean the medicine and lower the toxicity or soften the Chinese medicine to be cut easily	Rinsing, washing, soaking, splashing, and power-refining method with water (refining and getting the fine powder by grinding the insoluble and minerals in water)
Processing with fire	Fire processing is to warm the Chinese medicine directly or parch the Chinese medicine with little liquid or solid adjuvant	Parching, stir-frying with liquid, burning, calcining, and roasting in hot ashes
Processing with both water and fire	Both water and fire should be used in this method	Steaming, boiling, blanching, and stewing
Other processing method		Frost-like powder preparation and fermentation germination

1.4 Properties and Effects

The properties and effects of Chinese medicine also referred to as "medicinal preferences" by predecessors, which were highly summarized from the basic natures and characteristics of their effects relating to treatment, are the essential basis of the analyses and clinical usage of Chinese medicine. The basic principle of TCM treatment is to use medicinal preferences to rebalance the excess or deficiency of yin and yang, as well as the re-establish the functions of zang-fu viscera and meridians of the body, so as to achieve the therapeutic effects.

Properties and effects of the Chinese medicine include the five important aspects: four properties, five flavors, four directions (ascending, descending, floating, and sinking), meridian entry, and toxicity, which are of great significance in TCM practice.

1.4.1 Four Natures and Five Flavors

1.4.1.1 Four Natures

Four natures refer to the four properties of Chinese medicals, cold, hot, warm, and cool and are also called the "four xing" in TCM. Cold and cool or hot and warm are only varying in intensity, and cold-cool and warm-hot are two completely different

Table 1.5 Four natures and effects of Chinese medicine

Natures	Effects		Examples
Hot	Alleviate or eliminate cold syndrome	Superior at dispersing cold	Fuzi, Ganjiang (Rhizoma Zingiberis)
Warm		Weaker at dispersing cold	Mahuang, Guizhi (Ramulus Cinnamomi)
Cold	Alleviate or eliminate heat syndrome	Superior at clearing heat	Shigao (Gypsum Fibrosum), Huanglian
Cool		Weaker at clearing heat	Bohe (Herba Menthae), Danshen (Radix Salviae Miltiorrhizae)

categories of nature. Cool is inferior to cold, and cold-cool belonging to yin, whereas warm is inferior to hot, and warm-hot belonging to yang. In addition, sometimes some medicine are marked as extremely cold or hot, cold or hot, and slightly cold or hot.

Four natures are summarized mainly from the body's response after different Chinese medicines are taken, which can reflect the properties, cold or hot of the diseases treated. Medicines with cold-cool property can clear heat, purge fire, and remove heat toxin, which are mainly used for heat syndrome. On the contrary, medicines with warm-hot property can disperse cold and warm the middle and assist yang, which are mainly used for cold syndrome (Table 1.5).

When you apply medicine to treat heat or cold syndromes, respectively, with hot or cold medicine, you cannot achieve desired results of treatment and even bring about harmful results if you do not consider the properties of Chinese medicines, cold or hot.

In addition, there are also some Chinese medicines of neutral nature, medicinal preference of which for cold or hot are not so remarkable, and their properties and effects are relatively mild. But actually, they still have differences in the tendency to cool or warm, so they are still in the range of four natures.

1.4.1.2   Five Flavors

Five flavors refer to the five different medicinal tastes in a prescription—sour, bitter, sweet, pungent, and salty. As the characteristic of Chinese medicines, five flavors are summarized by ancient people not only from the actual and true taste of the Chinese medicine by the tongue, but more importantly from the clinical effect of Chinese medicine. So, five flavors demonstrate the basic range of effects of the medicine. Chinese medicines with same flavor mostly possess similar effects, while the Chinese medicines with different flavors show different effects in the treatment.

1. Pungent

    It has the functions of dispersing and promoting the circulation of qi and activating blood. Pungent medicines are generally indicated for exterior syndromes, syndromes of qi stagnation, and syndromes of blood stasis. For example, Shengjiang (Rhizoma Zingiberis Recens) and Bohe can produce the effects of inducing sweating to expel the exogenous pathogenic factors from the exterior, and Muxiang (Radix Aucklandiae) and Chenpi can circulate qi, and Chuanxiong and Honghua (Flos Carthami) can activate blood circulation.

2. Sweet

It has the effects of nourishing, harmonizing, and moderating. Sweet medicines are generally utilized for deficiency syndromes, spasm or pain in epigastric abdomen and limbs, and spleen-stomach disharmony syndrome. It can moderate toxic and violent property of other medicinal and blend taste. So, it is widely used in many prescriptions. For example, Huangqi (Radix Astragali seu Hedysari) and Renshen have nourishing effect, and Fengmi (Mel) and Gancao (Radix Glycyrrhizae) can moderate emergency and relieve spasm and pain and moderate toxic and violent property of many medicine.

3. Sour

It has the effects of consolidating, contracting, and astringing. Sour medicines are often used to treat collapse syndromes which are for the loss of essence due to deficiency of right qi, such as spontaneous sweating, night sweating, chronic cough, chronic diarrhea, seminal emission, and enuresis. For example, Wumei (Fructus Mume) and Wuweizi are used to relieve cough and diarrhea, and Shanzhuyu (Fructus Corni) are used to relieve emission and enuresis.

4. Bitter

It has the effects of purging and drying. Purging medicines are often used for clearing heat and purging fire, descending and purging, and purging and rushing down the bowels, heat syndromes, cough, vomit, and hiccup due to adverse rising of lung qi or stomach qi and constipation. For example, Huanglian, Huangqin (Radix Scutellariae), and Zhizi (Fructus Gardeniae) can clear away heat, Kuxingren (Armeniacae Semen Amarum) and Banxia can lower and disperse lung qi or stomach qi, and Dahuang and Mangxiao (Natrii Sulfas) can cause downward discharge. Drying means drying dampness and is used for damp syndromes, including cold-damp syndrome and dampness-heat syndrome. For example, Cangzhu (Rhizoma Atractylodis) and Yinchen (Herba Artemisiae Scopariae) are able to remove dampness.

5. Salty

It has the effects of purging and softening. Purging means that it is able to relieve constipation, while softening means that it can soften hardness and dissipate nodules. Salty medicines are often used to treat constipation and hard nodes or masses syndromes, such as scrofula, goiter, and phlegm nodule. For example, Mangxiao can relieve constipation by purgation, and Muli and Kunbu (Thallus Eckloniae) can disperse scrofula.

Five flavors are the basic tastes of medicine, and actually, the tastes are more than five kinds (Table 1.6). There are also astringent and bland flavors. Astringent flavor has the same effects with sour flavor. Bland flavor has the effects of promoting urination and draining dampness. But they are still included in the range of five flavors. People in ancient times held that bland flavor falls under the sweet and astringent

Table 1.6 Five flavors and effects of Chinese medicine

Flavor	Effects		Indications	Examples
Pungent	Disperse	Disperse	Exterior syndromes	Shengjiang and Bohe
	Promote	Promote the circulation of qi	Syndromes of qi stagnation	Muxiang and Chenpi
		Activate blood	Syndromes of blood stasis	Chuanxiong and Honghua
Sweet	Nourish	Tonify and replenish	Deficiency syndromes	Huangqi and Renshen
	Harmonize and moderate	Moderate toxic and violent property	Widely used in many prescriptions	Fengmi and Gancao
		Blend taste		Fengmi and Gancao
		Harmonize the middle energizer, moderate emergency, and relieve spasm and pain	Spasm or pain epigastric abdomen and limbs	Fengmi Gancao
Sour/astringent	Contract and astringe	Astringe and consolidate	Collapse syndromes	Shanzhuyu and Wuweizi
Bitter	Purge	Clear and expel the fire and heat pathogens	Heat syndromes	Huangqin and Zhizi
		Descend and purge	Cough, vomit, and hiccup	Kuxingren and Banxia
		Purge and rush down the bowels	Constipation	Dahuang and Mangxiao
	Dry	Dry the dampness	Dampness syndromes	Cangzhu and Yinchen
Salty	Purge	Purge	Constipation	Mangxiao
	Soften	Soften hardness and dissipate nodules	Tumor, phlegm nodule, and goiter	Muli and Kunbu
Bland	Drain and promote	Drain dampness and promote urination	Dampness syndromes such as edema and dysuria	Fuling and Yiyiren (Semen Coicis)

flavor falls under the sour flavor category, for the purpose to integrate the five flavors with five elements theory. In five flavors, they can be divided into two parts: pungent, sweet, and bland belong to yang property, while bitter, sour, and salty to yin property.

Due to the fact that both the four properties and the five flavors can only reveal one of the basic characteristics of Chinese medicinal herbs from different angles, the relationship between four properties and five flavors is very close. The clinical application of medicine must combine their specific individual property with flavor in order to obtain a comprehensive and correct understanding.

1.4.2 Four Directions (Ascending, Descending, Floating, and Sinking)

Ascending, descending, floating, and sinking are the four directions that the specific embodiment of qi movement, which is presented as the activities of ascending, descending, exiting, and entering. They indicate the directional effects of medicines on the human body when they are taken.

Different diseases often appear to show a tendency to move upward, downward, and toward, the exterior or the interior because of various pathogenic factors. To correct the disorder of the body functions and restore them to the normal, the directions of effects of Chinese medicines on human body also have the ascending, descending, floating, and sinking distinction. When treating diseases, doctors should select corresponding Chinese medicines and make the best use of their ascending, descending, floating, or sinking effects to help dispel pathogenic factors.

The four directions of medicine are opposite to the pathogenic tendencies and correspond with syndrome locations. Generally speaking, for syndromes in the upper and superficial part of the body, it is appropriate to choose medicines of ascending or floating direction. For the syndromes in the lower and interior part of the body, medicines of descending or sinking direction should be used. Medicine of descending direction is more suitable for syndromes of upward tendency, while medicine of ascending for syndromes of sinking tendency.

Chinese medicines of "ascending" have the effect toward the upper parts, which are utilized for the diseases in lower and deeper parts. For instance, Huangqi and Shengma (Rhizoma Cimicifugae) are able to raise splenic qi and are indicated for syndrome of visceroptosis with hyposplenic qi such as chronic diarrhea and lingering dysentery, prolapse of the rectum, prolapse of uterus, and gastroptosis. Chinese medicines of "descending" have the function toward the lower parts and possess the effect of descending adverse qi and are utilized for the disease due to adverse ascending of pathogenic factors. For example, Daizheshi, Xuanfuhua (Flos Inulae), Banxia, and Kuxingren can descend adverse flow of qi, subdue exuberant rang of the liver, and descend adverse qi of the lung and stomach and are indicated for dizziness due to hyperactivity of liver yang, cough, and dyspnea due to adverse rising of lung qi, nausea and vomiting and eructation due to adverse rising of stomach qi. Chinese medicines of "floating" have the function toward the upper and outward parts, generally exert the effects of sweating and dispersing, and are indicated for the disease in the upper and superficial parts. For example, Mahuang medicine, Fangfeng (Radix saposhnikoviae), and Qianghuo (Rhizoma et Radix Notopterygii) can dispel wind-cold and dampness from the exterior and are indicated for syndrome of exterior tightened by wind-cold, wind-dampness type of impediment disease, etc. Chinese medicines of "sinking" have the function toward the lower and inward parts, have the effects of lowering the adverse flow of qi and relaxing bowels and promoting diuresis, and are indicators for the disease in the lower and interior. For instance, Dahuang and Mutong (Caulis Akebiae) separately have the effects of relaxing the bowels and promoting diuresis and are used to treat constipation, abdominal distention and pain, dysuria, etc. (Table 1.7).

Table 1.7 Four directions and effect of Chinese medicine

Directions	Effects		Indication	Examples
Ascending	Move toward the upper parts of the body	Elevate yang, relieve superficies, dispel wind and cold, cause vomiting, induce emetic, etc.	Diseases in lower and deeper parts, such as syndrome of visceroptosis with hyposplenic qi such as chronic diarrhea and lingering dysentery, prolapse of the rectum, prolapse of uterus, and gastroptosis	Huangqi and Shengma
Floating	Move toward the outward parts		Disease in the upper and surficial parts, such as syndrome of exterior tightened by wind-cold, wind-dampness type of impediment disease, etc.	Mahuang and Qianghuo
Sinking	Move toward the inward parts	Lower the adverse flow of qi, clear heat, purge, promote diuresis, suppress the hyperactive yang, stop wind, etc.	Disease in the lower and interior, such as constipation, dysuria, etc.	Dahuang and Mutong
Descending	Move toward the lower parts		Diseases due to adverse ascending of liver fire or liver yang, and lung and stomach qi, such as dizziness, cough and dyspnea, nausea, and vomiting	Daizheshi, Xuanfuhua, Banxia and Kuxingren

The ascending and descending, floating, and sinking of Chinese medicine are often mentioned as two opposite pairs. Ascending and floating, descending, and sinking are, respectively, similar in their effects and often mentioned concurrently. The former belongs to yang, and the later belongs to yin. The ascending and floating Chinese medicines move in ascending and outward directions, generally exert the effects of elevating yang, relieve superficies, dispel wind and cold, cause vomiting, move qi, and relieve depression, induce emetic, etc. The descending and sinking Chinese medicines move in descending and inward directions generally have the effects of lowering the adverse flow of qi, clear heat, purge, promote diuresis, suppress the hyperactive yang, stop wind, etc.

The ascending, descending, floating, and sinking of Chinese medicines are having a close relationship with the four properties, five flavors, medicinal parts, and qualities. Generally speaking, Chinese medicines of pungent and sweet in flavor, of warm or heat in property, are mostly ascending and floating in their effects, while those of bitter, sour, and salty in flavor and of cold or cool in property are mostly descending and sinking in their effects. Chinese medicines of flowers, leaves, branches, etc., which are light in quality are mostly ascending and floating in their effects while those of fruits, seeds, minerals, etc., which are heavy in quality are mostly descending and sinking. But it should be noted that this is not always the case. There is an additional small number of Chinese medicine, for instance, Houpo (Cortex Magnoliae Officinalis), a bark kind, pungent, bitter, and warm in its flavor and nature can lower qi and relieve dyspnea. Xuanfuhua, a flower kind, can lower qi.

In addition, the ascending, descending, floating, and sinking effects of Chinese medicine can be affected or even altered by some medicinal processing or medicinal combination. For example, the descending or sinking Chinese medicine can turn into the ascending and floating ones when they are stir-baked with wine; in the same way, the ascending or floating Chinese medicine will turn into the ascending or sinking ones, which enter the kidney when they are stir-baked with a salt solution. And when they are used in combination with a variety of strong descending or sinking ones, and their ascending or floating effects are changed into obscurity.

1.4.3   Meridian Entry

Meridian entry refers to that Chinese medicine may often produce their therapeutic effects on some portion of a human body in preference; in other words, their therapeutic effect is mainly related to some specific zang-fu viscera or meridians or some meridians in predominance, while it may seem to produce fewer effects on or seem not related to the other zang-fu viscera and meridians.

Meridian entry takes the theory of zang-fu and meridians and the indication of syndromes as bases. So generally speaking, meridian entry has close relations with defining the location of the syndromes; in other word, what meridian or meridians a Chinese medicinal herb is attributed to is just related to the certain meridian or meridians on which the Chinese medicinal herb may work. For example, Mahuang and Xingren effective in syndromes of the disorder of the lung meridian marked by cough and dyspnea are attributed to the lung meridian. Chaihu (Pericarpium Citri Reticulatae), Qingpi (Pericarpium Citri Reticulatae Viride), and Xiangfu (Rhizoma cyperi) indicated syndromes of the disorder of the liver meridian of foot jueyin marked by distending pain in breast and hypochondrium and hernia pain are attributed to the liver meridian. From above, we can see that meridian entry of Chinese medicine is summarized from the therapeutic effects through a long time of clinical observation, and being practiced repeatedly gradually develops into a theory. In addition, when the theory of meridian entry is used, the relationships between zang-fu viscera and meridians must be taken into full consideration.

Mastery of meridian entry is essential for improving clinical practices, because the theory of meridian entry plays an important role in clinical selection of Chinese medicinal herbs according to syndromes, improving the pertinence of direction and strengthening the therapeutic effects. For instance, Chinese medicines which are cold in nature all have effects of clearing away heat, but with the differences in tendency toward clearing away heat in the heart, lung, stomach, liver, or kidney. Those hot in nature can all warm the interior to expel cold, but their effects also have the differences in warming the lung, spleen, stomach, or kidney. Medicine for tonifying yin is sweet in flavor and cold in nature, Shashen (Radix Adenophorae, Radix

Glehniae) is attributed to lung meridian, while Guiban (Carapax et Plastrum Testudinis) is attributed to kidney meridian. So when we prescribe medicine, we should select those that work on the diseased zang-fu viscera or meridian or some zang-fu viscera or meridians in the light of their properties of meridian entry to achieve desired therapeutic effects.

The theories such as meridian entry, four natures and five favors, ascending, descending, floating, and sinking all explain the properties of Chinese medicine from various points of view, which jointly constitute their properties and effects.

Therefore, when we apply Chinese medicine in clinic, we must combine their various properties and effects to give them an all-round consideration so that we can select and apply them correctly and avoid one-said.

1.4.4 Toxicity

There are different implications of toxicity of Chinese medicine between ancient time and today. In the ancient, toxic medicine was the general name for all of the medicine, because the toxicity of medicine was regarded as medicinal deflection, by which pathological deflection could be treated. The basic principle of treating diseases was to revise the deflection of diseases with the deflection of medicine. Meanwhile, the ancients also took toxicity as an index to judge how the toxic and side effect was, which was caused by medicine. In modern times, toxicity only indicates the degree of toxic and side effects and refers to the harmful effects and injuries of a medicine on organism. The so-called toxicant refers to the material drastic or poisonous in nature that can do harm to the human body for the light and can cause death for the severe if used improperly. Close observation of the potential side effect of toxic reaction during the therapeutic process is beneficial to the early diagnosis and treatment of poisoning.

In addition, TCM always held that there is a theory of "treating virulent pathogen with poisonous agents"; that is, some poisonous Chinese medicine with obvious therapeutic effects, under the safety of administration, may be used properly for such serious intractable diseases as malignant boil with swelling, scabies, scrofula, goiter, cancer tumor, and abdominal mass.

Factors with close relation with toxic reaction can be summarized into the following five aspects. Dosage of poisonous Chinese medicine in the treatment is close to or the same as poisoning dosage, so the safety margin is small and poisoning is easily resulted. Whereas the dosage of nonpoisonous Chinese medicine in treatment is much farther from the poisoning dosage, the safety margin is also larger. But it is not absolute whether they can result in poisonous reaction or not. Toxicity also has a close relationship with processing, combination, preparation of medicine, ways, mount and the period of using them, the physical condition, age, and syndromes of the patient. Therefore, in order to ensure the safety in the use of Chinese medicine and bring therapeutic effects into play and avoid poisonous reaction, toxic medicine must be controlled according to the above facts to avoid poisoning when used. In particularly, we should pay more attention to the following.

1.4.4.1 Strictly Processing

The toxicity of Chinese medicine can be weakened by being processed. Therefore, we must strictly follow the process principles to minimize or eliminate the toxicity or side effects before use. For example, Badou (Fructus Crotomis), a kind of drastic purgatives that is poisonous, easily results in poisoning if not processed into Badoushuang (Semen Crotonis Pulzerataum) which is taken orally. After Fuzi is prepared through soaking, its toxicity decreases and it can be widely used.

1.4.4.2 Control of Dosage

Poisoning occurrence is related to the excessive dosage of treatment. So the dosage of toxic Chinese medicines especially those with extreme toxin must be controlled strictly and cannot be increased at will. Toxic medicine such as Pishuang (Arsenicum), Banmao (Mylabris), Maqianzi (Semen Strychni), and Fuzi should be used in small dose and increased according to the syndromes and reaction of the patient after they are taken. At the same time, administration time of medicines should be controlled strictly too. If Chinese medicines are taken for a long time, the body will be poisoned due to accumulation of toxicity.

1.4.4.3 Notes of Application

The poisonous Chinese medicine maybe be used in deferent ways. Some cannot be taken orally and can only be applied exteriorly, such as Shengyao (Coarsely prepared mercuric oxide) and Tianxianzi (Semen Hyoscyami); some can only be added to pill or bolus and powder, and not to decoction, such as Banmao and Chansu (Venenum Bufonis); other some cannot be prepared into pill or tablet with wine, such as Chuanwu. And still others should be decocted longer (about 0.5–1 h) and the toxins of which can be destroyed, such as Fuzi. If the boiling time is short, it will cause poisoning.

1.4.4.4 Reasonal Combination

If being put into a complex prescription, the toxicity of some medicines often can be reduced. And if taken singly, the toxicity will be severer. For instance, Banxia has a toxin if being taken singly, but its toxicity will decrease if being taken with

Shengjiang. On the other hand, using medicines with prohibited combinations may cause a strong side effect, for example, when the incompatible medicine Gancao and Gansui (Radix Euphorbiae Kansui) used together.

1.5 Compatibility and Contraindication

1.5.1 Compatibility

Compatibility refers to the combination of more than two Chinese medicines to lighten the clinical requirement such as specific syndromes and medicinal properties and effects. It is the main method of medicinal application and the basis of making up formulae of Chinese medicine.

In clinical practice, if a disease is simple and light, we can use a single medicine to treat it and achieve the therapeutic purpose. While a disease is complicated, accompanied by other diseases, with exterior and interior syndromes appearing simultaneously, or asthenic syndrome complicated with sthenic syndrome, or cold syndrome accompanied by heat syndrome, single-medicinal formula will fail. Furthermore, some medicines used in single form may produce toxic and side effects and be harmful to patients. Therefore, Chinese medicines are usually used in combination according to their specific properties so as to decrease or eliminate their toxic side effects, reinforce or increase their effects, and gain better therapeutic effects, whereas unreasonal combination may produce toxicity and poor reactions.

The relationship between medicines was generalized by the ancients as seven aspects, namely singular application, mutual reinforcement, mutual assistance, mutual restraint, mutual detoxication, mutual inhibition, and incompatibility.

1.5.1.1 Single Application

It means the use of a single Chinese medicine to treat a disorder and fulfill its therapeutic purpose. Usually, the case condition is simple and light, but sometimes is serious. For example, Dushen Tang uses Renshen to treat the syndrome of qi collapse. Strictly speaking, singular application means using a medicine alone, not denoting the relationship of compatibility between Chinese medicines.

1.5.1.2 Mutual Reinforcement

It means that two or more Chinese medicines with similar properties and effects are combined to reinforce each other's effect. For example, Dahuang and Mangxiao are both purgative and can reinforce each other's original purgative effect when they are used in combination; Mahuang and Guizhi are both pungent and warm-natured and are combined to reinforce their effect of sweating and relieving exterior syndrome.

1.5.1.3 Mutual Assistance

It means Chinese medicines that are not certainly similar but have some relationship in the aspect of medicinal properties and effects are used in combination, in which one medicine is taken as the dominating factor and the others as its assistant to raise its therapeutic effects. For example, Huangqi with the effect of tonifying qi and promoting the flow of water is used in combination with Fangji (Radix Stephaniae Tetrandrae) with the effects of promoting the flow of water and permeating the dampness, the latter reinforcing the former's effect of promoting the flow of water, so their combination can be used for edema due to spleen deficiency; Gouqizi and Juhua are combined to treat blurred vision due to liver and kidney deficiency. Gouqizi, which is able to nourish liver and kidney yin, supplement blood and essence, and improve vision, is the major medicine, while Juhua, which can remove liver heat, dispel wind-heat, and improve vision, acts as the assistant medicine.

The similarities between mutual reinforcement and mutual assistance are that by combination, medicine can cooperate to enhance the overall medicinal effect. The differences lie in the fact that the medicine in mutual reinforcement relationship are of equal importance, while in mutual assistant relationship, which are comprised of a major medicine and an assistant one.

1.5.1.4 Mutual Restraint

It means a combination in which one Chinese medicine's toxicity or side effects are reduced or removed by another one. For instance, the poisonous effect of Banxia or Nanxing (Rhizoma Arisaematis) may be decreased or eliminated by Shengjiang; therefore, we say there is mutual restraint between Banxia or Nanxing and Shengjiang.

1.5.1.5 Mutual Suppression

It means that one Chinese medicine can relieve or remove toxic properties and side effects of the other. A common example is that Shengjiang can be used to relieve or eliminate the toxicity or side effects of Banxia or Nanxing. Therefore, we say that Shengjiang can detoxicate the toxicity or eliminate the side effects of Banxia or Nanxing.

From the above, we can see that mutual restraint and mutual suppression actually refer to the same thing, but they are expressed in two different ways.

1.5.1.6   Mutual Inhibition

It means that when two Chinese medicines are used in combination, their original therapeutic effects or even their medicinal effects are weakened or loosed. For instance, the effect of tonifying qi of Renshen can be weakened by Laifuzi; therefore, we say there is mutual inhibition between Renshen and Laifuzi.

1.5.1.7   Mutual Antagonism

It means that when two incompatible Chinese medicines are used in combination, toxic reaction or side effects may result. There are 18 antagonisms of incompatible medicaments which are believed to give rise to serious side effects if given in combination. For instance, Gancao antagonizes Haizao (Sargassum), Daji (Radix Euphorbiae Knoxiae), Gansui, and Yuanhua (Flos Genkwa).

In conclusion, in clinical application of Chinese medicines, mutual reinforcement and mutual assistance medicines can improve their therapeutic effects, while mutual restraint and mutual suppression can suppress or neutralize each toxicity or side effect and make medicine safe and effective, so we should make the widest possible use of them. While mutual inhibition and incompatibility can decrease or lose the therapeutic effects and produce toxin and side effects, we should avoid using them as much as possible.

1.5.2   Contraindication of Medicine

Chinese medicines have not only effects of treating and preventing diseases, but also harmful effects on human body. So when learning medicinal properties, we should not only know their therapeutic effects but also master their harmful effects produced after being taken, which is essential to understanding the contraindications of Chinese medicine.

The properties of those medicines which have an unfavorable aspect on human body should be corrected or avoided. In order to decrease the risk of side effects and increase treatment efficacy, doctors must pay close attention to the contraindication of Chinese medicines. The contraindications mainly include prohibited combination, contraindication during pregnancy, syndrome medication contraindications, and dietary incompatibility.

1.5.2.1   Prohibited Combination

Prohibited combination means that medicine in specific combinations in a prescription that can reduce and neutralize efficacies or reinforce toxicity and increase side effects should be avoided. The prohibited combinations mainly include mutual inhibition and mutual antagonism, especially denoting "18 antagonisms" and "19 incompatibilities."

Eighteen antagonisms are as follows: Wutou (Radic Aconiti) being incompatible with Banxia, Gualou (Fructus Trichosanthis), Beimu (Bulbus Fritilariae), Bailian (Radic Ampelopsis), and Baiji (Rhizoma Bletinae); Gancao with Haizao, Daji, Gansui, and Yuanhua; and Lilu (Rhicoma et Radix Veratri) with Renshen, Shashen, Danshen, Xuanshen (Radic Scrophulariae), Kushen (Radix Sophorae Flavescentis), Xixin, and Shaoyao (Radic Paeoniae).

Nineteen incompatibilities are as follows: Liuhuang (Sulfur) being antagonistic to Puxiao (Mirabilite), Shuiyin (Hnydrargyrum) to Pishuang, Langdu (Stellera chamaejasme Linn) with Mituoseng (Lithargyrum), Badou with Qianniu (Semen Pharbitidis), Dingxiang (Rlos Caryorphglli) with Yujin (Radic Curcumae), Yaxiao (Crystallized Mirabilite) with Sanleng (Rhicoma Sparganii), Chuanwu and Caowu with Xijiao (Coral Ehinocerotis Asiatici), Renshen with Wulingzhi, Rougui (Corter Cimnamomi) with Chishizhi (Faeces Traopteroram).

As to "18 antagonisms" and "19 incompatibilities," they are regarded as medicine which are incompatible, but some of them were still used in combination by some doctors. The conclusion of "18 antagonisms" and "19 incompatibilities" got in modern experiments and research is not completely similar. Therefore, the conclusion has not been confirmed and further research will be made. So we should use them cautiously and generally we should avoid using them in combination.

1.5.2.2 Contraindication of Drugs in Pregnancy

Some medicines that are regarded as contraindicated should be used with cautions in pregnant women. Otherwise, negative effects on mother, fetus, or the growth and development of the born and the unborn child may occur, or induced abortion or miscarriage may be brought about.

Contraindication of medicines in pregnancy can be classified into two types according to the intensity of the medicinals effect as follows: to be avoided completely or to be given cautiously. The medicines to be avoided usually have severe toxicity and drastic property, such as Daji, Gansui, Shanglu, Badou, Qianniuzi, Banmao, Shuizhi (Hirudo), Wugong (Scolopendra), Sanleng, Ezhu (Rhizoma Curcumae), Yuanhua, Shexiang (Moschus Artifactus), Shuiyin, Chansu, and Xionghuang (Realgar). On the other hand, the medicines pertain to blood-activating and stasis-dispelling, qi-moving, purgative, and part of pungent-warm medicines should be given cautiously, such as Taoren (Semen Persicae), Honghua, Ruxiang (Olibanum), Moyao (Myrrha), Wangbuliuxing (Semen Vaccariae), Dahuang, Zhishi, Fuzi, Ganjiang, and Rougui.

No matter whether the medicines are regarded as forbidden herbs or cautiously used ones, they should be avoided in pregnancy if there is no special need so as to avoid unexpected results. But if the pregnant woman is dangerously ill, and no other choices are available, those mentioned above may be used with great care. If the patient in pregnancy has blood stasis, the medicine for blood-activating and stasis-dispelling regaining like Taoren may be still used.

1.5.2.3 Contraindication of Drugs in Syndrome

As it is said, "every medicinal contains toxicity in a certain degree." On account of the different properties and meridian entry of the Chinese medicine, one kind of Chinese medicine is only suitable to one certain or some specific syndromes, while invalid to other syndromes, even counteractive sometimes, and it is contraindication to the syndromes at the moment. Actually, each medicine has its prohibited syndrome. Most of the medicines have medication contraindications, which will be referred to below the category "prohibitions for use." For example, cold or cool medicines with the effect of clearing away heat may be likely to damage yang. For example, Huanglian cold in nature and bitter in flavor is indicated for diarrhea due to dampness-heat, but it is not suitable for diarrhea due to spleen yang deficiency. Warm or hot ones with the effect of dispersing pathogenic cold may damage yin. For example, Ganjiang hot in nature and pungent in flavor is indicated for cough due to lung cold, but contraindicated for dry cough due to lung heat.

1.5.2.4 Contraindication of Diet

In the period of medicine being taken, some foods are forbidden or limited to be eaten for therapeutic purpose during the treatment of illness, and this is known as forbidden food. Those foods have a negative influence on the absorption of stomach and spleen or decrease efficacies and reinforce toxicity side effects.

Generally speaking, while taking medicines a patient should abstain from raw, cold, greasy and spicy foods, and foods with a smell of fish or mutton. In addition, dietetic restraint differs in different diseases. Some foods should be avoided based on certain disease conditions. For example, for warm febrile disease, pungent, greasy, or fried foods are prohibited; for cold disease, raw and cold foods should be avoided; fatty or greasy foods, smoking, and drinking should be prohibited in a patient with such syndromes as retention of phlegm in the chest, chest distress, and cardiac pain; pungent foods should be avoided in a patient with syndromes of headache and dizziness due to hyperactivity of liver yang; fried and greasy foods should be prohibited in a patient with deficiency of the stomach and spleen; fish, shrimp, crab, and pungent foods should be prohibited in a patient with pathogenic infection and ulcerous disease of skin and other skin troubles.

Moreover, some foods are incompatible during medicine taking and not beneficial to the cure of a disease, and even toxic effects can be brought about. For example, Renshen with radish, Guanzhong (Rhizoma Dryopteris Crassirhizomatis) with greasy, Dihuang, and Heshouwu (Radix Polygoni Multiflori) with onion, garlic, and radish. We should take all the above for reference when we take Chinese medicines.

1.6   Dosage and Usage of Medicine

1.6.1   Dosage of Medicine

Dosage refers to the amount of each Chinese medicine to be taken, which signifies the daily amount of one particular medicine for one adult in making decoction or the daily amount of powder and secondly shows the comparative measurements of medicine in the same prescription and is also known as relative dosage. As to the amount of Chinese medicine to be taken, we mostly take weight as the unit of measurement and take quantity and capacity as the unit for the special ones. Now, we take the metric system (g) as the unit of measurement, which is now stipulated in the Mainland of China.

Exact dosage is an important factor to ensure the safety and efficacy of medicinal administration. As the dosage of a medicine has direct relationship with its therapeutic effect, a medicine when used below its level of effective dosage will not achieve desired results; the dose of a certain medicine when used beyond its limit may often damage the healthy qi and is also wasted. Some Chinese medicines are drastic or extremely poisonous, so their doses must be used properly to get the best therapeutic effects and meanwhile prevent patients from poisoning.

Exact dosage is based on the specific features of each medicine, its properties, aimed disease, and application methods, as well as consideration of the individual differences in patients.

1.6.1.1   Properties of Medicine

Generally speaking, the medicine moderate in nature such as Gouqizi and Shanyao can be used in a large dose; those drastic or toxic in nature such as Banxia and Gansui must be used in a small dose; those light in property such as flowers and leaves should be used in a small dose; those heavy in property, such as metals stones and shells but without toxin, can be used in a large dose, fresh plant medicine, since they contain water, should be used in a large dose. Medicine which are bitter and cold in nature cannot be used in a long time and large dosage to avoid injuring the spleen qi and stomach qi.

1.6.1.2   Compatibility and Prescription

In clinic, the dosage of one medicine varies according to the combination, formula, and aimed disease. Generally speaking, the dosage of a medicine used alone is usually larger than that applied in a prescription; the dosage of a main medicine in a prescription is larger than that of an accessory one. Under the same condition, the dosage of a medicine used in decoction is larger than that in pills or powder.

1.6.1.3 The Condition of Illness, the Patients' Constitution, and Age

The dosage varies greatly with differences in disease, ages, and gender of the patients. Generally speaking, based on disease trends, the dosage used in the treatment of the mild or chronic disease is comparatively smaller, while the dosage of a medicine used in the treatment of serious or acute disease must be fairly larger. Based on patients' constitution, the dosage used for those with strong physique must be larger while for those with weak physique, such as children, delivery women and the elders, the dose is generally smaller. Based on patients' ages, the dosage for children over 5 years is half of that given to an adult; for children below 5 years, the dose is one-fourth of that for adult; for an infant, the dose should be much smaller.

Furthermore, for expensive medications covered by insurance, the dosage should be kept small to ensure medicinal effectiveness. Examples of such medications include Shexiang (Musk) and Niuhuang (Calculus Bovis). This approach helps us to avoid unnecessary waste of medicinal resources and alleviate the economic burden on the patient.

1.6.2 Usage of Medicine

The common administration of Chinese medicine may be oral, external, or local. Forms of decoction, pill, powder, soft extract, wine, etc., are prepared for oral use, while application, moxibustion, pigmentum, lotion, laryngeal insufflation of medicinal powder, eye drops, thermotherapy, suppository, etc., are used exteriorly, whereas decoction is the most widely used form in clinic, which are generally prepared by patients. The correct method for decoction and administration is very important to ensure high quality of decoction and desired curative effect and medication safety; therefore, doctors should tell their patients or patient's relatives how to decoct medicine.

1.6.2.1 Methods of Decocting Chinese Medicine

First of all, choose an appropriate decocting utensil, such as a clay pot or earthen jar or a piece of enamelware as metal utensils such as iron and copper are forbidden to decoct medicine because metal tends to take chemical reactions with medicinal ingredients, which can reduce the treatment effect and may even cause toxicity or side effects. Then, the decocting water must be clean without peculiar smell.

Secondly, the decocting methods must be mastered. Put Chinese medicine into the enamelware and pour the water in it, the water being usually over the surface of the medicine. Before being decocted, the Chinese medicine need immersing in water for about half an hour in order to make their active ingredients easily dissolve in the solution. Usually, fire used in decocting the medicine should be controlled in the light of medicinal properties and qualities, because the method for decoction depends on the properties qualities and effect of the medicine. For example, the medicine with aromatic smell should be decocted with strong fire until the solution is boiled for several minutes, and then, mild fire is used until the decoction is finished. Otherwise, the medicinal effects will be reduced. These nourishing medicines should be decocted with mild fire for a long time because of their greasy qualities, or the effective factors are not easily dissolve out.

Because their properties and qualities are usually obviously different, different medicine should be given different decocting methods and time. When a prescription is made out, the decocted methods of some Chinese medicine should be noted. The chief methods are shown as follows.

1. To Be Decocted Earlier

    Some kinds of minerals and shell medicine such as Shigao, Muli, Longgu (Os Draconis), Shijueming (Concha Haliotidis), and Biejia (Carapax Triomgcis) should be broken and decocted first for 20–30 min; then, the other medicine are put in it, as their qualities are hard and their effective ingredients are not easily decocted out. Furthermore, the method is also indicated for decocting or boiling toxic medicine, in order to lessen or eliminate their poisonous effects and ensure the safety of administration. When some poisonous medicine such as Wutou and Fuzi is used, they should be decocted 30–60 min earlier before the others.

2. To Be Decocted Later

    Some aromatic medicine with volatile components such as Bohe, Sharen, and Qinghao (Herba Artemisiae Annuae) should be put in after the solution of the other medicine has been boiled 10–30 min and then boiled together for another 5 min or so. Furthermore, the method is also indicated for decocting some medicine such as Gouteng (Ramulus Uncariaecum Uncis) and Shengdahuang (Radie et Rhizoma Rhei), because their active ingredients tend to be destroyed easily during the decocting.

3. To Be Wrap-Decocted

    Some medicine such as Cheqianzi (SemenPlantaginis) and Xuanfuhua, Chishizhi, Huashi (Talcum), which have strong glutinosity, in powder form, or are small seeds, must be wrapped in a piece of cloth or of gauze with floss and then put together with others in an enamelware into which water is added. These medicines, if decocted directly in water, will make their decoction turbid, and thus, it is difficult to be taken orally, and some small seed medicine will float on the decoction after being boiled, which cannot be removed easily; some downy medicine will make their decoction mixed with soft hairs, if decocted directly, which cannot be removed easily and can irritate the throat when the decoction is taken.

4. To Be Decocted Separately

    Some expensive medicine, such as Renshen and Lingyangjiao (Cornu Saigae Tataricae), must be decocted or boiled alone, because when they are decocted or boiled with others, their ingredients may be absorbed by other medicine. We should avoid waste of medicinal materials and economic burden on the patient.

And on the other time, some expensive medicine should be decocted separately about 2–3 h to ensure the active components can be fried out.

5. Melting

Some glue-like medicines, such as Ejiao, Guibanjiao (Colla PlastriTestudinis), Fengmi, and Yitang (Saccharum Granorum), which have a lot of mucilage and easily soluble ones, must be melted first with water or yellow rice or millet wine until they are melted well and then mixed with the decoction for oral administration. If decocted directly together with other medicine in water, they will be deposited at the bottom of the pot and easy to stick to the pot and the other ingredients and be uneasily filtered.

6. Infusions for Oral Taking

Some medicines are dissolved quickly when they are put in liquid, such as Mangxiao; some kinds of juice medicine such as Zhuli (Succus Phyllostachydis Henonis) and juice of Xiandihuang and Shengjiang; those that are got by grinding such as Lingyangjiao, Sanqi and Chenxiang (Ligmaum Aquilariae Resinatum) with water do not need decoction and must be mixed directly with water or the decocted juice for oral administration.

1.6.2.2 Methods of Taking Chinese Medicine

Generally speaking, decoction must be taken warm. A dose of Chinese medicine in a prescription is usually decocted twice daily, while nourishing medicine may be decocted three times. The decocted juice is about 150–200 mL every time. When the decocting is finished, squeeze the Chinese medicine in order to obtain all the liquid of the decoction, then mix the decoction, and divide it into 2 or 3 parts for daily use.

An acute patient must take twice a day or even three times, that is, once every 4 h. A chronic patient may take a dose a day or 2 days. Those used for stopping vomiting should be taken frequently in small amount. The decoction should be fed through nose for the patients who are unconsciousness or trismus. Diaphoretics should be taken warmly, and after taking medicine, patients should tuck in the quilt or drink some hot porridge in order to promote the medicinal effects until sweating. Purging medicine must be taken until reducing diarrhea or vomiting. Wan or powder can be taken with warm water. As far as treatments are concerned, Chinese medicine warm in nature should be taken in cold or those cold in nature should be taken in warm. As for the time of taking medicine, tonics that are greasy and tend to be digested and absorbed should be taken before meals in the morning and evening and those irritant to the stomach and intestine should be taken after meals. Paraciticides and purging medicine should be taken when stomach is empty, and those for calming the mind should be taken before sleeping and those for stopping malaria should be taken 2 h ahead when the disease has an attack. Medicine should be taken at a regular time for chronic diseases, while a patient with an acute and severe disease can take medicine at any time. In addition, when disease is in the chest and diaphragm above such as headache, dizziness, and sore throat, it should be taken after meals. When disease is below chest and stomach such as liver, kidney, and stomach, it should be taken before meals.

Pills can be delivered directly with warm water. The big honeyed pill can be divided into small ones. Powder can be mixed with honey or encapsulated to avoid stimulating the throat. Paste should be taken after mixing with water.

1.7 Classification and Common Used Medicine

1.7.1 Exterior-Releasing Medicine

Exterior-releasing medicines refer to the medicines with the main effects of releasing the exterior and treating the exterior syndrome. They are also considered to be diaphoretic medicinal herbs. These kinds of medicines mainly have the pungent taste and the quality of lightly floating, and they are mainly attributed to the lung and bladder meridians, with the function of promoting sweating and dispersing exogenous pathogenic factors. They are mainly used for the treatment of exterior syndrome, manifested as aversion to cold, fever, headache, no sweat, floating pulse, etc. Parts of the medicine also can be used for the edema, cough, measles, rubella, and rheumatic pain at the early stage with the exterior syndrome.

Exterior-releasing medicines are divided into two kinds: wind-cold-dispersing medicine and wind-heat-dispersing medicine. The former are used for the treatment of wind-cold syndrome, and the latter are used for the wind-heat syndrome. When we use these kinds of medicines, the dosage should not be too large to avoid excessively sweating and consumption of yin. The application should be stopped as soon as the syndrome disappears. Therefore, these kinds of medicines do not apply to the interior deficiency syndrome, strangury, and blood lost patients. Most exterior-releasing medicines have active volatile oil. If added to decoction, they should not be decocted for a long time to prevent effective constituents from volatilizing and decrease the clinical efficacy.

In addition, they can dry dampness and harmonize stomach, so they are effective for disharmony of stomach and restlessness when combined with Shumi in Banxia Shumi Tang.

In addition, they can be used to treat gastroptosis, prolapse of rectum, and uterus, but they must be combined with Chaihu, Shengma, and Huangqi, in order to get good therapeutic effect, and they have the effect of raising blood pressure as well.

In addition, they could also be used in the treatment of coronary heart disease with angina pectoris and various stagnant blood syndromes of gynecology.

In addition, they can replenish qi and strengthen yang, and it is used to treat impotence. When combined with pathogen-expelling such as exterior-releasing, cathartic drugs, they have the efficacy to reinforce the healthy and dispel the pathogenic. They are used to treat excessive pathogens with healthy qi being deficient, such as in the case of qi deficiency with external contraction or with heat accumulation of interior excess.

1.7.1.1   Mahuang (Ephedra, Herba Ephedrae)

Properties and Tastes: pungent, slightly bitter, and warm
   Meridian Entry: lung and bladder meridians
   Effects

1. Promote sweating to release the exterior
2. Diffuse the lung to calm panting
3. Induce diuresis to alleviate edema

Application

1. The common cold due to wind-cold
   The medicinal herb has the nature of pungent and warm and attributive to the lung meridian; therefore, it can diffuse the lung qi and strongly promote sweating. It is often used for superficial asthenia syndrome due to wind-cold, which is manifested as aversion to cold, fever without sweating, headache and pain all over the body, nasal obstruction, and a floating and tense pulse. It is often used in combination with Guizhi in order to strengthen the work of promoting sweating to releasing the exterior, such as Mahuang Tang.
2. Cough and dyspnea
   It is majorly used for the cough and dyspnea due to stagnation of lung qi which belongs to excessive syndrome. But after combination, it can be used in all kinds of cough and dyspnea. For example, when it is combined with Gancao and Xingren, it can be used to treat cough and dyspnea due to wind-cold attacking lung. When it is combined with Shigao, Xingren and Gancao, it can be used to treat the cough and asthma due to lung heat. The former is called Sanao Tang, and the latter is called Mahuang Xingren Shigao Tang.
3. The wind edema
   The wind edema is a type of edema especially of the face and head, ascribed to attack on the lung by pathogenic wind, manifested by sudden onset of edema accompanied by fever with aversion to wind, aching joints, and oliguria. The medicinal herb can promote sweating and diffuse the lung qi, so it can be used to treat the wind edema, such as Yuebi Jia Zhu Tang, which is consisting of Mahuang, Shengjiang, and Baizhu.

Usage and Dosage: 2–10 g for decoction. When it is used to relieve exterior, the herb is fresh. When used to control asthma, the honey-Mahuang is often used.

1.7.1.2 Guizhi (Cassia Twig, Ramulus Cinnamomi)

Properties and Tastes: pungent and sweet in flavor, warm in nature
  Meridian Entry: heart, lung, and bladder meridians
  Effects

1. Promote sweating to release the flesh
2. Warm and free the meridian
3. Reinforce yang and promote the flow of qi

   Application

1. The common cold due to wind-cold
     The medicinal herb has the nature of pungent, sweet, and warm, and it can disperse yang qi and promote blood to flow in the body surface and muscles; therefore, it has the function of promoting sweating to release the flesh. It is used for the exterior syndrome due to wind-cold whether the syndrome is deficiency or sufficiency. It is often used in combination with Mahuang in order to strengthen the work of promoting sweating to releasing the exterior, such as Mahuang Tang. For the wind-cold syndrome with spontaneous perspiration due to superficial deficiency, it is often used in combination with Baishao, such as Guizhi Tang.
2. The stomach duct cold pain, blood cold amenorrhea, joint pain caused by impediment
     The medicinal herb can warm and free the meridian, so it can be used in all kinds of pain resulting from the syndrome of congealing cold with blood stasis. When it is used in combination with Zhishi and Xiebai, it can treat the patient with chest impediment and heart pain, such as Zhishi Xiebai Guizhi Tang. When it is used in combination with Baishao and Yitang, it can warm spleen and stomach for dispelling cold and relieve pain, such as Xiaojianzhong Tang. If a woman has the syndrome of congealing cold with blood stasis and the symptoms of dysmenorrhea, amenorrhea, irregular menstruation, and postpartum abdominal pain, it can be used in combination with Danggui, Wuzhuyu, such as Wenjing Tang. When it is used in combination with Fuzi, it can be beneficial to the patient with impediment, such as Guizhi Fuzi Tang.
3. Phlegm syndrome and edema
     Because of the nature of pungent, sweet, and warm, it can not only warm spleen yang to promote the transportation of water, but also warm kidney yang to promote the qi transformation of bladder. It is often used in the phlegm, fluid retention, and edema, such as Wuling San.
4. Palpitation and renal mass due to retention of fluids
     Because of the nature of pungent, sweet, and warm, it warms heart yang and promotes blood circulation to stop throbbing, such as Zhigancao Tang, which is combined with Gancao, Renshen, and Maidong.

Usage and Dosage: 3–10 g for decoction

1.7.1.3   Bohe (Peppermint, Herba Menthae)

Properties and Tastes: pungent and cold
  Meridian Entry: lung and liver meridians
  Effects

1. Disperse wind-heat
2. Clear heat from the head and eyes
3. Soothe the throat
4. Outthrust rashes
5. Soothe the liver and move qi

  Application

1. The common cold due to wind-heat and early stage of seasonal febrile disease
    For the syndrome manifested as fever and anhidrosis, slight aversion to wind and cold and headache, it is often combined with Jingjie, Niubangzi, Jinyinhua, Lianqiao, etc., such as Yinqiao San.
2. Headache and redness of eyes, swollen and painful throat
    The drug has light texture and fragrant odor, so it is usually for the syndrome of wind and heat attacking upward manifested as headache and redness of eyes; it is used together with Sangye, Juhua, and others that can clear away heat from head and eye. For the swollen and painful throat, it is often used with Jiegeng, Gancao, and Jiangcan, such as Liuwei Tang.
3. Unsmooth eruption of measles and itching due to rubella
    It is usually used together with Chantui, Niubangzi, etc., so as to promote eruption of measles, such as Zhuye Liubang Tang; it can be combined with Kushen, Baixianpi, Fangfeng, etc., to expel wind and relieve itching and treat rubella with itching, too.
4. The syndrome of stagnation
    Especially for stagnation of liver qi, oppressed feeling in the chest and hypo-chondriac pain, or swollen pain in breast and irregular menstruation, it can be used together with Chaihu, Baishao, and Danggui, such as Xiaoyao San.

  Usage and Dosage: 3–6 g for decoction and decoct later

1.7.1.4   Niubangzi (Great Burdock Achene, Fructus Arctii)

Properties and Tastes: pungent, bitter and cold
  Meridian Entry: spleen and stomach meridians
  Effects

1. Disperse wind-heat
2. Diffuse the lung and outthrust rashes
3. Detoxify and soothe the throat

Application

1. The common cold due to wind-heat and the early stage of seasonal febrile disease
   The medicine has the nature of cold and the taste of pungent and bitter. Therefore, it can be used for exterior syndrome of wind and heat type with sore and swollen throat, together with Bohe, Jinyinhua, and Lianqiao, etc., such as Yinqiao San, for those with sore and swollen throat, usually used together with Dahuang, Huangqin, and other herbs that can clear away heat and remove toxic materials.
2. Itching due to rubella
   Also, it can be used for unsmooth eruption of measles. At this time, usually combined with Bohe, Jingjie, Chantui, etc.
3. The urticaria and sores
   It is often used together with Dahuang, Mangxiao, and Zhizi, etc. It is combined with Xuanshen, Huangqin, Banlangen, etc., to treat mumps and pharyngalgia.

Usage and Dosage: 6–12 g for decoction. It is pounded into pieces that are used in decoction, and the stir-baked one can reduce its cold nature.
Other Exterior-releasing medicines (Table 1.8).

1.7.2 Heat-Clearing Medicine

Heat-clearing medicines refer to the medicinal herbs that have the main effect of clearing away interior heat.

These kinds of medicines are mostly cold and cool in nature, have sinking effect, and work toward the inward parts. They have the effects of clearing away heat, draining dampness, cooling the blood, detoxifying, relieving malnutrition fever, etc. They are often used for various internal heat syndromes, manifesting as high fever, excessive thirst and dampness-heat diarrhea and dysentery, jaundice with dampness heat pathogen, carbuncle, maculae due to warm toxin, and fever due to yin deficiency.

According to different effects and on different types of qi aspect, xuefen, yingfen, sthenia, and asthenia of the internal heat syndrome, these kinds of medicines are divided into five types, that is, heat-clearing and fire-purging medicine, heat-clearing and dampness-drying medicine, heat-clearing and detoxicating medicine, heat-clearing and blood-cooling medicine, and deficiency heat-clearing medicine.

Heat-clearing medicinal herbs are cold and cool in nature, so they easily injure the spleen and stomach qi. When heat-clearing medicines are applied, we must pay attention to the patients with deficiency of spleen and stomach or yin deficiency. Firstly, we must distinguish the exterior from the interior and be sure of the position of heat. If the heat is at qi aspect with high fever, thirst, sweat, and restlessness,

Table 1.8 Simple list of other exterior-releasing medicines

Name	Properties and tastes	Meridian entry	Effects	Application	Dosage
Zisu (Folium Perillae)	Pungent and warm	Lung and spleen meridians	(1) Release the exterior and dissipate cold (2) Move qi and smooth the middle (3) Prevent abortion	(1) The common cold due to wind-cold (2) Stagnation of spleen qi and stomach qi and vomitus gravidarum (3) Poisoning from fish and crabs	5–10 g for decoction. Do not overcook
Shengjiang (Rhizoma Zingiberis Recens)	Pungent and slightly warm	Lung, spleen, and stomach meridians	(1) Release the exterior and dissipate cold (2) Warm the middle energizer to arrest vomiting (3) Warm the lung to suppress cough	(1) The common cold due to wind-cold (2) Spleen and stomach cold syndromes (3) Vomiting due to stomach cold (4) Cough caused by lung cold (5) Poisoning of fish and crabs	3–10 g for decoction
Xiangru (Herba Moslae)	Pungent and slightly warm	Lung, spleen, and stomach meridians	(1) Promote sweating to release the exterior (2) Eliminate dampness and regulate the function of the spleen and stomach (3) Induce diuresis to alleviate edema	(1) The affection of exogenous wind-cold and internal injury by summer-damp, aversion to cold with fever, vomiting, and diarrhea (2) Edema, inhibited urination	3–10 g for decoction
Jingjie (Herba Schizonepetae)	Pungent and slightly warm	Lung and liver meridians	(1) Release the exterior and dissipate wind (2) Outthrust rashes (3) Disperse wounds (4) Stop bleeding	(1) The common cold and headache (2) The early stage of measles, urticaria, and sores (3) Blood disease	5–10 g for decoction. Do not overcook

(continued)

Table 1.8 (continued)

Name	Properties and tastes	Meridian entry	Effects	Application	Dosage
Fangfeng (Root Radix Saposhnikoviae)	Pungent, sweet and slightly warm	Bladder, liver, and spleen meridians	(1) Dispel wind and release the exterior (2) Dispel dampness and relieve pain (3) Relieve convulsive disease	(1) The exterior syndrome (2) Wind-cold-dampness impediment (3) Itching due to rubella (4) Urticaria	5–10 g for decoction
Qianghuo (Rhizoma et Radix Notopterygii)	Pungent, bitter, and warm	Bladder and kidney meridians	(1) Release the exterior and dissipate cold (2) Dispel wind and dampness (3) Relieve pain	(1) The common cold due to exogenous wind-cold (2) Wind-dampness impediment and pain in back and shoulder	3–10 g for decoction
Baizhi (Radix Angelicae Dahuricae)	Pungent and warm	Lung, stomach, and large intestine meridians	(1) Release the exterior and dissipate cold (2) Dispel wind and relieve pain (3) Relieve the stuffy nose (4) Dry dampness and stanch vaginal discharge (5) Disperse swelling and expel pus	(1) The common cold due to wind-cold (2) Headache, toothache caused by wind-cold-dampness (3) The allergic rhinitis, sinusitis and stuffy running nose (4) Vaginal discharge	5–10 g for decoction
Gaoben (Rhizoma Ligustici)	Pungent and warm	Bladder meridians	(1) Release the exterior and dissipate cold (2) Dispel dampness and relieve pain	(1) The common cold due to wind-cold (2) Wind-cold-dampness impediment	3–10 g for decoction

Table 1.8 (continued)

Name	Properties and tastes	Meridian entry	Effects	Application	Dosage
Xinyi (Flos Magnoliae)	Pungent and warm	Spleen and stomach meridians	(1) Release the exterior and dissipate cold (2) Relieve the stuffy nose	(1) The common cold due to wind-cold (2) The allergic rhinitis, sinusitis, and stuffy running nose	3–9 g for decoction. Wrap-decoction
Congbai (Fistular Onion Stalk)	Pungent and warm	Lung and stomach meridians	(1) Promote sweating to release the exterior (2) Dissipate cold and promote the yang qi	(1) The common cold due to wind-cold (2) The exuberant yin repelling yang	3–10 g for decoction
Sangye (Folium Mori)	Sweet, bitter cold	Lung and liver meridians	(1) Disperse wind-heat (2) Clear lung fire and moisten dryness (3) Pacify the liver yang (4) Clear the liver and improve vision	(1) The common cold due to wind-heat and early stage of seasonal febrile disease (2) The cough with lung heat or dryness-heat (3) The hyperactivity of liver yang, headache and dizziness (4) For the red eyes and dim sight	5–10 g for decoction
Chantui (Periostracum Cicadae)	Sweet and cold	Lung and liver meridians	(1) Dispersing wind-heat (2) Soothe the throat (3) Outthrust rashes (4) Remove nebula to improve vision (5) Relieve convulsion	(1) The wind-heat syndrome, seasonal febrile disease at the early stage, sore throat (2) Itching due to rubella and unsmooth eruption of measles (3) Conjunctivitis and pterygium (4) Tetanus and infantile convulsion	3–6 g for decoction

(continued)

Table 1.8 (continued)

Name	Properties and tastes	Meridian entry	Effects	Application	Dosage
Juhua (Flos Chrysanthemi)	Pungent, bitter, sweet, and slightly cold	Lung and liver meridians	(1) Dispersing wind-heat (2) Clear the liver and improve vision (3) Clear heat and detoxify	(1) The common cold due to wind-heat and early stage of seasonal febrile disease (2) Dizziness and headache due to hyperactivity of liver yang (3) Red, swollen, and painful eyes and blurred vision (4) Furuncle and especially for furunculosis	5–10 g for decoction
Manjingzi (Fructus Viticis)	Pungent, bitter, and slightly cold	Bladder, liver, and stomach meridians	(1) Disperse wind-heat (2) Clear heat from the head and eyes	(1) The common cold due to wind-heat (2) Red eyes and obscure eyes (3) For dizziness	5–10 g for decoction
Chaihu (Radix Bupleuri)	Pungent, bitter and slightly cold	Liver, gallbladder, and lung meridians	(1) Release the exterior and discharge heat (2) Sooth the liver and alleviate mental depression (3) Elevate yang qi	(1) Fever caused by exogenous pathogenic factors and alternating chills and fever (2) The liver qi stagnation, fullness and pain in chest and hypochondrium, irregular menstruation (3) Prolapses due to deficiency of qi, such as uterine prolapse and archoptosis	3–10 g for decoction

Table 1.8 (continued)

Name	Properties and tastes	Meridian entry	Effects	Application	Dosage
Shengma (Rhizoma Cimicifugae)	Pungent and slightly sweet	Lung, spleen, stomach, and large intestine meridians	(1) Release the exterior and outthrust rashes (2) Clear heat and detoxify (3) Uplift yang qi	(1) The common cold due to wind-heat (2) For itching due to rubella or unsmooth eruption of measles (3) Toothache and aphtha, swollen and throat pain (4) Prolapse due to qi deficiency manifested as shortness of breath, fatigue, prolapse of rectum due to chronic diarrhea, prolapse of uterus, flooding and spotting	3–10 g for decoction
Gegen (Radix Puerariae)	Sweet, pungent, and cold	Spleen, stomach, and lung meridians	(1) Release the flesh and bring down a fever (2) Engender fluid and relieve thirst (3) Outthrust rashes (4) Uplift yang and check diarrhea	(1) Fever and headache caused by exogenous factors (2) Thirst during febrile disease and internal heat with diabetes (3) For itching due to rubella with unsmooth eruption (4) Dampness-heat dysentery and spleen deficiency diarrhea	10–15 g for decoction
Dandouchi (Semen Sojae Preparatum)	Bitter, pungent, and cold	Spleen and stomach meridians	(1) Release the exterior (2) Relieve restlessness (3) Disperse stagnated heat	(1) The common cold (2) For irritability and chest tightness	6–12 g for decoction

heat-clearing and fire-purging medicine should be applied; if the heat in blood aspect, manifesting high fever at night, restlessness, and insomnia, heat-clearing and blood-cooling medicine should be used. There are differences in application of these five kinds of medicines. Secondly, we must distinguish the asthenia from sthenia. For the sthenic heat syndrome, those medicinal herbs of clearing away heat and purging fire, or clearing away heat from both qifen and xuefen, or clearing away heat from yingfen and cooling blood are used; for deficient heat syndrome, those medicinal herbs of cooling blood and clearing away heat or cooling blood to remove steaming fever or nourishing yin to clear away heat. In the meantime, according to syndromes accompanying with or following the above syndromes, antipyretic herbs must be used in combination with others. For example, for heat syndrome with exogenous pathogenic factors, exterior-releasing medicine and heat-clearing medicine are used together.

1.7.2.1   Shigao (Gypsum, Gypsum Fibrosum)

Properties and Tastes: sweet, pungent and extremely cold
   Meridian Entry: lung and stomach meridians
   Effects
   Hydrated gypsum

1. Clear heat and purge fire
2. Relieve restlessness and thirst

   Calcined gypsum

1. Induce astringent
2. Promote tissue regeneration and close wound

   Application

1. High fever and excessive thirst
   The medicinal herb has the nature of sweet, pungent, and extremely cold and is attributed to the lung and stomach meridians; therefore, it is most suitable to be used for clearing away heat and fire of the lung and stomach, which is manifested as high fever, excessive thirst, perspiration, and large and bounding pulse. It is often used in combination with Zhimuin order to strengthen the work of clearing away heat and fire such as Baihu Tang. For syndrome involving both xuefen and qifen with coma, high fever, maculae, and delirium, it is usually combined with Mudanpi, Shengdihuang, and others that can cool blood.
2. Cough and dyspnea due to heat in the lung
   It is attributed to the lung meridian, and it can clear away heat and fire of the lung; therefore, when it is used in combination with Mahuang, Guizhi, Gancao, etc., we will get a very good curative effect on such kind of disease as Mahuang Xingren Gancao Shigao Tang.

3. For excessive stomach fire, headache, toothache, and internal heat dispersion thirst

   Shigao can be used for clearing away heat and fire in the stomach. In clinical practice, it is often used in combination with Huanglian, Shengma, Zhimu, Shengdihuang, Maidong, etc., such as Qingwei San and Yunv Tang.
4. For the anabrosis, eczema, scald, and bleeding wound

   Calcined gypsum has the function of promoting tissue regeneration and closing wound. It is often used in combination with Shengyao for the treatment of anabrosis, such as Jiuyi Dan. When it is used with Huangbai, it can treat eczema, such as Shihuang San. Shigao together with Qingdai can used for scald.

Usage and Dosage: Hydrated gypsum, 15–60 g, decoct first. Calcined gypsum for external using spread the affected area with appropriate amount powder.
Zhimu (Common Anemarrhena Rhizome, Rhizoma Anemarrhenae)
Properties and Tastes: bitter, sweet, cold
Meridian Entry: lung, stomach, and kidney meridians
Effects

1. Clear heat and purge fire
2. Nourish the yin and moisturize dryness

Application

1. For high fever and excessive thirst

   The medicinal herb has the nature of bitter and cold; therefore, it can be used for clear away heat and fire, which is manifested as high fever, excessive thirst, perspiration, and large and bounding pulse. It is often used in combination with Shigao in order to strengthen the function of clearing away heat and fire, such as Baihu Tang.
2. The cough due to lung heat and dry cough due to yin deficiency

   The medicinal herb is attributed to the lung meridian and has the nature of bitter, sweet, and cold, and it can clear away heat and purge fire from the lung as well as nourish yin and moisten the lung; therefore, it can clear away heat and fire of lung meridian, which is manifested as cough or dry cough. For cough with yellow sputum due to lung heat, it is often used in combination with Huangqin, Zhizi, Gualou, etc., such as Qingjin Huatan Tang. For dry cough due to yin deficiency in lung, it is used together with Maimendong, Beishashen, and others that can nourish yin and moisten the lung.
3. For osteopyrexia and fever

   The medicinal herb is attributed to the kidney meridian and has the nature of bitter, sweet, and cold; therefore, it can nourish the kidney yin and clear away heat and fire of kidney meridian. It can be used for such diseases as hectic fever, night sweat, and restlessness. It is often used in combination with Huangbai, Di Huang, etc., such as Zhibai Dihuang Wan.

4. Internal heat dispersion thirst

It is often used in combination with Tianhuafen and Gegen to clear away heat and fire and nourish the yin and moisturize dryness, such as Yuye Tang.

5. For the constipation due to intestinal dryness

The medicinal herb can nourish the yin and moisturize dryness to purge. It is often used in combination with Shengdihuang, Xuanshen, Maidong, etc.

Usage and Dosage: 6–12 g for decoction. When it is used to clear away heat and fire, the herb is fresh. When used to nourish the yin and moisturize dryness, the herb is often processed with brine.

1.7.2.2 Zhizi (Cape Jasmine Fruit, Fructus Gardeniae)

Properties and Tastes: bitter and cold
Meridian Entry: heart, lung, and triple energizer meridians
Effects

1. Purge fire and relieve dysphoria
2. Cool the blood and detoxify
3. Clear heat and drain dampness
4. Cool the blood to stop bleeding

Application

1. Febrile disease with irritability

It can clear away fire from the triple energizer and heart and relieve vexation. For febrile diseases with irritability, it is often used combined with Dandouchi, such as Zhizichi Tang, for overabundance of heart heat with high fever, irritability, coma, and delirium; it is usually used together with Huanglian, Huangqin, Huangbai, and others that can clear away heat and purge fire, such as Huanglian Jiedu Tang.

2. Jaundice of dampness-heat syndrome

For stagnation of dampness and heat in the liver and gallbladder manifested as jaundice, fever, and oliguria with brownish urine, it is often combined with Yinchen, Dahuang, etc., such as Yinchenhao Tang.

3. Strangury disease due to dampness-heat

The medicine can cool the blood to stop bleeding, so it is mostly used for blood strangury. It is often used with Mutong, Cheqianzi, Huashi, and so on, such as Bazheng San.

4. Hematemesis, epistaxis caused by blood heat

For bleeding due to blood heat manifested as hematemesis, epistaxis, hematuria, etc., it is often combined with Baimaogen, Dahuang, Cebaiye, etc., such as Shi Hui San. Also, it can be used together with Huangqin, Huanglian, Huangbai, such as Huanglian Jiedu Tang.

5. Red, swollen, and painful eyes

It can be used for such symptoms due to heat of liver and gallbladder, usually with Dahuang, such as Zhizi Tang.

Usage and Dosage: 5–10 g for decoction

1.7.2.3   Huangqin (Baical Skullcap Root, Radix Scutellariae)

Properties and Tastes: bitter, cold
Meridian Entry: lung, gallbladder, spleen, large intestine and small intestine meridians
   Effects

1. Clear heat and dry dampness
2. Clear fire and detoxify
3. Stop bleeding
4. Prevent abortion

   Application

1. Dampness-warmth, summer heat-dampness, epigastric fullness due to dampness-heat, diarrhea, and jaundice.

   The medicinal herb has the nature of bitter and cold and is attributed to the lung, gallbladder, spleen, large intestine, and small intestine meridians; therefore, it can clear heat and eliminate dampness of them, especially effective in clearing away dampness-heat of the middle and upper energizers. For dampness-warmth manifested as perspiration, fever, chest oppression, and greasy fur, it is often combined with Tongcao, Huashi, Baidoukou, etc. For jaundice due to dampness-heat, it is used together with Zhizi, Yinchen, Dahuang, etc. For the treatment of diarrhea of dampness-heat type, it is often used in combination with Huanglian, Banxia, Ganjiang, etc., such as Banxia Xiexin Tang.
2. For cough due to heat in the lung and high fever and excessive thirst

   The medicinal herb as attributed to the lung meridian, so it can be used for clearing heat in lung and good at clearing away sthenic heat of the upper energizer. It is the important herb for cough caused by lung heat. It is often used in combination with Gualou, Sangbaipi, Kuxingren, etc., such as Qingqi Huatan Wan. On the other hand, it is suitable for clearing heat in qifen, which is manifested as high fever and excessive thirst, such as Liangge San. For Shaoyang syndrome of alternating episodes of chills and fever, it is often used in combination with Chaihu, and the representative formula is Xiaochaihu Tang having the effect of regulating the function of Shaoyang.
3. For sore and ulcer, swollen sore

   The medicinal herb has the effect of clearing fire and detoxicating, so it can be used to treat sore and ulcer. For example, Huanglian Jiedu Tang consists of Huanglian, Huangbai, and Zhizi.

4. Hemopyretic bleeding

   It can be used alone (Huangqin San) or combined with Dahuang (Dahuang Tang) for hemopyretic bleeding, which is manifested as hematemesis, hemoptysis, hematochezia, hemafecia, and metrorrhagia.

5. For threatened abortion

   It can be used for excessive fetal movement and gravid vaginal bleeding due to heat syndrome in pregnancy together with Baizhu, Danggui, such as Danggui San.

Usage and Dosage: 3–10 g for decoction. When it is used to clear heat and eliminate dampness and clear fire and detoxicate, the herb is fresh. When used to prevent miscarriage, the herb is often processed with wine.

1.7.2.4   Huanglian (Coptis chinensis Franch, Coptis Rhizome)

Properties and Tastes: bitter and cold
Meridian Entry: heart, spleen, stomach, liver, gallbladder and large intestine meridians
   Effects

1. Clear heat and dry dampness
2. Clear fire and detoxify

   Application

1. The stuffiness and fullness, vomiting, and acid regurgitation

   The medicinal herb has the nature of bitter and cold, and it has a stronger effect of clearing heat and eliminating dampness than Huangqin, especially specializing in clearing away dampness-heat of middle energizers. It serves as an essential medicinal herb for the treatment of diarrhea and dysentery of dampness-heat type. It can be combined with Muxiang for the patients with abdominal pain due to qi stagnation, such as Xianglian Wan. Gegen Qinlian Tang, combined with Gegen for the case with general fever. Shaoyao Tang, combined with Baishao, Muxiang, Binlang, etc., for dysentery with pus and blood. For dampness-heat stagnation in the middle energizer, it is used together with Ganjiang, Huangqin, Banxia, etc., such as Banxia Xiexin Tang.

2. High fever and coma, heart fire hyperactivity, vexation and sleeplessness, palpitation, and lusterless

   It can clear heat and is especially good at removing heart fire. Therefore, it can be used for the diseases with excessive fire and heat, which is manifested as high fever and restlessness, such as Huanglian Jiedu Tang, which is combined with Zhizi and Huangqin. For heart fire hyperactivity, manifested as vexation and sleeplessness, it can be used together with Danggui and Shichangpu, such as Huanglian Anshen Wan. For vexation and sleeplessness due to insufficiency of yin and blood, it can be used together with Ejiao and Baishao, such as Huanglian Ejiao Tang.

3. For Vomiting blood due to blood heat

    It has the effect of clearing fire and detoxicating, and it can be used together with Dahuagn and Huangqin, such as Xiexin Tang.

4. Vomiting due to stomach heat and toothache due to stomach fire

    It can be used together with Zhuru, Banxia, Jupi, etc., such as Huanglian Jupi Zhuru Tang, which can clear away stomach heat and relieve vomiting. To treat vomiting with acid regurgitation due to liver fire attacking the stomach, it is often used together with Wuzhuyu, such as Zuojin Wan. When used together with Shengdihuang, Shengma, and Mudanpi, it can treat the toothache due to stomach fire. For the syndrome of excessive stomach fire with polyorexia and diabetes manifested as excessive thirst and frequent drinking, it can be used together with Tianhuafen, Dihuang, and others that can clear away heat and promote the production of the body fluids.

Usage and Dosage: 2–5 g for decoction. The herb stir-baked with wine is especially effective in clearing away dampness-heat of the middle energizers. The one stir-baked with ginger is especially good at clearing away stomach heat and relieving vomiting.

1.7.2.5 Huangbai (Amur Cork-Tree, Cortex Phellodendri)

Properties and Tastes: bitter and cold
  Meridian Entry: kidney and bladder meridians
  Effects

1. Clear heat and dry dampness
2. Clear fire and detoxify
3. Relieve malnutrition fever and hectic fever due to yin deficiency

Application

1. Syndrome of dampness-heat in the lower energizer

    The medicinal herb has the nature of bitter and cold and is attributed to the kidney and bladder meridians, so it is effective in clearing away dampness and heat of the lower energizer. For dysentery due to dampness-heat, it is usually combined with Baitouweng, Huanglian, and Qinpi to clear heat and eliminate dampness, such as Baitouweng Tang.

    When combined with Zhizi, it can be used for jaundice and brownish urine due to dampness and heat, such as Zhizi Baipi Tang. For yellow and thick leucorrhea due to dampness and heat, often combined with Shanyao, Qianshi, Cheqianzi, etc., such as Yihuang Tang. For the oliguria and brownish urine due to dampness-heat in bladder, it is usually combined with Cheqianzi, Fuling,

Bixie, etc., such as Bixie Fenqing Yin. For beriberi, swelling, and pain in foot and knees due to dampness-heat in the lower energizer, it is usually combined with Cangzhu, Niuxi, such as Sanmiao Wan.

2. Hectic fever, night sweat, and spermatorrhea

    The medicinal herb is attributed to the kidney meridian and can relieve malnutrition fever and hectic fever due to kidney yin deficiency and excessive kidney fire. At this time, it is usually combined with Zhimu, Shengdihuang, Shanyao, such as Zhibai Dihuang Wan.

3. Carbuncle and swelling and sore of dampness type due to heat toxin

    It is often used orally and combined with Huangqin, Huanglian, Zhizi, etc., such as Huanglian Jiedu Tang.

Usage and Dosage: 3–12 g for decoction. A suitable amount used externally.

When it is used to clear heat, eliminate dampness, clear fire, and detoxicate, the herb is fresh. When used to relieve malnutrition fever and hectic fever due to yin deficiency, the herb is often processed with brine.

1.7.2.6 Jinyinhua (Honeysuckle Flower, Flos Lonicerae)

Properties and Tastes: sweet and cold
   Meridian Entry: lung, heart and stomach meridians.
   Effects

1. Clear heat and detoxify
2. Disperse wind-heat

   Application

1. Carbuncle and pyocutaneous disease, pharyngitis, and erysipelas

    It is the essential medicine to clear away heat and detoxify, so it is used for excessive yang syndrome, such as carbuncle, whether the carbuncle is ripe or not or the beginning of rupture, and pyocutaneous, pharyngitis, and erysipelas. It can be used orally or the fresh is pounded for external application. For carbuncle and pyocutaneous, it is often used in combination with Danggui, Chishao, Baizhi, etc., such as Xianfang Huoming Yin, and also combined with Yejuhua, Pugongying, etc., for the treatment of deep-rooted boil. When it is used in combination with Danggui, Diyu, and Huangqin, it can treat the abdominalgia with intestinal abscess, such as Qingchang yin. For abscess of lung, it is often combined with Yuxingcao, Lugen, Yiyiren, etc.

2. The common cold due to wind-heat and seasonal febrile disease, no matter whether the heat of seasonal febrile diseases is in weifen, qifen, or involving yingfen and xuefen

    For early stage of seasonal febrile disease which manifested as generalized heat, headache, sore throat, and thirst, it is often used in combination with Liaoqiao, Bohe, and Niubangzi, such as Yinqiao San. For pathogenic factors

being in weifen manifested as strong heat and polydipsia, it is combined with
Shigao, Zhimu, etc.

When the heat of seasonal febrile disease involves yingfen and xuefen, it is
often used in combination with Shengdihuang, Xuanshen, etc., to clear heat and
cool blood, such as Qingying Tang.

3. For blood and epidemic dysentery

The medicinal herb has the nature of cold, and it can be used for clearing
away heat and detoxicating, combined with Huanglian, Huangqin, and
Baitouweng to strengthen the effect of relieving dysentery.

4. For summer heat syndrome

Manifested as excessive thirst, sore throat, summer carbuncle, heat rash, etc.,
it can be steamed with water into Jinyinhua Distillate for oral or external use.

Usage and Dosage: 6–15 g for decoction. The fresh is better for clearing away
heat and detoxicating; the carbonized one is used for dysentery; and distillate
medicinal water is used for heat polydipsia.

1.7.2.7 Lianqiao (Weeping Forsythia Capsule, Forsythia Forsythia)

Properties and Tastes: bitter and slightly cold
Meridian Entry: lung, heart and small intestine meridians.
Effects

1. Clear heat and detoxify
2. Disperse swelling and nodules
3. Disperse wind-heat

Application

1. Carbuncle, crewels, acute mastitis, and erysipelas

The medicinal herb has the nature of bitter and slightly cold, and it is similar
to Jinyinhua in effects. It can also clear away heat and toxin and is accompanied
by expelling wind and heat as well, so it is usually used for heat syndrome due
to exogenous attack. It is often used in combination with Chuanshanjia and
Zaojiaoci in order to strengthen the work of clearing away heat and detoxicating,
such as Jiajian Xiaodu Yin. When combined with Mudanpi and Tianhuafen, it
can be used to treat conditions such as carbuncles with redness, swelling, and
ulceration, similar to the effects of Lianqiao Jiedu Tang. For erysipelas, it is
often combined with Xiakucao, Beimu, and Xuanshen. Since it is good at clearing away heart fire, it can also be used for febrile disease involving the pericardium with restless fever, coma, or delirium.

2. For the common cold due to wind-heat and early stage of seasonal febrile disease

The medicinal herb has the nature of bitter and slightly cold, and its effects
are similar to Jinyinhua. For early stage of seasonal febrile disease manifested as
fever, sore throat, and thirsty, it is often used in combination with Bohe,

Niubangzi, etc., such as Yinqiao San. For pathogenic factors being in xuefen manifested as high fever polydipsia and god faint spots, it is often combined with Shengdihuang, etc. Because it specializes in clearing away heart fire, it can also be used for febrile disease involving the pericardium manifested as fever, coma, or delirium.

3. For dysuria or dribbling urination with pain
   Usually, it is combined with Cheqianzi, Baimaogen, and Zhuye for the treatment of dysuria or dribbling urination with pain, such as Rusheng San.

Usage and Dosage: 6–15 g for decoction

1.7.2.8 Shengdihuang (Fresh Rehmannia Root, Radix Rehmanniae Recens)

Properties and Tastes: sweet and cold.
  Meridian Entry: heart, liver, and kidney meridians.
  Effects

1. Clear heat and cool the blood
2. Nourish yin and promote the production of body fluid

Application

1. Seasonal febrile disease involving xuefen and yingfen
   The medicinal herb has the nature of sweet and cold; it is good at clearing away heat in yingfen manifested as fever, restlessness, and crimson tongue, often combined with Xuanshen, Lianqiao and Huanglian and others that can cool the blood, promote the production of the body fluids, and clear away heat, such as Qingying Tang. If the heat in xuefen manifested as macules, it can be used in combination with Shuiniujiao, Chishao, Mudanpi, etc., such as Xijiao Dihuang Tang.
2. For hemorrhage due to blood heat
   The medicinal herb is effective in clearing away heat in yingfen and has the effect of cooling blood and hemostasis. For hematemesis and epistaxis, it is often used in combination with Cebaiye, Heye, and Aiye, etc., such as Sisheng Wan, and for hemafecia and hematuria, usually combined with Diyu, Yimucao, etc.
3. Febrile disease consuming yin
   The medicinal herb has the nature of sweet and cold and has the effect of clearing away heat and nourishing yin and promoting production of body fluid. When manifested as red tongue and oral dryness, it is combined with Maidong, Shashen, and Yuzhu to promote the production of body fluid, such as Yiwei Tang.
4. For constipation due to dryness of intestine
   It is usually used together with Xuanshen and Maimendong, such as Zengye Tang.

Usage and Dosage: 10–15 g for decoction. The fresh amount is doubled or the fresh is pounded into juice that is put in decoction. The fresh is very cold and with plenty of juice; it can clear away heat and promote the production of the body fluids and has effect of cooling blood and arresting bleeding, so the fresh is suitable for seasonal febrile diseases and bleeding due to blood heat; the cold nature of the dry is slightly-weak, while its effect of nourishing yin is better, so the dry is especially suitable for yin deficiency with interior heat.

Other heat-clearing medicines (Table 1.9).

1.7.3 Purgative Medicine

Purgative medicines refer to the drugs that can cause diarrhea or lubricate the intestine, help the bowels moving, and relieve constipation.

These kinds of medicines mainly have the functions of relaxing the bowels and purgation. Therefore, they are mainly used to treat constipation, various interior excess syndromes due to food and water retention, and interior excess heat syndrome, etc. According to the difference in the purgative drug's effects and application, they can be classified into three categories, that is, offensive purgative medicine, laxative medicine, and drastic water-expelling medicine. All these three kinds of medicines should be used with caution in cases of injuring healthy qi, especially for the pregnancy, menstruation, postpartum, and old and weak patients. As long as the conditions of disease get better, their application must be stopped and the large dosage must be avoided.

1.7.3.1 Dahuang (Rhubarb, Radix Et Rhizoma Rhei)

Properties and Tastes: bitter and cold

Meridian Entry: spleen, stomach, large intestine, liver and pericardium meridians.

Effects

1. Remove accumulation with purgation
2. Clear heat and purge fire
3. Cool the blood and detoxify
4. Break blood and expel stasis, unblock the meridian
5. Drain dampness and remove jaundice

Application

1. Constipation due to stagnation of heat

   With strong effects of removing stagnation by purgation, Dahuang is an essential medicine for the treatment of constipation. And the medicinal herb has

Table 1.9 Simple list of other heat-clearing medicines

Name	Properties and tastes	Meridian entry	Effects	Application	dosage
Lugen (Rhizoma Phragmitis)	Sweet and cold	Lung and stomach meridians	(1) Clear heat and purge fire (2) Engender fluid and relieve thirst (3) Relieve dysphoria (4) Check vomiting (5) Promote diuresis	(1) Fever with restlessness, thirsty (2) Cough due to lung heat and pulmonary abscess (3) Vomiting due to stomach heat (4) For pyretic stranguria with pain	15–30 g for decoction and 30–60 g of the fresh
Zhuye (Herba Lophatheri)	Sweet, pungent, and cold	Heart, stomach, and small intestine meridians	(1) Clear heat and purge fire (2) Engender fluid (3) Relieve dysphoria 4 Promote diuresis	(1) Fever with restlessness, thirsty (2) For tongue sore, dysuria, edema, and oliguria	6–15 g for decoction, 15–30 g of the fresh
Tianhuafen (Radix Trichosanthis)	Sweet, slightly bitter, and slightly cold	Lung and stomach meridians	(1) Clear heat and purge fire (2) Engender fluid and relieve thirst (3) Resolve swelling and drain pus	(1) Febrile disease with thirst, diabetes, and frequent drinking (2) Dry cough due to lung heat (3) Pyocutaneous disease of heat type whether the infection is ulcerous or not	10–15 g for decoction
Xiakucao (Spica Prunellae)	Bitter, pungent, and cold	Liver and gallbladder meridians	(1) Clear the liver and purge fire (2) Disperse swelling and nodules (3) Improve the vision	(1) Hyperactivity of liver fire with conjunctivitis, headache and dizziness (2) Scrofula and goiter (3) Acute mastitis and lump in breast	9–15 g for decoction

Table 1.9 (continued)

Name	Properties and tastes	Meridian entry	Effects	Application	dosage
Juemingzi (Semen Cassiae)	Sweet, bitter, salty, and slightly cold	Liver and large intestine meridians	(1) Clear the liver and improve the vision (2) Moisten the intestines and relax the bowels	(1) Redness, swelling and pain in the eyes due to liver heat or wind-heat (2) Headache and dizziness (3) Constipation due to dryness of the intestine	9–15 g for decoction
Longdan (Radix Gentianae)	Bitter and cold	Liver and gallbladder meridians	(1) Clear heat and dry dampness (2) Clear fire of liver and gallbladder	(1) Jaundice, brownish urine, pudendal swelling, vaginal discharge, eczema, etc. (2) For headache caused by liver fire, deafness, hypochondriac pain, and bitter taste in the mouth	3–6 g for decoction
Kushen (Radix Sophorae Flavescentis)	Bitter and cold	Heart, liver, stomach, large intestine, and bladder meridians	(1) Clear heat and dry dampness (2) Kill worms (3) Promote urination	(1) Dampness-heat diarrhea and jaundice (2) For vaginal discharge disease, eruption caused by dampness	5–10 g for decoction
Baixianpi (Cortex Dictamni)	Bitter and cold	Spleen, stomach and bladder meridians	(1) Clear heat and dry dampness (2) Dispel wind and detoxify	(1) Eruption caused by dampness (2) For dampness-heat jaundice, wind-heat-dampness impediment	5–10 g for decoction

(continued)

Table 1.9 (continued)

Name	Properties and tastes	Meridian entry	Effects	Application	dosage
Chuanxinlian (Herba Andrographis)	Bitter and cold	Heart, lung, large intestine, and bladder meridians	(1) Clear heat and detoxify (2) Cool the blood (3) Disperse swelling (4) Drain dampness	(1) The common cold due to wind-heat and seasonal febrile disease at the early stage (2) For sore throat, mouth sores (3) For abscess of lung (4) For stranguria due to heat and dribbling urination with pain	6–9 g for decoction
Daqingye (Folium Isatidis)	Bitter and cold	Heart and stomach meridians	(1) Clear heat and detoxify (2) Cool the blood and disperse maculae	(1) It is indicated for seasonal febrile diseases with fever, maculae, and papules (2) Abscess, erysipelas, aphtha, and mumps	9–15 g for decoction
Qingdai (Indigo Naturalis)	Salty and cold	Liver meridian	(1) Clear heat and detoxify (2) Cool the blood and disperse maculae (3) Purge fire and relieve convulsion	(1) For maculae due to warm toxin (2) Hematemesis and epistaxis due to blood heat	5–3 g for pill or powder
Pugongying (Herba Taraxaci)	Bitter, sweet, and cold	Liver and stomach meridians	(1) Clear heat and detoxify (2) Disperse swelling and nodules (3) Drain dampness and promote urination	(1) Carbuncle, furuncle, erysipelas, scrofula, and lung abscess (2) For dampness-heat jaundice and urination with pain	10–15 g for decoction
Zihuadiding (Herba Violae)	Bitter, pungent, and cold	Heart and liver meridians	(1) Clear heat and detoxify (2) Cool the blood and disperse swelling	(1) Carbuncle toxin (2) Acute mastitis (3) For jaundice caused by heat-damp and heat strangury	15–30 g for decoction

Table 1.9 (continued)

Name	Properties and tastes	Meridian entry	Effects	Application	dosage
Baitouweng (Radix Pulsatillae)	Bitter and cold	Stomach and large intestine meridians	(1) Clear heat and detoxify (2) Cool the blood and relieve dysentery	(1) Heat-blood dysentery (2) For vaginal discharge	9–15 g for decoction
Banlangen (Radix Isatidis)	Bitter and cold	Heart and stomach meridians	(1) Clear heat and detoxify (2) Cool the blood and soothe the throat	(1) It is indicated for seasonal febrile diseases with fever, sore throat, maculae and papules, carbuncle, sore toxin, etc.	9–15 g for decoction
Yuxingcao (Herba Houttuyniae)	Pungent and slightly cold	Lung meridian	(1) Clear heat and detoxify (2) Disperse swelling and nodules (3) Disperse abscess and expel pus	(1) It is indicated for cough due to lung heat and pulmonary abscess (2) For carbuncle toxin (3) For stranguria due to heat and dribbling urination with pain	15–25 g for decoction
Baijiangcao (Herba Patriniae)	Pungent, bitter, and slightly cold	Stomach, large intestine, and liver meridians	(1) Clear heat and detoxify (2) Disperse swelling and nodules (3) Dissipate blood stasis and relieve pain	(1) For intestinal abscess and lung's abscess (2) For postpartum abdominal pain and dysmenorrhea due to blood stasis	6–15 g for decoction
Lvdou (Green Gram)	Sweet and cold	Heart and stomach meridians	(1) Clear heat and detoxify (2) Release summer heat (3) Promote urination	(1) Swollen sore and ulcer (2) For thirst caused by summer heat (3) For drug and food poisoning (4) For edema	15–30 g for decoction

the nature of bitter and cold, so it is especially effective in treatment of constipation due to stagnation of heat. In order to strengthen the work of purging heat and removing accumulation, it is often used in combination with Mangxiao, Houpo, and Zhishi, such as Dachengqii Tang. If the constipation is accompanied by deficiency of qi and blood, Danggui and Renshen are always combined with, such as Huanglong Tang. For yin deficiency due to stagnation of heat, Maimendong and Shengdihuang are added to the prescription mentioned above, such as Zengye Chengqi Tang. For constipation due to insufficiency of spleen yang and stagnation of cold, Ganjiang and Fuzi are combined with, such as Wenpi Tang.

2. For redness of eye, sore throat, and hematemesis due to blood heat

   With significant effects of removing heat from the blood, clearing away heat and purging fire, it is combined with Huanglian and Huangqin for blood heat syndrome manifested as redness of eye, sore throat, oral ulcer, and hematemesis, such as Xie Xin Tang.

3. Pyocutaneous disease due to toxic heat and abdominalgia with intestinal abscess

   It is often used in combination with Jinyinhua, Pugongying, Lianqiao, etc., for carbuncle due to toxic heat, such as Banxia Xie Xin Tang. For abdominalgia with intestinal abscess, combined with Mudanpi, Taoren, Mangxiao, etc., such as Dahuang Mudan Tang.

4. For meniscus and postpartum abdominal pain caused by blood stasis

   With the effects of promoting blood circulation to relieve blood stasis, it can be used as a common medicine for syndrome of blood retention. For meniscus due to blood stasis, it is often used in combination with Taoren, Guizhi, etc., such as Taohe Chengqi Tang. For postpartum abdominal pain due to blood stasis, it is used combined with Taoren, Tubiechong, etc., such as Xiayuxue Tang.

5. Dysentery, stranguria due to dampness-heat

   It can be used alone or combined with Huanglian, Huangqin, and Baishao for dysentery due to stagnation. For stranguria resulting from dampness-heat, it is often used in combination with Mutong, Cheqianzi, Zhizi, etc., such as Bazheng San.

6. For burn and scald

   It can be used alone or combined with Diyu. When it is used for this kind of disease, it should be made into the type powder and then mixed with sesame oil for external application.

Usage and Dosage: 3–15 g for decoction, just right amount for external use, and the crude one with stronger purgative effect is used for downward discharging. It is later added to decoction or soaked in boiling water for oral use and is not decocted for a long time. That prepared with wine is suitable for blood stasis because of its better effect on circulating blood. The carbonized form is usually used for bleeding syndrome.

1.7.3.2   Mangxiao (Sodium Sulfate, Natrii Sulfas)

Properties and Tastes: salty, bitter, and cold
   Meridian Entry: stomach and large intestine meridians
   Effects

1. Relax the bowels with purgation
2. Moisten dryness and soften hardness
3. Clear heat and disperse swelling

Application

1. Constipation due to accumulation of heat in the stomach and intestine
      The medicinal herb has the nature of cold and is an essential medicinal herb
   to treat the constipation. It is especially effective in the treatment of constipation
   caused by dryness and usually used in combination with Dahuang in order to
   strengthen the work of relaxing the bowels, such as Dachengqi Tang
2. Abdominalgia with intestinal abscess
      Usually, it is used combined with Dahuang, Mudanpi, Taoren, etc., such as
   Dahuang Mudan Tang. For the early stage of intestinal abscess, it is often used
   in combination with Dahuang and Dasuan.
3. For acute mastitis, hemorrhoids, sore throat, aphthae, swelling, and pain in
   the eyes
      For the early stage of mastiffs, it can be dissolved in water for external appli-
   cation and wrapped with gauze. It also can be used alone for decoction to rinse
   for hemorrhoids. It is usually combined with Zhusha, Pengsha, and Bingpian to
   treat the sore throat and aphthae, such as Bingpeng San. For swelling and pain in
   the eyes, the solution form of Xuanmingfen can be used.

Usage and Dosage: 6–12 g dissolved in decoction or in boiling water for oral
using. Just appropriate amount is for external using.

1.7.3.3   Yuliren (Chinese Dwarf Cherry Seed, Semen Pruni)

Properties and Tastes: Pungent, bitter, sweet, and medium
   Meridian Entry: Spleen, large intestine, and small intestine meridians
   Effects

1. Moisten the intestines to relax the bowels
2. Induce diuresis to alleviate edema

Application

1. Constipation due to deficiency of blood and dryness of intestine
      The medicine can not only moisten the intestines, but also promote the circu-
   lation of large intestine qi. It is usually combined with Huomaren, Baiziren, and
   Xingren, such as Wuren Wan.

2. For edema, abdominal fullness, beriberi, and dysuria

   It can be used together with Sangbaipi, Chixiaodou, and so on, such as Yuliren Tang.

Usage and Dosage 6–12 g is used in decoction for oral use, broken, and then added to decoction.

1.7.3.4 Songziren (Pine Nut, Pinus Pinea)

Properties and Tastes: sweet and warm
  Meridian Entry: lung, liver, and large intestine meridians
  Effects

1. Moisten the intestines to relax the bowels
2. Moisten the lung to suppress cough

Application

1. Constipation due to dryness of intestine

   The medicine has the function of moistening the intestines, so it can be used for the constipation caused by intestine dryness due to consumption of fluid. It also can be used for the old man's constipation. Usually, it is used with Huomaren, Yuliren, and Baiziren, which made into the type of powder, taken with Huangqi Tang.
2. Dry cough due to lung dryness

   The medicine can moisten the lung, so it is better for the dry cough. It can be used with Hutaoren, mixed with honey, taken with rice water.

Usage and Dosage: 5–10 g for decoction
Other purgative medicines (Table 1.10).

1.7.4 Wind-Dampness-Dispelling Medicine

Wind-dampness-dispelling medicines refer to the drugs that mainly dispel the pathogens of wind and damp, which is for the treatment of impediment diseases.

These kinds of medicines are mainly pungent and bitter in nature. The pungent taste can dispel not only wind and damp, but also unobstructed meridians; therefore, they can dispel the wind-dampness staying in the muscles, meridians, and muscles. Wind-dampness-dispelling medicines mainly treat the impediment diseases caused by wind-dampness, manifesting as limb pain, swollen joints, and tendon spasm.

According to the difference in the natures and effects, the wind-dampness-dispelling medicines can be classified into three categories: wind-cold-dampness dispelling medicines, wind-heat-dampness dispelling medicines,

Table 1.10 Simple list of other purgative medicines

Name	Properties and tastes	Meridian entry	Effects	Application	Dosage
Fanxieye (Folium Sennae)	Sweet, bitter, and cold	Large intestine meridians	(1) Cool purgation and relax the bowels (2) Promote diuresis	(1) Constipation due to stagnation of heat (2) For edema	2–6 g for decoction and decoct later or soaked in warm boiled water for oral use
Luhui (Aaloe)	Bitter and cold	Liver, stomach, and large intestine meridians	(1) Relax the bowels (2) Clear fire of the liver (3) Kill worms	(1) Constipation due to heat stagnation (2) Overabundance of fire in the liver meridian (3) Infantile malnutrition and convulsion	2–5 g is added to pill or powder for oral using

wind-dampness-dispelling, and strengthening the bones and muscles medicines. The medicines with pungent taste and warm mature should be used carefully in cases of injuring blood and body fluid.

Most impediment diseases belong to chronic disease; therefore, this kind of medicine can be made into the type of pills or powder and processed with wine.

1.7.4.1 Duhuo (double Teeth Pubescent Angelica Root, Radix Angelicae Pubescentis)

Properties and Tastes: pungent, bitter, and slightly warm
Meridian Entry: kidney and bladder meridians
Effects

1. Dispel wind and dampness
2. Relieve pain in impediment diseases
3. Release the exterior

Application

1. Impediment diseases of wind-cold-dampness type

   The medicinal herb has the nature of pungent and warm, and it serves as an essential medicinal herb for wind-cold-dampness type of impediment diseases. It is attributed to the kidney meridian, so it is especially effective in the back and the lower half of the body with soreness and pain due to dampness. For the symptoms as muscle pain, back pain, hand, and foot pain, it can be used together with Danggui, Baizhu, Niuxi, etc., such as Duohuo Tang. For prolonged impediment diseases due to deficiency of qi and blood and insufficiency of the liver and kidney, it is often combined with Sangjisheng, Duzhong, Niuxi, etc., such as Duhuo Ji Sheng Tang.

2. For headache caused by wind-cold and dampness

   The medicinal herb has the effect of relieving exogenous pathogenic factors; therefore, it can be used together with Qianghuo, Gaoben and Fang Feng to treat the exterior syndrome, which is manifested as headache, general heavy sensation in body, such as Qianghuo Jisheng Tang.

Usage and Dosage: 3–10 g for decoction. Just appropriate amount is for external using.

1.7.4.2 Qinjiao (Largeleaf Gentian Root, Radix Gentianae Macrophyllae)

Properties and Tastes: pungent, bitter and medium
  Meridian Entry: stomach, liver, gallbladder meridians
  Effects

1. Dispel wind and dampness
2. Relieve pain in impediment diseases
3. Relieve asthenia heat
4. Clear heat and dampness

   Application

1. Impediment diseases, spastic muscles

   Qinjiao has the nature of pungent and bitter, but it is not dry. Therefore, it can be used for all kinds of impediment diseases and spastic muscles, especially for the heat impediment together with Fangji and Rendongteng. It also can be used together with Tianma, Qianghuo, and Chuanxiong to treat the impediment diseases of wind-cold-dampness type, such as Qinjiao Tianma Tang.
2. Jaundice with damp-heat pathogen

   The medicinal herb is attributed to the liver and gallbladder meridians, so it is better at clearing the heat and dampness of these two organs. When it is used for the jaundice, it can be alone or together with Yinchen, Zhizi, and Dahuang, such as Shanyinchen Wan.
3. Bone-steaming tidal fever

   The medicine is vital to the osteopyrexia and fever, usually together with Qinghao, Digupi, Zhimu, and so on, such as Qinjiaobiejia Tang.

Usage and Dosage: 3–10 g for decoction

1.7.4.3 Wujiapi (Acanthopanax, Cortex Acanthopanax Radicis)

Properties and Tastes: pungent, bitter and warm
  Meridian Entry: liver, kidney meridians

Effects

1. Dispel wind and dampness
2. Nourish the liver and kidney
3. Strengthen tendons and bones
4. Promote urination and disperse swelling

Application

1. Impediment diseases

    It is mostly used for the old people and the people with aeipathia because of its function of nourishing the liver and kidney. It can be soaked alone in wine, or used together with Danggui, Niuxi, etc., or with Mugua and Songjie.
2. Weakness of waist and knees or retarded ambulation of children

    The medicine can nourish the liver and kidney, so it can be used for yin deficiency of the liver and kidney with weakness of waist and knees or retarded ambulation of children, usually combined with Duzhong, Niuxi, and others that tonify the kidney and liver.
3. Edema

    It is usually in combination with Fulingpi, Dafupi, and Shengjiangpi, such as Wupi San.

Usage and Dosage: 5–10 g for decoction
Other wind-dampness-dispelling medicines (Table 1.11).

1.7.5 Dampness-Resolving Medicine

The medicines that resolve dampness, with fragrant odor, warming, and drying belong to dampness-resolving medicines.

The spleen does not function well with dampness. If turgid dampness blocks the middle-jiao internally, the transformation and transportation functions of the spleen become impaired. Dampness-resolving medicines are warm and dry. They facilitate the movement and functional activities of qi, dissipate turgid dampness, strengthen the spleen, and stimulate the stomach. They are especially useful when the spleen is blocked by dampness and its functions impaired, leading to such symptoms as abdominal distention, vomiting, acid regurgitation, diarrhea, anorexia, weariness, a sweet taste in the mouth with much salivation, and a white greasy tongue coating. They are also useful for treating illnesses due to dampness-heat and heatstroke.

Illnesses of dampness may be of cold-dampness or heat-dampness. When treating an illness caused by dampness, it is important to select an appropriate combination of herbs, for cold-dampness supplement with medicines that warm the interior and for heat-dampness supplement with herbs that cool heat and dry dampness.

Table 1.11 Simple list of other wind-dampness-dispelling medicines

Name	Properties and tastes	Meridian entry	Effects	Application	Dosage
Weilingxian (Radix Clematidis)	Pungent, salty, and warm	Bladder meridian	(1) Dispel wind and dampness (2) Free the collateral vessels and relieve pain in impediment diseases (3) Remove fishbone stuck in the throat	(1) Impediment disease due to wind-cold-dampness (2) Fishbone stuck in the throat	6–9 g for decoction
Mugua (Fructus Chaenomelis)	Sour and warm	Liver and spleen meridians	(1) Relax sinews and activate collateral (2) Resolve dampness and harmonize the stomach	(1) Wind-dampness impediment (2) Swelling of the foot (3) Vomiting, diarrhea, and twitch	6–9 g for decoction
Qingfengteng (Caulis Sinomenii)	Bitter and pungent	Liver and spleen meridians	(1) Dispel wind and dampness (2) Free the collateral vessels (3) Promote urination	(1) Wind-dampness impediment (2) Swelling of the foot	6–12 g for decoction
Fangji (Radix Stephaniae Tetrandrae)	Bitter and cold	Bladder and lung meridians	(1) Dispel wind and relieve pain (2) Promote urination and disperse swelling	(1) Wind-dampness impediment manifested as painful joints and stiffness (2) Edema, ascitic fluid, and dysuria (3) Eczema and carbuncle and sore toxin	5–10 g for decoction
Sangzhi (Ramulus Mori)	Slightly bitter medium	Liver meridian	(1) Dispel wind and dampness (2) Disinhibit the joints	Wind-dampness impediment with pains of general joints	9–15 g for decoction

Table 1.11 (continued)

Name	Properties and tastes	Meridian entry	Effects	Application	Dosage
Sangjisheng (Herba Taxilli)	Bitter, sweet and medium	Liver and kidney meridians	(1) Dispel wind and dampness (2) Nourish the liver and kidney (3) Strengthen tendons and bones (4) Prevent abortion	(1) Wind-cold-wetness type of arthralgia (2) For habitual abortion due to yin deficiency of the liver and kidney (3) Dizziness caused by yin deficiency of the liver and kidney	9–15 g for decoction
Gou Ji (Rhizoma Cibotii)	Bitter, sweet, and warm	Liver and kidney meridians	(1) Dispel wind and dampness (2) Nourish the liver and kidney (3) Strengthen waist and knee	(1) Wind-dampness impediment (2) For weakness of waist and knees and flaccidity of extremities due to yin deficiency of the liver and kidney	6–12 g for decoction

The nature of dampness is viscous and impeding. When it invades the meridians, qi movement becomes impeded. For this reason, when treating with dampness-resolving medicines, it is common to supplement them with medicines that promote qi movement. Also, weakening of the spleen can generate dampness. Treatment of dampness generated when the spleen is weakened should include medicines that nourish the spleen.

Some of the medicines are warm and dry in nature so they easily consume yin and blood; therefore, we must pay attention to these medicines to avoid insufficiency of yin, deficiency of blood, or consumption of the body fluids.

1.7.5.1 Huoxiang (Herba Agastaches, Wrinkled Gianthyssop Herb)

Properties and Tastes: pungent and slightly warm
Meridian Entry: spleen, stomach and lung meridians
Effects

1. Resolve dampness with aroma
2. Stop vomiting
3. Release summer heat

Application

1. The obstruction of dampness in the middle energizer

   The syndrome is manifested as fatigue of the body and spirits, loss of appetite and nausea, fullness in the chest, and epigastrium. It is often combined with Houpo, Cangzhu, etc., such as Buhuanjin Zhengqi San.
2. Vomiting

   It serves as an essential medicinal herb for the treatment of dampness-retention syndrome with vomiting. It is often used in combination with Banxia and Dingxiang, etc., such as Huo xiangbanxia Tang. For the vomiting caused by damp-heat, it is used with Huanglian and Zhuru, and for the vomiting caused by pregnancy, often it is used with Sharen and Sugeng. If the vomiting is caused by weakness of the spleen and the stomach, it is used with Dangshen, Baizhu, and so on.
3. Superficial syndrome of summer heat and damp type and early stage of seasonal febrile disease

   For the former, which is manifested as headache, fever, fullness and pain in the chest and epigastrium, vomiting, and diarrhea, it is often combined with Huangqin, Huashi, Yinchen, etc., such as Ganluxiaodu Dan and also combined with Zisuye, Houpo, etc., such as Huoxiangzhengqi San.

Usage and Dosage: 3–10 g for decoction. The amount of the fresh is doubled.

1.7.5.2   Cangzhu (Rhizoma Atractylodis, Atractylodes Rhizome)

Properties and Tastes: pungent, bitter, and warm
   Meridian Entry: spleen, stomach, and liver meridians
   Effects

1. Dry dampness to fortify the spleen
2. Dispel wind and dissipate cold
3. Improve vision

Application

1. Dampness-retention syndrome involving the middle energizer

   For such a syndrome manifested as abdominal fullness and distention, nausea and vomiting, and poor appetite, it is usually combined with Chenpi, Houpo, etc., such as Pingwei San. For the damp-retention due to deficiency of the spleen, it is often with Fuling, Zexie, and Zhuling, such as Zhuling Tang.
2. Wind-wetness type of arthralgia and wilting disease

   The medicinal herb has the nature of pungent and bitter; it is especially suitable for arthralgia with domination of dampness. It is often used in combination with Yiyiren, Duhuo, etc., such as Yiyiren Tang.

   For arthralgia of dampness-heat type, it is usually combined with Zhimu, Shigao, etc., such as Baihu Jia Cangzhu Tang. For wilting disease due to damp invasion of the lower energizer manifested as beriberi and swelling and pain in foot and knees and limp wilting, it is usually combined with Huangbai, Yiyiren, and Niuxi, such as Simiao San.

3. The common cold due to wind-cold, especially suitable for affection of exogenous wind-cold-dampness

    It is usually combined with Baizhi, Qianghuo, Fangfeng, etc., such as Shenzhu San.

4. Night blindness

    It can be used alone or combined with lamb liver and pork liver.

Usage and Dosage: 3–9 g for decoction

1.7.5.3 Houpo (Officinal magnolia bark, Cortex Magnoliae Officinalis)

Properties and Tastes: bitter, pungent, and warm
Meridian Entry: spleen, stomach, lung, and the large intestine meridians
Effects

1. Promote circulation of qi and dry dampness
2. Remove stagnation and relieve fullness
3. Descend qi and remove phlegm and asthma

Application

1. Abdominal distention and fullness due to stagnation of dampness or food

    It is often used in combination with Dahuang and Zhishi to remove the stagnation and relieve fullness, such as Houposanwu Tang.

2. Cough, asthma, and profuse sputum

    It is often used in combination with Zisuzi, Chenpi, and Banxia in order to strengthen the work of descending qi, removing phlegm and relieving asthma, such as Suzijiangqi Tang. For cough due to wind-cold, it is usually combined with Guizhi, Xingren, etc., such as Guizhijiahoupoxingzi Tang.

Usage and Dosage: 3–10 g for decoction.
Other dampness-resolving medicines (Table 1.12).

1.7.6 Dampness-Draining Diuretic Medicine

Dampness-draining diuretic medicines are herbs that have their principal actions of unblocking the water pathways and the dissipation of dampness (diuresis). They can increase the amount of urine, so that retained water and accumulated dampness can be excreted as urine.

Table 1.12 Simple list of other dampness-resolving medicines

Name	Properties and tastes	Meridian entry	Effects	Application	Dosage
Peilan (Herba Eupatorii)	Pungent	Spleen, stomach, and lung meridians	(1) Resolve dampness (2) Release summer heat	(1) The obstruction of dampness in the middle energizer (2) Affection of exogenous summer heat and dampness, the early stage of damp febrile disease	3–10 g for decoction. 6–20 g of the fresh
Sharen (Fructus Amomi Villosi)	Pungent and warm	Spleen, stomach, and kidney meridians	(1) Resolve dampness and move qi (2) Warm the middle to check diarrhea (3) Prevent abortion	(1) The obstruction of dampness in the middle energizer and stagnation of spleen qi and stomach qi (2) Vomiting and diarrhea due to asthenia-cold of the spleen and stomach (3) Vomiting due to pregnancy and threatened abortion due to stagnation of qi	3–10 g for decoction and decoct later
Doukou (Semen Myristicae)	Pungent and warm	Lung, spleen, and stomach meridians	(1) Resolve dampness and move qi (2) Warm the middle to check vomiting	(1) The obstruction of dampness in the middle energizer (2) Vomiting and hiccup due to cold and dampness	3–6 g for decoction and decoct later

Some of these medicines also act to clear dampness-heat and are especially suitable for such conditions as difficult and painful urination, edema, accumulated rheum and phlegm, jaundice, and exudative dermatitis. Dampness-draining diuretic medicines are sweet or bland in flavor and neutral, slightly cold, or cold in nature. Bland flavor is associated with ability to drain water and dissipate dampness. Cold nature is associated with the ability to cool heat. In addition to increasing the amount of urine, dampness-draining diuretic medicines of cold nature are especially effective in cooling heat and eliminating dampness from the lower-jiao. They are often prescribed for dysuria. When prescribing these medicines, pay attention to the character of the illness and add medicines as appropriate. For example, for acute edema associated with symptoms of the exterior, add medicines that soothe the lung and induce sweating. For chronic edema due to deficiency of spleen and kidney yang, add medicines that warm and nourish the spleen and the kidney. For illnesses of simultaneous dampness and heat, add medicines that cool heat and purge fire. For heat injury to blood vessels and hematuria, add medicines that cool blood and stop bleeding. When dampness-draining diuretic medicines are used inappropriately, they can easily damage yin fluids; hence, great care must be exercised when treating patients with yin deficiency or fluid insufficiency.

1.7.6.1   Fuling (Indian Bread, Poria)

Properties and Tastes: sweet and medium
  Meridian Entry: heart, lung, spleen, and kidney meridians
  Effects

1. Induce diuresis to drain dampness
2. Fortify the spleen
3. Nourish the heart to tranquilize

Application

1. Edema and dysuria
   It is an essential medicine to treat all kinds of edema. For edema caused by retention of water in the body, it is usually combined with Zexie, Zhuling, Baizhu, etc., such as Wuling San. For that with deficiency of spleen yang and kidney yang, it is usually combined with Ganjiang, Fuzi, etc., such as Zhenwu Tang. For accumulation of water with heat, manifested as anuresis and edema, it is often used with Huashi, Ejiao, and Zexie, such as Zhuling Tang.
2. Phlegm-fluid retention
   For that manifested as dizzy and palpitation, it is usually combined with Guizhi, Baizhu, Gancao, etc., such as Ling Gui Zhu Gan Tang. For that manifested as vomit, it is usually combined with Banxia and Shengjiang, such as Xiao Ban Xia Jia Fu Ling Tang.
3. Spleen deficiency syndromes
   The medicinal herb has the effect of invigorating the spleen and stopping diarrhea; it is especially effective in spleen deficiency with dampness. It is usually combined with Shanyao, Baizhu, and Yiyiren, such as Shenling Baizhu San. It is also combined with Renshen, Gancao, and Baizhu, such as Sijunzi Tang.
4. Restlessness, palpitation, and insomnia caused by deficiency of both the heart and spleen
   It is often combined with Huangqi, Danggui, Yuanzhi, etc., such as Guipi Tang. If it is caused by heart qi deficiency, usually with Renshen, Longchi, Yuanzhi, and so on, such as Anshendingzhi Wan.

Usage and Dosage: 10–15 g for decoction

1.7.6.2 Yiyiren (Coix Seed, Semen Coicis)

Properties and Tastes: pungent and cold
    Meridian Entry: spleen, stomach, and lung meridians
    Effects

1. Induce diuresis to drain dampness
2. Fortify the spleen to stanch diarrhea
3. Treat impediment manifested
4. Expel pus
5. Detoxify and disperse nodules

    Application

1. Dysuria, edema, beriberi
   The medicine has the function of inducing diuresis to drain dampness and fortifying the spleen. Therefore, it is used for spleen deficiency syndrome with accumulation of dampness manifested as dysuria, edema, and beriberi. For edema, it is usually combined with Fuling, Baizhu, Huangqi, etc.; for spleen deficiency with loss of appetite and diarrhea, it is usually used together with Dangshen and Baizhu.
2. Diarrhea due to spleen deficiency
   It is often used with Renshen, Fuling, and Baizhu, such as Shenling Baizhu San.
3. Impediment disease
   For impediment disease with dominant dampness manifested as bodily heaviness and soreness and rigidity of limbs, it is often used together with Mugua; for that with heat, it is combined with Dilong and Fangji; for the one with cold, combined with Mahuang and Guizhi; and for that with heavy dampness, usually combined with Cangzhu.
4. Pulmonary and intestinal abscess
   For the former that with cough and thick sputum, it is usually used with Weijing, Dongguaren, Taoren, etc., such as Weijing Tang; for the later, it is used together with Baijiangcao, Mudanpi, Fuzi, etc., such as Yiyi Fuzi Baijiang San.

    Usage and Dosage: 9–30 g for decoction

1.7.6.3 Zhuling (Chuling, Polyporus Umbellatus)

Properties and Tastes: sweet and medium
    Meridian Entry: kidney and bladder meridians
    Effects: Induce diuresis to drain dampness
    Application
Edema, dysuria, diarrhea, and turbid strangury
It can be used alone to treat edema caused by retention of water in the body. For dysuria and edema, it is often used in combination with Zexie, Fuling, and Baizhu, such as Siling San. For diarrhea due to cold and dampness in the stomach and

intestine, it is usually combined with Roudoukou, Huangbai, etc., such as Zhuling Wan. For dysuria and turbid strangury due to yin deficiency, it is usually combined with Ejiao, Zexie, etc., such as Zhuling Tang. In addition, it does not have the effect of invigorating the spleen. So, for edema syndrome due to spleen deficiency, it must be combined with other herbs of invigorating the spleen, such as Fuling, Baizhu, etc.

Usage and Dosage: 6–12 g for decoction

1.7.6.4   Zexie (Oriental Water Plantain Rhizome, Rhizoma Alismatis)

Properties and Tastes: sweet and cold
  Meridian Entry: kidney and bladder meridians
  Effects

1. Induce diuresis to drain dampness
2. Discharge heat
3. Eliminate turbid and reducing blood lipids

Application

1. Dysuria and edema
    It is often used with Fuling, Zhuling, and Guizhi, such as Wuling San. It also can be used for the diarrhea due to the cold of spleen and stomach, with Houpo, Cangzhu, Chenpi and so on, such as Weiling Tang; for the phlegm retention manifested as dizzy, it is used with Baizhu, such as Zexie Tang.
2. Stranguria caused by heat
    Zexie is especially effective in dampness-heat type in the lower energizer, usually with Mutong, Cheqianzi; for seminal emission, tidal fever caused by deficiency of kidney yin, it is used with Shudihuang, Shanzhuyu, Mudanpi, and so on, such as Liuweidihuang Wan.
3. Hyperlipidemia
    Studies have shown that the medicine can reduce blood lipids. It can be used in combination with Juemingzi, Heye, Heshouwu, and so on.

Usage and Dosage: 6–10 g for decoction.

1.7.6.5   Cheqianzi (Plantain Seed, Semen Plantaginis)

Properties and Tastes: sweet and cold
  Meridian Entry: liver, kidney, lung and small intestine meridians
  Effects

1. Clear heat and induced diuresis
2. Drain dampness to stanch diarrhea
3. Improve vision
4. Dispel phlegm

Application

1. Edema and stranguria
    It is especially suitable for stranguria of damp-heat types manifested as oligu-
ria with reddish urine, difficulty, and pain in micturition, and it is usually combined with Mutong, Huashi, and Bianxu, such as Bazheng San. For the edema
caused by retention of water-damp, it is used with Zhuling, Fuling, and Zexie;
for the kidney deficiency caused by aeipathia, it is used with Niuxi, Shudihuang,
Shanzhuyu, and so on, such as Jisheng Shenqi Wan.
2. Diarrhea due to summer heat-dampness
    It can promote the diuresis so does to make defecation forming; therefore, it
can be used for diarrhea due to domination of dampness. It can be used alone or
with Baizhu, Fuling, Zexie, etc.
3. Conjunctivitis due to flaring up of liver fire
    It is usually used combined with Juhua and Juemingzi; for deficiency of liver
yin and kidney yin manifested as dim eyesight and nebula, often used together
with Shudihuang, Tusizi, and Gouqizi.
4. Cough caused by lung heat
    It is usually combined with Gualou, Zhebeimu, Pipaye, etc.

Usage and Dosage: 9–15 g for decoction. Wrap-decoct.

1.7.6.6 Huashi (Talc, Talcum)

Properties and Tastes: sweet and cold
  Meridian Entry: bladder, lung, and stomach meridians
  Effects

1. Induce diuresis to treat stranguria
2. Release summer heat

Application

1. Strangury disease caused by heat
    Huashi is a commonly used medicine for the treatment of strangury, often
used with Mutong, Cheqianzi, Qumai, and so on, such as Bazheng San. For the
stone strangury, it is often used with Haijinsha, Jinqiancao, Mutong, and so on.
2. Summer heat syndrome with excessive thirst, dysuria. It can be used with
Gancao, such as Liuyi San. For the early stage of damp febrile disease manifested as headache, aversion to cold, heavy body, and chest tightness, it is used
with Yiyiren, Baikouren, Xingren, and so on, such as Sanren Tang.
3. Diarrhea due to dampness and heat
    It can promote the diuresis to make defecation forming, often used with
Zhuling, Cheqianzi, and Yiyiren.
    Besides, Huashi can astringe dampness and furuncle when it is being external
used, so it can be used for eczema, malaria, and so on.

Usage and Dosage: 10–30 g for decoction. Just appropriate amount of fresh for external using.

1.7.6.7 Yinchen (Virgate Wormwood Herb, Herba Artemisiae Scopariae)

Properties and Tastes: bitter, pungent and slightly cold
  Meridian Entry: spleen, stomach, liver and gallbladder meridians
  Effects

1. Clear heat and dampness
2. Normalize gallbladder to cure jaundice

   Application

1. Jaundice and dysuria
     It is an essential medicine to treat all kinds of jaundice; for that due to dampness and heat manifested as yellow tint of sclera and skin, it is usually combined with Zhizi, Dahuang, etc., such as Yinchenhao Tang; for that due to cold-dampness of spleen and stomach, usually combined with Fuzi, Ganjiang, etc., such as Yinchen Sini Tang.
2. Dampness-warmth syndrome and summer febrile disease, which is manifested as fever, malaise, stuffy chest, vomiting, and dysuria
     It is usually combined with Huashi, Huangqin, Mutong, etc., such as Ganlu Xiaodu Dan.
3. Eczema pruritus
     It can be used combined with Huangbai, Kushen, Difuzi, etc.

Usage and Dosage: 6–15 g for decoction. Just right amount is for external using.
Other dampness-draining diuretic medicines (Table 1.13).

1.7.7 Interior-Warming Medicine

These are herbs that have as their principal action the warming of and dispelling cold from interior. They are of pungent flavor and hot nature; these are the properties that make them so suitable for treating illnesses of interior cold.

There are two types of interior cold illnesses: those of exogenous cold invading the interior and suppressing yang qi of the spleen and the stomach and those of endogenous cold arising out of deficiency of yang qi or injury of yang qi by excessive sweating. In either case, interior-warming medicines are appropriate treatment.

When prescribing interior-warming medicines, it is appropriate to modify the combination of medicines depending on the clinical condition. For exogenous cold invading interior but associated with symptoms of exterior, add medicines that release the exterior. For qi stagnation due to congealing by cold, add medicines that

Table 1.13 Simple list of other dampness-draining diuretic medicines

Name	Properties and tastes	Meridian entry	Effects	Application	Dosage
Dongguapi (Exocarpium Benincasae)	Sweet, and cool	Spleen and small intestine meridians	(1) Induce diuresis to disperse swelling (2) Release summer heat	(1) Dysuria, edema (2) For summer heat syndrome with excessive thirst, dysuria	9–30 g for decoction
Tongcao (Medulla Tetrapanacis)	Sweet, and slightly cold	Lung and stomach meridians	(1) Clear heat and promote urination (2) Promote lactation	(1) Dysuria, edema, and stranguria caused by heat (2) For oligogalactia or agalactia	3–5 g for decoction
Qumai (Herba Dianthi)	Bitter and cold	Heart and small intestine meridians	(1) Induce diuresis to treat stranguria (2) Activate blood and unblock the meridian	(1) Heat strangury, blood strangury, stone strangury, and dysuria (2) Menstrual irregularities and amenorrhea caused by blood stasis	9–15 g for decoction
Bianxu (Herba Polygoni Avicularis)	Bitter and slightly cold	Bladder meridians	(1) Induce diuresis to treat stranguria (2) Kill worms (3) Relieve itching	(1) Heat strangury and oliguria with reddish urine (2) Abdominal pain due to parasitic infestation, eczema, and pruritus vulvae	9–15 g for decoction
Haijinsha (Spora Lygodii)	Sweet, salty, and cold	Bladder and small intestine meridians	(1) Clear heat and drain dampness (2) Induce diuresis to treat stranguria	Various stranguria	6–15 g for decoction. Wrap-decoction

Table 1.13 (continued)

Name	Properties and tastes	Meridian entry	Effects	Application	Dosage
Bixie (Rhizome Dioscoreae Hypoglaucae)	Bitter	Kidney and stomach meridians	(1) Eliminate dampness and turbidity (2) Expel wind	(1) Chyloid stranguria and whitish turbid urine (2) Wind-dampness impediment manifested as bodily heaviness, sore and painful waist, and knees	9–15 g for decoction
Jinqiancao (Herba Lysimachiae)	Sweet and slightly cold	Liver, gallbladder, kidney, and bladder meridians.	(1) Eliminate dampness to treat jaundice (2) Induce diuresis to treat stranguria (3) Detoxify and relieve swelling	(1) Jaundice due to dampness-heat (2) Strangury disease (3) Eczema and damp sore	15–60 g for decoction

mobilize qi. For accumulation of cold and dampness in interior, add medicines that strengthen the spleen and dissolve dampness. For yang deficiency in the spleen and the kidney, add warming medicines that strengthen the spleen and the kidney. For yang collapse and qi depletion, add medicines that can vigorously augment and support genuine qi.

The medicines in this group are pungency and hot, and they are drying. If applied improperly, they can easily injure body fluids. In illnesses of heat or yin deficiency and in pregnancy, they must be used with great care or are contraindicated.

1.7.7.1 Fuzi (Lateralis Preparata, Radix Aconiti Lateralis Praeparata)

Properties and Tastes: pungent, sweet, extremely hot, and toxic
  Meridian Entry: heart, kidney, and spleen meridians
  Effects

1. Recuperate the depleted yang for resuscitation
2. Supplement fire and strengthen yang
3. Expel cold to relieve pain

  Application

1. Syndrome of yang exhaustion

   It is used for yang exhaustion syndrome. It is an essential drug for the treatment of yang exhaustion syndrome manifested as clammy perspiration, faint breath, cold clammy limbs, indistinct, and faint pulse. It is usually used in combination with Ganjiang and Gancao, such as Sini Tang; for exhaustion of qi due to yang deficiency, it can be combined with Renshen to supplement qi to prevent collapse of qi, such as Shenfu Tang.

2. Syndrome of yang deficiency

   It is used to treat all kinds of syndromes of yang deficiency. For insufficiency of kidney yang with impotence, cold and painful waist and knees, and frequent micturition, it is usually combined with Rougui, Shanzhuyu, and Shudihuang, such as Yougui Wan; for insufficiency of spleen yang and kidney yang and interior domination of cold and dampness with coldness and pain in epigastric abdomen and loss of appetite and diarrhea, it is combined with Dangshen, Baizhu, and Ganjiang, such as Fuzilizhong Tang; for yang deficiency resulting in edema, and dysuria, it is usually used together with Baizhu, Fuling, and Shengjiang, such as Zhenwu Tang; for exogenous affection due to yang deficiency, it is combined with Mahuang and Xixin, such as Mahuang Fuzi Xixin Tang.

3. Syndrome of Cold B

   It is used to treat all pain syndromes of cold type. For arthralgia of wind-cold-dampness type, pain in general joints due to domination of cold and dampness, it is combined with Guizhi, Baizhu and Gancao, such as Gancao Fuzi Tang; for abdominal pain due to cold accumulation and qi stagnation, it is combined with Dingxiang and Gaoliangjiang.

Usage and Dosage: 3–15 g is used in decoction for oral use and decocted at first for about a half to 1 h until its narcotic-pungent taste is lost when its decoction is tasted by mouth. The raw medicinal material has a stronger toxicity and is generally used for external application.

Precautions: Contraindicated in a case with yin deficiency leading to hyperactivity of yang and pregnant women because of its pungent, hot, dry, and violent properties. It is incompatible with Banxia, Gualou, Beimu, Bailian, and Baiji. It must be soaked for oral use, decocted for a long time, and overdosage, and long-term treatment must be avoided.

1.7.7.2 Ganjiang (Zingiber Dried Ginger, Rhizoma Zingiberis)

Properties and Tastes: pungent and hot.
   Meridian Entry: spleen, stomach, kidney, heart, and lung meridians
   Effects

1. Warm the middle energizer to expel cold
2. Restore yang and dredge meridians
3. Warm the lung to resolve phlegm

Application

1. Stomachache, vomiting, and diarrhea

   It is used to treat spleen cold and stomach cold syndromes whether they are deficiency syndrome or excess syndrome. For stomach cold with vomiting and cold and painful epigastric abdomen, it is usually used in combination with Gaoliangjiang, such as Erjiang Wan; for deficiency and coldness of the spleen and stomach, it is usually combined with Dangshen and Baizhu, such as Lizhong Wan.

2. Syndrome of yang exhaustion

   For syndrome of yang exhaustion, it is usually combined with Fuzi for maximal effect to decrease the toxicity of Fuzi as well as to strengthen the effect of Fuzi in recuperating the depleted yang and rescuing the patient from qi collapse, such as Sini Tang.

3. Cough and asthma due to cold accumulation in the lung

   For cold accumulation in the lung manifested as cough and asthma, body's coldness, and profuse thin sputum, it is usually combined with Xixin, Wuweizi, and Mahuang, such as Xiao Qinglong Tang.

Usage and Dosage: 3–10 g is used in decoction for oral use.

Precautions: It must be used with caution when treating pregnant women, internal heat of yin deficiency, and blood heat. It is not suitable to be taken in large dosage and for a long time.

Other Interior-warming medicines (Table 1.14).

1.7.8 Qi-Regulating Medicine

These are medicines that have their principal actions of promoting the functional activities of qi and of facilitating qi movement. Qi-regulating medicines are generally aromatic and have pungent and bitter flavor and warm nature. They are efficacious in normalizing qi activities and movement, strengthening the spleen, and unblocking the liver and releasing stagnation and are particularly suitable for treating qi stagnation or suppressing abnormally ascending qi caused by impedance of qi movement.

Impedance of qi movement is manifested mainly through effects on the functions of the lung, the liver, the spleen, and the stomach. Qi stagnation generally shows tightness or an oppressed sensation, distention, and pain. Abnormal qi ascent generally shows hiccups, vomiting, or labored breathing.

Because of differences in location, progression, and severity, the actual symptoms may also differ. Hence, when prescribing qi-regulating medicines, the physician must choose them to suit the actual illness and supplement them appropriately. For example, for obstruction of qi caused by exogenous pathogenic evils, add medicines that ventilate the lung, dissolve sputum, and stop cough. For cough and dyspnea due to phlegm and heat in the lung, add medicines that cool heat and dissolve phlegm. For stagnation of spleen and stomach qi with associated dampness and

Table 1.14 Simple list of other interior-warming medicines

Name	Properties and tastes	Meridian entry	Effects	Application	Dosage
Rougui (Cortex Cinnamomi)	Pungent, sweet, and extremely hot	Spleen, kidney, liver, and heart meridians	(1) Supplement fire and strengthen yang (2) Expel cold and alleviate pain (3) Warm the meridians to promote the circulation of the blood	(1) It is used for insufficiency syndromes of kidney yang (2) It can be used to treat all pains due to accumulation of cold and stagnation of qi or stasis of the blood (3) Deficiency and coldness of lower energizer, and up-floating of deficiency yang (4) Yin abscess, carbuncle and sore that without being healed before suppuration or after rupture for a long time	1–5 g for decoction
Wuzhuyu (Fructus Evodiae)	Pungent, bitter, hot, and mild toxic	Liver, spleen, stomach, and kidney meridians	(1) Expel cold and relieve pain (2) Warm the spleen and stomach to stop vomiting (3) Strengthen yang and arrest diarrhea	(1) It is used to treat all syndromes due to cold accumulation in the liver meridian (2) Incoordination between the liver and stomach with acid regurgitation and vomiting (3) Diarrhea due to deficiency and cold	2–5 g for decoction
Xiaohui xiang (Fructus Foeniculi)	Pungent and warm	Liver, kidney, spleen, and stomach meridians	(1) Expel cold to alleviate pain (2) Regulate the stomach qi	(1) Colic of cold type, orchidoptosis and dysmenorrhea (2) Qi stagnation due to stomach cold with epigastric distention and pain, vomiting, and loss of appetite	3–6 g for decoction

Table 1.14 (continued)

Name	Properties and tastes	Meridian entry	Effects	Application	Dosage
Huajiao (Pericarpium Zanthoxyli)	Pungent and warm	Spleen, stomach, and kidney meridians	(1) Warm the middle energizer to alleviate pain (2) Kill worms to relieve itching	(1) It is used to treat syndrome of epigastric and abdominal cold pain, vomiting and diarrhea (2) It is used to treat abdominal pain due to worms (3) Eczema and pruritus vulvae	3–6 g for decoction
Dingxiang (Flos Caryophylli)	Pungent and warm	Spleen, stomach, lung, and kidney meridians	(1) Warm the middle energizer and descend adverse rising (2) Expel cold to alleviate pain (3) Warming the kidney and supporting Yang	(1) Vomiting, hiccup due to stomach cold (2) Cold pain in epigastric abdomen (3) Impotence due to kidney deficiency	1–3 g for decoction

heat, add herbs that cool heat and dissipate dampness. For cold and dampness blocking the spleen, add medicines that warm the middle-jiao and dry dampness. For food retention and indigestion, add medicines that promote digestion and relieve retention. For insufficiency of the spleen and the stomach, add medicines that augment qi and strengthen the spleen.

Many symptoms can accompany the stagnation of liver qi. Depending on the specific associated symptoms, it may be necessary to add medicines that nourish the liver, soften the liver, promote blood circulation, regulate the nutritive level, stop pain, or strengthen the spleen.

Most qi-regulating medicines are pungent and drying and can easily consume qi and injure yin. They must be used with great care in deficiency of both qi and yin.

1.7.8.1 Chenpi (Dried Tangerine Peel Pericarpium, Citri Reticulatae)

Properties and Tastes: pungent, bitter, and warm
   Meridian Entry: spleen and lung meridians
   Effects

1. Regulate qi and invigorate spleen
2. Eliminate dampness and resolve phlegm

Application

1. Stagnation of spleen qi and stomach qi

    It is used especially suitable for stagnation of spleen qi and stomach qi due to accumulation of cold and dampness in the middle energizer manifested as distention and fullness of epigastric abdomen, belching, nausea, and vomiting. It is usually used in combination with Cangzhu and Houpo, such as Pingwei San; for vomiting due to phlegm-heat, it is combined with Zhuru, Huanglian; for deficiency of spleen qi and stomach qi with abdominal pain that is reduced by pressure, fullness after meal, and loss of appetite, it is usually combined with Dangshen, Baizhu, and Fuling, such as Yigong San.
2. Retention of dampness, cough with profuse sputum

    It is used to treat cough with profuse sputum caused by dampness phlegm and cold phlegm. In the treatment of cough and dyspnea due to dampness phlegm, it is usually combined with Banxia and Fuling to deprive dampness and resolve phlegm, such as Erchen Tang; for cough due to cold phlegm, it is usually combined with Ganjiang, Xixin, and Wuweizi, such as Linggan Wuwei Jiangxin Tang.

Usage and Dosage: 3–10 g is used in decoction for oral use.

1.7.8.2 Zhishi (Immature Orange Fruit, Fructus Aurantii Immaturus)

Properties and Tastes: bitter, pungent, sour and warm
Meridian Entry: spleen, stomach, and large intestine meridians
Effects

1. Break stagnation of qi and remove food retention
2. Resolve phlegm and eliminate mass

Application

1. Food retention syndromes

    It is indicated for the treatment of indigestion, constipation due to accumulation of heat, and dysentery. For indigestion and fullness and pain in the chest and upper abdomen, it is used together with Shanzha, Maiya, and Shenqu, such as Qumai Zhizhu Wan; for constipation due to accumulation of heat, abdominal mass, and fullness and pain in the epigastrium, it can be combined with Houpo, Dahuang, Mangxiao, such as Dachengqi Tang; for stagnation of dampness and heat with dysentery and tenesmus, it is combined with Dahuang, Huanglian, and Huangqin, such as Zhishi Daozhi Wan.
2. Chest impediment and epigastric stuffiness

    It is used for turbid phlegm obstructing qi activity with fullness in the chest and epigastrium. For the syndrome due to deficiency of stomach yang and accumulation of cold phlegm, it can be combined with Xiebai, Guizhi, and Gualou, such as Zhishi Xiebai Guizhi Tang; for stagnation of dampness phlegm in the middle energizer, fullness in the epigastric abdomen, poor appetite, it is combined with Houpo, Banxia, and Baizhu, such as Zhishi Xiaopi Wan.

In addition, it can be used to treat gastroptosis, prolapse of rectum, and uterus, but it must be combined with Chaihu, Shengma, and Huangqi, in order to get good therapeutic effect, and it has the effect of raising blood pressure as well.

Usage and Dosage: 3–10 g is used in decoction for oral use and a large dosage is 30 g.

Precautions: It is used with caution in the cases with deficiency of the spleen and stomach and pregnant women.

Other qi-regulating medicines (Table 1.15).

1.7.9   Digestant Medicine

Any medicinal herb that acts to improve appetite and digestion or remove food stagnation is named digestant medicine.

These medicines mainly have the sweet taste and are mainly attributed to the spleen and stomach meridians, with the function of improving appetite and digestion and removing food stagnation. Besides, some of the medicines have the functions of regulating flow of qi and blood, etc.

They are mainly used for removing food stagnation, manifested as abdominal distension, eructation, acid regurgitation, nausea, and vomiting, irregular bowel movements.

Modern studies indicate that most of this category can promote gastrointestinal peristalsis and increase digestive juice, which helps digestion.

1.7.9.1   Shanzha (Hawthorn Fruit, Fructus Crataegi)

Properties and Tastes: sour, sweet, and slightly warm
   Meridian Entry: spleen, stomach, and liver meridians
   Effects

1. Promote digestion and invigorate the stomach
2. Move qi and dissipate blood stasis
3. Eliminate turbid and reducing blood lipids

   Application

1. Food stagnation
   It is especially effective in meat-type food accumulation, which is manifested as abdominal fullness and distention, belching and acid swallowing, abdominal pain, and diarrhea. It can be used alone or used in combination with Laifuzi, Shenqu, and so on.

Table 1.15 Simple list of other qi-regulating medicines

Name	Properties and tastes	Meridian entry	Effects	Application	Dosage
Qingpi (Pericarpium Citri Reticulatae Viride)	Bitter, pungent, and warm	Liver, gallbladder, and stomach meridians	(1) Soothe the liver to break qi stagnation (2) Eliminate mass and relieve dyspepsia	(1) It is indicated for liver qi stagnation manifested ashypochondriac distending pain, breast distending pain, and pain due to hernia (2) Distention and pain in the epigastrium due to indigestion	3–10 g for decoction
Muxiang (Radix Aucklandiae)	Pungent, bitter and warm	Spleen, stomach, large intestine, triple energizer, and gallbladder meridians	(1) Move qi to relieve pain (2) Regulate the middle energizer	(1) Syndromes of stomach and spleen qi stagnation (2) Dysentery due to dampness and heat with tenesmus (3) Syndromes of liver and gallbladder qi stagnation	3–6 g for decoction
Xiangfu (Rhizoma Cyperi)	Pungent, slightly bitter, slightly sweet, and neutral	Liver, spleen, and triple energizer meridians	(1) Soothe the liver and regulate qi (2) Regulate menstruation to relieve pain	(1) The syndromes of stagnation of liver qi with pain in the hypochondrium, distention and pain in epigastric abdomen and pain due to hernia (2) Irregular menstruation, dysmenorrhea and distension and pain in the breast	6–10 g for decoction
Foshou (Fructus Citri Sarcodactylis)	Pungent, bitter, and warm	Liver, spleen, and lung meridians	(1) Soothe liver to regulate qi flow (2) Harmonize stomach (3) Resolve phlegm	(1) Liver depression and qi stagnation (2) Spleen and stomach qi stagnation (3) Cough with profuse sputum	3–10 g for decoction

Table 1.15 (continued)

Name	Properties and tastes	Meridian entry	Effects	Application	Dosage
Wuyao (Radix Linderae)	Pungent and warm	Lung, spleen, kidney, and bladder meridians	(1) Promote the circulation of qi to relieve pain (2) Warm the kidney to disperse cold	(1) It is indicated for stagnation of cold and qi manifested as oppression and pain in the chest, fullness and pain in the epigastrium, hernia of cold type, and dysmenorrhea (2) Insufficiency of kidney yang, frequent urination, and enuresis due to deficiency and coldness of the bladder	6–10 g for decoction
Xiebai (Bulbus Allii Macrostemonis)	Pungent, bitter and warm	Lung, stomach, and large intestine meridians	(1) Activate yang and disperse lumps (2) Promote qi circulation and relieve the stagnation	(1) It is used to treat turbid phlegm and thoracic fullness due to deficiency of thoracic yang (2) Qi stagnation in the stomach and intestine manifested as dysentery with tenesmus	5–10 g for decoction
Shidi (Calyx Kaki)	Bitter, astringent, and neutral	Stomach meridian	Lower the adverse rising qi and relieve hiccup	It is used to treat syndrome of hiccup and can be combined with relevant medicinal herbs according to symptoms and signs	5–10 g for decoction

2. Diarrhea and bellyache

For this kind of syndrome, it is usually combined with Muxiang and Binglang.
3. Meniscus and postpartum abdominal pain due to blood stasis, chest stuffiness, and pains

Shanzha is usually used combined with Danggui, Xiangfu, Honghua, etc., to move qi and dissipate blood stasis, such as Tongyu Jian.
4. Hyperlipidemia studies have shown that the medicine can reduce blood lipids

The medicine can be used alone or combination with Danshen, Sanqi, and Gegen.

Usage and Dosage: 9–12 g for decoction. Charred Shanzha has stronger digestion-promoting effect than Shanzha.

1.7.9.2 Shenqu (Medicated Leaven, Massa Medicata Fermentata)

Properties and Tastes: sweet, pungent and warm
  Meridian Entry: spleen and stomach meridians
  Effects: Promote digestion and harmonize the stomach
  Application
Indigestion and retention food

It is often used in combination with Shanzha, Maiya, and Muxiang for syndromes manifested as abdominal fullness and distention, poor appetite, borborygmus, and diarrhea. This medicine also can relieve exterior syndrome, so it is more suitable for the dyspeptic retention with exterior syndrome in exopathy.

  Usage and Dosage: 6–15 g for decoction

1.7.9.3 Maiya (Germinated Barley, Fructus Hordei Germinatus)

Properties and Tastes: sweet
  Meridian Entry: spleen, stomach, and liver meridians
  Effects

1. Promote digestion and fortify the stomach
2. Terminate lactation

  Application

1. Food indigestion and retention

The medicine can promote the circulation of qi and promote digestion, fortify the spleen and stomach. It is better at promoting the digestion of starchy foods. So it is mainly used for the retention of rice, noodles, and yam, often used with Shanzha, Shengqu, Jineijin, and so on. For the anorexia caused by insufficiency of the spleen, it is usually used with Baizhu, Chenpi, such as Jianpi Wan.

2. Stagnation of qi

　　Maiya can smooth the liver and regulate the flow of qi, so it is used for the liver qi stagnation, marked by pain in lateral thorax and abdomen, often used together with Chaihu, Xiangfu, Chuanlianzi, and so on.

3. Milk stasis and breast pain

　　The medicine can terminate lactation; therefore, it can be used for the women's delectation and breast pain.

Usage and Dosage: 10–15 g for decoction. Stir-baked Maiya is used for delectation and the dosage is 60 g. Raw Maiya is used for promoting digestion and fortifying the stomach.

Other digestant medicines (Table 1.16).

1.7.10 Hemostatic Medicine

These are medicines that have their principal action of stopping bleeding. They are used mainly to treat bleeding conditions such as hemoptysis, epistaxis, hematemesis, hematuria, metrorrhagia, ecchymosis, and traumatic bleeding.

　　Hemostatic medicines come with a variety of associated properties, such as blood cooling, astringent, clot dissolving, and channel warming. When prescribing, the physician must select the most suitable medicines for the whole patient and combine them with appropriate supplementary medicines to enhance the therapeutic effect. For example, if the bleeding is due to heat in the blood driving it to flow erratically, add medicines that cool heat and blood. If it is due to yin deficiency with

Table 1.16 Simple list of other digestant medicines

Name	Properties and tastes	Meridian entry	Effects	Application	Dosage
Jineijin (Endothelium Corneum Gigeriae Galli)	Sweet and medium	Spleen, stomach, small intestine, and large intestine meridians	(1) Promote digestion and invigorate the stomach (2) Arrest seminal emission	(1) Dyspepsia, vomiting, diarrhea, especially effective in food accumulation of rice and noodles (2) Spermatorrhea, enuresis (3) Stone strangury	3–10 g for decoction
Laifuzi (Semen Raphani)	Pungent, sweet, and medium	Lung, spleen, and stomach meridians	(1) Promote digestion and relieve fullness (2) Descend qi and resolve phlegm	(1) Retention of indigested food and stagnation (2) Cough and dyspnea of retention of phlegm	5–15 g for decoction

hyperactive yang, add medicines that nourish yin and suppress yang. If it is due to blood stasis, add medicines that mobilize qi and blood. If it is due to deficiency cold, add medicines that warm yang, augment qi, or strengthen the spleen as appropriate for the clinical condition. If excessive bleeding has depleted qi and brought it to the verge of collapse, medicines that stop bleeding used alone are too slow in action for such an urgent situation; it is necessary to add medicines that augment genuine qi vigorously to avoid prostration.

When applying hemostatic medicines, the physician must take note whether there is blood stasis. If the clots that result from the stasis have not been completely reabsorbed, the physician must add medicines that mobilize blood and eliminate clots to avoid leaving residual clots.

1.7.10.1   Sanqi (Sanchi, Notoginseng Radix)

Properties and Tastes: sweet, slightly bitter and warm
   Meridian Entry: liver and stomach meridians
   Effects

1. Remove blood stasis to stop bleeding
2. Promote blood circulation and alleviate pain

   Application

1. Bleeding syndromes
   It is used for various kinds of internal and external bleedings, especially for bleeding with blood stasis, for it has the advantage of arresting bleeding without stasis and removing blood stasis while keeping healthy qi. For hematemesis, emptysis, metrorrhagia, and metrostaxis, it can be ground singly into powder to be swallowed or combined with Huaruishi, Xueyutan, such as Huaxue Wan; for bleeding due to trauma, its powder is applied externally in local area alone or combined with Longgu and Xuejie, such as Qibao San.
2. Trauma and painful swelling with blood stasis
   It is the primary medicinal material for wounds, for it has the effects of promoting blood circulation to remove blood stasis, relieving swelling, and alleviating pain. It could be taken orally or applied externally alone or combined with blood-activating, trauma-treating, and pain-relieving medicinal materials.
   In addition, it could also be used in the treatment of coronary heart disease with angina pectoris and various stagnant blood syndromes of gynecology.

Usage and Dosage: 3–9 g for decoction. 1–3 g of the powder to be taken orally. Appropriate amount for external application.
   Precautions: It is used with caution for pregnant women.

1.7.10.2   Baiji (Common Bletilla Rubber, Rhizoma Bletillae)

Properties and Tastes: bitter, sweet, astringent, and slightly cold
  Meridian Entry: lung, stomach, and liver meridians
  Effects

1. Stop bleeding by astringency
2. Remove swelling and promote regeneration

Application

1. Bleeding syndromes
    It is the primary astringent hemostatic and is used for various internal and external bleedings, especially for bleedings in the lung and stomach. It can be powdered and used alone or mixed with rice soup for oral use or in combination with other medicinal materials; for insufficiency of lung yin with dry cough and hemoptysis, it is usually combined with Pibaye, Oujie, Ejiao; for bleeding of stomach, it is combined with Haipiaoxiao, while for bleeding due to trauma, it can be ground into powder or combined with Duanshigao for external application.
2. Sores and carbuncle, and rhagades of hands and feet
    It is suitable for both oral and external uses. For the early stage of carbuncle, its powder could be used alone for external application, or combined with Jinyinhua and Tianhuafen to clear off carbuncle; for ulcerated and unhealed carbuncle, it is usually ground into powder together with Huanglian, Qingfen, and Wubeizi for external application; for rhagades of hands and feet, the powder can be mixed with sesame oil and then applied to the local area.

Usage and Dosage: 6–15 g. 3–6 g of the powder is used per time. Appropriate amount for external application.
  Precautions: It is incompatible with Wutou.
  Other hemostatic medicines (Table 1.17).

1.7.11   Blood-Activating and Stasis-Resolving Medicine

These are medicines that have their principal action of stimulating blood circulation and of removing blood stasis. They are especially efficacious at dispersion, including reversing stasis, dissolving hematomas, stimulating blood circulation, restoring menstrual flow, ameliorating dampness, reducing swelling, and stopping pain.

The main application of these medicines is the condition of blood stasis. This is a commonly seen condition with four major presentations: (1) aches, pain, or numbness, (2) masses in the interior or the exterior, or traumatic hematomas, (3) internal hemorrhage with dark purple blood clots, and (4) ecchymosis on the skin, mucous

Table 1.17 Simple list of other hemostatic medicines

Name	Properties and tastes	Meridian entry	Effects	Application	Dosage
Xiaoji (Herba Cirsii)	Bitter and cold	Heart and liver meridians	(1) Cool blood and stop bleeding (2) Eliminate toxic material to treat carbuncle	(1) Blood heat causing bleeding (2) Toxic heat causing sores and carbuncles	5–12 g for decoction
Diyu (Radix Sanguisorbae)	Bitter, astringent, and slightly cold	Liver, stomach, and large intestine meridians	(1) Cool the blood and stop bleeding (2) Eliminate toxic material and treat pyogenic infection	(1) Blood heat causing bleeding (2) Scald, eczema, sores and ulcers, swollen pains	9–15 g for decoction
Huaihua (Flos Sophorae)	Bitter and slightly cold	Liver and large intestine meridians	(1) Cool the blood and stop bleeding (2) Clear away liver heat and lower the fire	(1) Blood heat causing bleeding (2) Conjunctivitis and headache	5–10 g for decoction
Cebaiye (Cacumen Platycladi)	Bitter, astringent, and slightly cold	Lung, liver, and intestine meridians	(1) Cool the blood and stop bleeding (2) Eliminate phlegm and relieve cough	(1) Blood heat causing bleeding (2) Lung heat causing cough with sputum	6–12 g for decoction
Qiancao (Radix Rubiae)	Bitter and cold	Liver meridian	(1) Remove blood stasis and stop bleeding (2) Cool the blood and circulate the meridians	(1) Bleeding caused by blood stasis or blood heat (2) Stagnant blood syndromes	6–10 g for decoction
Puhuang (Pollen Typhae)	Sweet and neutral	Liver and pericardium meridians	(1) Stop bleeding and remove blood stasis (2) Promote diuresis	(1) Bleeding syndromes (2) Blood stasis causing pain (3) Blood stranguria	5–10 g for wrapped decoction

Table 1.17 (continued)

Name	Properties and tastes	Meridian entry	Effects	Application	Dosage
Xianhe cao (Herba Agrimoniae)	Bitter, astringent, and neutral	Liver meridian	(1) Stop bleeding by astringing (2) Relieve dysentery and kill trichomonad	(1) Bleeding syndromes (2) Chronic dysentery, sores, and carbuncles (3) Trichomoniases	6–12 g for decoction
Aiye (Folium Artemisiae Argyi)	Bitter, pungent, and warm	Liver, spleen, and kidney meridians	(1) Stop bleeding by warming meridians (2) Expel cold and alleviate pain	(1) Deficiency and cold causing bleeding (2) Irregular menstruation, menstrual pain and abdominal pain and cold	3–9 g for decoction
Paojiang (Rhizoma Zingiberis)	Bitter, astringent, and warm	Spleen and liver meridians	(1) Warm meridians to stop bleeding (2) Warm the middle energizer to alleviate pain	(1) Deficiency and cold causing bleeding (2) Abdominal pain and diarrhea	3–9 g for decoction

membranes, or the tongue. Blood stasis develops in the course of many illnesses, and itself is also the cause of further disease.

Since there are many causes of blood stasis, when prescribing medicines that stimulate blood circulation and remove blood stasis the physician must form a firm diagnosis and select and add medicines appropriate to the clinical requirements. For example, if the blood stasis is due to cold gelling qi and impeding blood flow, add medicines that warm the interior and dispel cold. If it is due to heat consuming yin and blood, add medicines that cool heat and blood. For dampness with pain due to wind-dampness, add medicines that dispel wind and dissipate dampness. For blood stasis associated with deficiency of genuine qi, add medicines that restore the deficient.

Qi and blood are intimately interrelated. When qi moves, so does blood, and when qi becomes impeded, then blood becomes static. Hence, when prescribing medicines that stimulate blood circulation and relieve stasis, it is appropriate to include medicines that stimulate qi movement. Doing so enhances the ability of the medicines to stimulate blood circulation and relieve stasis.

1.7.11.1   Chuanxiong (Szechwan Lovage Rhizome, Rhizoma Ligustici Chuanxiong)

Properties and Tastes: pungent and warm
   Meridian Entry: liver, gallbladder, and pericardium meridians
   Effects

1. Activate blood and move qi
2. Expel wind and alleviate pain

   Application

1. Stagnation of blood and qi
   For irregular menstruation, dysmenorrhea, and amenorrhea, this medicinal material is usually combined with Danggui and Xiangfu. In case of postpartum abdominal pain due to blood stasis, it is often combined with Yimucao and Taoren. For hypochondriac pain due to unsmooth circulation of blood caused by stagnation of liver qi, it is combined with Chaihu and Xiangfu. In the case of physical trauma, it is used with Chishao and Honghua. Also, for carbuncle, sore, purulence without ulceration, it is usually combined with Danggui and Chuanshanjia, such as Tounong San.
2. Headache and impediment disease pain in wind and damp
   For headache due to external contraction of wind-cold, it is usually combined with Baizhi, Fangfeng, and Xixin, such as Chuanxiong Chatiao San. If the headache is due to wind-heat, it should be combined with Juhua, Shigao, and Jiangchan, such as Chuanxiong San. If headache due to wind-dampness, it is often used with Qianghuo, Gaoben, and Fangfeng, for example, in the Qianghuo Shengshi Tang. If headache is due to blood stasis, then it is usually combined with Chishao, Honghua, and Danshen. For headache due to blood deficiency, it is often combined with Danggui and Baishao. For painful joints due to Impediment disease blockage, it is usually combined with Qianghuo, Duhuo, and Sangzhi.

Usage and Dosage: 3–9 g. For powder form, 1-(1) 5 g is used and taken for each time.
Precautions: It is pungent, warm, ascending, and dispersing, so it is contraindicated in cases with a reddish tongue and dryness of the mouth, caused by yin deficiency with hyperactivity fire. It should be used with caution in cases of excessive menstruation and with conditions with hemorrhagic disease.

1.7.11.2   Danshen (Danshen Root, Radix Salviae Miltiorrhizae)

Properties and Tastes: bitter and slightly cold
   Meridian Entry: heart and liver meridians
   Effects

1. Promote blood circulation to remove blood stasis
2. Clear heat from the blood and resolving swelling
3. Remove annoyance and tranquilize the mind

Application

1. Blood stasis Syndromes
   It is especially effective for women's syndromes of blood stasis with heat, such as irregular menstruation, amenorrhea, and postpartum abdominal pain. It can be taken in powder form together with aged wine or combined with Danggui and Yimucao. For angina pectoris and epigastric pain, caused by blood stasis and stagnation of qi, it is usually combined with Tanxiang and Sharen, such as, in the Danshen Tang. In cases of abdominal masses, it is combined with Sanleng, Ezhu, and Biejia. For trauma with pain due to blood stasis, it is combined with Danggui, Honghua, and Chuanxiong. In addition, for heat impediment with reddish, swollen, and painful joints, it should be combined with Rendongteng, Chishao, and Sangzhi.
2. Breast abscess with swelling and pain
   To treat breast abscess with swelling and pain, it is usually combined with Ruxiang, Jinyinhua, and Lianqiao, such as Xiaoru Tang.
3. Restlessness and insomnia
   For heat invading the Yingfen and Xuefen in the seasonal febrile disease, it is usually combined with Dihuang and Xuanshen, such as in the Qingying Tang. For blood failing to nourish the heart, it is usually combined with Suanzaoren and Yejiaoteng.

Usage and Dosage: 9–15 g. The stir-baked with wine form has the ability to strengthen the medicinal function of promoting blood circulation.
Precautions: It is incompatible with Lilu.

1.7.11.3   Yanhusuo (Yanhusuo, Rhizoma Corydalis)

Properties and Tastes: pungent, bitter, and warm
  Meridian Entry: liver, spleen, and heart meridians
  Effects

1. Activate blood
2. Move qi
3. Relieve pain

Application
Syndromes of stagnation of qi and blood stasis causing pain
For pains in the epigastric abdominal area, it can be taken orally alone, or ground into a powder, and mixed with warm liquor. Also, it can treat the above problems when combined with Chuanlianzi, such as, in the Jinglingzi San. In cases of abdominal pain during menstruation, it should be combined with Danggui, Chuanxiong,

and Xiangfu. If stuffiness and pains in the chest, it should be used together with Gualou, Xiebai, and Yujing. In cases of hypochondriac pain, it is usually combined with Qingpi and Xiangfu. For pain due to hernia, it is used with Xiaohuixiang and Wuzhuyu. In addition, for pain in the limbs, or general pain due to blood stasis, it is combined with Danggui, Guizhi, and Chishao. To treat physical trauma, it should be combined with Danggui, Ruxiang and Moyao.

Usage and Dosage: 3–9 g. 1.5–3 g of the powder to be swallowed per time.

1.7.11.4   Yimucao (Motherwort Herb, Herba Leonuri)

Properties and Tastes: pungent, bitter, and slightly cold
  Meridian Entry: liver, pericardium, and bladder meridians
  Effects

1. Activate blood and dispel stasis
2. Induce diuresis to alleviate edema

   Application

1. Syndromes of blood stasis
     To treat blood stasis causing irregular menstruation, dysmenorrheal, amenorrhea, postpartum abdominal pain, lochiorrhea, and trauma pain, it can be decocted alone into a paste or combined with Danggui, Chuanxiong, and Chishao, such as Yimu Wan.
2. **Dysuria and Edema**
     It can be decocted alone or combined together with Xianmaogen and Zelan.
     In addition, it can clear heat and relieve toxicity, for which it may be used for ulcer and carbuncle and itchy skin rash.

Usage and Dosage: 9–30 g. In the fresh form 12–40 g. It can be used decocted into a paste or processed into pills. The appropriate amount of the pounded fresh form is utilized for external application.
   Precautions: It is contraindicated in pregnant women.
   Other Blood-activating and stasis-resolving medicines (Table 1.18).

1.7.12   Phlegm-Dispelling, Cough-Suppressing, and Panting-Calming Medicine

This group actually comprises two subgroups of medicines: phlegm-dispelling medicines and cough-suppressing and panting-calming medicines. The phlegm-dispelling medicines act principally to dissolve phlegm and eliminate sputum. Cough is usually accompanied by sputum and phlegm usually causes cough. In

Table 1.18 Simple list of other blood-activating and stasis-resolving medicines

Name	Properties and tastes	Meridian entry	Effects	Application	Dosage
Yujin (Radix Curcumae)	Pungent, bitter, and cold	Liver, heart, lung, and gallbladder meridians	(1) Activate blood and relieve pain (2) Promote qi and disperse the stagnated qi (3) Clear heart and cool blood (4) Excrete bile and relieve jaundice	(1) Liver qi stagnation and blood stasis causing blockage (2) Mental confusion by phlegm heat (3) Blood heat causing bleeding as hematemesis, epistaxis, hematuria, and unsmooth menstruation (4) Dampness-heat jaundice and gallstone	3–10 g for decoction
Ruxiang (Olibanum)	Pungent, bitter, and warm	Liver, heart, and spleen meridians	(1) Activate blood and alleviate pain (2) Subside swelling and promote tissue regeneration	(1) Blood stasis causing pain (2) Trauma and sores and ulcers, abscess, and swelling	3–5 g for decoction
Moyao (Myrrha)	Bitter and neutral	Heart, liver, and spleen meridians	(1) Activate blood and alleviate pain (2) Subside swelling and promote tissue regeneration	(1) Blood stasis causing pain (2) Sores and ulcers after rupture	3–5 g for decoction
Taoren (Semen Persicae)	Bitter, sweet, and neutral	Heart, liver, and large intestine meridians	(1) Promote blood circulation by removing blood stasis (2) Lubricate the bowels to relieve constipation	(1) Syndromes of blood stasis causing dysmenorrhea, amenorrhea, postpartum abdominal pain, pain in chest and hypochondrium, and trauma pain (2) Blood stasis of heat type causing pulmonary and intestine abscess (3) Constipation due to dry intestine	5–10 g for decoction

(continued)

Table 1.18 (continued)

Name	Properties and tastes	Meridian entry	Effects	Application	Dosage
Honghua (Flos Carthami)	Pungent and warm	Heart and liver meridians	(1) Promote blood circulation by removing blood stasis (2) Regulate menstruation and relieve pain	(1) Blood stasis syndromes (2) Chest and hypochondriac pain and mass (3) Trauma pain and pains in joints (4) Stagnation of heat and blood stasis	3–10 g for decoction
Yimucao (Herba Leonuri)	Pungent, bitter, and slightly cold	Liver, pericardium, and bladder meridians	(1) Activate blood and dispel stasis (2) Induce diuresis to alleviate edema	(1) Syndromes of blood stasis (2) Dysuria and edema	10–15 g for decoction
Wangbuliuxing (Semen Vaccariae)	Bitter and neutral	Liver and stomach meridians	(1) Activate blood circulation and stimulate meridians (2) Promote lactation and cure abscess (3) Induce diuresis to relieve stranguria	(1) Blood stasis causing amenorrhea, dysmenorrhea, dystocia (2) Postpartum, agalactia, breast abscess, and swollen pain (3) Heat stranguria, blood stranguria, and urolithic stranguria	5–10 g for decoction
Ezhu (Rhizoma Curcumae)	Pungent, bitter, and warm	Liver and spleen meridians	(1) Break blood stasis and move qi (2) Eliminate stagnation and alleviate pain	(1) Stagnation of qi and blood stasis (2) Syndromes of food stagnancy and qi stagnation	6–9 g for decoction
Sanleng (Rhizoma Sparganii)	Pungent, bitter, and neutral	Liver and spleen meridians	(1) Break blood stasis and move qi (2) Eliminate stagnation and alleviate pain	(1) Stagnation of qi and blood stasis (2) Stagnation of food with fullness and pain in epigastric abdomen	5–10 g for decoction

general, phlegm-dispelling medicines also can stop cough and relieve asthma and cough-stopping and asthma-relieving medicines also can dissolve phlegm. The two groups are therefore usually discussed together. Phlegm-dispelling medicines are mainly used to treat illnesses of phlegm causing much sputum and cough, cough with labored breathing, or sputum that is difficult to expectorate. Cough-suppressing and panting-calming medicines are mainly used to treat cough and asthma due to either internal injury or exogenous pathogenic agent. Since both internal injury and exogenous illness can produce cough, asthma, or much sputum, it is important to select these medicines on the basis of the cause and properties of the clinical condition being treated and to add appropriate supplemental medicines.

For cough with associated hemoptysis, it is not appropriate to prescribe phlegm-dispelling medicines that are harsh and irritating, as these may aggravate the hemoptysis. For cough in the early stages of measles, the main medicines to use are in general those that clear and ventilate the lung rather than cough-stopping medicines. Cough-suppressing medicines that are warm or astringent are especially inappropriate as they may aggravate heat or affect the proper eruption of the measles rash.

1.7.12.1 Banxia (Pinellia Tuber, Pinelliae Rhizoma)

Properties and Tastes: pungent, warm, and toxic
  Meridian Entry: spleen, stomach, and lung meridians
  Effects

1. Dry dampness and eliminate phlegm
2. Direct qi downward to relieve vomiting
3. Relieve stuffiness and dissipate nodulation
4. Relieve swelling and pain for external use

Application

1. Damp-phlegm syndromes
   It is an important drug for clearing dampness to reduce phlegm. For failure of spleen to transport and transform water and obstruction by phlegm and dampness causing profuse sputum, cough, and adverse rise of qi, it is usually combined with Chenpi and Fuling in Erchen Tang. For that accompanied by cold, profuse, and clear sputum, Xixin and Ganjinag are combined. For that with fever and thick and yellowish sputum, it is used together with Huangqin, Zhimu, and Gualou. For dizziness due to damp-phlegm, it is combined with Baizhu and Tianma in Banxia Baizhu Tianma Tang.
2. Adverse rise of stomach qi manifested as nausea and vomiting
   For vomiting due to cold-fluid retention, it is usually combined with Shengjiang in Xiaobanxia Tang; for vomiting due to stomach deficiency, combined with Renshen and Baimi in Dabanxia Tang; for vomiting due to stomach heat, combined with Huanglian and Zhuru; for vomiting during pregnancy, com-

bined with Zisugeng and Sharen; and for vomiting due to stomach yin deficiency, combined with Shihu and Maidong.
3. Chest and epigastric fullness and stuffiness, globus hystericus, goiter, and subcutaneous nodule
    For chest and epigastric fullness and stuffiness with vomiting due to mixed accumulation of phlegm and heat, it is combined with Huanglian and Gualou in Xiaoxianxiong Tang; for epigastric oppression due to phlegm and heat, it is usually combined with Ganjiang, Huanglian, and Huangqin in Banxia Xiexin Tang; for globus hystericus without fever due to qi stagnation and phlegm accumulation, it is combined with Houpo, Zisuye, and Fuling in Banxia Houpo Tang; and for goiter and subcutaneous nodule, it is used together with Kunbu, Haizao, and Zhebeimu.
4. Large carbuncle, mammary sore, and bite by poisonous snake
    It can relieve swelling and pain by external use. It is ground into powder to apply on the affected parts.
    In addition, it can dry dampness and harmonize stomach, so it is effective for disharmony of stomach and restlessness when combined with Shumi in Banxia Shumi Tang.

Usage and Dosage: 3–9 g. It is made into powder and applied on the affected parts with appropriate amount. It is usually used after processing. For instance, Jiangbanxia is very effective for suppressing adverse rise of qi and stopping vomiting, and Fabanxia is usually used to dry dampness with mildly warm property.
Precautions: It is incompatible with Wutou. Since it is warm and dry, it is used with caution to treat dry cough due to yin deficiency, hemorrhagic diseases, dry-phlegm, and heat-phlegm.

1.7.12.2   Chuanbeimu (Tendrilleaf Fritillary Bulb, Bulbus Fritillariae Cirrhosae)

Properties and Tastes: bitter, sweet, and slightly cold
   Meridian Entry: lung and heart meridians
   Effects

1. Clear heat and resolve phlegm
2. Moisten lung and relieve cough
3. Dissipate mass and relieve swelling

Application

1. Nonurgency cough due to lung deficiency and dry cough due to lung heat
    It is slightly cold in nature and bitter in flavor and could relieve lung heat and resolve phlegm. Also, it is sweet and moist in flavor and could moisten the lung to relieve cough. Combined with Shashen and Maidong, it treats lung deficiency and yin deficiency causing chronic cough with phlegm. To treat lung heat resulting in dry cough, it is usually combined with Zhimu in Ermu San.

2. Scrofula, carbuncle, mammary abscess, and pulmonary abscess

It has the effect of clearing heat and congestion. For scrofula, it is usually combined with Xuanshen and Muli in Xiaoluo Wans; for carbuncle and mammary abscess, it is usually combined with Pugongying, Tianhuafen, and Lianqiao; and for pulmonary abscess, it is usually combined with Yuxingcao, Xianlugen and Yiyiren.

Usage and Dosage: 3–10 g. It is ground into powder with 1–2 g for each time.
Precautions: It is incompatible with Wutou.

1.7.12.3   Zhebeimu (Thunberg Fritillary Bulb, Bulbus Fritillariae Thunbergii)

Properties and Tastes: bitter and cold
  Meridian Entry: lung and heart meridians
  Effects

1. Clear heat and resolve phlegm
2. Remove stagnation and dissipate mass

Application

1. Cough caused by wind-heat, dryness-heat, and phlegm-heat

It is cold in flavor and has the effect of removing heat-phlegm and driving lung qi downward. For cough due to wind-heat, it is usually combined with Sangye, Niubangzi, and Qianhu; for cough due to phlegm-heat accumulation in lung, it is usually combined with Gualou and Zhimu.
2. Scrofula, goiter, carbuncle, and pulmonary abscess

It has the effect of clearing heat and congestion. For scrofula, it is combined with Xuanshen and Muli in Xiaoluo Wan; for goiter, it is usually combined with Haizao and Kunbu; for carbuncle, it is often used together with Lianqiao and Pugongying; and for pulmonary abscess, it is used together with Yuxingcao, Lugen, and Taoren.

Usage and Dosage: 5–10 g
Precautions: It is incompatible with Wutou.

1.7.12.4   Kuxingren (Bitter Apricot Seed, Semen Armeniacae Amarum)

Properties and Tastes: bitter, slightly warm, and mildly toxic
  Meridian Entry: lung and large intestine meridians
  Effects

1. Relieve cough and asthma
2. Moisten intestine and relax the bowels

Application

1. Cough and asthma

    It is an important drug to relieve cough and asthma. It treats cough due to wind-heat, combined with Sangye and Juhua, such as Sangju Tang; for cough due to wind-cold, combined with Mahuang and Gancao, such as Sanao Tang Tang; it treats cough caused by dry-heat with Sangye, Chuanbeimu and Shashen, such as Sangxing Tang; in cases of cough and asthma resulting from lung heat, it is usually combined with Mahuang and Shengshigao, such as Mahuang Xingren Gancao Shigao Tang.

2. Intestinal dryness causing constipation

    It is usually used together with Huomaren, Danggui and Zhiqiao, such as Runchang Wan, and usually combined with Baiziren, Yuliren, Taoren, and Songziren, such as Wuren Wan.

Usage and Dosage: 5–10 g. The raw medicinal material is decocted later.

Precautions: It is mildly toxic, so it must be used within the amount listed. It is used with caution when treating infants.

Other cough-suppressing and panting-calming medicines (Table 1.19).

1.7.13 Tranquilizing Medicine

These are medicines that have their principal action of tranquilization or calming the mind. Their principal application is the treatment of restlessness, agitation, palpitations of the heart, insomnia, excessive dreaming, as well as infantile convulsions, epilepsy, and dementia.

Most medicines in this category derive from minerals or the seeds of plants. In general, mineral medicines are heavy and lowering in nature; hence, many of them are sedating or tranquilizing. The seed medicines are moistening and restorative in nature; hence, many of them strengthen the heart and calm the mind.

When prescribing tranquilizing medicine the physician must take full stock of the patient's illness—not only select an appropriate medicine, but also supplement and complement it with appropriate other medicinals. For example, for yin deficiency and blood insufficiency, complement the mind-calming medicines with medicinals that generate blood and augment yin. For abnormal ascent of liver yang, complement with medicines that calm the liver and suppress yang. For the blazing of heart fire, complement with medicines that cool the heart and clear fire. In such conditions as epilepsy and infantile convulsion, the approach is usually to use medicines that dissolve phlegm and open orifices or those that calm the liver and extinguish wind as the main treatment; tranquilizing medicinals are used only as supplement.

Table 1.19 Simple list of other cough-suppressing and panting-calming medicines

Name	Properties and tastes	Meridian entry	Effects	Application	Dosage
Xuanfuhua (Inula Flower)	Bitter, pungent, salty, and slightly warm	Lung, spleen, stomach, and large intestine meridians	(1) Direct qi downward to resolve phlegm (2) Direct qi downward to relieve vomiting	(1) It is used for phlegm-fluid congestion in lung causing cough and asthma with profuse sputum, phlegm and retained fluid causing oppressing in chest and diaphragm (2) It is used for belching, vomiting	3–9 g for decoction. Wrap-decoction
Gualou (Snakegourd Fruit)	Sweet and cold	Lung, stomach, and large intestine meridians	(1) Clear heat and resolve phlegm (2) Loosen chest to remove stasis (3) Moisten intestine and relieve constipation	(1) It is used for phlegm-heat causing cough and asthma (2) It is used for chest impediment, thoracic accumulation (3) It is used for pulmonary abscess, intestinal abscess, mammary abscess (4) It is used for intestinal dryness with constipation	9–15 g for decoction
Zhuru (Bamboo Shavings)	Sweet and slightly cold	Lung, stomach, and gallbladder meridians	(1) Clear heat and resolve phlegm (2) Alleviate restlessness and relieve vomiting	(1) It is used for phlegm-heat causing cough, inner disturbance by phlegm-fire causing restlessness and insomnia (2) It is used for stomach heat causing vomiting	5–10 g for decoction

(continued)

Table 1.19 (continued)

Name	Properties and tastes	Meridian entry	Effects	Application	Dosage
Jiegeng (Platycodon Grandiflorus)	Bitter, pungent, and neutral	Lung meridian	(1) Disperse lung qi and resolve phlegm (2) Relieve sore throat and eliminate abscess	(1) It is used for failure of lung qi in dispersion manifested as cough with profuse sputum, oppression in chest (2) It is used for sore throat and aphonia (3) It is used for pulmonary abscess	3–10 g for decoction
Zisuzi (Perilla Fruit)	Pungent and warm	Lung and large intestine meridians	(1) Send the adverse qi downward (2) Clear phlegm, relieve cough and asthma (3) Relax the bowels to relieve constipation	(1) It is used for phlegm accumulation, adverse rise of lung qi, cough and asthma (2) It is used for intestinal dryness with constipation	3–10 g for decoction
Baibu (Stemona Root)	Sweet, bitter, and slightly warm	Lung meridian	(1) Moisten the lung and relieve cough (2) Kill worms and insects, including louse	(1) It is used for acute or prolonged cough, whooping cough, cough caused by pulmonary tuberculosis (2) It is used for enterobiasis, head louse, body louse, scabies	3–9 g for decoction
Ziwan (Tatarian Aster Root)	Pungent, bitter, and warm	Lung meridian	(1) Nourish the lung to send the adverse qi downward (2) Relieve cough and asthma	(1) It treats external contraction by wind-cold manifested as cough with profuse sputum (2) It is used for lung deficiency causing prolonged cough with hemoptysis	5–10 g for decoction

Table 1.19 (continued)

Name	Properties and tastes	Meridian entry	Effects	Application	Dosage
Kuandonghua (Flos Farfarae)	Pungent, slightly bitter, and warm	Lung meridian	(1) Moisten lung to send the adverse qi downward (2) Resolve phlegm and relieve cough	Cough and asthma	5–9 g for decoction
Pipaye (Loquat Leaf)	Bitter and slightly cold	Lung and stomach meridians	(1) Clear lung and relieve cough (2) Suppress adverse rise of qi to stop vomiting	(1) It is used for lung heat causing cough (2) It is used for stomach heat manifested as thirst, vomiting	6–10 g for decoction
Sangbaipi (White Mulberry Root Bark)	Sweet and cold	Lung meridian	(1) Purge lung heat to relieve asthma (2) Diuresis and eliminate edema	(1) It is used for lung heat causing cough and asthma (2) It is used for excess syndrome of fluid retention manifested as edema, difficult urination	6–12 g for decoction

Mineral herbs when taken as pills or powders can easily injure the stomach and impair stomach qi. They must be complemented with herbs that nourish the stomach and strengthen the spleen. Some of them are quite toxic and must be used only with great care.

1.7.13.1   Zhusha (Cinnabar, Cinnabaris)

Properties and Tastes: sweet, slightly cold and toxic
   Meridian Entry: heart meridian
   Effects

1. Relieve palpitation and calm spirit
2. Clear heat and remove toxin

   Application

1. Irritability, palpitation, insomnia
   For exuberance of heart fire causing irritability, restless fever in chest, palpitation, and insomnia, it is combined with Huanglian and Gancao; for those accompanied by deficiency of heart blood, Danggui and Shengdihuang are

added, such as Zhusha Anshen Wan; for palpitation due to fright or heart deficiency, it is put into a pig's heart and stewed for oral administration; for deficiency of yin and blood resulting in palpitation and insomnia, it is combined with Danggui, Baiziren and Suanzaoren.

2. Convulsion and epilepsy

   For high fever causing coma and convulsion, it is used with Niuhuang and Shexiang, such as Angong Niuhuang Wan; for infantile convulsion, it is combined with Niuhuang and Quanxie, such as Niuhuang San; for epilepsy, sudden coma and convulsion, it is combined with Cishi and Shenqu, such as Cizhu Wan.

3. Carbuncle, sore throat and aphthae

   To treat carbuncle, it is combined with Xionghuang and Daji, such as Zijin Troche; it treats sore throat and aphthae, with Bingpian and Pengsha in Bingpeng San for external application.

   In addition, it is also used as coat of pills and boluses, strengthening the effect of calming spirit and preventing decaying.

Usage and Dosage: 0.1–0.5 g is usually used in pill or powder form, not in decoction. It is used externally with appropriate dosage.

Precautions: Since it is toxic, it cannot be used in large amount or for a prolonged time. It contraindicates with abnormal function of liver and kidneys. It avoids being calcined, because mercury can be separated out, which is extremely toxic.

1.7.13.2   Suanzaoren (Spine Date Seed, Semen Ziziphi Spinosae)

Properties and Tastes: sweet, sour and neutral
   Meridian Entry: liver, gall bladder, and heart meridians
   Effects

1. Nourish heart and benefit liver
2. Clam mind
3. Arrest sweating

Application

1. Palpitation and insomnia

   For blood deficiency of heart and liver resulting in palpitation and insomnia, it is combined with Danggui, Baishao, and Heshouwu; for liver deficiency with heat causing vexation and insomnia, it is usually combined with Zhimu and Fuling, such as Suanzaoren Tang; for deficiency of heart and kidney and yin deficiency leading to hyperactive yang causing insomnia, palpitation, amnesia, it is combined with Shengdihuang, Xuanshen, and Baiziren, such as Tianwang Buxin Wan.

2. Weak constitution manifested as spontaneous sweating and night sweating
   To treat spontaneous sweating and night sweating caused by weak constitution, it is usually combined with Dangshen, Wuweizi, and Shanzhuyu.

Usage and Dosage: 9–15 g. It is ground into powder for oral administration with 1.5–3 g each time.
Other tranquilizing medicines (Table 1.20).

Table 1.20 Simple list of other tranquilizing medicines

Name	Properties and tastes	Meridian entry	Effects	Application	Dosage
Cishi (Magnetitum)	Salty and cold	Liver, heart, and kidney meridians	(1) Induce sedation and calm mind (2) Calm liver and suppress yang (3) Improve auditory and visual acuity (4) Improve inspiration and relieve dyspnea	(1) Irritability, fright palpitation, insomnia, and epilepsy (2) Liver yang hyperactivity manifested as dizziness and headache (3) Yin deficiency of liver and kidney causing tinnitus, deafness, and blurred vision (4) Dyspnea of kidney deficiency type	9–30 g for decoction first
Longgu (Os Draconis)	Sweet, astringent, and neutral	Heart, liver, and kidney meridians	(1) Induce sedation and calm mind (2) Pacify liver and subdue hyperactive yang (3) Astringe and arrest discharge	(1) Restlessness, palpitation, insomnia, fright epilepsy, and mania (2) Yin deficiency and yang hyperactivity manifested as irritability and dizziness (3) Loss and consumption syndromes	15–30 g for decoction
Baiziren (Semen Platycladi)	Sweet and neutral	Heart, kidney, and large intestine meridians	(1) Nourish heart and calm mind (2) Moisten intestines to release bowels	(1) Palpitation and insomnia (2) intestinal dryness with constipation	3–10 g for decoction

(continued)

Table 1.20 (continued)

Name	Properties and tastes	Meridian entry	Effects	Application	Dosage
Yuanzhi (Radix Polygalae)	Bitter, pungent, and warm	Heart, kidney, and lung meridians	(1) Calm heart and tranquilize mind (2) Eliminate phlegm for resuscitation (3) Dissipate swelling and carbuncles	(1) Fright palpitation, insomnia and amnesia (2) Confusion of mind by phlegm causing epilepsy and mania (3) Cough with profuse sputum (4) Large carbuncle causing swelling pain	3–10 g for decoction
Hehuan pi (Cortex Albiziae)	Sweet and neutral	Heart, liver, and lung meridians	(1) Calm mind and alleviate mental depression (2) Activate blood circulation and relieve swelling	(1) Emotional injury manifested as depression, insomnia, and amnesia (2) Fracture caused by trauma, abscess of internal organs, and carbuncle swelling	6–12 g for decoction

1.7.14 Tonifying and Replenishing Medicine

These medicines have their principal actions of replenishing the vital substances of the body and of strengthening its visceral organs. By doing so, they enhance the body's resistance to illness and eliminate the deficiencies.

There are four types of deficiency—qi, blood, yin, and yang. By their actions and applications restorative medicines fall into four categories: those that augment qi, those that generate blood, those that restore yin, and those that restore yang. Which medicine to prescribe will depend upon the type of deficiency. Moreover, in conditions of deficiency or damage of qi, blood, yin and yang often interact and affect one another. Hence, medicines from the different categories must often be prescribed together—restorative medicines for qi and yang together and restorative medicines for blood and yin together.

Tonifying and replenishing medicines are inappropriate in strength illnesses due to exogenous pathogenic evils. Also, if they are used incorrectly, restoratives can do more harm than good. When prescribing them the physician must take proper care of the spleen and the stomach. To avoid impairing digestion and absorption, as well as to obtain the desired therapeutic effects, the physician must include appropriate medicines that strengthen these organs.

1.7.14.1 Renshen (Ginseng, Radix Ginseng)

Properties and Tastes: sweet, slightly bitter and neutral
Meridian Entry: lung, spleen, and heart meridians
Effects

1. Replenish the primordial qi
2. Reinforce the spleen and nourish the lung
3. Promote fluid production
4. Induce tranquilization and improve intelligence

Application

1. Prostration syndrome of primordial qi
   It is a vital life-saving medicine and used to treat the crucial state due to prostration syndrome of primordial qi manifested as shortness of breath, listlessness, as well as a weak and faint pulse. It can be used alone such as in the Dushen Tang. For declination of yang qi manifested as cold extremities, it is used in combination with Fuzi, such as in the Shenfu Tang. For thirst due to deficiency of both qi and yin, it is used in combination with Maidong and Wuweizi, such as in the Shengmai San.
2. Lung qi deficiency syndrome
   For shortness of breath, dyspnea, and reluctance to speak and a low voice due to deficient lung qi, it is usually used in combination with Huangqi and Wuweizi. For dyspnea due to deficiency of both the lung and kidney, it is used in combination with Gejie and Wuweizi, such as in the Renshen Gejie San.
3. Spleen qi deficiency syndrome
   For lassitude, lack of strength, anorexia, and loose stools due to spleen qi deficiency, it is usually used in combination with Baizhu and Fuling, such as in the Sijunzi Tang. For various types of bleeding due to the failure of spleen to control blood, it is usually used in combination with Huangqi and Baizhu, such as in the Guipi Tang.
4. Thirst due to qi deficiency and consumption of fluid in febrile diseases and diabetes
   For febrile diseases with consumption of qi and body fluid manifested as thirst, large, and feeble pulse, it is usually combined with Zhimu, Shigao, such as in Baihu Jia Renshen Tang. For Xiaoke (similar to diabetes), it is used in combination with Tianhuafen and Shengdihuang.
5. Palpitation, insomnia, and dreamful sleep
   Due to its effect of replenishing heart qi, it is usually used in combination with Suanzaoren and Baizhiren to treat heart qi deficiency syndrome manifested as palpitation, fearful throbbing, insomnia, and dream-disturbed sleep.
   In addition, it can replenish qi and strengthen yang and it is used to treat impotence. When combined with pathogen-expelling medicine such as exterior-releasing medicinal and cathartic drugs, it has the efficacy to reinforce the healthy and dispel the pathogenic. It is used to treat excessive pathogens with

healthy qi being deficient, such as in the case of qi deficiency with external contraction or with heat accumulation of interior excess.

Usage and Dosage: 3–9 g. In case of prostration syndrome, the recommended dosage can be as much as 15–30 g. It should be simmered separately and later mixed with decoction of other medicinal herbs for oral administration. As to wild ginseng, it is ground into powder for swallows, 2 g each time, 2 times per day.

Precautions: It should not be used in combination with Lilu. Nonurgency administration of Renshen or Renshen preparations can cause diarrhea, rashes, insomnia, nervousness, increased blood pressure, melancholy, hypersexuality (or hyposexuality), headache, or palpitations. Bleeding is indicative of acute poisoning of Renshen.

1.7.14.2   Huangqi (Milkvetch Root, Radix Astragali seu Hedysari)

Properties and Tastes: sweet and slightly warm
  Meridian Entry: spleen and lung meridians
  Effects

1. Tonify qi and raise yang
2. Strengthen the defensive and superficial
3. Induce diuresis to alleviate edema
4. Expel toxin and promote tissue regeneration

Application

1. Spleen qi deficiency syndrome and syndrome of sinking of middle qi
    It is an essential medicine for invigorating the middle and replenishing qi. For lassitude, lack of strength, anorexia, and loose stool, due to spleen qi deficiency, it is often used in combination with Dangshen and Baizhi. In cases of proctoptosis due to prolonged diarrhea, prolapse of internal organs, which result from the sinking of middle qi, it is used with Renshen and Shengma, such as in the Buzhong Yiqi Tang. Furthermore, it functions to tonify qi and produce blood and treats blood deficiency syndrome in combination with Danggui, such as in the Danggui Buxue Tang. For loss of blood, which is due to the failure of spleen to control blood, it is combined with Renshen and Baizhu, such as in the Guipi Tang. To treat Xiaoke (similar to diabetes), which is due to the spleen failing to distribute fluid, it is usually combined with Tianhuafen and Gegen.
2. Lung qi deficiency syndrome and spontaneous sweating due to qi deficiency
    For chronic cough and dyspnea, shortness of breath, and listlessness, which is due to lung qi deficiency, it is used in combination with Ziyuan and Kuandonghua. To treat spontaneous sweating due to exterior deficiency, it is used with Muli and Mahuanggen. For those with exterior deficiency syndrome presenting as spontaneous sweating, and vulnerability to pathogenic wind, it is combined with Baizhu and Fangfeng, such as in the Yupingfeng San.

3. Edema due to qi deficiency

    It is an essential medicine to treat edema due to qi deficiency. In this case, it is usually combined with Baizhu and Fuling.
4. Deficiency syndrome of qi and blood, unruptured ulcers, or unhealed ulcers after rupture When the healthy qi is deficient and fails to expel interior toxins outwardly, there may appear even-shaped wide-rooted ulcers which fail to heal for a long period after rupturing. In this case, it is prescribed with Danggui and Shengma, such as in the Tounong San; for that due to deficiency of qi and blood, it is combined with Danggui and Rougui, such as in the Shiquan Dabu Tang

    Furthermore, with the function of tonifying qi to promote blood circulation, it treats arthralgia syndrome and sequela of apoplexy.

Usage and Dosage: 9–30 g. Honey-roasted, it is more effective for invigorating the middle and replenishing qi.

1.7.14.3   Danggui (Chinese Angelica, Radix Angelicae Sinensis)

Properties and Tastes: sweet, pungent and warm
  Meridian Entry: liver, heart and spleen meridians
  Effects

1. Tonify blood and activate blood
2. Regulate menstruation to relieve pain
3. Moisten the bowels to relieve constipation

Application

1. Blood deficiency syndrome

    It is the most essential medicine for treating blood deficiency syndrome. In this case, it is usually combined with Huangqi, as in the Danggui Buxue Tang
2. Irregular menstruation, amenorrhea and menorrhagia

    To treat irregular menstruation, amenorrhea, and menorrhagia due to blood deficiency or blood stasis, it is usually combined with Shudihuang, Baishao, and Chuanxiong, such as in the Siwu Tang. If it is accompanied by qi deficiency, it is combined with Renshen and Huangqi; if accompanied by qi stagnation, it is used combined with Xiangfu and Yanhusuo; and if by blood heat, it is combined with Huangqin and Huanglian. For amenorrhea due to blood stasis, it is used in combination with Taoren and Honghua; for that due to blood deficiency and cold stagnation, it is combined with Ejiao and Aiye.
3. Abdominal pain due to deficiency cold, injuries from falls, carbuncles and ulcers and sores, and arthralgia due to wind-cold

    It treats abdominal pain due to blood deficiency, blood stasis, or cold stagnation, it is used in combination with Guizhi, Shaoyao, and Shengjiang, such as in the Danggui Jianzhong Tang; for injuries from falls marked by pains and ecchymoma, it is combined with Ruxiang, Moyao, and Taoren, such as in the Fuyuan Huoxue Tang; in the case of early stage of ulcers with redness, swelling, and pain, it is combined with Jinyinhua, Chishao and Tianhuafen, such as in the Xianfang Huoming Tang; in the treatment of unhealed ulcers after rupture, it is combined with Huangqi, Renshen, and Rougui, such as in the Shiquan Dabu Tang. It also treats arthralgia due to wind-cold, combined with Qianghuo, Fangfen, and Huangqi.

4. Constipation due to blood deficiency with intestinal dryness

   In this case, it is usually used in combination with Roucongrong and Niuxi.

Usage and Dosage: 5–15 g.
Precautions: It is contraindicated in patients with excessive dampness with abdominal fullness and diarrhea.

1.7.14.4   Ejiao (Ass Hide Glue, Colla Corii Asini)

Properties and Tastes: sweet and neutral
   Meridian Entry: lung, liver, and kidney meridians
   Effects

1. Tonify blood
2. Nourish yin
3. Moisten the dryness
4. Stop bleeding

Application

1. Blood deficiency syndrome

   It is an essential medicine for treating blood deficiency. It is better at treating bleeding due to blood deficiency and usually prescribed with Shudihuang, Danggui, and Shaoyao, such as in the Ejiao Siwu Tang; for palpitations, fearful throbbing, knotted and intermittent pulse, due to deficiency of qi and blood, it is usually prescribed with Guizhi and Gancao, such as the Zhigancao Tang.

2. Hemorrhage

   For bloody urine during pregnancy, it is baked by itself and ground into powder for oral administration. In cases of hematemesis and hemorrhage due to yin deficiency with blood heat, it is combined with Puhuang and Shengdihuang. To treat hemoptysis, it is used together with Renshen and Tiandong. Also, for metrorrhagia and metrostaxis due to blood deficiency or blood cold, it is usually combined with Shudihuang and Danggui. To treat hemafecia or hematuria due to deficiency cold of spleen qi, it is combined with Baizhu and Zaoxintu in the Huangtu Tang.

3. Yin deficiency with dry cough

   For syndrome of lung heat with yin deficiency, manifested as dry cough with little phlegm, dry throat, and bloody sputum, it is used in combination with Madouling, Niubangzi, and Xingren. For syndromes of dryness injury to the

lung manifesting as dry cough without sputum, dry nose, and throat, it is combined together with Sangye, Xingren and Maidong.
4. Dysphoria and insomnia and clonic convulsions of the four extremities
   In combination with Huanglian and Baishao, such as in the Huanglian Ejiao Tang, it treats febrile disease with dysphoria and insomnia due to deficiency of kidney yin with exuberance of heart fire for clonic convulsions of the four extremities in the advanced stage of febrile disease encompassing exhaustion of true yin and yin deficiency stirring wind, and it is combined with Guijia and Hen Egg Yolk, such as in the Dadingfengzhu Tang or Xiaodingfengzhu Tang.

Usage and Dosage: 5–15 g, melted by heating for oral administration with water.
Precautions: It is sticky and greasy and may cause dyspepsia; therefore, it should be administered cautiously for patient with weakness of spleen and stomach.

1.7.14.5   Maidong (Dwarf Lilyturf Tuber, Radix Ophiopogonis)

Properties and Tastes: sweet, bitter slightly and cold slightly
   Meridian Entry: stomach, lung, and heart meridians
   Effects

1. Nourish Yin and moisten the lung
2. Tonify the stomach to promote the production of the body fluid
3. Dispel heat from the heart and relieve vexation

Application

1. Stomach yin deficiency syndrome
   In combination with Shengdihuang and Yuzhu, it treats deficiency of stomach yin due to heat, manifesting as dry mouth and tongue; for Xiaoke (similar to diabetes), it is combined with Tianhuafen and Wumei. It is combined with Banxia and Renshen to treat vomiting due to deficiency of stomach. To treat constipation due to pathogenic heat-damaging fluid, it is prescribed with Shengdihuang and Xuanshen, such as in the Zengye Tang.
2. Lung yin deficiency syndrome
   Prescribed with Ejiao, Shigao, and Sangye in Qingzao Jiufei Tang, it treats yin deficiency with dryness-heat in the lung, manifesting as dry nose and throat, dry cough with little phlegm, sore throat, and hoarse voice.
3. Heart yin deficiency syndrome
   To treat deficiency of heart yin, manifested as dysphoria, insomnia, dream-disturbed sleep amnesia, palpitations, and fearful throbbing, it is prescribed with Shengdihuang and Suanzaoren, such as in the Tianwang Buxin Wan. To treat dysphoria and hyposomnia, due to heat invading heart-nutrient level, it is used in combination with Huanglian and Shengdihuang.

Usage and Dosage: 6–12 g.

1.7.14.6   Gouqizi (Lycii Fructus Barbary, Wolfberry Fruit)

Properties and Tastes: sweet and neutral
   Meridian Entry: liver and kidney meridians
   Effects

1. Nourish liver and kidney
2. Replenish essence and improve vision

   Application
   Syndrome of liver-kidney yin deficiency
   It is indicated for dizziness, aching, and limpness in the loins and knees, spermatorrhea, deafness, loosened teeth, early graying of hair, insomnia, and dream-
disturbed sleep, due to insufficiency of essence and blood, tidal fever, night sweating,
and Xiaoke (diabetes), due to yin deficiency of liver and kidney. To treat xerotic
eyes, cataract, and blurry vision, it is prescribed with Shudihuang, Shanzhuyu,
Shanyao, and Juhua, such as in the Qiju Dihuang Wan.

   Usage and Dosage: 6–12 g
   Other tonifying and replenishing medicines (Table 1.21).

1.7.15   Astringent Medicine

These are medicines that have their principal actions of astringing and stabilizing.
Most of them are sour and astringent. Individual medicines have the ability to hold
back sweat, stop diarrhea, hold back semen, reduce diuresis, curtail vaginal discharge, stop bleeding, or stop cough. Hence, they are suitable for use in a patient in
whom the constitution has been weakened by chronic illness or genuine qi is infirm.
Such a patient may show symptoms of unrestrained flow, such as spontaneous
sweating, night sweat, chronic diarrhea, dysentery, spermatorrhea, premature ejaculation, enuresis, polyuria, chronic cough with labored breathing, persistent metrorrhagia, and persistent vaginal discharge.
   Astringent medicines treat only the appearance, not the root. They can prevent
exhaustion of genuine qi from the unrestrained and continual loss and avoid other
complications. However, the fundamental cause of illnesses with such unrestrained
loss is deficiency of genuine qi. Hence, complete treatment of both root and appearance requires the use of complementary restorative medicines. For example, for
spontaneous sweating due to qi deficiency or night sweat due to yin deficiency, add,
respectively, medicines that augment qi or nourish yin. For chronic diarrhea, dysentery and persistent vaginal discharge due to insufficiency of the spleen and the kidney, add medicinals that nourish and strengthen the spleen and the kidney. For
premature ejaculation, spermatorrhea, enuresis, and polyuria due to kidney insufficiency, add medicines that nourish and strengthen the kidney. For infirmity of the
Ren and Chong meridians causing metrorrhagia, add medicines that nourish the

Table 1.21 Simple list of other tonifying and replenishing medicines

Name	Properties and tastes	Meridian entry	Effects	Application	Dosage
Xiyang shen (Radix Panacis Quinquefolii)	Sweet, slightly bitter, and cool	Lung, heart, and kidney meridians	(1) Tonify qi and nourish yin (2) Clear heat and promote fluid production	(1) Syndrome of both qi and yin deficiency (2) Lung qi deficiency syndrome and lung yin deficiency syndrome (3) Thirst due to qi deficiency and consumption of fluid in febrile diseases and diabetes	3–6 g for decoction alone
Dangshen (Radix Codonopsis)	Sweet and neutral	Spleen and lung meridians	(1) Invigorate the middle energizer and replenish qi (2) Invigorate spleen and lung (3) Nourish blood and promote fluid production	(1) Insufficiency of middle qi (2) Lung qi deficiency syndrome (3) Qi and blood deficiency syndrome (4) Qi deficiency and fluid consumption syndrome	9–30 g for decoction
Taizishen (Radix Pseudostellariae)	Sweet, slightly bitter, and neutral	Spleen and lung meridians	(1) Tonify spleen qi (2) Promote fluid production and nourish lung	(1) Spleen deficiency syndrome (2) Insufficiency of qi and yin after disease (3) Dry cough due to lung insufficiency	9–30 g for decoction
Baizhu (Rhizoma Atractylodis Macrocephalae)	Sweet, bitter, and warm	Spleen and stomach meridians	(1) Invigorate spleen and replenish qi (2) Dry dampness and induced diuresis (3) Stop sweating (4) Prevent abortion	(1) Spleen qi deficiency syndrome (2) Edema and phlegm-fluid retention (3) Spontaneous sweating due to qi deficiency (4) Threatened abortion due to spleen deficiency	6–12 g for decoction

(continued)

Table 1.21 (continued)

Name	Properties and tastes	Meridian entry	Effects	Application	Dosage
Shanyao (Rhizoma Atractylodis Macrocephalae)	Sweet and neutral	Spleen, lung, and kidney meridians	(1) Nourish the spleen and stomach (2) Promote production of fluid and nourish lung (3) Tonify kidney and secure essence	(1) Spleen deficiency syndrome (2) Lung deficiency syndrome (3) Kidney deficiency syndrome (4) Xiaoke with deficiency of both qi and yin	15–30 g for decoction
Baibiandou (Semen Dalichoris Album)	Sweet and slightly warm	Spleen and stomach meridians	(1) Invigorate spleen and resolve dampness (2) Harmonize the middle and dispel summer heat	(1) Spleen qi deficiency syndrome (2) Syndrome of summer heat vomiting, and diarrhea	9-15g for decoction
Gancao (Radix Glycyrrhizae)	Sweet and neutral	Heart, lung spleen, and stomach meridians	(1) Tonify spleen and replenish qi (2) Dispel phlegm and arrest cough (3) Relive spasm and alleviate pain (4) Clear heat and relieve toxicity (5) Harmonize all medicine	(1) Spleen qi deficiency syndrome (2) Heart qi insufficient syndrome (3) Cough and dyspnea (4) Spasm in the abdomen and extremities (5) Heat toxin with ulcers, sore throat, medicinal or food poisoning (6) Moderating the properties of medicine	2–10 g for decoction
Dazao (Fructus Jujubae)	Sweet and warm	Spleen and stomach meridians	(1) Tonify the middle and replenish qi (2) Nourish blood and induce tranquilization	(1) Spleen qi deficiency syndrome (2) Sallowness due to blood deficiency, and hysteria	6–15 g for decoction

Table 1.21 (continued)

Name	Properties and tastes	Meridian entry	Effects	Application	Dosage
Lurong (Ccornu Cervi Pantotrichum)	Sweet, salty, and warm	Kidney and liver meridians	(1) Tonify kidney yang (2) Replenish essence and blood (3) Strengthen tendons and bones (4) Regulate Chong (Thoroughfare) and Ren (conception) vessels (5) Expel sores	(1) Kidney yang deficiency and essence blood deficiency (2) Kidney deficiency with bone weakness (3) Deficiency cold in thoroughfare and conception vessels (4) Unhealed chronic ulcers, deep-rooted yin abscess	1–2 g. It is ground into powder for swallows or used in pill for powder form
Yinyanghuo (Herba Epimedii)	Pungent, sweet, and warm	Kidney and liver meridians	(1) Tonify kidney yang (2) Strengthen tendons and bones (3) Expel wind-damp	(1) Declination of kidney yang (2) Wind-cold-damp arthralgia and numbness in limbs	6–10 g for decoction
Bajitian (Radix Morindae Officinalis)	Pungent, sweet, and slightly warm	Kidney and liver meridians	(1) Tonify kidney yang (2) Strengthen tendons and bones (3) Expel wind-damp	(1) Deficiency of kidney yang (2) Kidney deficiency limpness in the knees and lumbus, lumbago, and Impediment disease	3–10 g for decoction
Xianmao (Rhizoma Curculigins)	Pungent, hot, and toxic	Kidney, liver, and spleen meridians	(1) Tonify kidney yang (2) Strengthen tendons and bones (3) Expel wind-damp	(1) Deficiency of kidney yang (2) Pain and cold sensation in knees and lumbus, bone limpness, and chronic impediment disease	3–10 g for decoction

(continued)

Table 1.21 (continued)

Name	Properties and tastes	Meridian entry	Effects	Application	Dosage
Xuduan (Radix Dipsaci)	Bitter, pungent, and slightly warm	Liver and kidney meridians	(1) Tonify kidney and liver (2) Strengthen tendons and bones (3) Heal bone fracture (4) Stop metrorrhagia and metrostaxis	(1) Impotence, spermatorrhea, and enuresis (2) Soreness in knees and lumbus, arthralgia due to cold-dampness (3) Injuries from falls, soft tissue injuries and bone fracture (4) Metrorrhagia and metrostaxis, threatened abortion	9–15 g for decoction
Roucongrong (Herba Cistanches)	Sweet, salty, and warm	Kidney and large intestine meridians	(1) Tonify kidney yang (2) Replenish essence and blood (3) Moisten bowels to relieve constipation	(1) Impotence, spermatorrhea, and sterility (2) Constipation due to intestinal fluid consumption	6–10 g for decoction
Tusizi (Semen Cuscutae)	Sweet and warm	Liver, kidney, and spleen meridians	(1) Tonify kidney and replenish essence (2) Nourish liver to improve vision (3) Stop diarrhea and prevent abortion	(1) Kidney insufficiency with lumbago, impotence, spermatorrhea and frequent urination, and sterility due to cold uterus (2) Insufficiency liver and kidney, dim and blurred vision (3) Deficiency of spleen and kidney yang and diarrhea (4) Kidney insufficiency with threatened abortion and habitual abortion	6–12g for decoction

Table 1.21 (continued)

Name	Properties and tastes	Meridian entry	Effects	Application	Dosage
Hetaoren (Semen Juglandis)	Sweet and warm	Kidney, lung, and large intestine meridians	(1) Tonify kidney and warm lung (2) Moisten bowels to relieve constipation	(1) Declination of kidney yang, lumbago and feet flaccidity, and frequent urination (2) Deficiency of lung and kidney, cough, and dyspnea due to deficiency cold (3) Constipation due to intestinal dryness	6–9 g for decoction
Shudihuang (Radix Rehmanniae Preparata)	Sweet and slightly warm	Liver and kidney meridians	(1) Nourish yin and supplement blood (2) Replenish essence and marrow	(1) Blood deficiency syndromes (2) Deficiency syndromes of liver-kidney yin	9–15 g for decoction
Baishao (Radix Paeoniae Alba)	Sitter, sour, and slightly cold	Liver and spleen meridians	(1) Nourish blood and regulate menstruation (2) Suppress liver to relieve pain (3) Astringe yin to arrest sweating	(1) Irregular menstruation (2) Pain in the hypochondrium, stomach and abdomen, or spasm and pain in the extremities (3) Hyperactivity of liver yang with headache and vertigo (4) Sweating with aversion to wind, night sweating due to yin deficiency	6–15 g for decoction
Beishashen (Radix Glehniae)	Sweet, slightly bitter, and slightly cold	Lung and stomach meridians	(1) Nourish yin and clear lung heat (2) Reinforce the stomach and promote fluid production	(1) Lung yin deficiency syndrome (2) Stomach yin deficiency syndrome	5–12 g for decoction

(continued)

Table 1.21 (continued)

Name	Properties and tastes	Meridian entry	Effects	Application	Dosage
Baihe (Bulbus Lilii)	Sweet and cold	Heart and lung meridians	(1) Nourish yin and moisten lung (2) Clear heart to induce tranquilization	(1) Lung yin deficiency syndrome (2) Insomnia, palpitations, and lily disease	6–12 g for decoction
Tiandong (Radix Asparagi)	Sweet, bitter, and cold	Lung and kidney meridians	(1) Nourish yin and moisten dryness (2) Clear lung and promote fluid production	(1) Lung yin deficiency syndrome (2) Kidney yin deficiency syndrome (3) Febrile disease with consumption of fluid, anorexia, thirst, and constipation to intestinal dryness	6–12 g for decoction
Shihu (Herba Dendrobii)	Sweet and slightly cold	Stomach and kidney meridians	(1) Strengthen stomach and promote fluid production (2) Nourish yin and clear heat	(1) Stomach yin deficiency syndrome (2) Kidney yin deficiency syndrome	6–12 g for decoction
Yuzhu (Rhizoma Polygonati Odorati)	Sweet and slightly cold	Lung and stomach meridians	(1) Nourish yin and moisten dryness (2) Promote fluid production to relieve thirst	(1) Lung deficiency syndrome (2) Stomach yin deficiency syndrome	6–12 g for decoction
Huangjing (Rhizoma Polygonati)	Sweet and neutral	Spleen, lung, and kidney meridians	(1) Tonify qi and nourish yin (2) Invigorate the spleen (3) Moisten the lung (4) Reinforce the kidney	(1) Ling yin deficiency syndrome (2) Spleen deficiency syndrome (3) Deficiency of kidney essence	9–15 g for decoction
Mohanlian (Herba Ecliptae)	Sweet, sour, and cold	Liver and kidney meridians	(1) Nourish liver yin and kidney yin (2) Cool blood to stop bleeding	(1) Syndrome of liver-kidney yin deficiency (2) Hemorrhage due to yin deficiency with blood heat	6–12 g for decoction

Table 1.21 (continued)

Name	Properties and tastes	Meridian entry	Effects	Application	Dosage
Guijia (Carapax et Plastrum Testudinis)	Salty, sweet, and slightly cold	Liver, kidney, and heart meridians	(1) Nourish yin and suppress yang (2) Tonify kidney and strengthen bones (3) Nourish blood and replenish heart	(1) Syndrome liver-kidney yin deficiency (2) Kidney deficiency with flaccidity of the tendons and bones (3) Insufficiency of yin-blood with palpitations, insomnia, and amnesia	9–24 g for decoction first
Biejia (Carapax Trionycis)	Salty and cold	Liver and kidney meridians	(1) Nourish yin and suppress yang (2) Reduce bone-steaming fever (3) Soften hardness and dissipate nodulation	(1) Yin deficiency with internal heat, with wind stirring inside, with yang hyperactivity (2) Abdominal masses	9–24 g for decoction first

liver and the kidney and those that reinforce the Ren and Chong meridians. For chronic cough and labored breathing due to insufficiency of the lung and the kidney, add medicines that nourish the lung and enhance the kidney's capacity to receive qi.

Astringent medicine has the disadvantage of potentially retaining disease-causing evils. In general, if the exogenous pathogenic evil is still present in the exterior, if dampness has accumulated in the interior, or if interior heat has not been cleared, then it is inappropriate to prescribe these medicines.

1.7.15.1 Mahuanggen (Ephedra Root, Radix Ephedrae)

Properties and Tastes: sweet, slightly astringent, and neutral
  Meridian Entry: lung meridian
  Effects: strengthen superficies and stop sweating
  Application
  Spontaneous sweating and night sweating
  For spontaneous sweating due to deficiency of qi, it can be used combined with Huangqi and Muli, such as in Muli San. In cases of night sweating due to yin deficiency, it is usually used together with Shudihuang and Danggui. To treat frequent perspiration after delivery due to asthenia, it can be used in combination with Danggui and Huangqi. Also, it can be used with Muli and prepared as powder for external application, for any sweating syndrome, due to asthenia.

Usage and Dosage: 3–9 g is used for oral use. For external application, the amount should be appropriate

Precautions: It is contraindicated in those patients who are infected with exogenous pathogens.

1.7.15.2   Wuweizi (Magnolia Vine Fruit, Fructus Schisandrae Chinese)

Properties and Tastes: sour, sweet, and warm
  Meridian Entry: lung, heart, and kidney meridians
  Effects

1. Astringe and strengthen
2. Benefit qi and promote the production of body fluid
3. Tonify the kidney and calm the mind

Application

1. Nonurgency cough and dyspnea resulting from asthenia

    It is used for chronic cough and dyspnea resulting from asthenia. It is the essential medicine for the treatment of this kind of syndrome in treating chronic cough due to deficiency of the lung, and it is used in combination with Yingsuke such as in the formula Wuweizi Wan. To treat the syndrome of lung and kidney deficiency manifesting as heavy breathing, it is often used combined with Shanzhuyu and Shudihuang, such as in the formula Duqi Wan. In treating cough and asthma caused by lung cold, it should be used together with Mahuang and Xixin, such as in Xiao Qinglong Tang.
2. Spontaneous perspiration and night sweating

    It is used for spontaneous perspiration and night sweating, and it is often used in combination with Mahuanggen and Muli.
3. Emission and spermatorrhea

    In treating spermatorrhea, it can be used with Sangpiaoxiao, Fuzi, and Longgu. For treating emission while dreaming, it is often used together with Maidong and Shanzhuyu.
4. Nonurgency diarrhea

    It is indicated for chronic diarrhea, and it is often used together with Buguzhi, Roudoukou, and Wuzhuyu, such as in the formula Sishen Wan.
5. Thirst due to fluid loss and diabetes

    To treat thirst of fluid loss resulting from thermal injury qi and yin, it is often used in combination with Renshen and Maidong, such as Shengmai powder; it is used for polydipsia resulting from internal heat due to yin deficiency in diabetes, and it is usually used in combination with Shanyao and Zhimu.
6. Palpitation, insomnia, and dreaminess

    To treat deficiency of yin and blood, or heart-kidney imbalance manifesting as palpitation, insomnia, and dreaminess, it is usually used in combination with Maidong, Danshen, and Shengdihuang, such as Tianwang Buxin Wan.

Usage and Dosage: 3–6 g is taken orally. It is ground into powder 1–3 g.

Precautions: It is not suitable for those with exterior pathogen factors which have not been eliminated and sthenic heat in the interior, manifesting as cough and measles in the initial stage.

1.7.15.3 Wumei (Smoked Plum, Fructus Mume)

Properties and Tastes: sour, astringent, and neutral
  Meridian Entry: liver, spleen, lung, and large intestine meridians
  Effects:

1. Astringe the lung and relieve cough
2. Astringe the intestine and antidiarrheal
3. Promote the production of body fluid
4. Relieve ascaris colic

Application

1. Prolonged cough due to deficiency of the lung
    In treating prolonged cough with a small amount of sputum due to deficiency of the lung, or dry cough without sputum, it is often used together with Yingsuke and Kuxingren, such as in the formula Yifu San.
2. Prolonged diarrhea or dysentery
    For prolonged diarrhea or dysentery, it can be used together with Yingsuke and Hezi, such as in the formula Guchang Wan. In treating hygropyretic dysentery and purulent hematochezia, it can be combined with Huanglian, such as in the formula Wumei Wan.
3. Xiaoke (diabetes) due to deficiency heat
    Its single decoction is effective in treating Xiaoke (diabetes) due to heat of deficiency type, or used together with Tianhuafen, Maidong, and Renshen, such as in the formula Yuquan San.
4. Abdominal pain and vomiting caused by intestinal ascariasis
    Ascaris becomes sedated when it meets a sour flavor, as this medicine is quite sour. It is a good medicine for ascariasis in treating abdominal pain, vomiting, and cold extremities caused by intestinal ascariasis, and it is often combined with Chuanjiao and Huanglian, such as in the formula Wumei Wan.
    In addition, when carbonized it has the function of strengthening the chong vessel and stopping metrostaxis, it can treat metrorrhagia and metrostaxis and hemafecia. Also, it is able to eliminate sores accompanied by toxins by external application, such as pterygium and head sore.

Usage and Dosage: 3–10 g is taken orally, in a large dosage may be up to 30 g. For external application, the amount should be appropriate, and it can be pounded or carbonized and then ground into powder. In order to stop bleeding and diarrhea, the carbonized form is applicable.

Precautions: If taken orally, it is contraindicated for patients with exogenous factors or those with stagnation of sthenic heat.

1.7.15.4   Shanzhuyu (Asiatic Cornelian Cherry Fruit, Fructus Corni)

Properties and Tastes: sour, astringent, and slightly warm
   Meridian Entry: liver and kidney meridians
   Effects

1. Tonify liver and kidney
2. Astringe essence and strengthen collapse

   Application

1. Soreness of waist and knees, dizziness, tinnitus, and impotence
   It can be used for deficiency of the liver and kidney manifesting as dizziness, soreness of waist, and tinnitus, it is often combined with Shudihuang and Shanyao, such as in the formula Liuwei Dihuang Wan; it can be used for weak fire of Mingmen manifesting as cold pain in waist and knees, dysuria, combined with Rougui and Fuzi, such as in the formula Shenqi Wan; for impotence due to insufficiency of kidney yang, it is combined with Lurong, Buguzhi, and Bajitian.
2. Emission, spermatorrhea, enuresis, and frequent urination
   In treating emission, spermatorrhea due to kidney deficiency leading to essence not being consolidated, it is often used together with Shudihuang and Shanyao; in treating enuresis and frequent urination with deficiency of kidney leading to bladder loss restriction, it is often used together with Fupenzi, Jinyingzi, and Shayuanzi.
3. Metrorrhagia and metrostaxis and menorrhagia
   In treating metrorrhagia and metrostaxis and menorrhagia due to deficiency of liver and kidney, it is often used with Shudihuang and Baishao. In treating those due to deficiency of spleen, unconsolidation of thoroughfare, and conception meridians, it is often used with Longgu and Huangqi.
4. Profuse sweating and collapse due to weak constitution
   For profuse sweating and collapse due to weak constitution, it is often used with Renshen, Fuzi, and Longgu.
   In addition, it also can be used for Xiaoke (diabetes), and it is mostly combined with Shengdihuang and Tianhuafen.

Usage and Dosage: 3–10 g is used for oral use. Large dosage may be up to 20–30 g for emergency to strengthen collapse.
   Precautions: It is not suitable for patients with dribbling and astringent pain during urination due to damp-heat in normal timer.
   Other astringent medicines (Table 1.22).

Table 1.22 Simple list of other astringent medicines

Name	Properties and tastes	Meridian entry	Effects	Application	Dosage
Fuxiaomai (Fructus Tritici Levis)	Sweet and cool	Heart meridian	(1) Strengthen superficies and arrest sweating (2) Tonify healthy qi and eliminate heat	(1) Spontaneous sweating and night sweating (2) Hectic fever and overstrain fever	15–30 g for decoction
Wubeizi (Galla Chinensis)	Sour, astringent, and cold	Lung, large intestine, and kidney meridians	(1) Astringe lung and lower fire (2) Astringe intestines to stop diarrhea (3) Astringe perspiration and stop bleeding (4) Absorb dampness and heal sore	(1) Cough and emptysis (2) Prolonged diarrhea or dysentery (3) Spontaneous perspiration and night sweat (4) Metrorrhagia and metrostasis, hematochezia, and hemorrhoids with bleeding (5) Damp sore and swollen sore with toxicity	3–6 g for decoction
Hezi (Fructus Chebulae)	Bitter, sour, astringent, and neutral	Lung and large intestine meridians	(1) Astringe the intestines and lung (2) Drive fire downward and benefit the throat	(1) Prolonged diarrhea and dysentery (2) Prolonged cough and loss of voice	5–10 g for decoction
Roudoukou (Semen Myristicae)	Pungent and warm	Spleen, stomach, and large intestine meridians	(1) Astringe the intestine to stop diarrhea (2) Warm the middle energizer to promote flow of qi	(1) Diarrhea of deficiency type and cold dysentery (2) Stomach cold leading to distending pain, poor appetite, and vomiting	3–10 g for decoction
Chishizhi (Halloysitum Rubrum)	Sweet, sour, astringent, and warm	Large intestine and stomach meridians	(1) Astringe the intestine to stop bleeding (2) Promote tissue regeneration and healing of wounds	(1) Chronic diarrhea and dysentery (2) Metrorrhagia and metrostaxis, bloody stool, and leucorrhea (3) Unhealed chronic ulcer	9–12 g for decoction first

(continued)

Table 1.22 (continued)

Name	Properties and tastes	Meridian entry	Effects	Application	Dosage
Sangpiaoxiao (Oötheca Mantidis)	Sweet, salty, and neutral	Liver and kidney meridians	(1) Benefit kidney and astringe essence (2) Reduce the frequency of urination to stop turbidity	(1) Impotence, emission, and spermatorrhea (2) Enuresis and frequent urination and white turbidity	5–10 g for decoction
Jingyingzi (Fructus Rosae Laevigatae)	Sour, sweet, astringent, and neutral	Kidney, bladder, and large intestine meridians	(1) Astringe essence (2) Reduce the frequency of urination (3) Astringe the intestine to relieve diarrhea	(1) Nocturnal emission, spermatorrhea, enuresis, frequent micturition, and excessive leucorrhea (2) Chronic diarrhea and dysentery	6–12 g for decoction
Haipiaoxiao (Os Sepiellae seu Sepiae)	Salty, astringent, and warm	Spleen and kidney meridians	(1) Astringe to stop bleeding (2) Astringe essence and stop emission and leucorrhea (3) Control acid regurgitation (4) Promote sore healing	(1) Metrorrhagia and metrostasis, hematochezia, and hemorrhoids with bleeding due to trauma (2) Nocturnal emission, spermatorrhea, and leucorrhea (3) Stomachache with acid regurgitation (4) Skin pyogenic infection, eczema, and ulcer without being healed	5–10 g for decoction
Lianzi (Semen Nelumbinis)	Sweet, astringent, and neutral	Spleen, kidney, and heart meridians	(1) Invigorate the spleen and relieve diarrhea (2) Benefit the kidney to preserve the essence (3) Nourish the heart and tranquilize the mind	(1) Diarrhea due to deficiency of the spleen (2) Nocturnal emission, spermatorrhea, and leucorrhea (3) Palpitation and insomnia	6–15 g for decoction

Table 1.22   (continued)

Name	Properties and tastes	Meridian entry	Effects	Application	Dosage
Qianshi (Ssemen Euryales)	Sweet, astringent, and neutral	Spleen and kidney meridians	(1) Benefit the kidney to preserve the essence (2) Invigorate the spleen and relieve diarrhea (3) Dispel dampness to relieve leucorrhea	(1) Nocturnal emission and spermatorrhea (2) Prolonged diarrhea due to deficiency of the spleen (3) Leucorrhea	9–15 g for decoction

1.8   Summary

The common theory of Chinese medicines covers the habitat and collection, processing, properties and effects, compatibility, and contraindication.

The common Chinese medicines are classified according to the main effect, and several representatives are introduced in detail.

Questions

1. What are the concepts and functions of four natures and five flavors?
2. What are the concepts and functions of compatibility?
3. What are the concepts of contraindication?
4. What kind of drugs should be decocted first?
5. Please discuss the relationship between the drug's properties and the dosage.
6. What should be paid attention to when we decoct?
7. What are the concepts, properties, and functions of the exterior-releasing medicine?
8. Please discuss the similarities and differences between Shigao and Zhimu.
9. What are the matters that should be noticed when we use the Purgative medicine?
10. What are the medical properties, meridian entry, effects and application of Jinyinhua?
11. Describe the similarities and differences in the medicinal efficacies of Chuanbeimu and Zhebeimu.
12. Compare the similarities and differences between the efficacies and indications of Fuzi and Ganjiang.
13. Outline the medicinal properties and clinical applications of Chenpi and Zhishi.
14. Why is Sanqi signified as the most significant medicine for trauma and wounds?

15. State the reasons why Chuanxiong is the most significant medicine for headache.
16. Describe the tranquilizing features of Zhusha and Suanzaoren.
17. Combined with its medicinal efficacies, describe the clinical applications of Renshen.
18. List the medicinal properties, efficacies, and indications of Wuweizi.

Chapter 2
Basic Knowledge of Prescription

Mingmin Zhu and Yong Huang

Objectives

Master the formation and modification, and preparation form of TCM prescription. Know the commonly used prescriptions.

Guideline

Prescription, which is one of the important methods of TCM, is used for the prevention and treatment of diseases. Prescriptions are used under the guidance of TCM theory, upon syndrome differentiation, and according to different diseases. The application of prescription involves the combination of medicine, determination of dosage and preparation form, and the modification according to the syndrome development. This chapter starts with the basic theory of prescriptions and introduces the commonly used prescriptions in terms of main effect.

2.1 Introduction

Prescriptions are formed with appropriate combination of selected Chinese medicines according to the principle of prescription for the determination of dosage and preparation form of medicines. As the important measure of TCM treatment, prescriptions are the specific expression of treatment upon syndrome differentiation. Prescriptions are composed of Chinese medicines, and comprehensive application of Chinese medicines form prescriptions.

M. Zhu
Jinan University, Guangzhou, China

Y. Huang (✉)
School of Traditional Chinese Medicine, Southern Medical University, Guangzhou, China

© Zhengzhou University Press 2024
Y. Huang, L. Zhu (eds.), *Textbook of Traditional Chinese Medicine*,
https://doi.org/10.1007/978-981-99-5299-1_2

2.2 Formation and Modification of Prescription

Prescription comes from combination of the Chinese medicine. The efficacy and specific nature of each Chinese medicine are different. Therefore, only by following the certain principle and reasonable collocation, to enhance the original efficacy of Chinese medicine, harmonize the special aspects of their nature, and restrict their toxicity, can the integrated use of various Chinese medicine be fully utilized. At the same time, prescription has great flexibility. The ingredient, dosage, and preparation form must be adjusted during the clinical practice.

2.2.1 Forming Principles

The composition of each prescription must be confirmed by choosing appropriate combination and on the basis of syndrome differentiation and decision of therapeutic methods according to different conditions. The forming principles must be followed strictly during combination. In the prescription, different medicines play a different role with the help of special combination. According to the different roles and status of Chinese medicine, this combination relationship can be described as sovereign (jun), minister (chen), assistant (zuo), and courier (shi) medicines.

2.2.1.1 Sovereign Medicine

Sovereign medicine is the essential component of the prescription and its pharmacological effects stronger than others. Sovereign medicine plays a primary curative role aiming at the main disease or syndrome.

2.2.1.2 Minister Medicine

Minister medicine plays a supporting role to sovereign medicine, and its pharmacological effects are second on to the sovereign medicine. There are two different conditions. In one condition, the minister medicine helps sovereign medicine to enhance the curative effect of main disease or syndrome. In another, minister medicine plays a primary curative role aiming at the accompanying diseases or syndrome.

2.2.1.3 Assistant Medicine

Assistant medicine can be used in three conditions.

Promotion Assistant: It can help sovereign and minister medicine to enhance the curative effect or treat secondary accompanying diseases or syndrome directly.

Restriction Assistant: It is used to eliminate or slow the toxicity and potent nature of sovereign and minister medicine.

Counteracting Assistant: In this condition, the pathogenic factors of disease are too serious to make patients refuse the medicine. Thus, the medicine that has opposite nature and flavor to those of sovereign medicine but plays supplementing role in the treatment will be chosen.

2.2.1.4   Courier Medicine

There are two conditions for the courier medicine. One is used as meridian ushering medicine, guiding the medicine of the prescription into the pathogenic location. The other is used as harmonizing medicine, harmonizing all the medicine of the prescription.

In clinics, not all the prescription has the assistant medicine and courier medicine. In case of simple pathogenic condition, one or two ingredients of medicine can take effect. If there is not toxic or drastic or the sovereign and minister medicine, it is not necessary to add assistant medicine. The meridian entry of the sovereign and minister medicine can lead into the pathogenic location, and then, courier as meridian ushering medicine is not also necessary. In a general way, the ingredients of sovereign medicine should be fewer but with large dosage, while the minister medicine more than sovereign, and assistant medicine more than minister, and one or two courier medicines. In a word, the quantity of medicine ingredients and the application of sovereign, minister, assistant, and courier medicine should be basic on the condition of disease state and the treatment method.

2.2.2   Modification of Prescription

The composition of prescription has strict principle and also great flexibility. Forming prescription in clinical practice must be based on the specific condition and flexibility.

2.2.2.1   Modification of Ingredients

Ingredient is the main factor that determines efficacy of prescription. So, the increase or decrease in ingredients inevitably changes the efficacy of prescription. There are two cases of it. One is the increase or decrease in assistant medicine and courier medicine, which is applied to the cases that the main disease is unchanged but accompanying syndrome different, and this will not lead to a fundamental change in the prescription. For example, Yinqiao San is the commonly used prescription for wind-heat exterior syndrome. If there is also cough, it is due to lung qi failing to diffuse. Therefore, we can add Kuxingren to descending lung qi and relieve cough. The other is the increase or decrease in minister medicines. Due to the forming relation change of the prescription, it will make a fundamental change in the overall efficacy. For example, Mahuang Tang is a prescription for the treatment of wind-cold excess exterior syndrome. If the minister medicine Guizhi is removed, which leads to the weakening of sweating power, the prescription will become a treatment for cough and asthma in cold syndrome; if Baizhu is added, which is minister medicine as Guizhi, the effects of prescription will increase resolving dampness effect based on promoting sweating to release the exterior. The prescription becomes a treatment for wind-cold fixed impediment.

2.2.2.2   Increase and Decrease in Dosage

The dosage and pharmacological effects are directly related. (The dosage is directly related to the pharmacological effects.) Although the ingredients of prescription are the same, if one or more ingredients are changed, it will lead to the combination, and effects and main indications are different. For example, both Xiaochengqi Tang and Houpo Sanwu Tang contain same three kind herbs, Dahuang, Houpo, and Zhishi. Dahuang, the sovereign medicine with great effect of purging heat accumulation, has been used with a big dosage in Xiaochenqi Tang, in order to treat yangming fu viscera excess syndrome, while Houpo, the sovereign medicine with great effect of moving qi to resolve fullness, has been used with a big dosage in Houpo Sanwu Tang, for the treatment of constipation with qi stagnation syndrome.

2.2.2.3   Modification of Preparation Forms

Prescription can have a variety of preparation forms and different preparation form features. The same prescription with different preparation forms will lead to the strength and also the drastic and mile of the prescription and will lead to the treatment of disease with its priorities. For example, Lizhong Wan and Renshen Tang, both medicines and dosages are exactly the same, but Lizhong Wan is a pill that grinds the above into a fine powder and makes it into the pill, which is for mild deficiency cold syndrome in middle energizer with gentle effect, while Renshen Tang is a decoction boiled by medicines, with the features of fast absorption and taking effect quickly, which is the treatment of serious deficiency cold syndrome in upper and middle energizer.

2.3 Preparation Forms of Prescription

Preparation form of prescription is a particular form, which can be made according to the needs and characteristics of medicines after the combination of prescription, in order to make it easy to use or better for treatment of diseases. Traditional preparation forms of prescription include decoction, pill, powder, paste, pellet, wine preparation, soluble granule, and syrup. The commonly used preparation forms of prescription are introduced as follows.

2.3.1 Decoctions (Tang)

Decoction is the most commonly used and most traditional preparation form of prescription. After completing the medicines of prescription, soaked with water or wine, or a mixture of 50% of wine and 50% of water for a period of time (often for half an hour), boiled to certain amount of water or boiled after a certain of time, removed the slag, then the decoction is obtained. Decoction is mostly orally used or for external wash. For example, Mahuang Tang and Guizhi Tang are made this way. The characteristics of decoction are fast absorption and rapid action and especially facilitate with modification of preparation form according to the disease. It is the most widely used in clinical practice, which is suitable for patients with severe or unstable conditions. The disadvantage of decoction is that some of the effective medicines are not easy to decocte, and the dosage is large, and inconvenient to carry.

2.3.2 Pills (Wan)

Pills are a round solid fixed dosage form that grind the medicines of the prescription into fine powder and then add a proper amount of excipient. Pills have the advantages of slow absorption, lasting effect, and more convenient to be taken and carried. It is suitable for chronic disease and debilitating diseases such as Liuwei Dihuang Wan and Lizhong Wan. There are also pills for first aids such as Angong Niuhuang Wan, which made into pills, and thus can be easily stored for emergency use.

2.3.2.1 Honeyed Pill

Honeyed pill is made by grinding medicines into fine powder and adding honey as excipient. There are big honeyed pills and small honeyed pills with moderate and lasting effects.

2.3.2.2   Water-Bindered Pill

Water-bindered pill is made by grinding medicines into fine powder and adding cooled boiled water or distilled water as excipient. Compared to honeyed pills, water-bindered pills are fast disintegrated and easy to be absorbed.

2.3.2.3   Starched Pill

Starched pill is made by grinding medicines into fine powder and adding paste such as rice paste, panada, and leaven paste and so on as excipient. Starched pills are slowly disintegrated, which can prolong the effect of medicine and reduce adverse reactions when taken orally.

2.3.2.4   Condensed Pill

Condensed pill is made by decocting medicines into pastes and then mixed with other medicinal fine powders, and water or honey added, or decoction. It is easy to be accepted for its small size and low dosage.

2.3.3   Powders (San)

Powders are made by the medicines ground into fine powders and mixed evenly. There are two types of powders, for oral or external use. Oral use powders are divided into fine powder and coarser powder. Fine powders such as Qili San can be taken with water. Coarser powder such as Yinqiao San can be decocted and for oral use after subducting residue. Externally used powders such as Jinhuang San are generally used as external applications, which are applied to sore surface or to the wound. Others such as Bingpeng San are for throat sprinkle. The features of the powders are quick absorption, simple making, convenient for taking and caring, and saving the medicinal materials.

2.3.4   Pastes (Gao)

Pastes are made by medicines decocted with water or plant oil and removing slag, for oral and external use. Oral-use pastes such as Pipa Gao include three kinds, which are liquid pastes, semi-liquid pastes, and decocted pastes, while externally used pastes include ointment such as Sanhuang ointment. Liquid pastes and semi-liquid pastes are used by blending with other prescriptions. Decocted pastes are semi-liquid pastes made by medicines decocted with water and removing slag and added with honey or sugar. Decocted pastes are suitable for chronic diseases. The ointment made of fine powder and appropriate medicinal substrates with appropriate viscosity of semi-solid prescription for external use only, which is usually used for skins, mucosa, or the surface of the wounds. Plaster also known as hard paste can be used for orthopedics and traumatology and impediment disease.

2.3.5   Pellets (Dan)

There are two types of pellets. One is for oral used, and the other is for external use. Oral pallets do not have fixed prescriptions such as pills or powder. It is called "Dan" because the medicines are precious, such as Zhibao Dan. Pellets are medicines made of some mineral medicines under the high temperature, which is often ground into powder and sprinkled on the surface of the wound. They are mainly for surgery use.

2.3.6   Wine Preparation (Jiu)

Wine preparation also known as medicinal liquor is made of medicines soaked in wine, removing slag, and then taking the liquid for internal or external use. Wine has the characteristics of promoting blood circulation and promoting efficacy of the drug, which is suitable for impediment disease, weakness of nourishing and orthopedics and traumatology, and so on, such as Duzhong Hugu Jiu. Wine for external use has the ability for activating blood, resolving edema, and relieving pain, but not suitable for yin deficiency with excess fire syndrome.

2.3.7   Soluble Granules (Keli)

Soluble granules are granulated prescriptions made through the modern technology by extraction of active ingredients of medicines and then being mixed with appropriate number of excipients such as starch or some of the medicines fine powder. It is soluble in water, so it can be used by being dissolved in water. Soluble granules have the characteristic of storage, rapid effect, and convenience to take. There are compound granules such as Ganmao granules (granules for cold) and single granules with one medicine and then combined into prescriptions.

2.3.8   Syrup (Tangjiang)

Syrup is made by decocting medicine, removing slag, and concentrating and adding suitable sucrose in it. Syrup is characterized by sweet in taste and small in volume, especially suitable for children.

2.4 Classification and Commonly Used Prescriptions

2.4.1 Exterior-Releasing Prescriptions

2.4.1.1 Concept

Those that are mainly composed of medicines for relieving exterior syndrome and can promote sweating, release the flesh and outthrust eruption, used for exterior syndrome, and are known as exterior-releasing prescription.

2.4.1.2 Classification

Exterior syndrome generally includes two kinds of syndrome: wind-cold syndrome and wind-heat syndrome. Therefore, exterior-releasing prescription falls into two kinds as prescriptions for relieving the exterior syndrome with pungent-warm and those for relieving the exterior syndrome with pungent-cold accordingly. Prescriptions for relieving the exterior syndrome with pungent-warm are mainly formed with medicines of pungent-warm and have the effect of dispersing wind-cold, used for exterior syndrome of wind-cold. Contrarily, prescriptions for relieving the exterior syndrome with pungent-cold are mainly formed with medicines of pungent-cold and have the effect of dispersing wind-heat, used for exterior syndrome of wind-heat.

2.4.1.3 Notes

Exterior-releasing prescriptions should not be decocted too long; otherwise, the pharmacological effects of the prescriptions would be lost greatly with dissipating drug property. That is because the medicines for forming exterior-releasing prescriptions are those with light-textured property and pungent flavor and are easy to dissipate with long decocted. What is more, the decoction of exterior-releasing prescriptions must be taken warm. Keeping warm should also be paid attention to after taking the decoction in order to eliminate the pathogenic factors out of the body with sweating slightly.

Mahuang Tang (Ephedra Decoction)

Ingredients (Table 2.1)

Table 2.1 Ingredients of Mahuang Tang

Mahuang	Ephedrae Herba	9 g
Guizhi	Ramulus Cinnamomi	6 g
Kuxingren	Semen Armeniacae Amarum	6 g
Zhigancao	Radix Glycyrrhizae	3 g

Administration

All medicines above are decocted in water, for oral use.

Effects

Promote sweating to release the exterior, diffuse the lung to calm panting.

Application

This prescription is for the syndrome of wind-cold and exterior-excess, caused by externally contracted wind-cold. The syndrome of wind-cold and exterior-excess is characterized by aversion to cold, fever, headache, generalized pain, no sweating, dyspnea, thin and white tongue coating, floating, and tight pulse. It can be used for common cold, flu, acute bronchitis, bronchial dyspnea, and other diseases, main symptoms of which are aversion to cold without sweating, cough, and dyspnea, and belonging to syndrome of wind-cold and exterior-excess.

Analysis

The syndrome treated by this prescription is caused by externally contracted wind-cold, block of defensive qi and yang, tight striae, and failed diffusion of lung qi. This syndrome should be dealt with treatment methods as follows: Diffuse the lung to calm panting and promote sweating to release the exterior.

1. Sovereign medicine: Mahuang.
   Promote sweating to release the exterior in order to dispel wind-cold and diffuse the lung to calm panting.
2. Minister medicine: Guizhi.
   Warm the meridian to dissipate cold, assist Mahuang to promote sweating to release the exterior.
3. Assistant medicine: Kuxingren.
   Diffuse and descend lung qi, assist Mahuang to calm panting.
4. Courier medicine: Zhigancao.
   Harmonize all the medicines, not only ease the middle, but also restrict the oversweating of Mahuang and Guizhi.

Modification

If complicated with dampness pathogen characterized by arthrosis pain and heavy limbs and trunk, add Baizhu to dispel dampness. If mainly showed cough and panting but slight aversion to cold, get rid of Guizhi to concentrate on diffusing the lung to calm panting. If with heavy aversion to cold, no sweating and generalized pain, complicated with interior heat and vexation, double Mahuang to enhance the sweating to dispel pathogen, and then add Shigao to discharge interior heat.

Notes

Because this prescription is drastic in promoting sweating with pungent-warm and used to treat syndrome of wind-cold and exterior-excess, it is forbidden for exterior syndrome of wind-cold with sweating. It also should be caution for patient with serious yin deficiency, blood deficiency, and interior heat.

Guizhi Tang (Cinnamon Twig Decoction)

Ingredients (Table 2.2)

Administration

All medicines above are decocted in water, for oral use.

Effects

Release the flesh, and harmonize nutrient qi and defensive qi to release exterior syndrome.

Application

This prescription is for the syndrome of wind-cold and exterior deficiency, syndrome of nutrient-defense disharmony, and yin-yang disharmony after cure or after delivery. These syndromes are characterized by headache, fever, sweating and aversion to wind, thin and white tongue fur, and floating and relaxed pulse. It can be

Table 2.2 Ingredients of Guizhi Tang		
Guizhi	Ramulus Cinnamomi	9 g
Baishao	Radix Alba Paeoniae	9 g
Shengjiang	Rhizoma Zingiberis Recens	9 g
Dazao	Fructus Jujubae	3 pcs
Zhigancao	Radix Glycyrrhizae	6 g

used for common cold, flu, lichen, pruritus cutanea, agnogenic low-grade fever, after cure or after delivery low-grade fever, and other diseases belonging to syndrome of nutrient-defense disharmony and yin-yang disharmony.

Analysis

The syndrome treated by this prescription is caused by externally contracted wind-cold, weakness after cure or after delivery, disharmony of nutrient and defense, and yin-yang. This syndrome should be dealt with treatment methods as follows: Release the flesh and outthrust the exterior, and harmonize the nutrient qi and defensive qi.

1. Sovereign medicine: Guizhi.

   Release the flesh and dissipate cold, and warm the meridian to promote the yang qi and defensive qi.
2. Minister medicine: Baishao.

   Enrich yin and engender fluid, and secure the nutrient qi to stop sweating. Guizhi and Baishao combine equally in this prescription, one for dissipating, while the other securing can lead to dissipating wind-cold exterior, securing nutrient interior, harmonization of nutrient and defense, and yin and yang.
3. Assistant medicine: Shengjiang and Dazao.

   Shengjiang harmonizes the stomach and assists Guizhi to dissipate cold. Dazao tonifies the spleen and assists Baishao to enrich yin. These two medicines not only strengthen the sovereign and minister to harmonize nutrient and defense, but also regulate the stomach and tonify the spleen to supplement the source of generation and transformation of nutrient and defense.
4. Assistant and courier medicine: Zhigancao.

   On the one hand, as assistant, this medicine tonifies qi to harmonize the middle, combines with the sovereign in order to transform yang with pungent-sweet to release the flesh, and combines with the minister in order to transform yin with sour-sweet to harmonize the nutrient. On the other hand, as courier, it harmonizes all the medicines.

Modification

If complicated with painful stiff nape, add Gegen to release the flesh and exterior syndrome, and engender fluid to relax sinews. If complicated with cough and panting, add Houpo and Kuxingren to direct qi downward to suppress cough and to calm panting.

Table 2.3 Ingredients of
Xiaoqinglong Tang

Mahuang	Ephedrae Herba	9 g
Guizhi	Ramulus Cinnamomi	6 g
Ganjiang	Rhizoma Zingiberis	6 g
Xixin	Herba Asari	6 g
Baishao	Radix Paeoniae Alba	9 g
Wuweizi	Fructus Schisandrae Chinensis	6 g
Banxia	Pinelliae Rhizoma	9 g
Zhigancao	Radix Glycyrrhizae	6 g

Notes

Because this prescription is mild in promoting sweating, known as "release the flesh," it is unsuitable for exterior syndrome of wind-cold without sweating. After administration, the patient should have a bowl of warm congee and put on more clothes to promote sweating slightly.

Xiaoqinglong Tang (Small Blue Dragon Decoction)

Ingredients (Table 2.3)

Administration

All medicines above are decocted in water, for oral use.

Effects

Release the exterior and dispel cold, warm the lung, and resolve fluid retention.

Application

This prescription is for the syndrome of external contraction and internal fluid retention. This syndrome is characterized by aversion to cold, fever, headache without sweating, cough and dyspnea, excessive thin phlegm, inability to lie on back when serious, or limbs edema, white slippery tongue fur, and floating pulse. This treatment can be used for various conditions including acute exacerbation of chronic bronchitis, bronchial asthma, and senile emphysema. It is particularly effective for diseases that primarily exhibit symptoms such as an aversion to cold without sweating, coughing, and excessive phlegm. These symptoms are typically associated with the syndrome of external contraction of wind-cold and cold phlegm residing in the lung.

Analysis

The syndrome that this prescription treats is caused by two factors: the external contraction of wind-cold and the presence of cold phlegm in the lung. These conditions result in the lung's inability to properly diffuse and depurate. This syndrome should be dealt with treatment methods as follows: Release the exterior and dispel cold, warm the lung, and resolve fluid retention.

1. Sovereign medicine: Mahuang and Guizhi.
   Promote sweating to release the exterior cold, and diffuse the lung to calm dyspnea.
2. Minister medicine: Ganjiang and Xixin.
   Warm the lung to dispel cold, and tonify yang to resolve the phlegm fluid.
3. Assistant medicine: Baishao, Wuweizi, and Banxia.
   Baishao nourishes the blood and astringes the yin; Wuweizi astringes the lung to calm dyspnea. Both restrict the dryness nature of Mahuang, Guizhi, and Ganjiang consuming qi and fluid. Banxia dries dampness to dispel cold phlegm.
4. Courier medicine: Zhigancao.
   Tonify qi to regulate the middle, and harmonize all the medicines.

Modification

If complicated with thirst, subduct Banxia, add Tianhuafen to clear heat and generate fluid. If phlegm fluid transforms heat, complicated with vexation, add Shigao to clear heat and remove vexation.

Notes

This prescription is forbidden for patients with cough and yellow phlegm.

Yinqiao San (Lonicera and Forsythia Powder)

Ingredients (Table 2.4)

Table 2.4 Ingredients of Yinqiao San

Jinyinhua	Flos Lonicerae	30 g
Lianqiao	Fructus Forsythiae	15 g
Bohe	Herba Menthae	6 g
Niubangzi	Fructus Arctii	12 g
Jingjiesui	Spica Schizonepetae	12 g
Dandouchi	Semen Sojae Preparatum	12 g
Lugen	Rhizoma Phragmitis	30 g
Danzhuye	Herba Lophatheri	6 g
Jiegeng	Radix Platycodonis	12 g
Gancao	Radix Glycyrrhizae	6 g

Administration

All medicines above are decocted in water, for oral use.

Effects

Release the exterior with pungent-cool, clear heat, and detoxify.

Application

This prescription is for the exterior syndrome of wind-heat or defense aspect syndrome of warm disease. These syndromes are characterized by fever, aversion to wind and cold slightly, slight sweating or not, headache, thirst, cough, pharyngalgia, red tongue tip, thin and yellow tongue fur, and floating and rapid pulse. It can be used for common cold, flu, acute tonsillitis, upper respiratory infection, pneumonia, measles, epidemic meningitis, Japanese encephalitis, mumps, and other diseases belonging to exterior syndrome of wind-heat or defense aspect syndrome of warm disease. It is also can be used in some skin diseases, like rubella, urticaria, and sore carbuncle.

Analysis

The syndrome treated by this prescription is caused by externally contracted wind-heat, stagnant defensive qi, and lung qi ascending counterflow. This syndrome should be dealt with treatment methods as follows: Disperse wind to outthrust through the exterior, clear heat, and detoxify.

1. Sovereign medicine: Jinyinhua and Lianqiao.
   Large dose of these two medicines used in order to clear heat and detoxify, and outthrust through the exterior at the same time.
2. Minister medicine: Bohe, Nuibangzi, Jingjiesui, and Dandouchi.
   Bohe and Nuibanzi disperse wind-heat with pungent-cool nature, detoxify, and soothe the throat. Jingjiesui and Dandouchi disperse exterior with pungent-warm nature but not dry, not only promote the effect of disperse pathogenic qi and release exterior, but also avoid warm dryness to decrease fluid.
   All these four medicines assist the sovereign to promote the effect of disperse pathogenic qi and release exterior.
3. Assistant medicine: Lugen, Danzhuye, and Jiegeng.
   Lugen and Danzhuye generate the fluid to clear heat. Jiegeng diffuses the lung qi, suppresses cough, and soothes the throat.
4. Assistant and courier medicine: Gancao.
   On the one hand, as assistant, this medicine clears heat and detoxify and cooperates with Jiegeng to soothe the throat. On the other hand, as courier, it harmonizes all the medicines.

Modification

If heat syndrome is serious, complicated with high fever and thirst, add Shigao, Huangqin, and Daqingye to clear heat, purge fire, and detoxify. If complicated with stuffiness in the chest caused by turbid pathogen and foul turbidity, add Huoxiang and Yujin to resolve dampness with aroma, dispel filth, and resolve turbidity. If complicated with serious cough, add Kuxingren to direct qi downward to suppress cough.

Notes

Because this prescription is used for exterior syndrome of wind-heat with slight sweating, it is unsuitable for exterior syndrome of wind-heat with no sweating and aversion to cold, slight fever, and no thirst.

2.4.2 Heat-Cleaning Prescriptions

2.4.2.1 Concept

Those that are mainly composed of medicines for heat-clearing and can clear heat, purge fire, cool the blood aspect, detoxify, and used for interior heat syndrome are known as heat-cleaning prescription.

2.4.2.2 Classification

There are differences in the interior heat syndrome between qifen and blood aspect, between warm-heat and summer-heat, between excess heat and deficiency heat, and between zang viscera and fu viscera. Therefore, heat-cleaning prescription can be divided into six categories: qifen heat-cleaning prescription, clean nutrient and cool blood prescription, heat-cleaning and detoxify prescription, zang-fu viscera heat-cleaning prescription, deficiency heat-cleaning prescription, and summer-heat-cleaning prescription.

2.4.2.3 Notes

The nature and flavor of the medicines which form heat-cleaning prescription are mainly cold and bitterness. Therefore, heat-cleaning prescription should not to be used for a long time in case that cold and bitterness property might decline the stomach qi, yin and yang. What is more, add some fortify the spleen and invigorate the stomach medicines. It also should be cautious used for patient with weakness of spleen and stomach, torpid intake, and sloppy stool. If interior heat is flaming, the

Table 2.5 Ingredients of
Baihu Tang

Shigao	Gypsum Fibrosum	50 g
Zhimu	Rhizoma Anemarrhenae	18 g
Jingmi	Semen Oryzae Nonglutionosae	9 g
Zhigancao	Radix Glycyrrhizae	6 g

patient emesis immediately after taking heat-cleaning prescription so call "reject medicines." In these cases, methods of counteracting assistant that administering warm or adding a few pungent-warm ginger juice would be taken to relieve or eliminate these situations.

Baihu Tang (White Tiger Decoction)

Ingredients (Table 2.5)

Administration

All medicines above are decocted in water, for oral use.

Effects

Clear heat and generate fluid.

Application

This prescription is for the yangming meridian syndrome and exuberant heat in qifen. This syndrome is characterized by high fever, reddened complexion, vexation thirst, desire for cold drink, sweating and aversion to heat, yellow urine, hardbound stool, red tongue, and yellow fur, surging, and large pulse or slippery and rapid pulse. It can be used for common cold, flu, lobar pneumonia, epidemic encephalitis B, songo fever, gingivitis, and other diseases belonging to yangming meridian syndrome and exuberant heat in qifen. This syndrome would be recognized as four exuberant symptoms: Exuberant heat, extreme thirst, excessive sweating, surging, and large pulse.

Analysis

The syndrome treated by this prescription is caused by exuberant heat in yangming meridian or warm disease with qifen syndrome scorching body fluid. This syndrome should be dealt with treatment methods as cleaning heat and generating fluid.

1. Sovereign medicine: Shigao.
   This medicine can clear heat and purge fire while protecting fluid with the nature flavor of pungent-sweet and extremely cold.

2. Minister medicine: Zhimu.

   The nature flavor of this medicine that is bitter-cold but smooth assists the sovereign to clear heat and purge fire and enriches yin to engender fluid.
3. Assistant medicine: Jingmi.

   Invigorate the stomach, protect the fluid, and also prevent the extremely cold of sovereign to harm stomach.
4. Assistant and courier medicine: Zhigancao.

   On the one hand, as assistant, this medicine invigorates the stomach qi and protects the damage of fluid cooperated with Jingmi. On the other hand, as courier, it harmonizes all the medicines.

Modification

If there is excessive heat damaging the body fluid, and it's complicated by symptoms such as unquenchable thirst and a weak, large pulse, Renshen can be added to the treatment. Renshen is known to enrich qi and promote the generation of body fluid. If warm diseases manifested as blazing of both qi and blood, complicated with mental confusion and delirious speech, macula on the body, add Dihuang, Shuiniujiao to clear heat and cool the blood. If extreme heat engendering wind, complicated with limbs twitch, add Lingyangjiao, Gouteng to extinguish wind to arrest convulsions. If interior heat with dampness complication, or wind-dampness and heat arthralgia, add Cangzhu to dry dampness.

Notes

Because this prescription is used for yangming meridian syndrome and excess heat, it is unsuitable for deficiency heat syndrome characterized by surging and large pulse but weak and pale tongue.

Qingying Tang (Decoction for Cleaning Heat in Nutrient Aspect)

Ingredients (Table 2.6)

Table 2.6 Ingredients of Qingying Tang

Shuinuijiao[a]	Cornu Bubali[a]	30 g
Dihuang	Radix Rehmanniae	15 g
Xuanshen	Radix Scrophulariae	9 g
Maidong	Radix Ophiopogonis	9 g
Jinyinhua	Flos Lonicerae	9 g
Lianqiao	Fructus Forsythiae	6 g
Huanglian	Rhizoma Coptidis	5 g
Danshen	Radix Salviae Miltiorrhizae	6 g
Zhuyexin	Herba Lophatheri	3 g

[a]Decocted first

Administration

All medicines above are decocted in water, for oral use.

Effects

Clear heat and detoxify, expel heat, and nourish yin aspect.

Application

This prescription is for the nutrient aspect syndrome by heat pathogenic at the early stage. This syndrome is characterized by general fever worsening at night, delirious speech sometimes, thirst or not, macula seen indistinctly, crimson dry tongue, and fine and rapid pulse. It can be used for epidemic encephalitis B, epidemic cerebrospinal meningitis, septicemia, ileotyphus, and other heat diseases belonging to nutrient aspect syndrome by heat pathogenic at the early stage.

Analysis

The syndrome treated by this prescription is caused by that heat pathogenic just turn into nutrient aspect, damaging nutrient yin, affecting blood vessels. This syndrome should be dealt with treatment methods as cleaning heat and detoxify, expelling heat and nourishing yin aspect.

1. Sovereign medicine: Shuinuijiao.
   Clear the nutrient heat.
2. Minister medicine: Dihuang, Xuanshen, and Maidong.
   On the one hand, these three medicines can assist the sovereign to clear nutrient heat. On the other hand, they can enrich yin and engender fluid.
3. Assistant medicine: Jinyinhua, Lianqiao, Huanglian, and Danshen.
   Because of the outthrusting and pungent-cool nature, Jinyinhua and Lianqiao can clear the nutrient heat and expel heat from nutrient aspect to defense aspect. Huanglian assists the sovereign to clear heat and detoxify. Danshen can cool blood heat and activate blood to prevent heat accumulation in blood aspect.
4. Courier medicine: Zhuyexin.
   Clear heart and detoxify, and direct medicines to heart meridian.

Modification

If complicated with heat in qifen, administer this prescription with Baihu Tang in order to clear both qi and blood aspect. If complicated with heat block pericardium with mental confusion and delirious speech, administer this prescription with Angong Niuhuang Wan.

Table 2.7 Ingredients of Huanglian Jiedu Tang

Huanglian	Rhizoma Coptidis	9 g
Huangqin	Radix Scutellariae	6 g
Huangbai	Cortex Phellodendri	6 g
Zhizi	Fructus Gardeniae	9 g

Notes

Because of the nature of three minister medicines in this prescription is nutritious, so it is unsuitable for syndrome of dampness obstruction and heat hidden characterized as crimson tongue, white and slippery fur.

Huanglian Jiedu Tang (Decoction of Coptis for Detoxification)

Ingredients (Table 2.7)

Administration

All medicines above are decocted in water, for oral use.

Effects

Purge fire and detoxify.

Application

This prescription is for the syndrome of fire toxin and exuberant heat in triple energizer. This syndrome is characterized by high fever, vexation, thirst and desiring to drink, delirious speech, inability to sleep, or fever and diarrhea, or deep-rooted boil, red tongue, yellow fur, and powerful rapid pulse. It can be used for epidemic encephalitis B, epidemic cerebrospinal meningitis, septicemia, septicopyemia, dysentery, pneumonia, urinary infection, and other infection diseases belonging to syndrome of fire toxin and exuberant heat.

Analysis

The syndrome treated by this prescription is caused by exuberant heat binding in the triple energizer. This syndrome should be dealt with treatment methods as purging fire and detoxify with bitter-cold.

1. Sovereign medicine: Huanglian.
   Purge heart fire and middle energizer fire.

2. Minister and assistant medicines: Huangqin, Huangbai, and Zhizi.

   Huangqin purges upper energizer fire, Huangbai purges lower energizer fire, and Zhizi purges the whole triple energizer and directs medicines downward.

   All four medicines purge fire toxin with their nature of bitter-cold.

Modification

If complicated with constipation, add Dahuang to relax the bowels and purge fire and direct the heat toxin downward. If complicated with hematemesis, nosebleed, and macula, add Dihuang, Xuanshen, and Mudanpi to clear heat and cool blood.

Notes

The medicines of this prescription are all bitter-cold one. These medicines would damage the fluid and stomach, so this prescription just can be used in syndrome of exuberant heat toxin. It needs to stop once it takes effect. It is forbidden for patients with fluid deficiency.

2.4.3 Purgative Prescriptions

2.4.3.1 Concept

Those that are mainly composed of medicines for purgating, with the effects that induce relaxing the bowels, purgating heat, removing accumulation, and expelling water, and used for interior excess syndrome, are known as purgative prescription.

2.4.3.2 Classification

Interior excess syndrome would be different in heat accumulation, cold accumulation, dryness accumulation, and dampness accumulation, and healthy qi of human would be different in deficiency and excess. Accordingly, purgative prescription can be divided into five categories: cold-purgative prescription, warm-purgative prescription, lubricant laxation prescription, expelling water prescription, and tonifying to relax bowels prescription.

2.4.3.3 Notes

Purgative prescription would be easy to damage middle, consume fluid, interrupt blood, and induced abortion. Thus, it must stop once it takes effects and cannot be overused. It is caution or forbidden for patients who are worn with age, yin-blood deficiency, menstrual period, or pregnancy.

Table 2.8 Ingredients of Dachengqi Tang

Dahuang	Radix et Rhizoma Rhei	12 g
Houpo	Cortex Magnoliae officinalis	12 g
Zhishi	Fructus Aurantii Immaturus	9 g
Mangxiao	Natrii sulfas	9 g

Dachengqi Tang (Major Purgative Decoction)

Ingredients (Table 2.8)

Administration

Decocte Houpo and Zhishi first and Dahuang later. Decoction would be for oral use without medicine residues and dissolved with Mangxiao.

Effects

Drastic purge heat—accumulation.

Application

This prescription is for yangming fu viscera excess syndrome. This syndrome is characterized by constipation, abdominal pain with aversion to press, fever aggravated in the afternoon, thirst with great desire to drink, red tongue, yellow dry fur with prickly, or black, dry and cracked fur, and sunken replete pulse. It can be used for acute simple intestinal obstruction, adhesive intestinal obstruction, acute cholecystitis, acute pancreatitis, and constipation in heat diseases that complicated with high fever, delirious speech, unconsciousness, eclampsia, and even raving.

Analysis

The syndrome treated by this prescription is caused by heat pathogen accumulation in the large intestine and stoppage of fu qi. This syndrome should be dealt with treatment methods as follows: Purge heat accumulation and remove accumulation to relax the bowels.

1. Sovereign medicine: Dahuang.
   Purge heat and relax the bowels, and remove accumulation of intestines and stomach.
2. Minister medicine: Mangxiao.
   Soften hardness and moisten dryness, and assist the sovereign to purge heat and relax the bowels.
3. Assistant medicine: Houpo and Zhishi.
   Move qi to remove fullness, and assist Dahuang and Mangxiao to remove and purge heat accumulation.

Modification

If complicated with exuberant heat consuming qi, qi deficiency, and overstrain, add Renshen to tonify qi and prevent qi desertion with drastic purgation. If complicated with heat accumulation damaging yin, serious thirst with great desire to drink, red dry tongue, and less fur, add Xuanshen and Dihuang to tonify yin and generate fluid and moisten dryness to relax the bowels.

Notes

It is caution for yangming fu viscera excess syndrome but without exuberant heat accumulation or someone who has always dual deficiency of qi and yin, old age, weakness, and pregnancy.

Wenpi Tang (Warming Spleen Decoction)

Ingredients (Table 2.9)

Administration

All medicines above are decocted in water, for oral use.

Effects

Purge cold accumulation, and warm-tonify the spleen yang.

Application

This prescription is for syndrome of yang deficiency and cold accumulation. This syndrome is characterized by constipation and abdominal pain, or chronic diarrhea with pus and blood, cold of the extremities, pale tongue, thin white fur, and sunken string-like pulse. It can be used for acute simple intestinal obstruction, partial small-bowel obstruction, chronic dysentery, chronic appendicitis acute attack, and other diseases characterized by constipation and abdominal pain, spiritlessness and weakness, and aversion to cold and prefer warm, which belonging to syndrome of yang deficiency and cold accumulation.

Table 2.9 Ingredients of Wenpi Tang

Dahuang	Radix et Rhizoma Rhei	12 g
Fuzi	Radix Aconiti Lateralis Preparata	9 g
Ganjiang	Rhizoma Zingiberis	6 g
Renshen	Radix ginseng	6 g
Gancao	Radix Glycyrrhizae	6 g

Analysis

The syndrome treated by this prescription is caused by deficiency of spleen yang, internal generation of cold, and cold accumulation in the intestine. This syndrome should be dealt with treatment methods as follows: Purge cold accumulation, and warm-tonify the spleen yang.

1. Sovereign medicine: Dahuang and Fuzi.
      Dahuang removes accumulation with purgation and relaxes the bowels. Fuzi warm interior, support yang, and dispel cold. This combination can warm interior and dispel cold and removes cold accumulation.
2. Minister medicine: Ganjiang.
      Assist Fuzi to warm middle and dispel cold.
3. Assistant medicine: Renshen.
      Tonify qi and harmonize middle, combine Fuzi and Ganjiang to tonify qi, warm yang, and tonify spleen.
4. Assistant and courier medicines: Gancao.
      Tonify qi and harmonize middle, and harmonize all the medicines.

Modification

If complicated with serious abdominal pain, add Rougui and Muxiang to strengthen the effect of warming yang and moving qi to check pain. If complicated with vomiting, add Banxia and Sharen to harmonize stomach and direct qi downward. If complicated with chronic diarrhea and dampness-heat and yellow slimy tongue fur, add Jinyinhua and Huangqin to clear intestine and relax the bowels.

Jichuan Jian (Blood Replenishing Decoction)

Ingredients (Table 2.10)

Administration

All medicines above are decocted in water, for oral use.

Table 2.10 Ingredients of Jichuan Jian

Roucongrong	Herba Cistanches	9 g
Danggui	Radix Angelicae Sinensis	12 g
Niuxi	Radix Achyranthis Bidentatae	6 g
Zhike	Fructus Aurantii	3 g
Zexie	Rhizoma Alismatis	5 g
Shengma	Rhizoma Cimicifugae	3 g

Effects

Warm kidney and nourish blood and moisten the intestines to relax the bowels.

Application

This prescription is for constipation with kidney deficiency syndrome. This syndrome is characterized by constipation, clear urine in large amounts, soreness and weakness of waist and knees, pale tongue, thin white fur, sunken fine, and slow pulse. It can be used for habitual constipation and senile constipation which belonging to kidney deficiency, fluid depletion, and intestines dryness.

Analysis

The syndrome treated by this prescription is caused by deficiency of kidney qi, atony of transportation, depletion of blood, and loosing nutritious of intestines. This syndrome should be dealt with treatment methods as follows: Warm kidney and nourish blood and moisten the intestines to relax the bowels.

1. Sovereign medicine: Roucongrong.
   Warm kidney and tonify essence, warm waist and moisten intestines.
2. Minister medicine: Danggui and Niuxi.
   Danggui nourish blood to moisten intestines. Niuxi tonify kidney to strong waist.
3. Assistant medicine: Zhike, Zexie, and Shengma.
   Zhike directs qi downward. Zexie purges turbidity. Both assist large intestines to strengthen the effect of transportation. Shengma upraises clear yang, while Zhike and Zexie direct turbidity downward.

   All medicines combined, strengthen transportation through tonifying, upraise yang through purge turbidity, and warm-moisten to relax the bowels.

Modification

If complicated with qi deficiency and overstrain, add Renshen to tonify qi, strengthening the effect of transportation. If complicated with serious deficiency of kidney essence, dizziness, and tinnitus, add Shudihuang to tonify kidney essence and nourish yin to moisten the intestines.

Notes

It is forbidden for syndrome of kidney yin deficiency, characterized by dry constipation, dry mouth, and red tongue.

2.4.4 Wind-Dispelling Prescriptions

2.4.4.1 Concept

Those that are mainly composed of medicines with pungent in flavor and disperse in nature and medicines for extinguishing wind to arrest convulsions, used for wind diseases included internal wind syndrome and external wind syndrome, are known as wind-dispelling prescription.

2.4.4.2 Classification

Wind diseases are all those caused by wind pathogen. Wind pathogen can be divided into external wind and internal wind. Accordingly, wind-dispelling prescription would be divided into external wind-dispelling prescription and internal wind-extinguishing prescription.

2.4.4.3 Notes

When using wind-dispelling prescription, it is necessary to distinguish between external wind and internal wind, between cold, heat, deficiency, and excess. External wind would be dispersed while internal wind would be extinguished. If wind pathogen is complicated with cold, heat, dampness, and phlegm, combine with dispelling cold, cleaning heat, dispelling dampness, and resolving phlegm accordingly.

Chuanxiong Chatiao San (Ligusticum Powder)

Ingredients (Table 2.11)

Administration

Grind the above medicines into fine powder, and take 6 g each time and twice daily with tea. All medicines above are decocted in water, for oral use.

Table 2.11 Ingredients of Chuanxiong Chatiao San

Chuanxiong	Rhizoma Ligustici Chuanxiong	9 g
Qianghuo	Rhizoma et radix Notopterygii	6 g
Baizhi	Radix Angelicae Dahuricae	6 g
Xixin	Herba Asari	3 g
Bohe	Herba Menthae	9 g
Jingjie	Herba Schizonepetae	12 g
Fangfeng	Radix Saposhnikoviae	6 g
Zhigancao	Radix Glycyrrhizae	6 g

Effects

Dispel wind and relieve pain.

Application

This prescription is for headache with external contraction syndrome of wind pathogen. This syndrome is characterized by headache, or migraine, or parietal headache,
fever, aversion to cold, dizziness, stuffy nose, thin and white tongue fur, and floating
pulse. It can be used for migraine, vascular neuropathic headache, and headache in
chronic rhinitis that are complicated with rhinobyon and floating pulse, caused by
external contraction syndrome of wind pathogen.

Analysis

The syndrome treated by this prescription is caused by external contraction of wind
pathogen. Wind pathogen upward to invade the head along meridian, and hamper
lucid yang qi. This syndrome should be dealt with treatment methods as dispelling
wind and relieving pain.

1. Sovereign medicine: Chuanxiong, Qianghuo, and Baizhi.
   All these three medicines can dispel wind and relieve pain. Chuanxiong is
   good at relieving pain, particularly relieving headache in shaoyang, Jueyin
   meridian (vertex and tempus). Qianghuo is good at relieving headache in taiyang
   meridian (occiput). Baizhi is good at relieving headache in yangming meridian
   (forehead).
2. Minister medicine: Xixin and Bohe.
   Xixin can dispel cold and relieve pain, while Bohe dispels wind and refreshes
   the mind. Both assist the sovereigns to dispel wind pathogen.
3. Assistant medicine: Jingjie and Fangfeng.
   Jingjie and Fangfeng can dispel wind pathogen, enhancing the power of sovereign and minister.
4. Courier medicine: Zhuyexin.
   Harmonize all the medicines.

Modification

If caused by external contraction of wind-cold, complicated with obvious aversion
to cold, increase the dosage of Chuangxiong, and add Zisuye and Shengjiang to
enhance the effect of dispelling wind-cold. If caused by external contraction of
wind-heat, complicated with obvious fever, dry mouth, and red tongue, subtract
Qianghuo and Xixin, and add Manjingzi, Juhua to dispel wind-heat. In case of long
treatment of headache, add Quanxie, Jiangcan, and Taoren to seek wind, activate
blood, and relieve pain.

Notes

It is forbidden for headache caused by deficiency of qi and blood or stirring wind due to hyperactivity of yang.

Duhuo Jisheng Tang (Pubescent Angelica and Taxillus Decoction)

Ingredients (Table 2.12)

Administration

All medicines above are decocted in water, for oral use.

Effects

Dispel wind-dampness, relieve impediment-pain, benefit liver and kidney, and tonify qi and blood.

Application

This prescription is for syndrome of wind-cold-dampness obstructing arthralgia. This syndrome is characterized by arthralgia in long treatment, depletion of liver and kidney, deficiency of qi and blood, cold pain and flaccid in waist and knee, unsmooth bend and stretch of limbs, or numbness, aversion to cold, flavor warm, pale tongue, white fur, and fine and week pulse. It can be used for chronic arthritis, rheumatoid arthritis, ischialgia, lumbar muscle degeneration, osteoproliferation, poliomyelitis, and other diseases belonging to syndrome of wind-cold-dampness obstructing arthralgia.

Table 2.12 Ingredients of Duhuo Jisheng Tang

Duhuo	Rhizoma Ligustici Chuanxiong	9 g
Qinjiao	Radix Gentianae Macrophyllae	9 g
Fangfeng	Radix Saposhnikoviae	9 g
Rougui	Cortex Cinnamomi	6 g
Xixin	Herba Asari	3 g
Sangjisheng	Herba Taxilli	15 g
Duzhong	Cortex Eucommiae	9 g
Niuxi	Radix Achyranthis Bidentatae	9 g
Renshen	Radix ginseng	6 g
Fuling	Poria	9 g
Danggui	Radix Angelicae Sinensis	9 g
Chuanxion	Rhizoma Ligustici chuanxiong	6 g
Dihuang	Radix Rehmanniae	9 g
Baishao	Radix Paeoniae Alba	9 g
Gancao	Radix Glycyrrhizae	6 g

Analysis

The syndrome treated by this prescription is caused by arthralgia in long treatment, consumption of liver, kidney, qi, and blood, pathogen retaining in the arthrosis. So this syndrome is manifested as co-occurrences of agonizing-fixed arthralgia and depletion of liver and kidney.

1. Sovereign medicine: Duhuo.
   Dispel wind-cold-dampness pathogen in lower body, dredge arthralgia, and relieve pain.
2. Minister medicine: Qinjiao, Fangfeng, Rougui, and Xixin.
   Qinjiao and Fangfeng dispel wind and dampness. Rougui dispel cold and relieve pain, and warm through blood vessels. Xixin dispel cold and relieve pain with its pungent-warm nature.
3. Assistant medicine: Sangjisheng, Duzhong, Niuxi, Renshen, Fuling, Danggui, Chuanxion, Dihuang, and Baishao.
   Sangjisheng, Duzhong, and Niuxi tonify liver and kidney, and strengthen the sinews and bones. Danggui, Chuanxion, Dihuang, and Baishao nourish blood and activate blood. Renshen and Fuling tonify qi to fortify the spleen and strengthen health qi.
4. Assistant and courier medicines: Gancao.
   As assistant, strengthen health qi. As courier, harmonize all the medicines.

Modification

If complicated with serious arthralgia pain, add Zhichuanwu, Zhicaowu, Baihuashe, Dilong, and Honghua to seek and dispel wind pathogen to free collateral vessels, activate blood, and relieve pain. If complicated with serious cold pathogen, add Fuzi and Ganjiang to warm yang qi and dispel cold. If complicated with serious dampness pathogen, subtract Dihuang, and add Fangji and Yiyiren to drain dampness to alleviate edema.

Tianma Gouteng Yin (Gastrodia and Uncaria Decoction)

Ingredients (Table 2.13)

Table 2.13 Ingredients of Tianma Gouteng Yin

Tianma	Rhizoma Gastrodiae	9 g
Gouteng	Ramulus Uncariae cum Uncis	12 g
Shijueming	Concha Haliotidis	18 g
Chuanniuxi	Radix Cyathulae	12 g
Huangqin	Radix Scutellariae	9 g
Zhizi	Fructus Gardeniae	9 g
Yimucao	Herba Leonuri	9 g
Duzhong	Cortex Eucommiae	9 g
Sangjisheng	Herba Taxilli	9 g
Shouwuteng	Caulis Polygoni Multiflori	9 g
Fushen	Poria contain pine root	9 g

Administration

All medicines above are decocted in water, for oral use.

Effects

Pacify the liver to extinguish wind, clear heat and cool blood, and tonify liver and kidney.

Application

This prescription is for syndrome of ascendant hyperactivity of liver yang and syndrome of liver wind disturbing upward. These syndromes are characterized by headache, dizziness, inability to sleep, red tongue, yellow fur, and string-like pulse. It can be used for hypertension with above syndromes.

Analysis

The syndrome treated by this prescription is caused by deficiency of liver and kidney, ascendant hyperactivity of liver yang, internal stirring of liver wind, and disquieted heart spirit. This syndrome should be dealt with treatment methods that pacify the liver to extinguish wind, clear heat and cool blood, and tonify liver and kidney.

1. Sovereign medicine: Tianma and Gouteng.
     Pacify the liver to extinguish wind.
2. Minister medicine: Shijueming and Chuanniuxi.
     Shijueming pacifies the liver to subdue yang. Chuanniuxi directs the blood downward. Both strengthen the effect of sovereigns to subdue yang, pacify the liver, and extinguish wind.
3. Assistant medicine: Huangqin, Zhizi, Yimucao, Duzhong, Sangjisheng, Shouwuteng, and Fushen.
     Huangqin and Zhizi clear heat and purge fire to subdue liver heat. Yimucao cools blood and induces diuresis to subdue liver yang. Duzhong and sangjisheng tonify liver and kidney to treat the origin. Shouwuteng and Fushen nourish the heart to tranquilize.

2.4.5 Dampness-Draining Prescriptions

2.4.5.1 Concept

Prescriptions based on clearing heat and removing dampness medicines, which have the effectof inducing dampness and clearing drenchingand are used for diseases caused by dampness, are called dampness-dispelling prescriptions.

2.4.5.2 Classification

About dampness pathogen, the generation would include external contraction and internal generation; the location would be different in exterior, interior, upper, and lower; the nature also would be cold or heat. Therefore, dampness-draining prescription would be divided into five categories: Dry dampness to harmonize stomach prescription, clear heat and dispel dampness prescription, induce diuresis to drain dampness prescription, warm-dispel dampness prescription, and dispel wind and drain dampness prescription.

2.4.5.3 Notes

The prescription would damage the yin fluid with the medicines of aroma dry-warm or sweet-tasteless draining. Thus, it is unsuitable for those who always have deficiency of yin fluid, weakness, or for pregnant women.

Huoxiang Zhengqi San (Patchouli Qi-Restoring Powder)

Ingredients (Table 2.14)

Administration

Grind the above medicines into fine powder, take 6 ~ 9 g each time, and add Shengjiang three slices, Dazao one piece, decocted in water, for oral use.

Effects

Release the exterior with resolve dampness, and regulate qi and harmonize the middle.

Table 2.14 Ingredients of Huoxiang Zhengqi San

Huoxiang	Herba Pogostemonis	9 g
Zisuye	Folium Perillae	6 g
Baizhi	Radix Angelicae Dahuricae	6 g
Banxia	Rhizoma Pinelliae	9 g
Houpo	Cortex Magnoliae officinalis	6 g
Chenpi	Pericarpium Citri Reticulatae	6 g
Dafupi	Pericarpium Arecae	9 g
Baizhu	Rhizoma Atractylodis Macrocephalae	9 g
Fuling	Poria	9 g
Jiegeng	Radix Platycodonis	9 g
Zhigancao	Radix Glycyrrhizae	6 g

Application

This prescription is for external contraction of wind-cold combine internal damaging of dampness syndrome. These syndromes are characterized by aversion to cold, fever, headache, stomach and abdominal pain, vomiting, diarrhea, white slimy tongue fur, and floating or soggy pulse. It can be used for acute gastroenteritis, gastrointestinal influenza, and other diseases that characterized by exterior cold and interior dampness.

Analysis

The syndrome treated by this prescription is caused by externally contracted wind-cold, stagnant defensive qi, internal obstruction of dampness-turbidity, unharmonization of spleen-stomach, and abnormality of upward and downward. This syndrome should be dealt with treatment methods as follows: Release the exterior with resolve dampness, regulate qi, and harmonize the middle.

1. Sovereign medicine: Huoxiang.
    Dispel wind-cold, resolve dampness-turbidity, harmonize the middle, and check vomiting.
2. Minister medicine: Zisuye and Baizhi.
    Assist the sovereign to dispel wind-cold and resolve dampness with the nature of pungent aroma.
3. Assistant medicine: Fuling, Baizhu, Banxia, Chenpi, Houpo, Dafupi, and Jiegeng.
    Fuling and Baizhu fortify spleen to transport dampness and harmonize middle jiao to stop diarrhea. Banxia and Chenpi dry dampness and harmonize stomach and direct the qi downward to check vomiting. Houpo and Dafupi move qi to resolve dampness. Jiegeng diffuse the lung to relieve the exterior and resolve the dampness.
4. Courier medicine: Zhigancao.
    Harmonize all the medicines.

Modification

If exterior syndrome is serious, complicated aversion to cold and no sweating, add Xiangru to support the effect of relieving exterior. If complicated with qi stagnation and serious distending pain in stomach and abdominal, add Muxiang and Yanhusuo to move qi and check pain.

Notes

Because the aroma and pungent dispelling are nature, the medicines of this prescription would not be decocted too long.

Table 2.15 Ingredients of
Yinchenhao Tang

Yinchen	Herba Artemisiae Scopariae	19 g
Zhizi	Fructus Gardeniae	9 g
Dahuang	Radix et Rhizoma Rhei	6 g

Yinchenhao Tang (Oriental Wormwood Decoction)

Ingredients (Table 2.15)

Administration

All medicines above are decocted in water, for oral use.

Effects

Clear heat and drain dampness to resolve jaundice.

Application

This prescription is for jaundice with dampness-heat syndrome. These syndromes are characterized by bright yellow on whole body, face, and eyes, slight abdominal fullness, thirst, inhibited urination, yellow slimy tongue fur, and sunken rapid pulse. It can be used for acute icterohepatitis, cholecystitis, cholelithiasis, leptospirosis, and other diseases that characterized by jaundice with bright yellow, yellow slimy tongue fur, and internal dampness-heat syndrome.

Analysis

The syndrome treated by this prescription is caused by internal stagnation with dampness-heat and stasis-heat, heat without outthrust, and dampness without purgation. This syndrome should be dealt with treatment methods as follows: Clear heat and drain dampness to resolve jaundice.

1. Sovereign medicine: Yinchen.
   The important medicine for resolving jaundice, cleaning heat and draining dampness.
2. Minister medicine: Zhizi.
   Clear heat and purge fire, drain through triple energizer, and direct the dampness-heat expelling with urinate.
3. Assistant medicine: Dahuang.
   Expel stasis and purge heat, and direct the stasis-heat purging with stool.
   All three medicines combine, expelling dampness-heat out with urinate and stool separately. As a result, jaundice would be resolved follow clearing of dampness-heat and purgation of stasis-heat.

Modification

If complicated with serious dampness syndrome, add Fuling and Zexie to induce diuresis to drain dampness. If complicated with serious heat syndrome, add Huangbai and Longdancao to clear heat and resolve dampness. If complicated with hypochondriac pain, add Chaihu and Chuanlianzi to soothe the liver and regulate qi.

Notes

It is unsuitable for yin jaundice syndrome.

Wuling San (Five Poria Powder)

Ingredients (Table 2.16)

Administration

Grind the above medicines into fine powder; take 6 g each time and thrice daily with warm water. All medicines above are decocted in water, for oral use.

Effects

Induce diuresis to drain dampness, warm yang, and form qi.

Application

This prescription is for water retention syndrome. These syndromes are characterized by edema, diarrhea, inhibited urination, pale tongue, white slippery fur, and soggy pulse. It can be used for edema caused by nephritis and liver cirrhosis, acute enteritis, uroschesis, hydrocephalus, and other diseases belonging to water retention syndrome.

Table 2.16 Ingredients of Wuling San

Zexie	Rhizoma Alismatis	15 g
Fuling	Poria	9 g
Zhuling	Polyporus Umbellatus	9 g
Baizhu	Rhizoma Atractylodis Macrocephalae	9 g
Guizhi	Ramulus Cinnamomi	6 g

Analysis

The syndrome treated by this prescription is caused by spleen failing in transportation, water retention, and inhibited qi transform of bladder. This syndrome should be dealt with treatment methods as follows: Induce diuresis to drain dampness, warm yang, and form qi.

1. Sovereign medicine: Zexie.
   Heavy dose of Zexie to induce diuresis to drain dampness.
2. Minister medicine: Fuling and Zhuling.
   Drain dampness with the sweet-tasteless nature and flavor. Besides, Fuling also can fortify spleen to drain dampness. Both assist the sovereign to induce diuresis to alleviate edema.
3. Assistant medicine: Baizhu and Guizhi.
   Baizhu combines Fuling to strengthen the effect of fortifying spleen to drain dampness. Guizhi fortifies bladder forming qi.
   All the medicines focus on fortify spleen to disperse dampness. It is suitable for all water retention syndrome.

Modification

If water retention syndrome is serious, use Wupi San (Chenpi, Fulingpi, Shengjiangpi, Sanbaipi, Dafupi) together to strengthen the effect of inducing diuresis to drain dampness.

Notes

The nature of this prescription is warm. So it is not suitable for water-dampness transforming heat.

2.4.6 Digestant Prescriptions

2.4.6.1 Concept

Those that are mainly composed of medicines for improving appetite and digestion, with the effect of promote digestion and remove food stagnation, fortify spleen, and harmonize stomach, used for indigestion with food stagnation, are known as digestant prescription.

2.4.6.2   Classification

The cause of retained food is always due to overeating and spleen-stomach failing in transportation. Therefore, digestant prescription can be divided into two categories: Promote digestion and remove food stagnation prescription and fortify spleen to promote digestion prescription.

2.4.6.3   Notes

Internal stagnation of retained food can induce inhibited qi movement and easily generate dampness and heat. Therefore, the degree of food, qi, heat, and dampness stagnation will be distinguished when forming the prescription. Meanwhile, appropriate medicines will be added necessarily in different conditions. If accumulation formed with retained food and dampness-heat, induced abdominal pain, constipation, and diarrhea, medicines for purgating will be used in order to remove food stagnation and purge accumulation.

Baohe Wan (Harmony-Preserving Pill)

Ingredients (Table 2.17)

Administration

For pills, take 6 ~ 9 g each time and twice or thrice daily. All medicines above are decocted in water, for oral use.

Effects

Promote digestion and harmonize stomach.

Table 2.17 Ingredients of Baohe Wan

Shanzha	Fructus Crataegi	18 g
Shenqu	Massa Medicata Fermentata	6 g
Laifuzi	Semen Raphani	6 g
Banxia	Rhizoma Pinelliae	9 g
Chenpi	Pericarpium Citri Reticulatae	9 g
Fuling	Poria	9 g
Lianqiao	Fructus Forsythiae	6 g

Application

This prescription is for food accumulation syndrome. This syndrome is character-ized by stuffiness and fullness and distending pain in the stomach and abdominal, belching, acid regurgitation, anorexia, and vomiting, or diarrhea, thick slimy tongue fur, and slippery pulse. It can be used for acute gastritis, chronic gastritis, acute enteritis, chronic enteritis, dyspepsia, infantile diarrhea, and other diseases belong-ing to food accumulation syndrome.

Analysis

The syndrome treated by this prescription is caused by dietary irregularities, over-eat, food stagnation, inhibited qi movement, and spleen-stomach disharmony, gen-erating dampness-heat. This syndrome should be dealt with treatment methods as follows: Promote digestion and harmonize stomach.

1. Sovereign medicine: Shanzha.
   Shanzha can digest every food accumulation, even meat, and greasy food.
2. Minister medicine: Shenqu and Laifuzi.
   Shenqu promotes digestion and fortifies stomach, good at digesting wine and stained food. Laifuzi directs qi downward to promote digestion, good at digest-ing grain food.
   The combination of sovereign and minister can digest every stained food.
3. Assistant medicine: Banxia, Chenpi, Fuling, and Lianqiao.
   Banxia and Chenpi move qi to dispel accumulation, harmonize stomach to check vomiting. Fuling can drain dampness and fortify spleen and harmonize middle jiao to stop diarrhea. Lianqiao clears heat and dispels accumulation.

Modification

If complicated with serious food accumulation, add Zhishi and Binglang (Arecae Scmcn) to strengthen the effect of promoting digestion and removing food stagna-tion. If complicated with exuberant heat, add Huangqin and Huanglian to clear heat. If complicated with spleen deficiency and sloppy diarrhea, add Baizhu to fortify spleen and promote transportation.

Notes

The power of this prescription is slight with the effect of promoting digestion and harmonizing stomach. It is unsuitable for constipation with abdominal distend-ing pain.

2.4.7   Phlegm-Dispelling and Cough-Suppressing Prescriptions

2.4.7.1   Concept

Those that are mainly composed of medicines for treating phlegm, cough, and asthma, with the effect of dispelling phlegm-retained fluid, relieving cough and asthma, used for kinds of phlegm and cough diseases, are known as phlegm-dispelling and cough-suppressing prescription.

2.4.7.2   Classification

Phlegm diseases would be different in dampness phlegm, heat phlegm, dry phlegm, and cold phlegm, according to disease cause. Therefore, phlegm-dispelling and cough-suppressing prescription can be divided into five categories: Dry dampness to resolve phlegm prescription, clear heat to resolve phlegm prescription, moisten dryness to resolve phlegm prescription, warm cold to resolve phlegm prescription, and relieve cough and dyspnea prescription.

2.4.7.3   Notes

The phlegm generated from dampness accumulation and spleen moving and transforming dampness. Therefore, spleen is known as the source of the phlegm generation. What is more, as a tangible pathogen, phlegm is easy to block qi movement. Phlegm-dispelling prescription is always used combining medicines for fortifying spleen to treat the source of phlegm generation, combining medicines for regulating qi to move qi and dispel phlegm. The medicines for drying dampness to dispel phlegm are always warm dryness of their nature, easy to interrupt blood, so it is caution for hemoptysis tendency.

Erchen Tang (Two Old Ingredients Decoction)

Ingredients (Table 2.18)

Table 2.18 Ingredients of Erchen Tang

Banxia	Rhizoma Pinelliae	15 g
Juhong	Exocarpium Citri rubrum	15 g
Fuling	Poria	9 g
Zhigancao	Radix Glycyrrhizae	5 g

Administration

Add Shengjiang seven slices, Wumei 1 pcs, decocted all in water, for oral use.

Effects

Dry dampness to dispel phlegm, and regulate qi to harmonize middle.

Application

This prescription is for cough or vomiting with dampness-phlegm syndrome. This syndrome is characterized by cough with much phlegm which is white and easily expectorated, stuffiness and stuffiness in the chest, nausea and vomiting, lack of strength, or dizziness and palpitations, white slimy tongue fur, and slippery pulse. It can be used for chronic bronchitis, pulmonary emphysema, chronic gastritis, vomitus gravidarum, nervous vomiting, and other diseases belonging to dampness-phlegm syndrome with much white phlegm.

Analysis

The syndrome treated by this prescription is caused by spleen failing in transportation, dampness pathogen retention, dampness accumulation forming phlegm, and inhibited qi movement. This syndrome should be dealt with treatment methods as follows: Dry dampness to dispel phlegm, and regulate qi to harmonize middle.

1. Sovereign medicine: Banxia.
    Banxia can dry dampness to dispel phlegm and check cough, lower adverse qi, and harmonize stomach to check vomiting, with pungent-warm and dryness in flavor nature.
2. Minister medicine: Juhong.
    Assist the sovereign to strengthen the effect of dispelling phlegm and harmonize stomach. What is more, move qi to smoothen the phlegm expectoration.
3. Assistant medicine: Fuling.
    Fortify spleen to drain dampness, treating the source of phlegm generation. Combine with the sovereign and minister, treating both symptoms and root causes
4. Courier medicine: Zhigancao.
    Harmonize middle and fortify spleen, and harmonize all the medicines.
    When decocted, add Shengjiang to assist sovereign and minister, strengthening the effect of moving qi to dispel phlegm and harmonizing stomach to check vomiting and restrict the toxicity of Banxia in the meantime. Combine 1 pcs of Wumei to astringe lung qi avoid damaging the healthy qi. It is the basic method for phlegm-dispelling. Therefore, this prescription is known as commonly used phlegm-dispelling prescription.

Modification

This prescription is the basic prescription for dispelling phlegm, which can be used combining relevant medicines for kinds of phlegm diseases. If complicated with heat phlegm, add Huangqin and Dannanxing to clear heat and dispel phlegm. If complicated with cold phlegm, add Ganjiang and Xixin to warm-dispel cold phlegm. If complicated with wind phlegm, add Tiannanxing and Zhuli to extinguish wind and dispel phlegm. If complicated with food phlegm, add Laifuzi and Shenqu to digest food stagnation and dispel phlegm.

Notes

Because the warm dryness nature, it is forbidden for the patients with yin deficiency and lung dryness syndrome.

Qingqi Huatan Wan (Clear Heat and Dispel Phlegm Pill)

Ingredients (Table 2.19)

Administration

For pills with ginger juice, take 6 g each time with warm water. All medicines above are decocted in water, for oral use.

Effects

Clear heat to dispel phlegm, and regulate qi to check cough.

Table 2.19 Ingredients of Qingqi Huatan Wan

Dannanxing	Rhizoma Pinelliae	15 g
Gualouzi	Semen Trichosanthis	9 g
Huangqin	Radix Scutellariae	9 g
Zhishi	Fructus Aurantii Immaturus	9 g
Juhong	Exocarpium Citri rubrum	9 g
Fuling	Poria	9 g
Kuxingren	Semen Armeniacae Amarum	9 g
Banxia	Rhizoma Pinelliae	15 g

Application

This prescription is for cough with heat-phlegm syndrome. This syndrome is characterized by cough with yellow thickness phlegm which is difficult to expectorate, stuffiness and stuffiness in the chest, or dysphoria, red tongue, yellow slimy fur, and slippery rapid pulse. It can be used for acute and chronic bronchitis, pneumonia, and other diseases belonging to heat-phlegm syndrome with yellow thickness phlegm.

Analysis

The syndrome treated by this prescription is caused by that lung heat burning fluid and converting it into phlegm, intermingled phlegm and heat, inhibited qi movement, and lung failing to diffuse and depurate. This syndrome should be dealt with treatment methods as follows: clear heat to dispel phlegm, and regulate qi to check cough.

1. Sovereign medicine: Dannanxing.
   Clear heat to dispel phlegm.
2. Minister medicine: Huangqin and Gualouzi.
   Huangqin clear lung and purge heat. Gualouzi clear lung and dispel phlegm. This combination purge lung fire, and dispel phlegm-heat.
3. Assistant medicine: Zhishi, Juhong, Fuling, Kuxingren, and Banxia.
   Zhishi and Juhong move qi to dispel phlegm. Fuling fortify the spleen to drain dampness, treating the source of phlegm generation. Kuxingren can direct qi downward to calm cough. Banxia can dry dampness to dispel phlegm.

Modification

If complicated with exuberant lung heat, add Shigao and Zhimu to purge lung heat. If complicated with much phlegm, add Tianhuafeng and Yuxingcao to strengthen the effect of cleaning heat and dispelling phlegm. If complicated with heat constipation, add Dahuang to purge heat with relaxing the bowels, directing heat downward.

Notes

Because of its cold nature, it is forbidden for the patients always with spleen deficiency and sloppy stool.

Suzi Jiangqi Tang (Perilla Fruit Decoction for Directing Qi Downward)

Ingredients (Table 2.20)

Table 2.20 Ingredients of
Suzi Jiangqi Tang

Zisuzi	Fructus Perillae	15 g
Banxia	Rhizoma Pinelliae	15 g
Houpo	Cortex Magnoliae officinalis	6 g
Qianhu	Radix Peucedani	6 g
Rougui	Cortex Cinnamomi	9 g
Danggui	Radix Angelicae Sinensis	9 g
Zhigancao	Radix Glycyrrhizae	12 g

Administration

Add two slices of Shengjiang, 1 pcs Dazao, and Zisuye 3 g, all medicines above are decocted in water, for oral use.

Effects

Direct qi downward to calm dyspnea, and dispel phlegm to check cough.

Application

This prescription is for cough-dyspnea syndrome due to upper excess and lower deficiency. This syndrome is characterized by cough, dyspnea, with much white phlegm, stuffiness and stuffiness in the chest, or pain and flaccid in waist and knee, or limbs edema, white slimy or slippery fur, slippery, and string-like pulse. It can be used for chronic bronchitis, pulmonary emphysema, bronchial asthma, and other diseases belonging to chest stuffiness, much white phlegm with white slimy or slippery fur.

Analysis

The syndrome treated by this prescription is caused by that phlegm accumulation in the lung, lung failing to diffuse and depurate, complicated with kidney yang deficiency, failing to receive qi. Thus, this syndrome is called as upper excess and lower deficiency syndrome. According to principle of treating symptoms when an acute attack occurs, this syndrome should be dealt with treatment methods as follows: Direct qi downward to calm dyspnea, and dispel phlegm to check cough.

1. Sovereign medicine: Zisuzi.
   Direct qi downward and dispel phlegm, check cough, and calm dyspnea.
2. Minister medicine: Banxia, Houpo, and Qianhu.
   Banxia drain dampness to dispel phlegm, and direct qi downward. Houpo direct qi downward to calm dyspnea. Qianhu diffuse lung to dispel phlegm and

check cough. All these three medicines assist sovereign direct qi downward to dispel phlegm and calm dyspnea.

Sovereign combine minister to treat upper excess syndrome.

3. Assistant medicine: Rougui and Danggui.

Rougui warm tonify kidney qi, and receive qi to calm dyspnea. Danggui nourish blood and moisten the dryness.

The combination of assistant treats the lower deficiency syndrome.

4. Courier medicine: Zhigancao.

Harmonize all the medicines.

Modification

If cough and dyspnea complicated with inability to lie on back, add Chenxiang to strengthen the effect of directing qi downward to calm dyspnea. If complicated with exterior syndrome, aversion to cold and fever, add Mahuang and Kuxingren to diffuse lung and calm dyspnea. If complicated with qi deficiency, add Renshen and Wuweizi to tonify lung qi. If without lower deficiency, subduct Rougui and Danggui.

Notes

Because of the warm dryness nature, it is forbidden for the patients with yin deficiency of lung and kidney, or lung heat and phlegm-dyspnea.

2.4.8 Interior-Warming Prescriptions

2.4.8.1 Concept

Those that are mainly composed of medicines for warming the interior, with the effect of warming the interior and tonify yang, dissipating cold and freeing collateral vessels, used for interior cold syndrome are known as interior-warming prescription.

2.4.8.2 Classification

Regarding interior cold syndrome, the location would be different in zang-fu viscera and meridian. Therefore, interior-warming prescriptions can be divided into three categories: prescriptions of warming middle jiao to dissipate cold, prescriptions of restoring yang from collapse, and prescriptions of warming the meridian to dissipate cold.

2.4.8.3 Notes

The pungent-warm and dryness-heat nature of interior-warming prescription are easy to damage yin, assist heat, and interrupt blood; therefore, it is caution for those who are always yin deficiency with interior heat and on menstrual period.

Lizhong Wan (Middle-Regulating Pill)

Ingredients (Table 2.21)

Administration

For pills with honey, take 6 g each time and thrice 1 day with warm water. All medicines above are decocted in water, for oral use.

Effects

Warm the middle to dissipate cold, tonify qi, and fortify the spleen.

Application

This prescription is for deficiency cold syndrome of spleen-stomach. This syndrome is characterized by stomach and abdominal pain with preferring warm and pressure, aversion to cold, limb cold, inappetence, vomiting and diarrhea, or bleeding due to yang deficiency with little dark blood, pale tongue, white fur, and sunken fine pulse. It can be used for acute gastroenteritis, chronic gastroenteritis, stomach and duodenal ulcer, chronic colitis, and other diseases main symptoms of which are shown as vomiting, diarrhea, cold, and pain, belonging to deficiency cold syndrome of spleen-stomach.

Table 2.21 Ingredients of Lizhong Wan

Ganjiang	Rhizoma Zingiberis	9 g
Renshen	Radix ginseng	9 g
Baizhu	Rhizoma Atractylodis Macrocephalae	9 g
Zhigancao	Radix Glycyrrhizae	9 g

Analysis

The syndrome treated by this prescription is caused by deficiency of middle yang, deficiency cold of spleen and stomach, and failing in transportation and transformation. This syndrome should be dealt with treatment methods as follow: Warm the middle to dissipate cold, tonify qi, and fortify the spleen.

1. Sovereign medicine: Ganjiang.
    Warm middle, promote yang qi, and dissipate cold.
2. Minister medicine: Renshen.
    Tonify qi, fortify spleen, and promote the transportation.
3. Assistant medicine: Baizhu.
    Tonify qi, fortify spleen, and drain dampness. On the one hand, combine sovereign to warn-transport spleen yang; on the other hand, combine minister to tonify qi and fortify spleen.
4. Assistant and courier medicines: Zhigancao.
    As assistant, tonify middle with pungent-warm nature, assisting above three medicines to warm and tonify the spleen. As courier, harmonize all the medicines.

Modification

If complicated with serious cold, use heavy dosage of Ganjiang or add Fuzi to promote the effect of warming middle and assisting yang. If used for yang deficiency bleeding syndrome, change Ganjiang to Paojiang. If complicated with serious deficiency, use heavy dosage of Renshen, to strengthen the effect of tonifying qi and fortifying spleen. If complicated with serious diarrhea, use heavy dosage of Baizhu to fortify spleen and promote transport to check diarrhea. If complicated with serious vomiting, add Wuzhuyu and Shengjiang to warm stomach and check vomiting. If complicated with dampness phlegm, add Banxia and Fuling to warm-dispel phlegm.

Sini Tang (Resuscitation Decoction)

Ingredients (Table 2.22)

Table 2.22 Ingredients of Sini Tang

Fuzi	Radix Aconiti Lateralis Preparata	15 g
Ganjiang	Rhizoma Zingiberis	9 g
Zhigancao	Radix Glycyrrhizae	9 g

Administration

All medicines above are decocted in water, for oral use.

Effects

Restore yang to save from collapse.

Application

This prescription is for the syndrome of yin exuberance with yang debilitation. This syndrome is characterized by reversal cold of the extremities, aversion to cold with cowered in bed, vomiting with no sweating, abdominal pain, diarrhea, lassitude of spirit, somnolence, white slippery tongue fur, and faint fine pulse. It can be used for myocardial infarction, acute heart failure, acute or chronic gastroenteritis with over exhaling, or shock due to over sweating disease belonging to syndrome of yin exuberance with yang debilitation, even yang collapse.

Analysis

The syndrome treated by this prescription is caused by yin exuberance with heart and kidney yang debilitation. This syndrome should be dealt with treatment methods as restoring yang to save from collapse.

1. Sovereign medicine: Fuzi.
   Warm interior to dissipate cold and restore yang to save from collapse with great pungent heat.
2. Minister medicine: Ganjiang.
   Warm middle to dispel cold, combine Fuzi to strengthen the effect of restoring yang and dissipating cold. That is called as Fuzi do not heat without Ganjiang.
3. Assistant and courier medicines: Zhigancao.
   As assistant, assist the sovereign and minister with tonifying qi to warm middle, and relieve the toxic substances and dryness nature of Fuzi and Ganjiang. As courier, harmonize all the medicines.

Modification

If complicated with exuberant yin repelling yang, reddened complexion, which is known as true cold with false heat, use heavy dosage of Fuzi and Ganjiang to strengthen the effect of restoring yang to save from collapse. If complicated with water internal retention due to yang deficiency and limb edema, add Dangshen, Zexie, and Fuling to fortify spleen, drain dampness, and alleviate edema.

Notes

Syndrome of deficiency cold of spleen-stomach is always shown as true cold with false heat with exuberant yin repelling yang or upcast yang syndrome. In this case, do not misuse the heat-cleaning prescription. Emesis immediately after taking this prescription is called as "reject medicines." In these cases, method of counteracting assistant like adding a few cold medicines into the prescription would be taken to relieve or eliminate these situations.

2.4.9   Qi-Regulating Prescriptions

2.4.9.1   Concept

Those that are mainly composed of medicines for regulating qi, with the effect of regulating qi movement, used for disordered qi movement syndrome known as qi-regulating prescription.

2.4.9.2   Classification

Disordered qi movement syndrome includes qi stagnation and qi counterflow in a general way. Accordingly, qi-regulating prescription can be divided into two categories: qi-moving prescription and directing qi downward prescription. Qi-moving prescription can be used for qi stagnation in liver and spleen syndrome and qi stagnation in liver syndrome with the effect of moving qi to resolve stagnation and dispersing stuffiness and removing fullness. Directing qi downward prescription can be used for lung qi counterflow syndrome and stomach qi counterflow syndrome with the effect of directing qi downward, and calm dyspnea and check vomiting. The directing qi downward prescription for treating lung qi counterflow is described in the section of phlegm-dispelling and cough-suppressing prescription.

2.4.9.3   Notes

The nature and flavor of the medicines which form qi-regulating prescription are mainly pungent-warm and dryness. Therefore, qi-regulating prescription should not to be used for a long time in case the property might damage fluid and consume qi. It is also caution for senile people, pregnant woman, and someone with syndrome of yin deficiency with effulgent fire.

Table 2.23 Ingredients of Yueju Wan

Xiangfu	Rhizoma Cyperi	9 g
Chuanxiong	Rhizoma Ligustici chuanxiong	9 g
Cangzhu	Rhizoma Atractylodis	9 g
Zhizi	Fructus Gardeniae	9 g
Shenqu	Massa Medicata Fermentata	9 g

Yueju Wan (Relieving Stagnation Pill)

Ingredients (Table 2.23)

Administration

For pills, take 6 ~ 9 g each time and twice 1 day with warm water. All medicines above are decocted in water, for oral use.

Effects

Move qi to resolve stagnation.

Application

This prescription is for six stagnations syndrome such as qi, blood, phlegm, fire, dampness, and food stagnation. This syndrome is characterized by stuffiness in the chest and diaphragm, distending pain in stomach and abdominal, acid regurgitation and vomiting, and food accumulation. It can be used for gastroneurosis, chronic gastritis, stomach and duodenal ulcer, cholelithiasis, cholecystitis, hepatitis, intercostal neuralgia, dysmenorrhea, irregular menstruation, and other diseases belonging to six stagnations syndrome.

Analysis

The syndrome treated by this prescription is caused by qi stagnation in liver and spleen. Qi stagnation in the liver or constrained liver qi for long, lead to liver qi invading the spleen, spleen failing to transport, dampness accumulation generating phlegm, food accumulation not digested, or blood flow being not smooth, stagnation transforming into fire, result in qi, blood, phlegm, fire, food, and dampness stagnation appearing at the same time. Because qi stagnation appearing first in the six stagnations, this syndrome will be dealt with treatment methods mainly as moving qi to resolve stagnation.

1. Sovereign medicine: Xiangfu.
   Moving qi to resolve stagnation, in order to treat qi stagnation.

2. Minister and assistant medicines: Chuanxiong, Cangzhu, Zhizi, and Shenqu.

Chuanxiong promotes blood circulation for removing blood stasis in order to treat blood stagnation, and also assists Xiangfu to move qi to resolve stagnation. Zhizi clear heat and purge fire, in order to treat fire stagnation. Cangzhu dries dampness to fortify spleen, in order to treat dampness stagnation. Shenqu digests food to treat food stagnation. Phlegm stagnation is always due to spleen dampness and is related to qi, fire, and food stagnation. Thus, phlegm stagnation will be resolved with the other stagnation gone.

Modification

If complicated with obvious qi stagnation syndrome, use heavy dosage of Xiangfu and add Muxiang and Zhike to strengthen moving qi. If complicated with obvious blood stagnation syndrome, use heavy dosage of Chuanxiong and add Taoren and Honghua to promote blood circulation. If complicated with obvious dampness stagnation syndrome, use heavy dosage of Cangzhu and add Fuling and Zexie to drain dampness. If complicated with obvious food stagnation syndrome, use heavy dosage of Shenqu and add Shanzha and Maiya to promote digestion. If complicated with obvious fire stagnation syndrome, use heavy dosage of Zhizi and add Huangqin and Huanglian to purge fire. If complicated with obvious phlegm stagnation syndrome, add Banxia and Gualouzi to dispel phlegm.

Notes

Although this prescription can treat all the six stagnations, it just shows the basic method for treating the stagnation syndrome. In the clinical practice, modification will be taken flexibly in accordance with the syndrome.

Chaihu Shugan San (Bupleurum Soothing Liver Powder)

Ingredients (Table 2.24)

Table 2.24 Ingredients of Chaihu Shugan San

Chaihu	Radix Bupleuri	6 g
Chuanxiong	Rhizoma Ligustici chuanxiong	5 g
Xiangfu	Rhizoma Cyperi	5 g
Zhike	Fructus Aurantii	5 g
Juhong	Exocarpium Citri rubrum	6 g
Baishao	Radix Paeoniae Alba	5 g
Gancao	Radix Glycyrrhizae	3 g

Administration

All medicines above are decocted in water, for oral use.

Effects

Soothe liver to resolve stagnation, and move qi to check pain.

Application

This prescription is for liver qi stagnations syndrome. This syndrome is characterized by distending pain in lateral thorax, stomach, and abdominal, belching and sighing, and string-like pulse. It can be used for hepatitis, chronic gastritis, intercostal neuralgia, and other diseases belonging to liver qi stagnations syndrome.

Analysis

The syndrome treated by this prescription is caused by emotion depression, liver failing to free flow and rise of qi, and qi stagnation in liver. This syndrome will be dealt with treatment methods mainly as soothing liver to resolve stagnation, moving qi to check pain.

1. Sovereign medicine: Chaihu.
     Soothe liver to resolve stagnation.
2. Minister medicine: Chuanxiong and Xiangfu.
     Chuanxiong moves qi and promotes blood circulation. Xiangfu regulates qi to soothe liver. This combination supports sovereign to resolve stagnation and check pain.
3. Assistant medicine: Zhike, Juhong, and Baishao.
     Zhike and Juhong regulate qi and move stagnation. Baisho nourishes blood to soothe liver and check pain.
4. Assistant and courier medicines: Gancao.
     As assistant, combine Baishao to nourish blood and soothe liver. As courier, harmonize all the medicines.

Modification

If complicated with serious pain, add Danggui and Yujin to strengthen the moving qi, activating blood, and checking pain effect. If liver stagnation transforms to fire, with dryness of mouth and red tongue, add Zhizi and Chuanlianzi to clear liver and purge fire.

Table 2.25 Ingredients of
Banxia Houpo Tang

Banxia	Rhizoma Pinelliae	9 g
Houpo	Cortex Magnoliae officinalis	9 g
Fuling	Poria	9 g
Shengjiang	Rhizoma Zingiberis Recens	9 g
Zisuye	Folium Perillae	9 g

Banxia Houpo Tang (Pinellia and Magnolia Decoction)

Ingredients (Table 2.25)

Administration

All medicines above are decocted in water, for oral use.

Effects

Move qi to disperse nodules, and lower counterflow to resolve phlegm.

Application

This prescription is for plum-pit qi with syndrome of qi stagnation and congealing phlegm. This disease is characterized by subjective feeling that something seems to be obstructed in the throat unable to be thrown out or swallowed down, stuffiness and fullness in the chest and diaphragm, or cough, or vomiting, white slimy tongue fur, and slippery and string-like pulse. It can be used for chronic pharyngitis, hysteria, chronic bronchitis, gastroneurosis, and other diseases belonging to syndrome of qi stagnation and congealing phlegm.

Analysis

The syndrome treated by this prescription is caused by phlegm and qi congealed in the throat, lung and stomach failing to diffuse and depurate. This syndrome will be dealt with treatment methods mainly as moving qi to disperse nodules, lowering counterflow to resolve phlegm.

1. Sovereign medicine: Banxia and Houpo.
   Banxia disperse nodules and resolve phlegm, lowering counterflow to harmonize stomach. Houpo move qi to disperse stagnation, and direct qi downward to resolve fullness. In this combination, one disperse phlegm-congelation, when the other move qi stagnation.
2. Minister medicine: Fuling and Zisuye.
   Fuling fortifies spleen to drain dampness and also assists Banxia to resolve phlegm. Zisuye assists Houpo to regulate qi movement with its nature.

3. Assistant medicine: Shengjiang.

   Shengjiang harmonize stomach to check vomiting, assist Banxia to harmonize middle, and lower the counterflow.

Modification

If complicated with obvious qi stagnation syndrome, add Xiangfu and Yujin to strengthen moving qi. If complicated with chest and hypochondrium pain, add Chuanlianzi and Yanhusuo to soothe the liver and regulate qi to check pain. If complicated with throat pain, add Xuanshen and Jiegeng to detoxify and disperse nodules, and diffuse lung to smooth throat.

Notes

Because the warm dryness nature, it is forbidden for plum-pit qi with heat syndrome or due to deficiency of fluid.

2.4.10 Blood-Regulating Prescriptions

2.4.10.1 Concept

Those that are mainly composed of medicines for regulating blood, with the effect of promoting blood circulation or stopping bleeding, used for blood stasis syndrome and bleed syndrome, are known as blood-regulating prescription.

2.4.10.2 Classification

In a general way, blood disorder syndrome includes blood stasis and bleed. Blood stasis syndrome come from blood flow being suffocated, and then, blood stagnation transforms into stasis. Bleed syndrome due to blood go out from the vessels. Accordingly, blood-regulating prescription can be divided into two categories: Activate blood and resolve stasis prescription and stop bleeding prescription.

2.4.10.3 Notes

The nature of the medicines which form blood-regulating prescription is mainly drastic and purgative. These prescriptions are easy to consume blood and damage healthy qi and liable to disturb blood circulation and fetus. The dosage of the prescription will not be too heavy in case it might damage healthy qi or add some medicines for tonifying. It is also caution for hypermenorrhea patient and pregnant woman. Because the astringent nature of stop bleeding prescription, the medicines

Table 2.26 Ingredients of
Xuanfu Zhuyu Tang

Taoren	Semen Persicae	12 g
Honghua	Flos Carthami	9 g
Chishao	Radix Paeoniae Rubra	6 g
Chuanxiong	Rhizoma Ligustici chuanxiong	6 g
Niuxi	Radix Achyranthis Bidentatae	9 g
Dihuang	Radix Rehmanniae	9 g
Danggui	Radix Angelicae Sinensis	9 g
Chaihu	Radix Bupleuri	3 g
Jiegeng	Radix Platycodonis	6 g
Zhike	Fructus Aurantii	6 g
Gancao	Radix Glycyrrhizae	3 g

for promoting blood circulation will be combined to prevent stasis retention. What is more, whether the blood stasis syndrome or bleed syndrome, the pathogenesis will be different in cold and heat, excess, and deficiency. Therefore, the incidental and fundamental, primary and secondary, are necessary to be distinguished in clinical.

Xuanfu Zhuyu Tang (Expelling Chest Stasis Decoction)

Ingredients (Table 2.26)

Administration

All medicines above are decocted in water, for oral use.

Effects

Activate blood to expel stasis, and move qi to relieve pain.

Application

This prescription is for the syndrome of blood stasis in the chest. This syndrome is characterized by prolonged chest pain and headache, pain like being pricked at fixed location, or hiccup in chronic process, or internal heat with vexation, or palpitation and inability to sleep, impatience and be fractious, tidal fever at night, dark lip, deep red tongue even with ecchymosis, and rough or tight string-like pulse. It can be used for stenocardia of coronary heart disease, rheumatic heart disease, chest pain of chest trauma and costal chondritis, headache, dizzy, and depression of concussion sequela, and other diseases belonging to syndrome of blood stasis and qi stagnation of upper location.

Analysis

The syndrome treated by this prescription is caused by blood stasis obstructing in the chest and qi movement stagnation. This syndrome should be dealt with treatment methods as activating blood to expel stasis, moving qi to relieve pain.

1. Sovereign medicine: Taoren and Honghua.

   Taoren and Honghua are both importance medicines for activating blood to expel stasis. This combination brings out the best in each other with the effect of activating blood to expel stasis.
2. Minister medicine: Chishao, Chuanxiong, and Niuxi.

   Chishao activate blood to expel stasis. Chuanxiong moves qi to activate blood. Niuxi directs blood stasis downward. This combination strengthens the effect of activating blood to expel stasis.
3. Assistant medicine: Zhike, Jiegeng, and Chaihu.

   Zhike and jiegeng move qi to soothe the chest, and Chaihu soothes the liver to resolve stagnation. This combination regulates the qi movement, moving qi to promote blood circulation and expel the stasis. Dihuang and Danggui nourish blood and tonify yin, and clear heat of the blood.
4. Courier medicine: Gancao.

   Harmonize all the medicines.

Modification

If complicated with mass and nodules in coastal region, add Yujin and Danshen to activate blood to expel stasis and disperse mass and nodules.

Buyang Huanwu Tang (Tonifying Yang and Returning Five Decoction)

Ingredients (Table 2.27)

Table 2.27 Ingredients of Buyang Huanwu Tang

Huangqi	Radix Astragali seu Hedysari	120 g
Danggui	Radix Angelicae Sinensis	6 g
Chishao	Radix Paeoniae Rubra	6 g
Chuanxiong	Rhizoma Ligustici chuanxiong	3 g
Taoren	Semen Persicae	3 g
Honghua	Flos Carthami	3 g
Dilong	Lumbricus	5 g

Administration

All medicines above are decocted in water, for oral use.

Effects

Tonify qi, activate blood, and regulate the collateral vessels.

Application

This prescription is for sequela of stroke with syndrome of qi deficiency and blood stasis. This disease is characterized by hemiplegia, deviation of eyes and mouth, salivation, frequent micturition or incontinence of urinary, dark pale tongue, thin white fur, and moderate pulse. Hemiplegic paralysis, paraplegia, flaccidity syndrome of upper or lower limbs, and other diseases due to sequela of stroke belonging to syndrome of qi deficiency and blood stasis can be treated by this prescription.

Analysis

The syndrome treated by this prescription is caused by qi deficiency that cannot move blood and induce to stasis stagnation in the vessels, tendons, and muscle failing to be nourished. This syndrome should be dealt with treatment methods as tonifying qi, activating blood, freeing the collateral vessels.

1. Sovereign medicine: Huangqi.
   Use heavy dosage of Huangqi to greatly tonify original qi, for qi being exuberant to move blood.
2. Minister medicine: Danggui.
   Activate blood to expel stasis, for freeing the collateral vessels.
3. Assistant medicine: Chishao, Chuanxiong, Taoren, Honghua, and Dilong.
   The combination of Chishao, Chuanxiong, Taoren, and Honghua assists Danggui to activate blood to expel stasis. Dilong unblocks the meridian and activate collateral, for expelling the stasis in the vessels.

Modification

If complicated with much phlegm, add Banxia and Tianzhihua to resolve phlegm. If complicated with unsmooth speech, add Shichangpu, Yuanzhi, and Yujin to open the orifices and free the collateral vessels. If complicated with yang deficiency, aversion to cold, and cold limbs, add Fuzi to warm yang to dispel cold. If complicated with serious lower limbs flaccidity syndrome, add Duzhong and Niuxi to tonify liver-kidney, and strong the tendons and bones.

Notes

In this prescription, the dosage of Huangqi are generally starting from 30 ~ 60 g and will be increasing little by little when it did not work. What is more, it will be taken for a while after cure, for consolidating curative effect.

2.4.11   Tranquilizing Prescriptions

2.4.11.1   Concept

Those that are mainly composed of medicines for mental disease, with the effect of tranquilizing and settling will, used for mind disturbed and metal disorder diseases, are known as tranquilizing prescription.

2.4.11.2   Classification

Mind disturbed diseases are characterized by restless syndrome of heart spirit such as palpitation, inability to sleep, dysphoria, and manic psychosis. The basic mechanisms of these diseases are that heat damaging heart spirit and heart blood deficiency. Accordingly, tranquilizing prescription can be divided into two categories: Tranquilize by heavy settling prescription, and nourish the heart to tranquilize prescription.

2.4.11.3   Notes

The tranquilization and mental controlling prescription should not be administered for long time because mineral medicines are used, which would damage stomach qi if taken too mach.

Suanzaoren Tang (Wild Jujube Seed Decoction)

Ingredients (Table 2.28)

Table 2.28 Ingredients of Suanzaoren Tang

Suanzaoren	Semen Ziziphi Spinosae	15 g
Fuling	Poria	9 g
Zhimu	Rhizoma Anemarrhenae	9 g
Chuanxiong	Rhizoma Ligustici chuanxiong	6 g
Gancao	Radix Glycyrrhizae	6 g

Administration

All medicines above are decocted in water, for oral use.

Effects

Nourish the blood to tranquilize, and clear heat to relieve vexation.

Application

This prescription is for deficiency vexation syndrome with inability to sleep. This syndrome is characterized by inability to sleep, palpitation, restlessness in heart, dizziness, dryness of mouth and throat, red tongue, and fine and string-like pulse. It can be used for neurasthenia, cardiac neurosis, climacteric syndrome, and other diseases belonging to deficiency restlessness syndrome with inability to sleep.

Analysis

The syndrome treated by this prescription is caused by liver-blood deficiency, deficiency heat disturbing interior, and restlessness of heart spirit. This syndrome should be dealt with treatment methods as follow: Nourish the blood to tranquilize, and clear heat to relieve vexation.

1. Sovereign medicine: Suanzaoren.
   Tonify the liver to nourish blood, and calm heart to tranquilize.
2. Minister medicine: Fuling and Zhimu.
   Fuling calms heart to tranquilize. Zhimu nourishes yin to clear heat. This combination strengthens the relieve vexation and tranquilization effect of the sovereign.
3. Assistant medicine: Chuanxiong.
   Regulate the qi movement, and soothe liver qi. Chuanxiong soothe liver qi, while Suanzaoren nourishes liver-blood. Chuanxiong combines Suanzaoren, meaning opposite and supplementary to each other.
4. Courier medicine: Gancao.
   Gancao clears heat and regulates middle jiao and harmonizes all medicines.

Modification

If complicated with deficiency fire syndrome, heat vexation, and inability to sleep with dreaminess, subduct Chuanxiong, add Dihuang, Baishao, and Huanglian to nourish yin, clear heat, and remove vexation. If complicated with serious night sweating, add Muli and Fuxiaomai to astringe yin and calm heart. If complicated with frequent fright waking-up, palpitation with dreaminess, pale tongue, and fine and string-like pules, which are the symptoms of the qi deficiency of heart and gall-bladder, add Dangshen and Zhenzhumu to tonify qi and settle fright.

Notes

It is unsuitable for serious liver fire syndrome manifested as vexation and inability to sleep, headache with reddened complexion, bitter taste in the mouth, dry throat, and strong string-like and rapid pules.

2.4.12   *Tonifying and Replenishing Prescriptions*

2.4.12.1   Concept

Those that are mainly composed of medicines for tonifying deficiency, with the effect of tonify and nourish qi, blood, yin, and yang, used for kinds of deficiency syndromes, are known as tonifying and replenishing prescription.

2.4.12.2   Classification

In a general way, deficiency syndromes include qi deficiency syndrome, blood deficiency syndrome, yin deficiency syndrome, and yang deficiency syndrome. Accordingly, tonifying and replenishing prescription can be divided into four categories: tonifying qi prescription, tonifying blood prescription, tonifying yin prescription, and tonifying yang prescription.

2.4.12.3   Notes

Tonifying and replenishing prescription should not be administered for long because with the thick and greasy flavor damaging the spleen-stomach and not easy to be digested. It is also caution for patients always with spleen-stomach deficiency, eating less and sloppy stool. For preventing that, medicines for tonifying and replenishing spleen-stomach and regulating qi to promote transportation should be added when using tonifying and replenishing prescription. For patients with deficiency syndrome and intolerance of tonifying and nourishing, spleen-stomach must be regulated first. What is more, tonifying and replenishing prescription should be decocted slowly with mild fire, administrated before the meal for promoting the absorption and digestion.

Table 2.29 Ingredients of Sijunzi Tang

Renshen	Radix Ginseng	9 g
Baizhu	Rhizoma Atractylodis Macrocephalae	9 g
Fuling	Poria	9 g
Zhigancao	Radix Glycyrrhizae	6 g

Sijunzi Tang (Four Gentlemen Decoction)

Ingredients (Table 2.29)

Administration

All medicines above are decocted in water, for oral use.

Effects

Tonify qi and fortify the spleen.

Application

This prescription is for the spleen-stomach qi deficiency syndrome. This syndrome is characterized by sallow white complexion, speaking in a low and week voice, qi shortage and lack of strength, torpid intake and sloppy stool, pale tongue, white fur, and find and week pule. It can be used for chronic gastritis, stomach and duodenal ulcer, and other diseases belonging to spleen-stomach qi deficiency syndrome with mainly symptoms shown as above.

Analysis

The syndrome treated by this prescription is caused by qi deficiency of spleen-stomach and lack of strength for transportation. This syndrome should be dealt with treatment methods as tonifying qi and fortifying the spleen.

1. Sovereign medicine: Renshen.
   Tonify qi to fortify spleen and nourish stomach.
2. Minister medicine: Baizhu.
   Tonify qi to fortify spleen and drain dampness.
3. Assistant medicine: Fuling.
   Drain dampness and fortify spleen for promoting transportation.
4. Courier medicine: Zhigancao.
   On the one hand, tonify qi with nourish the middle. On the other hand, harmonize all the medicines.
   All four medicines combine, tonify but not accumulate, and warm but not dry, to form a neutral supplementation prescription for spleen-stomach.

Modification

If complicated with qi stagnation, stuffiness, and fullness in the chest, add Chenpi to move qi and resolve stagnation. If complicated with phlegm-dampness obstructing the lung and cough with much phlegm, add Chenpi and Banxia to drain dampness and resolve phlegm, namely Liujunzi Tang (Six Gentlemen Decoction). If complicated with dampness syndrome, with symptoms shown as limbs lack of strength, emaciation, food accumulation, vomiting or diarrhea, stuffiness and fullness in the stomach and abdominal, sallow complexion, pale tongue, white slimy fur, and vacuous and moderate pulse, add Lianzi, Yiyiren, Sharen, Jiegeng, Baibiandou, and Shanyao to tonify qi and fortify spleen, drain dampness, and check diarrhea, namely Shen Ling Baizhu San (Ginseng, Poria, and Bighead Atractylodes Powder).

Buzhongyiqi Tang (Tonify and Replenish Middle Qi Decoction)

Ingredients (Table 2.30)

Administration

All medicines above are decocted in water, for oral use.

Effects

Tonify and replenish the middle qi, and upraise the sunken qi.

Application

This prescription is for the qi deficiency and sunken middle qi syndrome. This syndrome is characterized by torpid intake, lack of strength, sloppy stool, fever, spontaneous sweating, thirst with desire for hot drink, rectocele or prolapse of uterus, chronic diarrhea or dysentery, metrorrhagia and metrostaxis, pale and enlarged tongue, and thin and white fur. It can be used for organ prolapse, chronic

Table 2.30 Ingredients of Buzhongyiqi Tang			
	Huangqi	Radix Astragali seu Hedysari	18 g
	Renshen	Radix ginseng	6 g
	Baizhu	Rhizoma Atractylodis Macrocephalae	9 g
	Zhigancao	Radix Glycyrrhizae	9 g
	Danggui	Radix Angelicae Sinensis	3 g
	Chenpi	Pericarpium Citri Reticulatae	6 g
	Shengma	Rhizoma Cimicifugae	6 g
	Chaihu	Radix Bupleuri	6 g

gastroenteritis, chronic dysentery, myasthenia gravis, chronic hepatitis, chronic low fever of undetermined origin, hypermenorrhea, and other diseases belonging to qi deficiency and sunken middle qi syndrome.

Analysis

The syndrome treated by this prescription is caused by qi deficiency of spleen-stomach, bright yang failing to raise, even with middle qi sunken. This syndrome should be dealt with treatment methods as tonifying qi and raising yang.

1. Sovereign medicine: Huangqi.
   A heavy dosage of Huangqi for tonifying and replenishing the middle qi, raising yang qi.
2. Minister medicine: Renshen, Baizhu, and Zhigancao.
   Tonify qi to fortify spleen, strengthen the tonifying and replenishing middle qi effect of Huangqi.
3. Assistant and courier medicines: Danggui, Chenpi, Shengma, and Chaihu.
   Danggui nourish blood to tonify deficiency, assist Huangqi to tonify qi and generate blood. Chenpi regulate qi to harmonize stomach, preventing tonifying from stagnation. Combine some Shengma and Chaihu, and raise the sunken middle qi when tonifying.

Modification

If used for organ prolapse or myasthenia gravis, add Zhishi to assist the raising qi effect. If used for hypermenorrhea with syndrome of qi failing to control the blood, add Haipiaoxiao to constrain and stop bleeding. If complicated with abdominal pain, add Baishao to smooth liver and check pain.

Notes

It is forbidden for patients who with dampness pathogen and deficiency heat.

Siwu Tang (Four-Ingredient Decoction)

Ingredients (Table 2.31)

Table 2.31 Ingredients of Siwu Tang

Shudihuang	Radix Rehmanniae Praeparata	12 g
Danggui	Radix Angelicae Sinensis	9 g
Baishao	Radix Paeoniae Alba	9 g
Chuanxiong	Rhizoma Ligustici chuanxiong	6 g

Administration

All medicines above are decocted in water, for oral use.

Effects

Nourish and harmonize the blood.

Application

This prescription is for the deficiency and stagnation of nutrient blood syndrome. This syndrome is characterized by palpitation and inability to sleep, dizzies, pale complexion, or irregular menstruation, scanty menstruation or amenorrhea, dull pain in abdominal, pale tongue, and fine pulse. It can be used for irregular menstruation, chronic skin diseases like chronic eczema and lichen, orthopedics diseases, anaphylactoid purpura, nerve headache, and other diseases belonging to deficiency and stagnation of nutrient blood syndrome.

Analysis

The syndrome treated by this prescription is caused by deficiency of nutrient blood and blood moving unsmooth. This syndrome should be dealt with treatment methods as nourishing and harmonize the blood.

1. Sovereign medicine: Shudihuang.
     Nourish the yin and blood.
2. Minister medicine: Danggui.
     Tonify blood and nourish the liver, harmonize the blood, and regulate the vessels.
3. Assistant medicine: Baishao and Chuanxiong.
     Baishao nourishes blood, soothes the liver, and harmonizes the nutrient. Chuanxiong activates blood and moves qi, preventing nourishing from stagnation.
     In this prescription, the sovereign and the minister focus on nourishing nutrient blood, while the assistants on nourishing with moving the blood and qi. All medicines combine; on the one hand, nourish the blood but not stagnate. On the other hand, move blood but not damage the blood.

Modification

If complicated with qi deficiency, lassitude of spirit, and shortage of qi, add Renshen and Huangqi to tonify qi for nourishing blood. If complicated with obvious stasis, dysmenorrhea, change Baishao to Chishao, add Taoren and Honghua to strengthen the activating blood and relieving stasis effect, namely Taohong Siwu Tang. If complicated with cold syndrome, abdominal pain and desire for warm, add Rougui,

Paojiang, and Wuzhuyu to warm and free the meridian. If complicated with heat syndrome and dryness of mouth and throat, change Shudihuang to Dihuang, add Huangqin and Mudanpi to clear heat, and cool the blood.

Notes

It is forbidden for irregular menstruation with serious stasis, stabbing pain in abdominal, or collapse of blood and qi.

Guipi Tang (Fortifying Spleen Decoction)

Ingredients (Table 2.32)

Administration

Grind the above medicines into coarser powder, decocted 12 g each time with Shengjiang 6 g and Dazao 3 pcs, for oral use.

Effects

Supplement qi and tonify blood, fortify spleen, and nourish heart.

Application

This prescription is for the syndrome of dual deficiency of qi and blood of spleen and heart or syndrome of spleen failing to control the blood. This syndrome is characterized by palpitation, amnesia and inability to sleep, torpid intake, lack of strength, sallow complexion, or metrorrhagia and metrostaxis, hemafecia, premature menstruation in large amount and pale color, pale tongue, thin and white fur, and fine and weak pulse. It can be used for neurasthenia, insomnia, and cardiovascular disease belonging to syndrome of dual deficiency of qi and blood of spleen

Table 2.32 Ingredients of Guipi Tang

Huangqi	Radix Astragali seu Hedysari	12 g
Longyanrou	Arillus Longan	12 g
Renshen	Radix ginseng	6 g
Baizhu	Rhizoma Atractylodis Macrocephalae	9 g
Danggui	Radix Angelicae Sinensis	9 g
Fushen	Poria contain pine root	9 g
Suanzaoren	Semen Ziziphi Spinosae	12 g
Yuanzhi	Radix Polygalae	6 g
Muxiang	Radix Aucklandiae	6 g
Zhigancao	Radix Glycyrrhizae	3 g

and heart, hemorrhage of stomach and duodenal ulcer, functional uterine bleeding, thrombocytopenic purpura, and other diseases belonging to syndrome of spleen failing to control the blood.

Analysis

The syndrome treated by worry beyond measure, fatigue damaging heart and spleen, spleen failing to transport, and heart loosing nourished. This syndrome should be dealt with treatment methods as supplementing qi and tonifying blood, fortifying spleen, and nourishing heart.

1. Sovereign medicine: Huangqi and Longyanrou.
   Huangqi supplements qi and fortifies spleen. Longyanrou nourishes blood and tranquilizes. This combination can dually tonify the qi and blood.
2. Minister medicine: Renshen, Baizhu, and Danggui.
   Renshen and Baizhu support Huangqi to tonify qi. Danggui support Longyanrou to nourish blood.
3. Assistant medicine: Fushen, Suanzaoren, Yuanzhi, and Muxiang.
   Fushen, Suanzaoren, and Yuanzhi calm heart to tranquilize. Muxiang regulate qi to invigorate spleen.
4. Courier medicine: Zhigancao.
   On the one hand, tonify qi with harmonize the middle. On the other hand, harmonize all the medicines.
   When decocted this prescription, add Shengjiang and Dazao to regulate spleen and stomach, for support the generating and transforming.

Modification

If complicated with serious blood deficiency, add Shudihuang to strengthen the nourishing blood effect. If bleed syndrome complicated with cold, add charcoals of Aiye and Paojiang to warm the vessels and check bleeding. If bleed syndrome complicated with heat, add charcoals of Dihuang and Zonglv to cool blood and check bleeding.

Liuwei Dihuang Wan (Six Ingredients with Rehmanniae Pill)

Ingredients (Table 2.33)

Table 2.33 Ingredients of Liuwei Dihuang

Shudihuang	Radix Rehmanniae PRAEPARATA	24 g
Shanzhuyu	Fructus Corni	12 g
Shanyao	Rhizoma Dioscoreae	12 g
Zexie	Rhizoma Alismatis	9 g
Fuling	Poria	9 g
Mudanpi	Cortex Moutan Radicis	9 g

Administration

For pills with honey, take 6 ~ 9 g each time and thrice 1 day with warm water or light salt brinc. All medicines above are decocted in water, for oral use.

Effects

Nourish yin and tonify kidney.

Application

This prescription is for the kidney yin deficiency syndrome. This syndrome is characterized by soreness and weakness of waist and knees, dizziness, tinnitus or deafness, night sweating, emission, wasting-thirst, bone steaming and tidal fever, feverishness in palms and soles, tongue dryness and throat pain, gomphiasis, heel pain, dribbling urination, infant fontanel not closed, red tongue, little fur, and fine and rapid pulse. It can be used for chronic nephritis, hypertension, diabetes, tuberculosis, nephrotuberculosis, hyperthyroidism, anovulia functional uterine bleeding, climacteric syndrome, and other diseases belonging to kidney yin deficiency syndrome.

Analysis

The syndrome treated by this prescription is caused by deficiency of kidney yin and deficiency fire flaming upward. This syndrome should be dealt with treatment methods as nourishing yin and tonifying kidney.

1. Sovereign medicine: Shudihuang.
   Nourish the yin and tonify kidney, and strengthen and nourish marrow and essence.
2. Minister medicine: Shanzhuyu and Shanyao.
   Shanzhuyu tonifies liver and kidney and astringes essence. Shanyao tonifies spleen and kidney and secures essence.
3. Assistant medicine: Zexie, Mudanpi, and Fuling.
   Zexie drains dampness and purges turbidity, preventing Shudihuang from greasy. Mudanpi clears liver and purges fire, countering the warm nature of Shanzhuyu. Fuling drains spleen dampness, assisting Shanyao to promote transportation.
   In this prescription, three tonics combine three purgation to be a treatment method as nourishing and tonifying yin with purging fire. Spleen, liver, and kidney would be tonified at the same time, but mostly the kidney yin.

Modification

If yin deficiency complicated with flame fire, add Zhimu and Huangbai to strengthen the cleaning heat and purging fire effect, namely Zhibai Dihuang Wan. If complicated with liver-yin deficiency and blurred vision, add Gouqizi and Juhua to nourish

Table 2.34 Ingredients of Shenqi Wan

Fuzi	Radix Aconiti Lateralis Preparata	3 g
Guizhi	Ramulus Cinnamomi	3 g
Shudihuang	Radix Rehmanniae Praeparata	24 g
Shanzhuyu	Fructus Corni	12 g
Shanyao	Rhizoma Dioscoreae	12 g
Zexie	Rhizoma Alismatis	9 g
Fuling	Poria	9 g
Mudanpi	Cortex Moutan Radicis	9 g

liver and clear eyes, namely Qiju Dihuang Wan. If complicated with lung yin deficiency, cough and dyspnea, add Maidong and Wuweizi to nourish yin and astringe lung qi, namely Maiwei Dihuang Wan.

Shenqi Wan (Kidney Qi Pill)

Ingredients (Table 2.34)

Administration

For pills with honey, take 6 ~ 9 g each time and twice 1 day with warm water or light salt brine. All medicines above are decocted in water, for oral use.

Effects

Nourish yang and tonify kidney.

Application

This prescription is for the kidney yang deficiency syndrome. This syndrome is characterized by soreness and weakness of waist and knees, sense of coldness in lower body, lower abdominal contracture, inhibited urination, or spontaneous urination, pale and enlarged tongue, and weak pulse with sunken and fine in chi. Phlegm fluid, edema, wasting-thirst, dermatophytosis, and shifted bladder can be seen in this syndrome. This prescription can be used for chronic nephritis, renal edema, diabetes, hypothyroidism, neurasthenia, hypoadrenocorticism, repeated attack of bronchial asthma, climacteric syndrome, and other diseases belonging to kidney yang deficiency syndrome.

Analysis

The syndrome treated by this prescription is caused by deficiency of kidney yang, failing to transform qi to move water. This syndrome should be dealt with treatment methods as nourishing the kidney yang.

1. Sovereign medicine: Fuzi and Guizhi.
   Warm-tonify kidney yang.
2. Minister medicine: Shudihuang, Shanzhuyu, and Shanyao.
   Nourish kidney yin. The combination of sovereign and minister is aimed at pursuing yang from yin, for strengthen the tonifying yang effect. Less medicines for tonifying yang with more medicines for nourishing yin, meaning that generating fire slightly to encourage the kidney qi.
3. Assistant medicine: Zexie, Mudanpi, and Fuling.
   The assistant combination induces diuresis to drain dampness and promote blood circulation and prevents tonic from greasy.

   All medicines combine, warm but not dryness, nourishing but not greasy, for encouraging kidney yang, recovering qi transformation, and then all syndromes gone.

Modification

In this prescription, Guizhi and changed to Rougui, for strengthening the warm yang effect. If complicated obvious edema, add Cheqianzi and Niuxi to induce diuresis to alleviate edema. If complicated with impotence, add Yinyanghuo, Buguzhi, and Bajitian to invigorate yang and raise impotence.

Notes

It is forbidden for patients who with dryness of mouth and throat, red tongue, and little fur.

2.4.13 Astringent Prescriptions

2.4.13.1 Concept

Those that are mainly composed of astringent medicines, with the effect of securing and astringing, used for consumption and prostration syndrome of qi, blood, essence, fluid, and liquid, are known as astringent prescription.

2.4.13.2 Classification

Kinds of consumption and prostration syndromes of qi, blood, essence, fluid, and liquid are different in pathogenic factor and location, even the clinical manifestation. Accordingly, astringent prescription can be divided into four categories: securing the exterior to check sweating prescription, astringing the intestines and check diarrhea prescription, securing essence to check emission prescription, and securing the chong vessel and stanching vaginal discharge prescription.

2.4.13.3   Notes

It is caution that pathogenic factor would be astringed when using astringent pre-scription. This kind of prescription is forbidden for prostration syndrome such as sweating with heat diseases, diarrhea with food accumulation, emission with fire interruption, and metrorrhagia with blood heat. In case of deficiency complicated by excess, it is necessary to combine medicines for expelling pathogenic factor, do not use medicines for astringing only.

Muli San (Oyster Shell Powder)

Ingredients (Table 2.35)

Administration

Grind the above medicines into fine powder, and decoct 9 g each time and twice 1 day with Xiaomai 30 g, for oral use in warm without residue.

Effects

Enrich qi to secure the exterior, and astringent yin and check sweating.

Application

This prescription is for qi deficiency and exterior insecurity syndrome of spontane-ous sweating and night sweating. This syndrome is characterized by always sweat-ing, worsen in sleeping, palpitation and feeling apprehensive, lack of strength, vexation, pale red tongue, and fine and week pules. It can be used for spontaneous sweating and night sweating caused by weak after the illness, operation, and childbirth.

Analysis

The syndrome treated by this prescription is caused by qi deficiency and defense-exterior insecurity, leakage of yin fluid, and heart yang damaging heart yin. This syndrome should be dealt with treatment methods as follow: Enrich qi to secure the exterior, and astringent yin to check sweating.

Table 2.35 Ingredients of Muli San

Duanmuli	Calcined Concha Ostreae	30 g
Huangqi	Radix Astragali seu Hedysari	30 g
Mahuanggen	Radix Ephedrae	30 g

1. Sovereign medicine: Duanmuli.
   Astringe yin to check sweating, and suppress yang.
2. Minister medicine: Huangqi.
   Enrich qi to secure the exterior, for checking sweating.
3. Assistant medicine: Mahuanggen and Xiaomai.
   Mahuanggen is specialized in astringing to check sweating. Xiaomai nourish heart to remove vexation.

Modification

If complicated with limbs cold, aversion to cold, and desiring for warm, add Fuzi to enrich yang to expel cold. If complicated with lack of strength, worsening after movement, use heavy dosage of Huangqi and add Renshen and Baizhu to enrich qi and tonify deficiency. If complicated with serious yin deficiency, dryness of mouth, and red tongue, add Dihuang and Baishao to nourish yin and astringe fluid.

Notes

Because the astringing nature, it is caution for patients who with interior heat or phlegm dampness.

2.4.14 Harmonizing Prescriptions

2.4.14.1 Concept

Those that are with the effect of harmonizing and regulating, used for cold damage disease in shaoyang meridian, unharmonization of liver and spleen, cold-heat complex, and dual disease of the exterior and interior, are known as harmonizing prescription.

2.4.14.2 Classification

According to pathogen location, the harmonizing prescription can be divided into four categories: harmonizing shaoyang prescription, regulating liver and spleen prescription, regulating cold and heat prescription, and dually releasing exterior-interior prescription.

2.4.14.3   Notes

When using the harmonizing prescription, the dosage of medicine is going to be weighed based on distinguishing of primary and secondary syndrome between zang and fu, and exterior and interior.

Xiaochaihu Tang (Minor Bupleurum Decoction)

Ingredients (Table 2.36)

Administration

All medicines above are decocted in water, for oral use.

Effects

Harmonize and regulate shaoyang.

Application

This prescription is for cold damage disease with shaoyang syndrome. This syndrome is characterized by alternating chills and fever, fullness and discomfort in chest and hypochondrium, vexation in heart, vomiting, bitter taste in mouth, dryness in throat, thin and white tongue fur, and string-like pulse. It can be used for common cold, flu, chronic hepatitis, acute and chronic cholecystitis, pleuritis, nephropyelitis, gastric ulcer, postpartum infection, and other diseases belonging to shaoyang syndrome.

Table 2.36 Ingredients of Xiaochaihu Tang

Chaihu	Radix Bupleuri	9 g
Huangqin	Radix Scutellariae	6 g
Banxia	Rhizoma Pinelliae	6 g
Shengjiang	Rhizoma Zingiberis Recens	6 g
Renshen	Radix ginseng	6 g
Zhigancao	Radix Glycyrrhizae	3 g
Dazao	Fructus Jujubae	4 pcs

Analysis

The syndrome treated by this prescription is caused by pathogenic factor in the shaoyang meridian, heathy qi, and pathogenic qi conflicting in half-exterior and half-interior. This syndrome should be dealt with treatment methods as harmonizing and regulating shaoyang.

1. Sovereign medicine: Chaihu.
    Expel the pathogenic factor of half-exterior, and regulate and free the qi stagnation of shaoyang.
2. Minister medicine: Huangqin.
    Clear and purge the heat of half-interior. The combination of Chaihu and Huangqin is expelling and the other cleaning, reliving the pathogenic factor of shaoyang together, known as the important combination of harmonizing and regulating shaoyang.
3. Assistant medicine: Banxia, Shengjiang, Renshen, and Dazao.
    Banxia and Shengjiang harmonize the stomach to check vomiting. Renshen and Dazao tonify qi to support the health qi, enriching interior to prevent pathogen entering the interior.
4. Assistant and Courier medicine: Zhigancao.
    On the one hand, tonify qi to assist the Renshen and Dazao. On the other hand, harmonize all the medicines.

Modification

If complicated with vexation but not vomiting, that is, heat stagnation in the chest, subduct Banxia and Renshen, add Gualou to clear heat and regulate qi movement to free chest. If heat damaging fluid, complicated with thirst, subduct Banxia and add Tianhuafen to generate fluid to check thirst. If liver qi invading the spleen, complicated with abdominal pain, subduct Huangqin and add Baishao to emolliate the liver and check pain.

Notes

It is caution for shaoyang syndrome with deficiency of yin and blood because of Chaihu dispelling, and Huangqin and Banxia drying.

Xiaoyao San (Ease Powder)

Ingredients (Table 2.37)

Table 2.37 Ingredients of Xiaoyao San

Chaihu	Radix Bupleuri	9 g
Baishao	Radix Paeoniae Alba	9 g
Danggui	Radix Angelicae Sinensis	9 g
Baizhu	Rhizoma Atractylodis Macrocephalae	9 g
Fuling	Poria	9 g
Zhigancao	Radix Glycyrrhizae	6 g

Administration

Grind the above medicines into fine powder, taken 9 g each time and twice 1 day with decoction of little Weishengjiang and Bohe for oral use. All medicines above are decocted in water, for oral use.

Effects

Soothe liver to relive stagnation, and nourish blood to fortify spleen.

Application

This prescription is for liver depression and deficiency of spleen and blood syndrome. This syndrome is characterized by hypochondrium pain, headache and dizziness, dryness of mouth and throat, lassitude of spirit, or alternating chills and fever, or irregular menstruation, distending pain in the breast, pale red tongue, and fine and string-like pulse. It can be used for chronic hepatitis, cholelithiasis, stomach and duodenal ulcer, chronic gastritis, gastrointestinal neurosis, premenstrual tension, lobules of mammary gland, climacteric syndrome, chronic pelvic inflammatory disease, and other diseases belonging to liver depression and deficiency of spleen and blood syndrome.

Analysis

The syndrome treated by this prescription is caused by liver stagnation for long, consumption of yin-blood, liver stagnation invading the spleen, and spleen failing to transport. This syndrome should be dealt with treatment methods as soothing liver to relive stagnation, nourishing blood to fortify spleen.

1. Sovereign medicine: Chaihu.
    Soothe liver to relive stagnation.
2. Minister medicine: Baishao and Danggui.
    Nourish blood and astringent yin, soothe liver, and relive urgency.
3. Assistant medicine: Fuling and Baizhu.
    Enrich qi to tonify the middle, fortify spleen to support transportation, and enrich spleen to prevent liver invading, for nourishing the generating source of qi and blood.
4. Assistant and Courier medicine: Zhigancao.
    As assistant, tonify qi to support the assistant. As courier, harmonize all the medicines.

Modification

If liver stagnation transformed to fire, complicated with bitter taste and dryness in mouth, add Mudanpi and Zhizi to purge liver fire, namely Jiawei Xiaoyao San. If complicated with serious deficiency of blood, pale complexion, dizziness, and pale tongue, add Shudihuang to nourish yin and blood, namely Heixiaoyao San.

Table 2.38 Ingredients of
Banxia Xiexin Tang

Banxia	Rhizoma Pinelliae	12 g
Ganjiang	Rhizoma Zingiberis	9 g
Huanglian	Rhizoma Coptidis	3 g
Huangqin	Radix Scutellariae	9 g
Renshen	Radix ginseng	9 g
Dazao	Fructus Jujubae	4 pcs
Zhigancao	Radix Glycyrrhizae	9 g

Banxia Xiexin Tang (Pinellia Heart-Draining Decoction)

Ingredients (Table 2.38)

Administration

All medicines above are decocted in water, for oral use.

Effects

Mildly regulate cold and heat, and relieve stuffiness and masses.

Application

This prescription is for stuffiness syndrome of cold and heat inter-stagnation. This syndrome is characterized by stuffiness and fullness but no pain in the upper abdomen, retching or vomiting, borborygmus and diarrhea, thin yellow and slimy tongue fur, and rapid and string-like pulse. It can be used for acute and chronic gastroenteritis, chronic colitis, nervous gastritis, chronic hepatitis, chronic cholecystitis, and other diseases belonging to excess deficiency and cold-heat complex, manifested as stuffiness, vomiting, and diarrhea.

Analysis

The syndrome treated by this prescription is caused by deficiency of middle yang, inter-stagnation of cold and heat, and disorder of upward and downward qi movement. This syndrome should be dealt with treatment methods as mildly regulating cold and heat, relieving stuffiness and masses.

1. Sovereign medicine: Banxia.
   Relieve stuffiness and masses, harmonize stomach, and descend adverse qi.
2. Minister medicine: Ganjiang, Huanglian, and Huangqin.
   Ganjiang combine Banxia to relive stuffiness, harmonize middle and dispel cold. Huanglian and Huangqin purge and clear heat.

3. Assistant medicine: Renshen and Dazao.

 Renshen and Dazao tonify qi to support the health qi, combine Ganjiang to warm middle and tonify deficiency, fortify spleen, and nourish stomach.
4. Assistant and Courier medicine: Zhigancao.

 On the one hand, tonify qi to assist the Renshen and Dazao. On the other hand, harmonize all the medicines.

 The medicines in this prescription include the functions of warming and clearing and the effects of tonify and reduction. Pungent medicines can dispel while bitter ones can descend, and then, cold-heat will be driven out and qi's up-downward movement recovered. Finally, stuffiness and fullness will be resolved, and vomiting and diarrhea are treated.

Modification

If stuffiness with vomiting, while the deficiency syndrome is not so serious, subduct Renshen and Dazao and add Zhishi and Shengjiang to regulate qi and harmonize stomach to stop vomiting.

Notes

It is forbidden for stomach stuffiness and fullness due to qi stagnation or food accumulation.

2.4.15 Resuscitative Prescriptions

2.4.15.1 Concept

Those that are mainly composed of medicines for causing resuscitation with aromatics, with the effect of opening the orifices and resuscitating, used for syndrome of orifice block with unconsciousness, are known as resuscitative prescription.

2.4.15.2 Classification

In a general way, syndrome of orifice blocks with unconsciousness includes two kinds such as heat block and cold block. Accordingly, resuscitative prescription can be divided into two categories: Cold resuscitative prescription and warm resuscitative prescription.

2.4.15.3 Notes

Orifice block syndrome is mainly caused by pathogenic factors such as warm-heat, phlegm-heat, qi stagnation, and turbid phlegm, blocking the heart orifices. Unconsciousness characterizes orifice block syndrome, but it is not all caused by heart orifice block. Therefore, when using the resuscitative prescription, unconsciousness due to collapse syndrome or heat accumulation in yangming must be excluded. What is more, aromatics medicines cannot be decocted to prevent the volatilizing of active ingredients and declining of curative effect. So resuscitative prescription is always made into power and pills. Finally, the pungent nature of the prescription is easy to damage original qi and fetus qi. For this reason, resuscitative prescription is mainly used as first aid and will be stopped immediately when it takes effect. It will not be taken for long, also caution for pregnant women.

Angong Niuhuang Wan (Peaceful Palace Bezoar Pill)

Ingredients (Table 2.39)

Administration

Grind the above medicines into fine powder made into pills with honey, weighing 3 g each. Take one pill each time and once or twice 1 day.

Effects

Clear heat and open orifices, sweep phlegm, and detoxify.

Table 2.39 Ingredients of Angong Niuhuang Wan

Niuhuang	Calculus Bovis	30 g
Shexiang	Moschus	7.5 g
Shuiniujiao	Cornu Bubali	30 g
Huanglian	Rhizoma Coptidis	30 g
Huangqin	Radix Scutellariae	30 g
Zhizi	Fructus Gardeniae	30 g
Bingpian	Borneolum Syntheticum	7.5 g
Yujin	Radix Curcumae	30 g
Zhenzhu	Margarita	15 g
Zhusha	Cinnabaris	30 g
Xionghuang	Realgar	30 g

Application

This prescription is for heat pathogen inward invading into pericardium syndrome. This syndrome is characterized by high fever, agitation, unconsciousness with delirious speech, dryness of mouth and tongue, exuberant phlegm accumulation, red or crimson tongue, and rapid pulse. It can be used for stroke, epidemic encephalitis B, epidemic cerebrospinal meningitis, toxic dysentery, uremia, hepatic coma, and other diseases belonging to heat pathogen inward invading into pericardium syndrome.

Analysis

The syndrome treated by this prescription is caused by warm-heat pathogen inward invading into pericardium and orifices confused by phlegm-heat. This syndrome should be dealt with treatment methods as cleaning heat and opening orifices, sweeping phlegm, and detoxifying.

1. Sovereign medicine: Niuhuang and Shexiang.

   Niuhuang clears heart and detoxifies, extinguishes wind to tranquilize fright, sweeps phlegm, and opens orifices. Shexiang frees the twelve meridians, opens orifices, and induces resuscitation. This combination aims at cleaning heart and opening orifices.
2. Minister medicine: Shuiniujiao, Huanglian, Huangqin, Zhizi, Bingpian, and Yujin.

   Shuiniujiao, Huanglian, Huangqin, and Zhizi clear heat, purge fire, and detoxify, supporting the Niuhuang to clear pericardium heat. Bingpian and Yujin repel foulness and open the block, supporting Shexiang to open orifices and induce resuscitation.
3. Assistant medicine: Zhusha, Zhenzhu, and Xionghuang.

   Zhusha and Zhenzhu settle the heart to tranquilize, for reliving vexation. Xionghuang assist the Niuhuang to sweep phlegm and detoxify.
4. Courier medicine: honey.

   For pills with honey, harmonize the stomach and regulate the middle.

Modification

If complicated with replete and strong pulse, take it with decoction of Jinyinhua and Bohe for strengthening the effect of cleaning heat and expelling the pathogenic factor. If complicated with week pulse, take it with decoction of Renshen for strengthening the effect of supporting healthy qi to expel pathogenic factor. If complicated with yangming fu viscera excess syndrome, unconsciousness, and constipation, dissolve two pills and take with powder of Dahuang 9 g, namely Niuhuang Chengqi Tang.

2.5   Summary

Prescription is the important part of the mode of thinking for Chinese medicine (theory, principle, prescription, and medicine). The forming of one prescription is based on the treatment method of Chinese medicine and the structure of sovereign, minister, assistant, and courier. Most prescriptions are only used for the specific syndrome and disease.

When using prescriptions to treat diseases, it is necessary to comprehensively analyze the data gained by the four methods of diagnosis, accurately differentiate the syndrome, and then select the appropriate prescription, and add or subtract ingredients according to the syndrome and the course of disease.

The combination and effect of some prescriptions are similar, but they all have obvious differences, and they need to be identified when they are used. At the same time, many prescriptions have clear contraindications and should be used carefully.

Questions
1. What is the forming principles of the prescriptions?
2. What is the effect of changes in the combination of the prescriptions on the effect?
3. Which prescription should be selected to be basic prescription when treating cold with wind-cold and wind-heat? Why?
4. What are the differences in the combination, effect, and application of Liuwei Dihuang Wan and Shenqi Wan?
5. What are the similarities and differences between Sijunzi Tang and Buzhongyiqi Tang?
6. What is the role of Chaihu in Xiaochaihu Tang and Xiaoyao San?

Chapter 3
Basic Knowledge of Acupuncture and Moxibustion

Zhonghua Yang, Liang Zhang, Lilong Tang, Wenzhan Tu, Shanshan Qu, and Yong Huang

Objectives

Master the concepts of meridian, collateral, and acupoint.

Master the regularities of the 12 meridians, methods for locating acupoints, locations, indications, and manipulations of frequently used acupoints.

Master manipulations, indications, and precautions of filiform needle therapy, moxibustion therapy, cupping therapy, three-edged needle therapy, skin needle therapy, intradermal needle therapy, electroacupuncture, scalp acupuncture, and auricular acupuncture.

Master the principles of acupuncture and moxibustion treatment.

Familiar with the components of the meridian and collateral system, functions and contents of the special points, and the courses of the 12 meridians, governor vessel, and conception vessel.

Know the effects of the 8 extra meridians, the 15 collaterals, the 12 divergent meridians, tendons along the 12 meridians and the 12 skin regions.

Z. Yang · L. Zhang
Guangzhou University of Chinese Medicine, Guangzhou, China

L. Tang
Ningxia Medical University, Yinchuan, Ningxia, China

W. Tu
Wenzhou Medical University, Wenzhou, China

S. Qu
Southern Medical University, Guangzhou, China

Y. Huang (✉)
School of Traditional Chinese Medicine, Southern Medical University, Guangzhou, China

© Zhengzhou University Press 2024
Y. Huang, L. Zhu (eds.), *Textbook of Traditional Chinese Medicine*,
https://doi.org/10.1007/978-981-99-5299-1_3

Guideline

There are three parts in this chapter. Part one is an introduction to the meridians and acupoints, including the basic concepts and the functions of the meridian system and acupoints, the courses of the meridians, locations and indications of the acupoints. Part two introduces various techniques of acupuncture and moxibustion, including filiform needle therapy, moxibustion therapy, cupping therapy, and other frequently used acupuncture techniques. Part three is clinical application of acupuncture and moxibustion, including the function and the principles of acupuncture and moxibustion treatment, selections of acupoints, selections of acupuncture and moxibustion techniques clinically.

3.1 Introduction

Acupuncture and moxibustion discipline is a subject using meridian theory and techniques of acupuncture and moxibustion to prevent and cure diseases, which is guided by the theory of traditional Chinese medicine. As an important component of traditional Chinese medicine, after a long process of development, acupuncture and moxibustion discipline has gradually become an independent subject with rich theoretical contents and high clinical application value.

Acupuncture and moxibustion have the following characteristics. Firstly, they are widely used in various clinical diseases and have significant curative effect. Secondly, adverse reactions happen infrequently if standardized manipulations of acupuncture and moxibustion are strictly followed. Thirdly, necessary instruments such as needles, moxa, and disinfection materials are small in size and convenient for the doctor to carry. So acupuncture and moxibustion are suitable for emergency treatment especially. Acupuncture and moxibustion originated in China. They not only play an important role in reproduction and prosperity of the Chinese nation, but also make a great contribution to the development of the world medicine. Today, acupuncture and moxibustion are applied in more and more countries and regions.

3.2 General Introduction to Meridians and Collaterals

3.2.1 The Basic Concepts of Meridians and Collaterals

Meridians and collaterals are pathways that transport qi and blood, and connect the zang-fu viscera with the surface and other parts of the body. Meridians mean main paths or straight lines. Collaterals refer to branches that separate from the meridians and distribute throughout the body like a net.

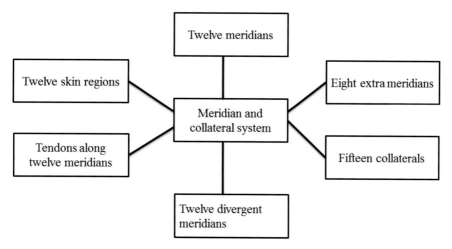

Fig. 3.1 The meridian and collateral system

The meridian and collateral system consists of the 12 meridians, the 8 extra meridians, the 15 collaterals, the 12 divergent meridians, tendons along the 12 meridians, and the 12 skin regions as listed in Fig. 3.1.

3.2.2   The 12 Meridians

3.2.2.1   The Nomenclature of the 12 Meridians

The nomenclature of the 12 meridians comprises 3 elements: hand and foot, yin and yang, and viscera viscera. Hand and foot refers to the external distribution and origin or termination of a meridian on upper or lower limb. Yin and yang designates the nature of the meridian. There are three hand and foot pairs of yin and three hand and foot pairs of yang meridians. Those with the most abundant yin are called taiyin; those with a lesser amount are called shaoyin; those with the least are called jueyin. Similarly those with the most abundant yang are called yangming; those with a lesser amount are called taiyang; those with the least are called shaoyang. Each yin meridian is also paired with its corresponding yang meridian to form six interior and exteriorly related pairs: hand taiyin and hand yangming; foot yangming and foot taiyin; hand shaoyin and hand taiyang; foot taiyang and foot shaoyin; hand jueyin and hand shaoyang; foot shaoyang and foot jueyin.

In the 12 meridians, qi circulates cyclically; beginning with the lung meridian of hand taiyin, it moves through the meridians one by one. After the 12th, the liver meridian of foot jueyin, it reenters the lung meridian to circulate again.

3.2.2.2 The Distribution Regularities of the 12 Meridians

1. Exterior distribution
   (a) The four limbs: The three yin meridians of hand run sequentially on the medial or palmar aspect of the upper limb; from anterior to posterior, the order is hand taiyin, hand jueyin, and hand shaoyin. The three yang meridians of hand run sequentially on the lateral or dorsal aspect of the upper limb; from anterior to posterior, the order is hand yangming, hand shaoyang, and hand taiyang. The three yin and three yang meridians of foot are similarly distributed on the lower limb, with the three yin meridians of foot ordered on the medial portion from anterior to posterior and the three yang meridians of foot on the lateral aspect from anterior to posterior. In an exception to this arrangement, the liver meridian of foot jueyin runs anterior to the spleen meridian of foot taiyin until the two meridians intersect eight cun above the medial malleolus where the liver meridian of foot jueyin returns to its regular position between the spleen meridian of foot taiyin and the kidney meridian of foot shaoyin.
   (b) The head, face, and trunk: The three yin meridians of hand run from the chest to the medial or palmar aspect of the hand. The three yin meridians of foot begin at the foot and end at the abdomen and the chest region. All the yang meridians either begin or end at the head and face region; as the saying goes, "the head is the convergence of all yang meridians." The three yang meridians of hand are not externally distributed on the trunk. They begin at the lateral aspect of the hand and end at the head or face. The 3 yang meridians of foot travel from head to the foot and are the longest of the 12 meridians. The stomach meridian of foot yangming travels on the anterior aspect of the body; the gallbladder meridian of foot shaoyang, on the lateral aspect; the bladder meridian of foot taiyang, on the posterior aspect.

2. Interior distribution
   Interior distribution of the 12 meridians refers to the portion of each meridian that enters the chest and abdomen internally to connect with the related zang-fu viscera and tissues. Each of the 12 meridians belongs to its respective zang-fu organ. As zang-viscera belong to yin and fu-viscera belong to yang, the three yin meridians of hand connect with the chest and belong respectively to the lung, the pericardium and the heart. The three yin meridians of foot connect with the abdomen and belong to the spleen, the liver, and the kidney. The three yang meridians of foot belong to the stomach, the gallbladder, and the urinary bladder. The three yang meridians of hand belong to the large intestine, the triple energizer, and the small intestine.

3. Exterior-Interior relationships of the 12 meridians
   The zang and fu-viscera have exterior-interior relationships with each other. Because the 12 meridians belong to the zang-fu viscera internally, each shares an exterior-interior relationship with its corresponding zang or fu-viscera. The yin

Table 3.1 Exterior-interior relationships of the 12 regular meridians

Interior meridian (yin meridian)	Exterior meridian (yang meridian)
Lung meridian of hand taiyin	Large intestine meridian of hand yangming
Heart meridian of hand shaoyin	Small intestine meridian of hand taiyang
Pericardium meridian of hand jueyin	Triple energizer meridian of hand shaoyang
Spleen meridian of foot taiyin	Stomach meridian of foot yangming
Kidney meridian of foot shaoyin	Bladder meridian of foot taiyang
Liver meridian of foot jueyin	Gallbladder meridian of foot shaoyang

meridians belong to the interior and to zang-viscera; the yang meridians, to the exterior and to fu-viscera. The exterior and interior relationships of yin and yang meridians share pertaining and connecting relationships within the body. Each yin meridian pertains to a zang-viscera and connects to a fu organ, each yang meridian pertains to a fu-viscera and connects to a zang-viscera. For example, the lung meridian of hand taiyin pertains to the lung and connects to the large intestine, the exterior-interior related viscera of the lung; conversely, the large intestine meridian of hand yangming pertains to the large intestine and connects to the lung. According to these exterior-interior, pertaining and connecting relationships, the 12 meridians are divided into 6 pairs (Table 3.1).

The exterior-interior relationships of the 12 meridians are also strengthened by the divergent meridians and collaterals, which facilitate communication and strengthen the connections between the exterior-interior related viscera and the relevant parts and regions of the body.

3.2.2.3 Flow and Entry of Qi and Blood into the 12 Meridians

Movement of qi and blood inside a meridian is known as "flow"; influx of qi and blood from one meridian to another is known as "entry." The general rule is that the three yin meridians of hand travel from chest to hands; the three yang meridians of hand, from hands to head; the three yang meridians of foot, from head to feet; the three yin meridians of foot, from feet to abdomen or chest. The connections between the 12 meridians also follow a pattern:

1. The exterior-interiorly related meridians connect at the extremities; e.g., the lung meridian of hand taiyin and the large intestine meridian of hand yangming connect at the tip of the radial side of the index finger.
2. Yang meridians with the same nomenclature connect at the head and facial region; e.g., the hand and foot yangming meridians connect next to the nose.
3. Yin meridians connect inside the chest; e.g., the spleen meridian of foot taiyin connects with the heart meridian of hand shaoyin inside the heart.

Based on their distribution and conjunction, the 12 meridians connect with each other to form a closed system (Fig. 3.2).

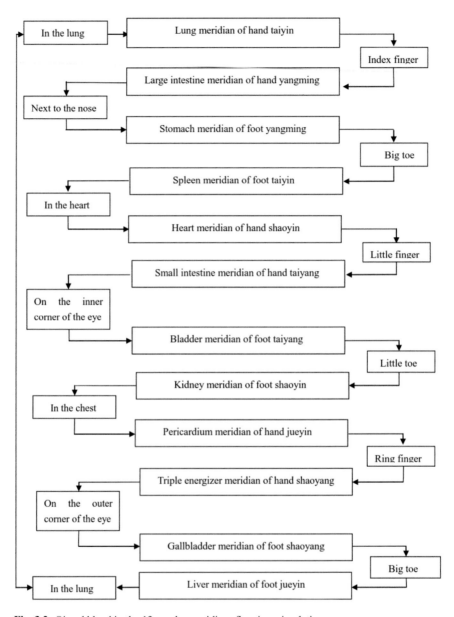

Fig. 3.2 Qi and blood in the 12 regular meridians flow in a circulation

Qi and blood flows continuously inside the closed loop formed by the connection of the 12 meridians in a circulation affected by the patterns of nature. For example, the day may be divided into 12 2-h intervals: the flow of qi and blood in each meridian correlates to one interval, after which it moves to the next meridian following the natural cycle of the earth's movement around the sun. This concept is the foundation of stem-branch acupuncture. In the 8 extra meridians, the conception vessel and the governor vessel were later incorporated into the loop system to form the circulation of the 14 meridians.

3.2.3   The Eight Extra Meridians

The eight extra meridians, governor vessel, conception vessel, chong vessel, belt vessel, yang heel vessel, yin heel vessel, yang link vessel, and yin link vessel, have unique functions, including governing, connecting, and regulating qi and blood within the meridians. They differ from the 12 meridians in that they do not belong directly to zang-fu viscera and have no exterior-interior relationships. However, they are closely related to extraordinary fu-viscera such as the uterus, the brain, and the marrow, and they intersect the 12 meridians. Governor vessel runs along the posterior midline; conception vessel travels the anterior midline. Like the 12 meridians, the governor vessel and conception vessel have points of their own. Thus they are often grouped with the 12 meridians into the arrangement known as the 14 meridians. With no points of their own, the remaining 6 meridians connect with the 12 meridians at various points throughout the body. Chong vessel runs along the first lateral line on the abdomen, where it connects with the kidney meridian of foot shaoyin. The conception vessel, governor vessel, and chong vessel all originate in the uterus (uterus in females; essence chamber in males). These three meridians emerge at the perineum and separate thereafter; hence the saying, "one origin and three divisions." The belt vessel encircles the waist and abdomen like a belt and intersects points on the gallbladder meridian of foot shaoyang. Yang heel vessel runs laterally on the lower limbs and ascends to the shoulder and head; it intersects points on meridians such as the bladder meridian of foot taiyang. Yin heel vessel travels on the medial aspect of the lower limbs and ascends to the head, face, and eye; it intersects the kidney meridian of foot shaoyin. Yang link vessel travels laterally on the lower limbs and ascends to the shoulder, head, and nape of the neck; it intersects points on meridians such as the bladder meridian of foot taiyang and the governor vessel. Yin link vessel travels on the medial aspect of the lower limbs and along the third lateral line of the abdomen to the neck; it intersects points on meridians such as the kidney meridian of foot shaoyin and the conception vessel (Table 3.2).

3.2.4   The 15 Collaterals

The 15 collaterals consist of the 12 collaterals which branch out from the 12 meridians on the limbs; 1 collateral for the conception vessel on the front, 1 collateral for the governor vessel on the back, and the major collateral of the spleen on the lateral side of the trunk. The 12 collaterals strengthen qi and blood communication between exterior-interior related meridians. The 12 collaterals start from the connecting

Table 3.2 Distribution and intersection of the eight extra meridians

Eight extra meridians	Distribution	Intersecting meridians
Governor vessel	Posterior midline	Conception vessel chong vessel, belt vessel, yang link vessel, kidney meridian of foot shaoyin, liver meridian of foot jueyin, three yang meridians of hand, three yang meridians of foot
Conception vessel	Anterior midline	Governor vessel, chong vessel, belt vessel, three yin meridians of foot, triple energizer meridian of hand shaoyang, small intestine meridian of hand taiyang, stomach meridian of foot yangming
Chong vessel	First lateral line on the abdomen	Conception vessel, governor vessel, belt vessel, kidney meridian of foot shaoyin, stomach meridian of foot yangming
Belt vessel	Around the waist	Governor vessel, gallbladder meridian of foot shaoyang, etc.
Yang heel vessel	The lateral aspect of lower limbs, shoulders, and head	Yin heel vessel, bladder meridian of foot taiyang, gallbladder meridian of foot shaoyang, small intestine meridian of hand taiyang, large intestine meridian of hand yangming, stomach meridian of foot yangming
Yin heel vessel	The medial aspect of lower limbs and eyes	Yang heel vessel, bladder meridian of foot taiyang, small intestine meridian of hand taiyang, stomach meridian of foot yangming, kidney meridian of foot shaoyin
Yang link vessel	The lateral aspect of the lower limbs, shoulder, head, and nape	Governor vessel, bladder meridian of foot taiyang, gallbladder meridian of foot shaoyang, small intestine meridian of hand taiyang, triple energizer meridian of hand shaoyang
Yin link vessel	The medial aspect of the lower limbs, the third lateral line on the abdomen, and the neck	Conception vessel, three yin meridians of foot

points on the 12 meridians and go toward their exterior-interiorly paired meridians. The three collaterals on the trunk infuse qi and blood to the anterior, posterior, and the lateral side of the body.

3.2.5 The 12 Divergent Meridians

The 12 divergent meridians are the divergent passages of the 12 meridians which travel deep inside the body in order to strengthen connection between exterior-interior related meridians. Their traveling characteristics can be summarized as "leaving," "entering," "exiting," and "merging." They "leave" from the 12 meridians in the areas above elbow or knee, "enter" thoracic and abdominal cavities, connect with their pertaining and connecting zang-fu viscera, "exit" at the neck or the face, then the yang divergent meridians "merge" with the yang meridians they leave from, while yin divergent meridians "merge" with their exterior-interior related yang meridians. For example, divergent meridian of foot taiyang and divergent meridian of foot shaoyin branch out from bladder meridian and kidney meridian at the popliteal fossa; they enter the body and connect with the kidney and the bladder, exit at the nape, and merge with the bladder meridian.

3.2.6 Tendons Along 12 Meridians

Tendons along 12 meridians refer to corresponding muscles and tendons around the 12 meridians. Each bundle of tendons corresponds to a meridian and is nourished by the meridian. All tendons along 12 meridians start from the tips of the fingers or toes, accumulate at joints, travel along the superficial part of the body, and finally reach the trunk or head. They do not connect the internal viscera. The tendons along three yang meridians of foot start from the tips of the toes and arrive at the face. The tendons along three yin meridian of foot start from the tips of the toes and reach the external genitalia. The tendons along three yang meridian of hand start from the tips of the fingers and reach the head. The tendons along three yin meridians of hand start from the tips of the fingers and end at the chest. The 12 meridians distribute, retain, and accumulate qi and blood in their respective tendon area.

3.2.7 Twelve Skin Regions

Twelve skin regions are the regions of the skin reflecting the functional condition of the 12 meridians. One skin region reflects the functional condition of one meridian. Like tendons along 12 meridians, the 12 skin regions also need the nourishment of qi and blood from the corresponding meridians.

3.2.8 Effects of Meridians and Collaterals

3.2.8.1 Linking the Interior with the Exterior Throughout the Body

The tissues and viscera in the human body, including the zang-fu viscera and extraordinary fu-viscera, five sensory viscera, nine orifices, skin, muscles, tendons, and bones, have individual physiological functions. Nevertheless, they are interconnected and coordinated via the meridian system. The 12 meridians form the main body; the 12 divergent meridians and the 15 collaterals are the large branches; the 12 skin regions and tendons along 12 meridians correspond to the 12 meridians on the skin, muscles, and tendons. The 8 extra meridians traverse, intersect, and connect the 12 meridians. The meridians and collaterals are independent of each other, but they interconnect and converge to form a network that integrates the whole body into a complete organism.

The 12 meridians connect the body surface with the internal viscera and strengthen communication among the zang-fu viscera. The 12 divergent meridians strengthen connection between yin and yang meridians and connection among meridians, zang-fu viscera, and the head and facial region. The 15 collaterals strengthen the relationship between the surface and the meridians. The 8 extra meridians strengthen the relationship among the 12 meridians.

3.2.8.2   Circulating Qi and Blood, Coordinating Yin and Yang

The *Miraculous Pivot* says, "The meridians move qi and blood, nourish yin and yang, and lubricate the joints and tendons." Qi and blood are the material foundation of all activities in the human body. The yang fu viscera and tissues conduct their normal physiological functions relying on the nourishment provided by qi and blood, which are transported by the meridians and collaterals throughout the body. Yin and yang differ throughout the human body. Meridians and collaterals connect the whole body to facilitate yin-yang balance, harmony, and normal physiological functions.

3.2.8.3   Resisting Pathogenic Qi, Reflecting Signs and Symptoms of Disorders

External pathogens usually attack the body through the meridians and collaterals, penetrating from the exterior to the interior via collaterals, meridians, fu-viscera, and zang-viscera. If meridian qi is robust, it can defend the body and prevent pathogenic qi from penetrating deeply into the body; if it is weak, it cannot withstand the attack, and pathogenic qi remains, lingering at different levels of the meridian and collateral system and ultimately penetrating the zang-fu viscera.

Because meridians and collaterals communicate with the interior and exterior of the body, pathological changes within the zang-fu viscera can be reflected on the body's surface through the meridians and collaterals. Internal disorders can manifest as tenderness, nodules, depressions, and saturated blood vessels on the body surface. Such signs and symptoms serve as important evidence for diagnosing internal disorders.

3.2.8.4   Transmitting Sensation, Regulating Deficiency and Excess

Meridians and collaterals play an important role during treatment, as they react to acupuncture, moxibustion, and massage. The transmission of the needling sensation along the meridians is shown in such phenomena as the arrival, movement, and spreading of qi to affected areas. Needling sensation is the key to therapeutic efficacy in acupuncture; it is conducted through the meridians to diseased areas to regulate deficiencies and excesses. Notably, acupuncture's regulating effects are optimizing: stimulating a point using the same method under different conditions can produce opposite therapeutic effects, but acupuncture always moves the body toward homeostasis and almost never has effects on healthy individuals. Hence needling Neiguan (PC 6) increases the heart rate in bradycardia and reduces it in tachycardia, and needling Tianshu (ST 25) can relieve constipation as well as diarrhea.

3.3 General Introduction on Acupoints

3.3.1 Nomenclature of Acupoints

The name of an acupoint usually has its specific meaning. Ancient scholars assigned names based on variety of subjects ranging from astronomy, geography, daily life, natural objects and anatomy to distribution characteristics, functions and indications of acupoint. Nomenclature of acupoint is summarized below.

3.3.1.1 Nomenclature Based on Astronomy and Geography

Acupoints named for the sun, moon or stars: Riyue (GB 24) refers to the sun and the moon. Shangxing (GV 23), Xuanji (CV 20), Taiyi (ST 23), and Taibai (SP 3) are all names of stars.

Acupoints named for the mountains, hills or valleys: Chengshan (BL 57) means supporting the mountains. Daling (PC 7) means a large mound. Liangqiu (ST 34) refers to a ridge in the hill. Hegu (LI 4) means the junction of valleys.

Acupoints named for seas, rivers, streams or ponds: Shaohai (HT 3) means the smaller sea. Sidu (SJ 9) is the four rivers. Houxi (SI 3) means the back stream. Quchi (LI 11) refers to a crooked pond.

Acupoints named for roads, paths or passes: Qichong (ST 30) means the pathway of qi. Shuidao (ST 28) means the pathway of water. Neiguan (PC 6) is an internal pass.

3.3.1.2 Nomenclature Based on Activities of Human Beings and Objects

Acupoints named for animals and plants: Jiuwei (CV 15) is the tail of a turtledove. Futu (ST 32) means a crouching rabbit. Cuanzhu (BL 2) means a clump of bamboo.

Acupoints named for buildings: Kufang (ST 14) is a warehouse. Tianchuang (SI 16) is a skylight. Zigong (CV 19) means royal palace.

Acupoints named for commonly used tools: Xuanzhong (GB 39) refers to a suspended bell. Dazhu (BL 11) is a larGeshuttle. Quepen (ST 12) is a basin.

Acupoints named for human affairs: Guilai (ST 29) means returning to the original place. Yanglao (SI 6) means providing for the aged.

3.3.1.3 Nomenclature Based on Acupoint Location and Function

Acupoints named for their anatomical locations: Dazhui (GV 14) is a large vertebra. Wangu (SI 4) is the carpus. Rangu (KI 2) is the navicular bone.

Acupoints named for the functions of zang-fu viscera: Shentang (BL 44) means the palace of mind. Pohu (BL 42) means the door of the corporeal soul. Hunmen (BL 47) is the door of the soul. Yishe (BL 49) is the house of thought. Zhishi (BL 52) is the room of will.

Acupoints named for meridians, collaterals, and yin-yang: Sanyinjiao (SP 6) is the intersection of the three yin meridians of foot. Sanyangluo (TE 8) is the junction of three yang meridians of hand.

Acupoints named according to the functions of acupoint: Guangming (GB 37) is for clear vision. Yingxiang (LI 20) is for sense of smell. Tinggong (SI 19) and Tinghui (GB 2) are for hearing.

3.3.2 Classification of Acupoints

Acupoints are classified as meridian points, extra points, and ashi points.

3.3.2.1 Meridian Points

The acupoints distributed along the course of the 14 meridians (12 regular meridians plus the governor vessel and the conception vessel) are called "acupoints of the 14 meridians," or "meridian points" for short. A meridian point has its definite name, fixed location, and specific indication. *The Source of Acupuncture and Moxibustion*, compiled in 1871 AD, recorded 361 acupoints, which is the number of meridian points still used today.

3.3.2.2 Extra Points

The acupoints that have fixed locations but do not belong to the 14 meridians are called "extra points." They have specific names and indications, and most of them are used for specific disorders. For example, Dingchuan (EX-B 1) is used for asthma; Yaotongdian (EX-UE 7) is used for acute lumbar muscle sprain; Dannang (EX-LE 6) is effective for acute cholecystitis.

3.3.2.3   Ashi Points

Ashi points refer to tender points or other sensitive spots due to diseases. They have neither definite names nor fixed locations. Most of them are located near the affected part, but some are distal to the affected part.

3.3.3   Rules for the Effects and Indications of Acupoints

3.3.3.1   Rules for the Effects of Acupoints

Acupoints are reaction points of diseases. They receive various stimulation including acupuncture and moxibustion. They prevent and treat diseases and are sites where qi and blood are transported and pathogenic qi invades. Acupoints are stimulated by acupuncture and moxibustion in order to strengthen healthy qi and remove pathogenic qi through dredging the meridians, regulating the flow of qi and blood, harmonizing yin and yang with each other and harmonizing zang-fu viscera functions. The rules for the effects of acupoints are classified as follows.

1. Local therapeutic effects

   Local therapeutic effect is a characteristic of all acupoints, including meridian points, extra points, and ashi points. All points can treat disorders of their adjacent locations. For example, Quchi (LI 11) located near the elbow is used to treat pain of the elbow. Zusanli (ST 36) and Yanglingquan (GB 34) located on the leg are effective for pain and paralysis of the lower limbs.

2. Remote therapeutic effects

   Remote therapeutic effects is a characteristic of meridian points, especially those of the 12 meridians located blow the elbow and the knee. They are effective not only for local disorders but also for disorders of remote locations on the course of their pertaining meridians. This is what the saying "the indications of the acupoints extend to where their pertaining meridians reach" means. For example, Zusanli (ST 36) is used to treat gastrointestinal disorders according to the course of the stomach meridian of foot yangming.

3. Special therapeutic effects

   In addition to local and remote therapeutic effects, some acupoints have special therapeutic effects such as bidirectional regulation, general regulation, and other specific effects. Many acupoints have the effects of bidirectional regulation. For instance, Tianshu (ST 25) and Zusanli (ST 36) relieve diarrhea or constipation. Neiguan (PC 6) decreases heart rate in patients with tachycardia but increases it in bradycardia. Some acupoints, especially in yangming meridians, governor vessel, and conception vessel, have effects of general regulation. For example, Hegu (LI 4), Quchi (LI 11), and Dazhui (GV 14) are used to treat fever caused by external pathogenic qi. Guanyuan (CV 4) and Zusanli (ST 36) have the effects of tonification and preserving health. Some acupoints have relatively specific effects, for example, Shaoze (SI 1) treats mastitis, and Zhiyin (BL 67) corrects malpresentation.

3.3.3.2 Rules for Indications of Acupoints

Each acupoint has wide range of indications directly related to its location and meridian. Acupoints from different meridians have some common indications in addition to their own characteristics. Acupoints located in the same region also have some common indications. The rules for acupoint indications in different meridians and regions are summarized in Tables 3.3, 3.4, and 3.5.

Table 3.3 Indications for acupoints of the 14 meridians

Meridians	Indications of the meridian	Common indications	
Lung meridian of hand taiyin	Disorders of the lung and throat		Disorders of the chest
Pericardium meridian of hand jueyin	Disorders of the heart and stomach	Disorders of the mind	
Heart meridian of hand shaoyin	Disorders of the heart		
Large intestine meridian of hand yangming	Disorders of the forehead, nose, mouth, and teeth		Disorders of the eyes and throat, fever
Triple energizer meridian of hand shaoyang	Disorders of the temporal region and hypochondrium	Disorders of the ears	
Small intestine meridian of hand taiyang	Disorder of the occipital region, scapula, and mind		
Stomach meridian of foot yangming	Disorders of the forehead, mouth, teeth, throat, stomach, and intestine		Disorders of the mind, fever
Gallbladder meridian of foot shaoyang	Disorders of the temporal region, ear, neck, gallbladder, and hypochondrium	Disorders of the eyes	
Bladder meridian of foot taiyang	Disorders of the occipital region, neck and back, anorectal disorders, and zang-fu viscera disorders		
Spleen meridian of foot taiyin	Disorders of the spleen and stomach		Disorders in the abdomen, gynecological disorders
Liver meridian of foot jueyin	Disorders of the liver	Disorders of the externalia	
Kidney meridian of foot shaoyin	Disorders of the kidney, lung, and throat		
Governor vessel	Fever, disorders of the head	Stroke, disorders of the mind and zang-fu viscera	
Conception vessel	Deficiency cold syndrome, disorders of lower energizer		

Table 3.4 Indications for acupoints of the head, face, and neck

Regions	Indications
Forehead and temporal region	Disorders of the eyes and nose
Occipital region	Disorders of the head and mind
Nape	Disorders of the mind, throat, eyes, head, and nape
Eyes	Disorders of the eyes
Nose	Disorders of the nose
Neck	Disorders of the tongue, throat, trachea, and neck

Table 3.5 Indications for acupoints of the chest, abdomen, and back

The front	The back	Indications
Chest	Upper back	Disorders of the lung and heart (upper energizer)
Hypochondrium and upper abdomen	Lower back	Disorders of the liver, gallbladder, spleen, and stomach (middle energizer)
Lower abdomen	Lumbosacral region	Disorders of the externalia and anus, kidney, intestine, and bladder (lower energizer)

3.3.4 Specific Points

Specific points refer to those acupoints of the 14 meridians that have special thera-peutic effects and are classified as specific categories. Specific points make up a considerable proportion of the acupoints of the 14 meridians and play an important role in the basic theory and clinical application of acupuncture and moxibustion.

3.3.4.1 Five Transport Points

Five transport points refer to five groups of points distal to elbow or knee, namely well, spring, stream, river, and sea points. The ancient doctors described qi flowing in the meridians as water flowing from a spring to the sea, from shallow to deep. The qi of meridians flows from the distal extremities to the elbows or knees, from well point, to spring, stream, river, and sea point in sequence. Most well points are located at the tips of the fingers or toes where the meridian qi starts to bubble like water coming out of a well. The spring points are distal to metacarpal-phalangeal or metatarsophalangeal joints where meridian qi starts to rush like a spring. The stream points are proximal to the metacarpal-phalangeal or metatarsophalangeal joints where meridian qi flows like a stream. The river points are proximal to the wrist or ankle where meridian qi pours abundantly like a river. Finally, sea points are near the elbows and knees where meridian qi enters the body and gathers in the zang-fu viscera like rivers converging to the sea.

Five transport points are widely applied clinically corresponding to the five elements. The details of the five transport points and their attributes of five elements are listed in Tables 3.6 and 3.7.

Based on ancient documents and contemporary clinical practice, the five transport points are applied as follows.

1. Selecting the five transport points according to their characteristics
   The indications of the five transport points are various in ancient documents. As stated in *Miraculous Pivot*, "well points are selected for diseases of zang-

Table 3.6 Five transport points of the six yin meridians

Six yin meridians		Well points (wood)	Spring points (fire)	Stream points (earth)	River points (metal)	Sea points (water)
Three yin meridians of hand	Lung (metal)	Shaoshang (LU 11)	Yuji (LU 10)	Taiyuan (LU 9)	Jingqu (LU 8)	Chize (LU 5)
	Pericardium (ministerial fire)	Zhongchong (PC 9)	Laogong (PC 8)	Daling (PC 7)	Jianshi (PC 5)	Quze (PC 3)
	Heart (fire)	Shaochong (HT 9)	Sha fu (HT 8)	Shenmen (HT 7)	Lingdao (HT 4)	Shaohai (HT 3)
Three yin meridians of foot	Spleen (earth)	Yinbai (SP 1)	Dadu (SP 2)	Taibai (SP 3)	Shangqiu (SP 5)	Yinling quan (SP 9)
	Liver (wood)	Dadun (LR 1)	Xingjian (LR 2)	Taichong (LR 3)	Zhongfeng (LR 4)	Ququan (LR 8)
	Kidney (water)	Yongquan (KI 1)	Rangu (KI 2)	Taixi (KI 3)	Fuliu (KI 7)	Yingu (KI 10)

Table 3.7 Five transport points of the six yang meridians

Six yang meridians		Well points (metal)	Spring points (water)	Stream points (wood)	River points (fire)	Sea points (earth)
Three yang meridians of hand	Large intestine (metal)	Shangyang (LI 1)	Erjian (LI 2)	Sanjian (LI 3)	Yangxi (LI 5)	Quchi (LI 11)
	Triple energizer (ministerial fire)	Guanchong (TE 1)	Yemen (TE 2)	Zhongzhu (TE 3)	Zhigou (TE 6)	Tianjing (TE 10)
	Small intestine (fire)	Shaoze (SI 1)	Qiangu (SI 2)	Houxi (SI 3)	Yanggu (SI 5)	Xiaohai (SI 8)
Three yang meridians of foot	Stomach (earth)	Lidui (ST 45)	Neiting (ST 44)	Xiangu (ST 43)	Jiexi (ST 41)	Zusanli (ST 36)
	Gallbladder (wood)	Zuqiaoyin (GB 44)	Xiaxi (GB 43)	Zulingqi (GB 41)	Yangfu (GB 38)	Yanglingquan (GB 34)
	Bladder (water)	Zhiyin (BL 67)	Zutonggu (BL 66)	Shugu (BL 65)	Kunlun (BL 60)	Weizhong (BL 40)

viscera, spring points for diseases with changes in colors, stream points for intermittent conditions, river points for abnormality in voice, and sea points for stomach disorders caused by irregular diet." *Classic of Difficult Issues* states, "well points are indicated for epigastric fullness, spring points for fever, stream points for heaviness of the body and pain of the joints, river points for asthma, cough, chill, and fever, and sea points for reversed flow of qi and diarrhea." This statement mainly focuses on therapeutic effects of the five transport points from the perspective of relation between the attributes of the five transport points of yin meridians and attributes of their internally related zang-viscera.

2. Selecting the five transport points according to mutual relations of generation and restraint

The five transport points follow the law of five element theory. According to the principle for reinforcing and reducing established by *Classic of Difficult Issues*: "Reinforce the mother when the son is deficient and reduce the son when the mother is excessive," the mother or son point from the five transport points on the diseased meridian is selected. For instance, the lung corresponds to metal, whose son is water and mother is earth. When the lung is excessive, Chize (LU 5), the sea point of the lung meridian corresponding to water, is reduced. When the lung is deficient, Taiyuan (LU 9), the stream point of the lung meridian corresponding to earth, is reinforced. These are typical examples of application of the mother or son point on diseased meridian.

In addition, the mother point from the mother meridian and the son point from the son meridian are also applied clinically. For example, when the lung is excessive, Yingu (KI 10), the sea point corresponding to water from the kidney meridian corresponding to water too, is reduced. When the lung is deficient, Taibai (SP 3), the stream point corresponding to earth from the spleen meridian corresponding to earth too, is reinforced.

3.3.4.2 Back Transport Points and Alarm Points

Back transport points are the points on the back where the qi of the respective zang-fu viscera is infused. Alarm points are the points on the chest or abdomen where the qi of the respective zang-fu viscera infuses and converges.

All back transport points are located on the first lateral line of the bladder meridian of foot-taiyang. All alarm points are located close to their corresponding zang-fu viscera. Each of the six zang and six fu viscera has one alarm point and one back transport point on each side of the spine (Table 3.8).

In general, back transport points are more often used for yin diseases including disorders of zang-viscera, cold or deficiency syndrome. Alarm points are more often used for yang diseases including disorders of fu-viscera, heat or excess syndrome. For example, Shenshu (BL 23), the back transport point of kidney, is indicated for kidney deficiency syndrome. Tianshu (ST 25), the alarm point of large intestine, is used to treat disorders of intestines, such as abdominal distension or pain, diarrhea, constipation, and so on.

Table 3.8 Back transport and alarm points of the zang-fu viscera

Zang-fu viscera	Back transport points	Alarm points
Lung	Feishu (BL 13)	Zhongfu (LU 1)
Pericardium	Jueyinshu (BL 14)	Danzhong (CV 17)
Heart	Xinshu (BL 15)	Juque (CV 14)
Liver	Ganshu (BL 18)	Qimen (LR 14)
Gallbladder	Danshu (BL 19)	Riyue (GB 24)
Spleen	Pishu (BL 20)	Zhangmen (LR 13)
Stomach	Weishu (BL 21)	Zhongwan (CV 12)
Triple energizer	Sanjiaoshu (BL 22)	Shimen (CV 5)
Kidney	Shenshu (BL 23)	Jingmen GB 25)
Large intestine	Dachangshu (BL 25)	Tianshu (ST 25)
Small intestine	Xiaochangshu (BL 27)	Guanyuan (CV 4)
Bladder	Pangguangshu (BL 28)	Zhongji (CV 3)

Back transport points and alarm points can be used either alone or in combination. The latter is called "back transport and alarm point combination method." For example, Danshu (BL 19) and Riyue (GB 24) are both selected to treat gallbladder diseases.

3.3.4.3 Source Points and Connecting Points

Source points are a group of 12 meridian points located near the wrist or ankle where the original qi of zang-fu viscera and meridians passes and gathers. Source point of a yin meridian is identical to its stream point, whereas source point of a yang meridian is independent of its stream point.

Connecting points are locations where the 15 collaterals branch out from the meridians. There is one-connecting point on each of the 12 meridians, the governor vessel, the conception vessel, and the major collateral of the spleen. Therefore, they are called "15 connecting points" (Table 3.9).

Source points and connecting points can be used either alone or in combination. When a source point of a primary diseased meridian is combined with connecting point of the interior-exterior related meridian which is affected subsequently, it is called "source-connecting points combination" or "host-guest points combination." For example, when the liver meridian is diseased first and the gallbladder meridian is affected subsequently, Taichong (LR 3) which is the source point of the liver meridian, and Guangming (GB 37) which is the connecting point of the gallbladder, are used in combination.

Table 3.9 Source points and connecting points of the meridians

Meridians	Source points	Connecting points
Lung meridian	Taiyuan (LU 9)	Lieque (LU 7)
Pericardium meridian	Daling (PC 7)	Neiguan (PC 6)
Heart meridian	Shenmen (HT 7)	Tongli (HT 5)
Spleen meridian	Taibai (SP 3)	Gongsun (SP 4)
Liver meridian	Taichong (LR 3)	Ligou (LR 5)
Kidney meridian	Taixi (KI 3)	Dazhong (KI 4)
Large intestine meridian	Hegu (LI 4)	Pianli (LI 6)
Triple energizer meridian	Yangchi (TE 4)	Waiguan (TE 5)
Small intestine meridian	Wangu (SI 4)	Zhizheng (SI 7)
Stomach meridian	Chongyang (ST 42)	Fenglong (ST 40)
Gallbladder meridian	Qiuxu (GB 40)	Guangming (GB 37)
Bladder meridian	Jinggu (BL 64)	Feiyang (BL 58)
Governor vessel		Changqiang (GV 1)
Conception vessel		Jiuwei (CV 15)
Major collateral of the spleen		Dabao (SP 21)

3.3.4.4 Confluence Points of the Eight Extra Meridians

The confluence points of the 8 extra meridians are the 8 points on the 4 limbs where the 12 meridians communicate with the 8 extra meridians (Table 3.10).

In clinical practice, each confluence point is effective for diseases of its related extra meridian. For instance, Houxi (SI 3), a confluence point communicating with the governor vessel, is applicable for diseases of the governor vessel such as stiffness or pain of the spine.

The eight confluence points are usually used in pairs according to the relationship of the eight extra meridians and areas where two extra meridians meet. For example, Gongsun (SP 4) and Neiguan (PC 6) are the confluence points of the chong vessel and yin link vessel, respectively; they are used in combination to treat diseases of the heart, chest, and stomach, where the two meridians both distribute.

3.3.4.5 The Eight Meeting Points

The eight meeting points are eight points corresponding respectively to eight kinds of viscera and tissues, including zang-viscera, fu-viscera, qi, blood, sinew, vessels, bones, and marrow. Each of points treats diseases of its corresponding viscera or tissue. For example, Danzhong (CV 17), the meeting point of qi, is applicable for qi disorders. Yanglingquan (GB 34), the meeting point of sinew, treats sinew disorders (Table 3.11).

Table 3.10 Confluence points of the eight extra meridians

Eight confluence points and their related extra meridians	Indications
Gongsun (SP 4) (chong vessel) Neiguan (PC 6) (yin link vessel)	Problems of the stomach, heart, and chest
Houxi (SI 3) (governor vessel) Shenmai (BL 62) (yang heel vessel)	Problems of the inner canthus, nape, ear, and shoulder
Zulinqi (GB 41) (belt vessel) Waiguan (TE 5) (yang link vessel)	Problems of the outer canthus, cheek, neck, the posterior of the ear, and shoulder
Lieque (LU 7) (conception vessel) Zhaohai (KI 6) (yin heel vessel)	Problems of the chest, lung, diaphragm, and throat

Table 3.11 The eight meeting points

Eight meeting points	Viscera or tissues
Zhangmen (LR 13)	Zang-viscera
Zhongwan (CV 12)	Fu-viscera
Danzhong (CV 17)	Qi
Geshu (BL 17)	Blood
Yanglingquan (GB 34)	Tendons
Taiyuan (LU 9)	Vessels
Dazhu (BL 11)	Bones
Xuanzhong (GB 39)	Marrow

Table 3.12 Cleft points of the meridians

Yin meridians	Cleft points	Yang meridians	Cleft points
Lung meridian	Kongzui (LU 6)	Large intestine meridian	Wenliu (LI 7)
Spleen meridian	Diji (SP 8)	Stomach meridian	Liangqiu (ST 34)
Heart meridian	Yinxi (HT 6)	Small intestine meridian	Yanglao (SI 6)
Kidney meridian	Shuiquan (KI 5)	Bladder meridian	Jinmen (BL 63)
Pericardium meridian	Ximen (PC 4)	Triple energizer meridian	Huizong (TE 7)
Liver meridian	Zhongdu (LR 6)	Gallbladder meridian	Waiqiu (GB 36)
Yin link vessel	Zhubin (KI 9)	Yang link vessel	Yangjiao (GB 35)
Yin heel vessel	Jiaoxin (KI 8)	Yang heel vessel	Fuyang (BL 59)

3.3.4.6 Cleft Points

Cleft points are locations where the meridian qi is deeply converged and accumulated in the limbs. Most cleft points are situated distal to elbow or knee. Each of the 12 meridians and the 4 extra vessels, yin and yang link vessel, yin and yang heel vessel, has 1 cleft points. There are 16 cleft points in all (Table 3.12).

Cleft points are frequently used for acute diseases of their respective meridians and their internally connected zang-fu viscera. Specifically, cleft points of yin meridians are effective for bleeding, while those of yang meridians are more frequently used for acute pain. For example, Kongzui (LU 6), the cleft point of the lung meridian, is applicable for hemoptysis. Liangqiu (ST 34), the cleft point of the stomach meridian, is effective for stomachache. In addition, cleft points are often used in combination with the eight meeting points, hence the name "cleft-confluent points combination." For instance, Geshu (BL 17), the meeting point of blood, is combined with Kongzui (LU 6) to treat hemoptysis. Zhongwan (CV 12), the meeting point of fu-viscera, is used in combination with Liangqiu (ST 34) for stomachache.

3.3.4.7 Lower Sea Points

The lower sea points, also called lower sea points of the six fu viscera, are the six points where the qi of the six fu viscera flows down toward the three yang meridians of foot. The lower sea points of the stomach, gallbladder, and bladder are identical to sea points of respective meridian, while the lower sea points of the large intestine, small intestine, and triple energizer are independent of sea points in respective meridian (Table 3.13).

As stated in *Miraculous Pivot*, "the lower sea points treat diseases of the fu-viscera." For example, Zusanli (ST 36), the lower sea point of stomach, is the main point to treat vomiting, stomach bloating, and pain. Weizhong (ST 40), the lower sea point of bladder, is effective for uroschesis and enuresis.

3.3.4.8 Crossing Points

Crossing points are those at which two or more meridians intersect. Most crossing points are distributed on the head, face, and trunk.

A crossing point is indicated for diseases of its pertaining meridian and the meridians that intersect at the point. For instance, Sanyinjiao (SP 6), a crossing point where three yin meridians of foot cross, is used not only for diseases of the spleen meridian, but also for diseases of the liver meridian and the kidney meridian. Chengjiang (CV 24), the crossing point of the conception vessel, the governor vessel, the large intestine meridian, and the stomach meridian, treats diseases of these four meridians.

Table 3.13 Lower sea points of six fu viscera

The six fu viscera	Lower sea points
Stomach	Zusanli (ST 36)
Large intestine	Shangjuxu (ST 37)
Small intestine	Xiajuxu (ST 39)
Triple energizer	Weiyang (BL 39)
Bladder	Weizhong (BL 40)
Gallbladder	Yanglingquan (GB 34)

3.3.5   Methods for Locating Acupoints

In general, commonly used methods for locating acupoints include anatomical land-marks measurement, proportional bone measurement, cunfinger cun measurement, and simplified measurement.

3.3.5.1   Location of Acupoints According to Anatomical Landmarks on Body Surface

The anatomical landmarks used to locate acupoints are divided into fixed landmarks and moving landmarks.

1. Fixed anatomical landmarks
   Fixed anatomical landmarks refer to prominences and depressions formed by the joints and muscles, contours of the eyes, ears, nose, and mouth, fingernails and toenails, the nipples, the umbilicus, and so on. For example, Cuanzhu (BL 2) is in the depression at the medial end of the eyebrow. Danzhong (CV 17) is between the nipples. Chengshan (BL 57) is on the posterior aspect of the leg where the calcaneal tendon connects with the two muscle bellies of the gastroc-nemius. Yanglingquan (GB 34) is in the depression anterior and distal to the head of the fibula.
   Commonly used anatomical landmarks on the back for locating acupoints are listed in Table 3.14.
2. Moving landmarks
   Moving landmarks refer to the depressions and folds on the joints, muscles, and skin with reference to specific body movements. For instance, Ermen (TE 21), Tinggong (SI 19), and Tinghui (GB 2) are located with the mouth open. Xiaguan (ST 7) is located when the mouth closed. Jiache (ST 6) is at the promi-nence of the masseter muscle when teeth are clenched.

Table 3.14 Commonly used anatomical landmarks on the back

Anatomical landmarks	Notes
The sternal angle	At the same level as the second rib
The nipples in males	At the same level as the fourth intercostal space
The spinous process of the seventh cervical vertebra	The most prominent spinous process on the posterior median line of the neck
The medial ends of the two spines of the scapula	At the same level as the spinous process of the third thoracic vertebra
The inferior angles of the scapula	At the same level as the spinous process of the seventh thoracic vertebra
The spinous process of the 12th thoracic vertebra	At the same level as the midpoint of the line connecting the inferior angle of the scapula with the highest point of the iliac crest
The highest points of the iliac crests	At the same level as the spinous process of the fourth lumbar vertebra

3.3.5.2 Location of Acupoints by Bone Proportional Cun

Location of acupoints by bone proportional cun refers to a method that using bones and joints as landmarkers to measure the length and width of various parts of the body and then convert them into proportional units for locating points. This method is based on the patient's own body: the length of a given bone or the distance between two joints is divided into equal units, and each unit is considered as one cun. This method of measurement is applicable for locating points on patients of different sexes, ages, and body types. The proportional bone measurements of different parts of body are shown in Table 3.15.

3.3.5.3 Location of Acupoints by Cun Measurement

Finger cun measurement refers to a method using the length or width of the patient's fingers for locating acupoints. Commonly used cunfinger cun measurement methods include middle finger cun, thumb cun, and fingerbreadth cun.

1. Middle finger cun: The distance between the ends of the two radial creases of the interphalangeal joints of the middle finger is taken as one cun when the middle finger is bent.
2. Thumb body cun: The width of the interphalangeal joint of the thumb is taken as one cun.

Table 3.15 Standards for bone proportional cun

Portion of the body	Distance	Proportional bone measurement	Method	Notes
Head and face	From the midpoint of the anterior hairline to the midpoint of the posterior hairline	12 cun	Longitudinal measurement	If the anterior and posterior hairlines are indistinguishable, the distance from the glabella to Dazhui (GV 14) is measured as 18 cun. The distance from Dazhui (GV 14) to the posterior hairline is 3 cun
	From the glabella to the midpoint of the anterior hairline	3 cun		
	Between the bilateral corners of the anterior hairline on the forehead	9 cun	Transverse measurement	
	Between the bilateral mastoid processes	9 cun		

(continued)

Table 3.15 (continued)

Portion of the body	Distance	Proportional bone measurement	Method	Notes
Chest and abdomen	From the suprasternal fossa to the midpoint of the xiphisternal symphysis	9 cun	Longitudinal measurement	
	From the midpoint of the xiphisternal symphysis to the center of the umbilicus	8 cun		
	From the center of the umbilicus to the superior border of the pubic symphysis	5 cun		
	Between the bilateral medial borders of the coracoid	12 cun	Transverse measurement	
	Between the two nipples	8 cun		For female, the distance between the two nipples may be substituted by the two mid-clavicular lines
Back	From the medial border of the scapula to the posterior midline	3 cun	Transverse measurement	
Upper limbs	From the anterior or posterior axillary fold to the cubital crease	9 cun	Longitudinal measurement	
	From the cubital crease to the wrist crease	12 cun		

Table 3.15 (continued)

Portion of the body	Distance	Proportional bone measurement	Method	Notes
Lower limbs	From the superior border of the pubic symphysis to the base of patella	18 cun	Longitudinal measurement	
	From the base of the patella to the apex of the patella	2 cun		
	From the apex of the patella (the center of the popliteal fossa) to the prominence of the medial malleolus	15 cun		
	From the inferior border of medial condyle of the tibia to the prominence of the medial malleolus	13 cun		
	From the prominence of the greater trochanter of femur to the popliteal crease	19 cun		
	From the gluteal fold to the popliteal crease	14 cun		
	From the popliteal crease to the prominence of the lateral malleolus	16 cun		
	From the prominence of medial malleolus to the sole	3 cun		

3. Fingerbreadth cun: When the patient's four fingers (the index, middle, ring, and little finger) are extended and closed together, the width of the four fingers at the level of the crease of the proximal interphalangeal joint of the middle finger is taken as three cun. This method is also called "four-finger measurement."

3.3.5.4 Simplified Measurement

Simplified measurement is a simple method to locate acupoints. For example, when the index fingers and thumbs of both hands are crossed with one index finger in extending position, Lieque (LU 7) is under the tip of the index finger. When a loose fist is made, Laogong (PC 8) is just under the tip of the middle finger. Baihui (GV 20) is located at the center of the line between the ear apexes. Simplified measurement is usually applied as an auxiliary to other methods of point locating.

3.4 Meridians and Acupoints

3.4.1 Frequently Used Acupoints on the 12 Meridians

3.4.1.1 Frequently Used Acupoints on Lung Meridian of Hand Taiyin

Lung meridian of hand taiyin originates from the middle energizer, and descends to connect with the large intestine. It then returns to connect the lung and exits transversely from lung system where the lung communicates with the throat. It descends along the anterior side of forearm and the upper arm and enters the cun kou. It then passes through the major thenar eminence, goes out to terminate at the medial side of the tip of the thumb. A branch of this meridian splits from the styloid process of the wrist and runs to the radial side of the tip of the index finger (Fig. 3.3).

1. **Zhongfu (LU 1)** Alarm Point of the Lung
   Location: On the upper lateral chest, 6 cun lateral to the anterior midline and at the same level of the first intercostal space (Fig. 3.4).
   Indications: (1) Cough, asthma, fullness in the chest, chest pain. (2) Upper back pain.
   Manipulation: Insert the needle obliquely into the lateral side of the chest, 0.5–0.8 cun deep. Deep perpendicular insertion toward the medial aspect is prohibited in order to avoid puncturing the lung and causing pneumothorax.
2. **Chize (LU 5)** Sea Point
   Location: On the transverse crease of the elbow, in the radial depression of the tendon of the biceps muscle (Fig. 3.5).
   Indications: (1) Cough, asthma, coughing up blood, sore throat, tidal fever. (2) Spasm and pain in the upper arm. (3) Acute vomiting and diarrhea. (4) Infantile convulsion.
   Manipulation: Insert the needle perpendicularly by 0.5–0.8 cun deep or prick to allow bleeding.

Fig. 3.3 The course of
lung merdian of hand
taiyin

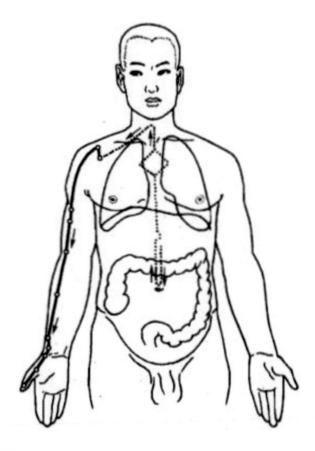

3. **Kongzui (LU 6)** Cleft Point

   Location: On the medial side of the forearm, along the line linking Taiyuan
   (LU 9) and Chize (LU 5), 7 cun above the transverse crease of the wrist (Fig. 3.5).

   Indications: (1) Cough, coughing up blood, asthma, nosebleed, sore throat.
   (2) Spasm and pain in the arm.

   Manipulation: Insert the needle perpendicularly by 0.5–1.0 cun deep.

4. **Lieque (LU 7)** Connecting Point; One of the Eight Confluence Points Associating
   with the Conception Vessel

   Location: On the radial aspect of the forearm between the extensor pollicis
   brevis tendon and the abductor pollicis longus tendon in the groove of the abductor pollicis longus tendon, 1.5 cun superior to the palmar wrist crease (Fig. 3.6).

   Indications: (1) Lung system diseases like cough, asthma, sore throat, etc.
   (2) Craniofacial diseases like rigidity of nape with headache, deviated mouth and
   eyes, toothache, etc. Pain in the wrist.

   Manipulation: Insert the needle obliquely upward by 0.3–0.8 cun deep.

Fig. 3.4 Location of
LU1, LU2

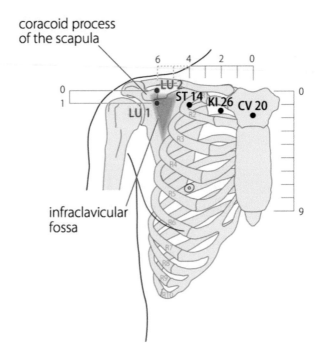

5. **Taiyuan (LU 9)** Stream Point, Source Point, One of the Eight Meeting Points
   (Vessels Convergence)
   Location: Between the radial styloid process and the scaphoid, in the depression ulnar to the abductor pollicis longus tendon, on the radial side of the transverse crease of the wrist where radial artery pluses (Fig. 3.7).
   Indications: (1) Cough, asthma, coughing blood, chest pain, sore throat. (2) Acrotism. (3) Pain in the wrist.
   Manipulation: Keep away from artery and insert the needle perpendicularly by 0.2–0.3 cun deep.
6. **Yuji (LU 10)** Spring Point
   Location: On the midpoint of the first metacarpal bone, on the junction of the red and white skin (Fig. 3.8).
   Indications: (1) Cough, asthma, coughing up blood, sore throat, sudden loss of voice. (2) Palm hot. (3) Infantile malnutrition.
   Manipulation: Insert the needle perpendicularly by 0.5–0.8 cun deep. Subcutaneous tissue resection therapy to treat infantile malnutrition is available.

Fig. 3.5 Location of LU 5, LU 6

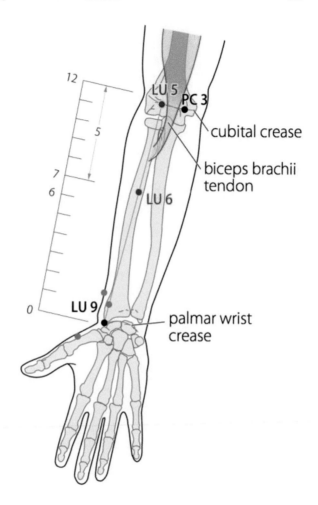

7. **Shaoshang (LU 11)** Well Point

   Location: On the radial side of the thumb, about 0.1 cun from the corner of the fingernail.

   Indications: (1) Swollen and sore throat, cough, nosebleed, high fever, unconsciousness. (2) Psychosis.

   Manipulation: Insert the needle superficially by 0.1 cun, or prick to allow bleeding.

8. **Other points on lung meridian of hand taiyin** (Table 3.16).

Fig. 3.6 Location of LU 7

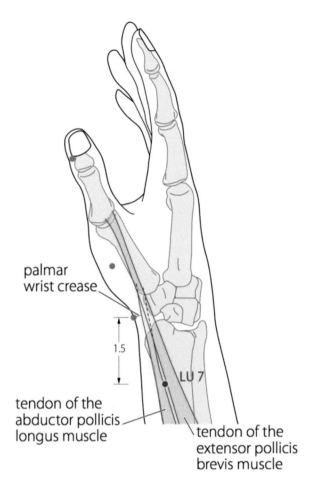

palmar
wrist crease

1.5

tendon of the
abductor pollicis
longus muscle

LU 7

tendon of the
extensor pollicis
brevis muscle

3.4.1.2 Frequently Used Acupoints on Large Intestine Meridian of Hand Yangming

Large intestine meridian of hand yangming starts from the tip of the index finger, proceeding upward along the radial side of the index finger, then goes upwards along the anterior aspect of the forearm and the lateral anterior aspect of the upper arm and reaches the anterior upper aspect of the shoulder joint. It then goes backward crossing Dazhui (GV 14) and descents to the supraclavicular fossa and enters into chest to connect with the lung, and then it goes downwards to connect the pertaining large intestine. Its branch splits from the supraclavicular fossa and runs upwards to the head.

It splits from the supraclavicular fossa and runs upwards along the neck, passes through the cheek, and enters the gingiva of the lower teeth. It then curves around the corner of the mouth and intersects at the philtrum with the opposite side of the same meridian, with this intersection the meridian on the right hand proceeds to the

Fig. 3.7 Location of LU 9

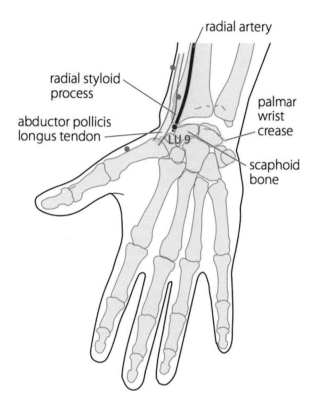

radial artery

radial styloid process

abductor pollicis longus tendon

palmar wrist crease

LU 9

scaphoid bone

Fig. 3.8 Location of LU10, LU 11

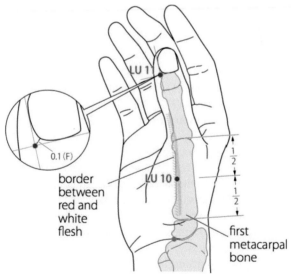

LU 11

0.1 (F)

border between red and white flesh

LU 10

first metacarpal bone

$\frac{1}{2}$

$\frac{1}{2}$

Table 3.16 Other points on lung meridian of hand taiyin

Points	Code	Location	Indication	Manipulation
Yunmen	LU 2	On the upper lateral chest, superior to the coracoid process of the scapula, in the depression of the infraclavicular fossa, 6 cun lateral to the anterior midline	(1) Cough, asthma, pain in the chest. (2) Shoulder and upper back pain	0.5–0.8 cun oblique insertion toward lateral side of the chest. Deep perpendicular insertion toward the medial aspect is prohibited in order to avoid puncturing the lung and causing pneumothorax
Tianfu	LU 3	On the radial border of the biceps muscle, 3 cun below the front end of the axillary fold	(1) Cough, asthma, nosebleed, goiter. (2) Pain in the upper arm	0.5–1.0 cun perpendicular insertion
Xiabai	LU 4	On the radial side of the tendon of the biceps muscle, 4 cun below the front end of the axillary fold	(1) Cough, asthma, nausea. (2) Pain in the upper arm	0.5–1.0 cun perpendicular insertion
Jiingqu (river point)	LU 8	In the depression between the styloid process of the radius and the radial side, 1 cun above the transverse crease of the wrist	(1) Cough, asthma, chest pain. (2) Swelling and pain in the throat. (3) Pain in the wrist	0.2–0.3 cun perpendicular insertion, keeping away from the radial artery

left while the left to right. It finally terminates on the lateral side of the nose (Fig. 3.9).

1. **Shangyang (LI 1)** Well Point
   Location: 0.1 cun lateral to the radial nail corner of the index finger (Fig. 3.10).
   Indications: (1) Swollen and sore throat, toothache. (2) Loss of consciousness, sunstroke. (3) Febrile diseases.
   Manipulation: Insert the needle superficially by 0.1 cun deep, or prick to induce bleeding.

2. **Hegu (LI 4)** Source Point
   Location: Between the first and second metacarpal bones, approximately in the middle of the second metacarpal bone on the radial side (Fig. 3.11).
   Indications: (1) Headache, deviated mouth and eye, toothache, conjunctival congestion, nosebleed, deafness. (2) Fever, aversion to cold, with or without sweating. (3) Amenorrhea, delayed labor. (4) Paralysis of the forearm, unable to move voluntarily, painful wrist, and forearm.
   Manipulation: Insert the needle perpendicularly by 0.5–1.0 cun deep. It is contraindicated for pregnant women.

Fig. 3.9 The course of large intestine meridian of hand yangming

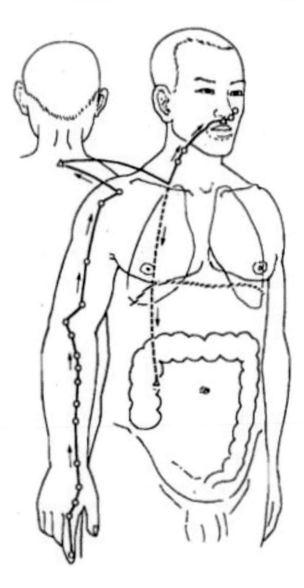

3. **Yangxi (LI 5)** River Point

    Location: At the radial side of the dorsal wrist crease, distal to the radial styloid process in the depression of the anatomical snuffbox, between the tendons of the extensor pollicis longus and extensor pollicis brevis (Fig. 3.11).

    Indications: (1) Headache, toothache, sore throat. (2) Pain in the wrist.

    Manipulation: Insert the needle perpendicularly by 0.3–0.5 cun deep.

Fig. 3.10 Location of LI 1

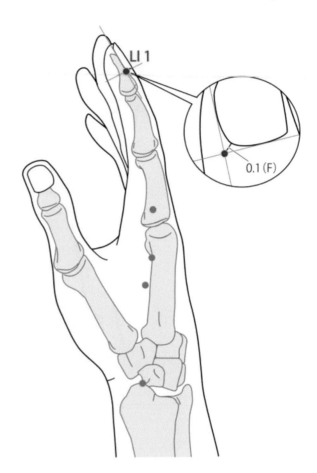

4. **Pianli (LI 6)** Connecting Point

    Location: With the elbow slightly flexed, on the radial side of the dorsal surface of the forearm and on the line connecting Yangxi (LI5) and Quchi (LI11), 3 cun above the crease of the wrist (Fig. 3.12).

    Indications: (1) Nosebleed, tinnitus, deafness. (2) Pain in the forearm. (3) Abdominal distending pain. (4) Edema.

    Manipulation: Insert the needle perpendicularly by 0.3–0.5 cun deep.

5. **Shousanli (LI 10)**

    Location: On the line linking the *Yangxi* (LI 5) and *Quchi* (LI 11) points, 2 cun below Quchi (LI 11) (Fig. 3.13).

    Indications: (1) Paralysis of the forearm, pain, and numbness in the elbow and arm. (2) Toothache, swollen cheek. (3) Abdominal pain, diarrhea.

    Manipulation: Insert the needle perpendicularly by 0.8–1.2 cun deep.

Fig. 3.11 Location of LI 4, LI 5

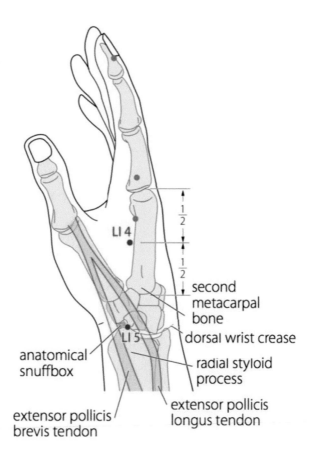

second metacarpal bone

dorsal wrist crease

radial styloid process

extensor pollicis longus tendon

anatomical snuffbox

extensor pollicis brevis tendon

6. **Quchi (LI 11)** Sea Point

   Location: With the elbow flexed, at the lateral end of the transverse cubital crease, midway between Chize (LU 5) and the lateral epicondyle of the humerus (Fig. 3.14).

   Indications: (1) Swollen and sore throat, toothache, redness, and pain in the eyes. (2) Febrile diseases. (3) Rubella, eczema. (4) Hypertension. (5) Paralysis of the arm, pain, and weakness in the elbow. (6) Psychosis. (7) Abdominal pain, diarrhea.

   Manipulation: Insert the needle perpendicularly by 0.8–1.5 cun deep.

7. **Binao (LI 14)**

   Location: On the lateral side of the arm anterior to the border of the deltoid muscle, 7 cun superior to *Quchi* (LI 11) (Fig. 3.15).

   Indications: (1) Painful upper arm and shoulder, impaired arm movement. (2) Eye diseases. (3) Scrofula.

   Manipulation: Insert the needle perpendicularly or obliquely upward by 0.8–1.5 cun deep.

Fig. 3.12 Location of LI
6, LI 7

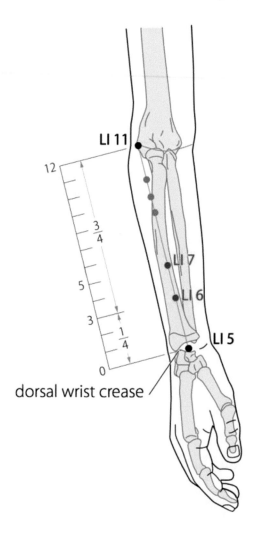

8. **Jianyu (LI 15)**

  Location: On the shoulder girdle in the depression between the anterior end of the lateral border of the acromion and the greater tubercle of the humerus (Fig. 3.15).

  Indications: (1) Pain and numbness in the upper arm and shoulder, impaired movement of arm. (2) Scrofula.

  Manipulation: Insert the needle perpendicularly or obliquely downward by 0.8–1.5 cun deep.

9. **Yingxiang (LI 20)**

  Location: 0.5 cun beside the lateral border of the nasal ala, in the nasolabial groove (Fig. 3.16).

Fig. 3.13 Location of LI
8, LI 9, LI 10

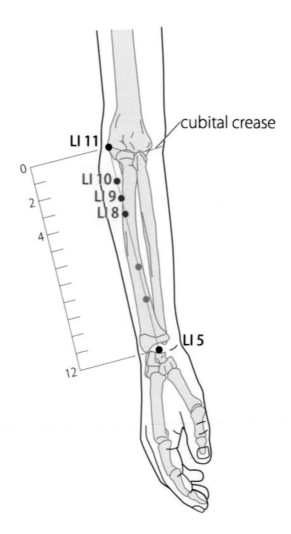

Indications: (1) Nasal obstruction, nosebleed, sinusitis. (2) Facial paralysis, facial itchiness. (3) Ascariasis of the biliary tract.

Manipulation: 0.2–0.5 cun deep perpendicular or oblique insertion.

10. **Other points on large intestine meridian of hand yangming** (Table 3.17).

3.4.1.3   Frequently Used Acupoints on Stomach Meridian of Foot Yangming

The stomach meridian of foot yangming starts from the lateral side of the nose. It travels upward to the root of the nose where it meets the foot taiyang meridian. Turning downward along the lateral side of the nose, it enters the upper gingiva.

Fig. 3.14 Location of
LI 11

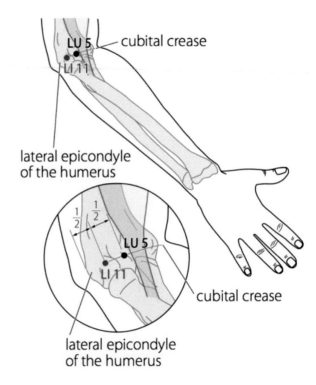

Fig. 3.15 Location of LI
12–LI 15

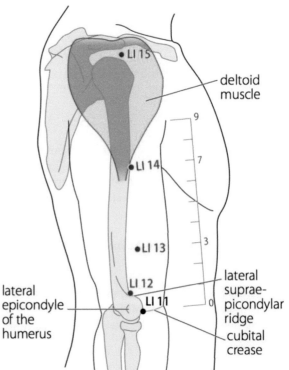

Fig. 3.16 Location of
LI 20

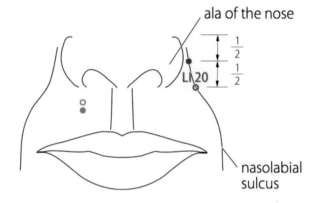

Table 3.17 Other points on large intestine meridian of hand yangming

Points	Code	Location	Indication	Manipulation
Erjian (spring point)	LI 2	In the depression of the radial side, distal to the second metacarpophalangeal joint when a loose fiat is made	(1) Nosebleed, toothache, red and swollen eyes, deviated mouth and eye. (2) Febrile disease	0.2–0.3 cun perpendicular insertion
Sanjian (stream point)	LI 3	In the depression of the radial side and proximal to the second metacarpophalangeal joint	(1) Toothache, nosebleed, sore throat. (2) Fever	0.3–0.5 cun perpendicular insertion
Wenliu (cleft point)	LI 7	With the elbow flexed, on the line linking the Yangxi (LI 5) and Quchi (LI 11) points, 5 cun above the wrist crease	(1) Headache, swollen of the face, sore throat. (2) Aching shoulders and back. (3) Abdominal pain, borborygmus	0.5–1.0 cun perpendicular insertion
Xialian	LI 8	On the line connecting Yangxi (LI 5) and Quchi (LI 11), 4 cun below the cubital crease	(1) Headache, vertigo, and pain in the elbow. (2) Abdominal distention, abdominal pain, pain in the elbow and arm	0.5–1.0 cun perpendicular insertion
Shanglian	LI 9	On the line connecting Yangxi (LI 5) and Quchi (LI 11), 3 cun below the cubital crease	(1) Pain and numbness in the elbow and arm, paralysis of the forearm, headache. (2) Borborygmus, abdominal pain	0.5–1.0 cun perpendicular insertion

(continued)

Table 3.17 (continued)

Points	Code	Location	Indication	Manipulation
Zhouliao	LI 12	With the elbow flexed, 1 cun above the Quchi (LI 11) point, on the border of the humerus	Aching, numbness, and spasm of the elbow and arm	0.5–1.0 cun perpendicular insertion
Shouwuli	LI 13	On the line connecting Quchi (LI 11) and Jianyu (LI 15), 3 cun above Quchi (LI 11)	(1) Spasm and pain in the elbow and arm. (2) Scrofula	0.5–1.0 cun perpendicular insertion
Jugu	LI 16	In the upper portion of the shoulder, in the depression between the acromial extremity of the clavicle and the scapular spine	(1) Pain of the shoulder and upper back. (2) Scrofula, goiter	0.5–0.8 cun oblique insertion toward lateral side of the chest. Deep perpendicular insertion is prohibited in order to avoid puncturing the lung and causing pneumothorax
Tian ding	LI 17	On the lateral side of the neck, on the posterior border of M. sternocleidomastoideus, at the midpoint of the line linking the Futu (LI 18) and Quepen (ST 12) points	(1) Sore throat, sudden loss of voice. (2) Scrofula, goiter	0.3–0.5 cun perpendicular insertion
Futu	LI 18	3 cun lateral to the tip of the Adam's apple, between the sternal head and clavicular head of musculus sternocleidomatoideus	(1) Sore throat, sudden loss of voice. (2) Scrofula, goiter. (3) Cough and asthma	0.5–0.8 cun perpendicular insertion
Kou he liao	LI 19	On the upper lip, directly below the lateral border of the nostril, on the level of Shuigou (GV 26)	Nosebleed, nasal obstruction, deviated face, trismus	0.3–0.5 cun perpendicular or oblique insertion

Curving around the lips, it meets Chengjiang (CV 24) in the mentolabial groove. It then travels to the posterior aspect of the mandible passing through the facial artery, ascending in front of the ear and following the anterior hairline, it reaches the forehead at last.

Cheek Branch: Its cheek branch splits from the front of the Daying (ST5) and passes through the carotid artery. Passing along the throat, it enters the supraclavicular fossa. It further descends and passes through the diaphragm, and then enters its pertaining organ, the stomach, and connects to the spleen, the related organ.

The stomach meridian descends from face to throat and enters the supraclavicular fossa, then enters its pertaining organ, the stomach, and connects to the spleen, the related organ. The straight branch of the meridian emerges from the supraclavicular fossa, which passes through the nipple descends along the lateral side of umbilicus and enters *Qichong* (ST30) which is located in the lower abdomen.

The branch starts from the lower orifice of the stomach, and descends inside of the abdomen, reaching Qichong (ST30). From here, it further descends to Biguan (ST31) and goes downward to the knee. From the knee, it continues further down along the anterior border of the lateral aspect of the tibia to the dorsum of the foot and reaches the lateral side of the tip of the second toe.

The tibial branch of the meridian splits from the place 3 cun below the knee and runs downward and ends at the lateral side of the middle toe. Another branch on the foot emerges from the dorsum of the foot to enter the medial side of the tip of big toe (Fig. 3.17).

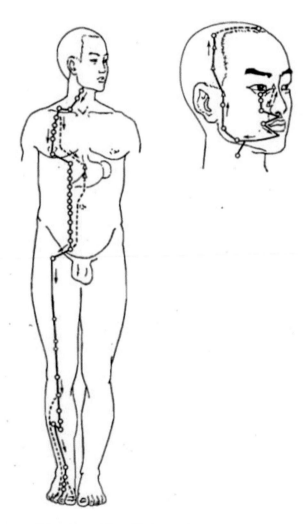

Fig. 3.17 The course of stomach meridian of foot yangming

Fig. 3.18 Location of ST 1

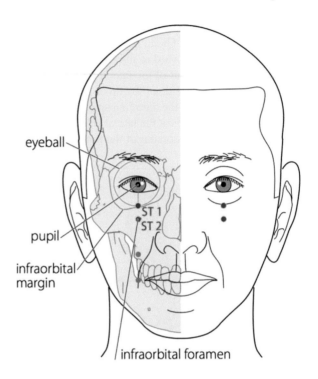

1. **Chengqi (ST 1)**

    Location: On the face, directly below the pupil with the eyes looking straightforward, between the eyeball and the infraorbital ridge (Fig. 3.18).

    Indications: (1) Trembling eyelids, red and swollen eyes, night blindness, lacrimation upon exposure to wind. (2) Deviation of the mouth and eyes, prosopospasm.

    Manipulation: With the eyes closed, push the eyeball upward slightly with the left thumb and puncture perpendicularly and slowly by 0.5–1 cun along the infraorbital ridge. It is not advisable to manipulate the needle with a large amplitude, compress the needling hole after withdrawing the needle.

2. **Sibai (ST 2)**

    Location: On the face, directly below the pupil with the eyes looking straightforward, in the depression of the infraorbital foramen (Fig. 3.18).

    Indications: (1) Red and painful eyes, lacrimation upon exposure to wind, superficial visual obstruction, blurred vision. (2) Deviation of the mouth and eye, twitching of the eyelids, facial pain and itchiness. (3) Vertigo.

    Manipulation: 0.3–0.5 cun deep perpendicular insertion. It is not advisable to manipulate the needle with large amplitude.

3. **Dicang (ST 4)**

    Location: On the face, 0.4 cun beside the corner of the mouth (Fig. 3.19).

    Indications: Deviation of the mouth and eyes, trembling lips, lacrimation.

    Manipulation: 0.5–0.8 cun horizontal insertion toward J*ia che* (ST 6).

Fig. 3.19 Location of ST 3, ST 4

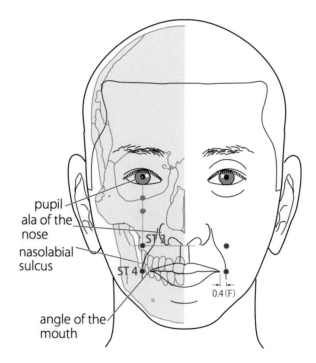

pupil
ala of the nose
nasolabial sulcus
ST 3
ST 4
0.4 (F)
angle of the mouth

4. **Jiache (ST 6)**

    Location: On the cheek, one finger width anterior and superior to the mandibular angle, in the depression where the masseter muscle is prominent (Fig. 3.20).

    Indications: Deviation of the mouth and eyes, swollen cheeks, toothache, locked jaw, spasm of facial muscles.

    Manipulation: 0.3–0.5 cun deep perpendicular insertion or 1.3–1.5 cun oblique insertion toward Di cang (ST 4).

5. **Xiaguan (ST 7)**

    Location: On the face, anterior to the ear, in the depression between the zygomatic arch and mandibular notch (Fig. 3.21).

    Indications: (1) Lower mandible pain, locked jaw, deviated mouth and eyes, toothache, swollen cheek, facial pain. (2) Deafness, tinnitus, ear infection.

    Manipulation: 0.5–1 cun deep perpendicular insertions. It is not advisable to open mouth when retaining the needle so as to avoid curving or breaking the needle.

6. **Touwei (ST 8)**

    Location: On the lateral side of the head, 0.5 cun above the anterior hairline, and 4.5 cun lateral to the anterior midline of the forehead (Fig. 3.21).

    Indications: Headache, vertigo, lacrimation upon exposure to wind, eyes pain.

    Manipulation: 0.5–1.0 cun horizontal insertions backward.

Fig. 3.20 Location of ST
5, ST 6

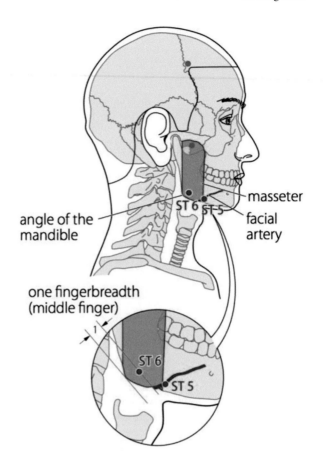

7. **Liangmen (ST 21)**

Location: On the upper abdomen, 4 cun above the center of the umbilicus, 2 cun lateral to the anterior midline of the abdomen (Fig. 3.22).

Indications: Stomachache, vomiting, poor appetite, and abdominal distension.

Manipulation: Puncture perpendicularly by 0.8–1.2 cun. Needling is not advisable for people with hepatomegaly or who have recently had a great feed. It is not advisable to manipulate the needle with large amplitude.

8. **Tianshu (ST 25)** Alarm Point of the Large Intestine

Location: 2 cun lateral to the center of the umbilicus (Fig. 3.22).

Indications: (1) Abdominal pain, abdominal distension, borborygmus, diarrhea, dysentery, constipation, intestinal abscess. (2) Irregular menstruation, dysmenorrhea.

Manipulation: 1.0–1.5 cun perpendicular insertion.

Fig. 3.21 Location of ST 7, ST 8

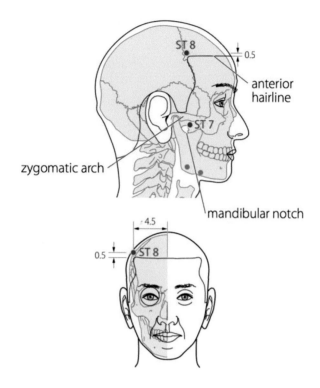

Fig. 3.22 Location of ST 19–ST 25

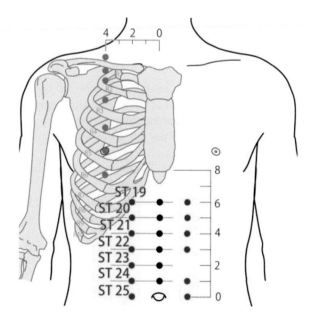

Fig. 3.23 Location of ST
26–ST 30

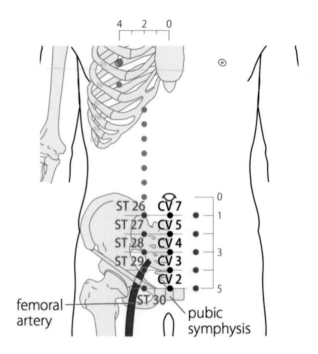

9. **Guilai (ST 29)**

   Location: 4 cun below the umbilicus, 2 cun lateral to the anterior midline of the abdomen (Fig. 3.23).

   Indications: (1) Amenia, prolapse of the uterus, dysmenorrheal, leucorrhea, irregular menstruation. (2) Lower abdominal pain, hernia.

   Manipulation: 0.8–1.2 cun perpendicular insertion.

10. **Futu (ST 32)**

    Location: On the anterolateral aspect of the thigh on the line connecting the lateral end of the base of the patella with the anterior superior iliac spine, 6 cun superior to the base of the patella (Fig. 3.24).

    Indications: (1) Pain and paralysis of the legs. (2) Hernia. (3) Abdominal distention.

    Manipulation: 1.0–2.0 cun perpendicular insertion.

11. **Liangqiu (ST 34)** Cleft Point

    Location: On the anterolateral aspect of the thigh 2 cun superior to the base of the patella between the vastus lateralis muscle and the rectus femoris tendon (Fig. 3.24).

    Indications: (1) Stomach pain. (2) Pain in the knee, atrophy, and paralysis of the legs. (3) Mastitis.

    Manipulation: 1.0–1.5 cun perpendicular insertion.

12. **Zusanli (ST36)** Sea Point; Lower Sea Point of the Stomach

    Location: 3 cun inferior to Dubi (ST 35), on the line connecting Dubi (ST 35) and Jiexi (ST 41) (Fig. 3.25).

Fig. 3.24 Location of ST
31–ST 34

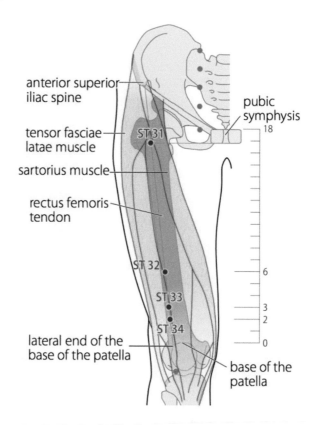

anterior superior
iliac spine

pubic
symphysis
18

tensor fasciae
latae muscle

ST 31

sartorius muscle

rectus femoris
tendon

ST 32

ST 33

6

3
2

ST 34

lateral end of the
base of the patella

0

base of the
patella

Indications: (1) Stomach pain, vomiting, abdominal pain and distension, diarrhea, dysentery, constipation, intestinal abscess. (2) Consumptive diseases, palpitation, shortness of breath. (3) Atrophy and paralysis of the legs, edema. (4) Psychosis and epilepsy. (5) This point has the function to strengthen the body. It is an important point for health care.

Manipulation: 1.0–2.0 cun perpendicular insertion, moxibustion is applicable.

13. **Shangjuxu (ST37)** Lower Sea Point of the Large Intestine

Location: 6 cun inferior to Dubi (ST 35), on the line connecting Dubi (ST 35) and Jiexi (ST 41) (Fig. 3.25).

Indications: (1) Abdominal pain and distension, dysentery, constipation, intestine abscess, stroke, paralysis. (2) Atrophy and pain of the legs.

Manipulation: 1.0–2.0 cun perpendicular insertion.

14. **Xiajuxu (ST39)** Lower Sea Point of the Small Intestine

Location: 9 cun inferior to Dubi (ST 35), on the line connecting Dubi (ST 35) and Jiexi (ST 41) (Fig. 3.25).

Indications: (1) Lower abdominal pain, borborygmus, diarrhea. (2) Atrophy and paralysis of the legs. (3) Mastitis.

Manipulation: 1.0–1.5 cun perpendicular insertion.

Fig. 3.25 Location of ST
36–ST 40

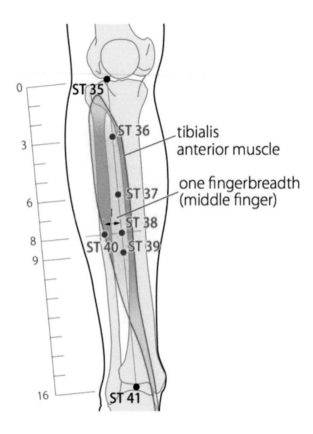

15. **Fenglong (ST40)** Connecting Point

Location: 8 cun superior to the prominence of the lateral malleolus at the lateral border of the tibialis anterior muscle, one fingerbreadth lateral to Tiaokou (ST 38) (Fig. 3.25).

Indications: (1) Headache, vertigo. (2) Psychosis, epilepsy. (3) Cough with phlegm. (4) Atrophy and paralysis of the legs. (5) Abdominal distension, constipation.

Manipulation: 1.0–1.5 cun perpendicular insertion.

16. **Jiexi (ST 41)** River Point

Location: On the anterior aspect of the ankle in the depression between the extensor hallucis longus tendon and the extensor digitorum longus tendon (Fig. 3.26).

Indications: (1) Atrophy and paralysis of the legs, pain in the ankle and wrist. (2) Abdominal distension, constipation. (3) Headache, vertigo. (4) Psychosis, epilepsy.

Manipulation: 0.5–1.0 cun perpendicular insertions.

Fig. 3.26 Location of
ST 41

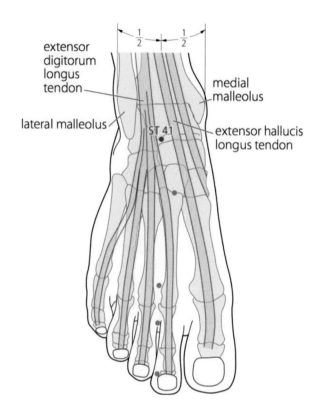

17. **Neiting (ST 44)** Spring Point
    Location: On the instep of the foot, at the junction of the red and white skin proximal to the margin of the web between the second and third toes (Fig. 3.27).
    Indications: (1) Toothache, swollen and sore throat, nosebleed, deviated mouth. (2) Febrile diseases. (3) Stomach pain with sour regurgitation, diarrhea, dysentery, constipation. (4) Swelling and pain in the dorsum of the foot.
    Manipulation: 0.5–0.8 cun perpendicular insertion.
18. **Lidui (ST 45)** Well Point
    Location: On the lateral side of the distal segment of the second toe, 0.1 cun from the corner of the toenail (Fig. 3.27).
    Indications: (1) Toothache, nosebleed, swollen and sore throat. (2) Febrile diseases. (3) Profuse dreaming, nightmares, psychosis.
    Manipulation: Puncture superficially by 0.1 cun.
19. **Other points on Stomach Meridian of Foot Yangming** (Table 3.18).

Fig. 3.27 Location of ST 42–ST 45

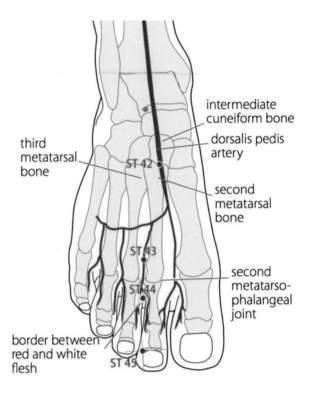

Intermediate cuneiform bone

dorsalis pedis artery

third metatarsal bone

ST 42

second metatarsal bone

ST 43

second metatarso-phalangeal joint

ST 44

border between red and white flesh

ST 45

Table 3.18 Other points on stomach meridian of foot yangming

Points	Code	Location	Indication	Manipulation
Juliao	ST 3	With the eyes looking straightforward, the point is vertically below the pupil, at the level of the lower border of the ala nasi, on the lateral side of the nasolabial groove	Deviation of the mouth and eye, twitching at the angle of the mouth, nosebleed, toothache	0.3–0.5 cun deep perpendicular insertion
Daying	ST 5	Anterior to the mandibular angle, on the anterior border of the masseter muscle, where the pulsation of the facial artery is palpable	Toothache, deviation of the mouth and eye, swollen cheeks, facial pain, twitching of the facial muscles	0.3–0.5 cun deep perpendicular or horizontal insertion, and avoid the artery
Renying	ST 9	In the anterior region of the neck, level with the superior border of the thyroid cartilage, anterior to the sternocleidomastoid and above the common carotid artery	(1) Swollen and sore throat. (2) Scrofula, goiter. (3) Hypertension. (4) Asthma	0.3–0.8 cun perpendicular insertion, avoiding needling the artery

Table 3.18 (continued)

Points	Code	Location	Indication	Manipulation
Shuitu	ST 10	On the neck, on the anterior border of M. sternocleidomastoideus, at the midpoint of the line linking the Renying (ST 9) and Qishe (ST 11) points	(1) Sore throat. (2) Cough, gasp. (3) Scrofula, goiter	0.3–0.5 cun deep perpendicular insertion
Qishe	ST 11	On the neck and on the upper border of the medial end of the clavicle between the sternal and clavicular heads of the stemocleidomastoid muscle	(1) Swollen and sore throat, scrofula. (2) Hiccup. (3) Goiter, gasp. (4) Pain and rigidity of the neck	0.3–0.5 cun deep perpendicular or horizontal insertion, and avoid the artery
Quepen	ST 12	In the midpoint of the supraclavicular fossa, 4 cun lateral to the anterior midline of the chest	(1) Cough, asthma. (2) Swollen and sore throat. (3) Pain in the supraclavicular fossa. (4) Scrofula	0.3–0.5 cun deep perpendicular or horizontal insertion, and avoid the artery
Qihu	ST 13	At the lower border in the center of the clavicle, 4 cun laterals to the anterior midline of the chest	(1) Cough, asthma, hiccups. (2) Pain in the chest	0.2–0.4 cun deep perpendicular or horizontal insertion, and avoid deep insertion so as to prevent puncturing the lung
Kufang	ST 14	In the first intercostal space, 4 cun lateral to the anterior midline of the chest	(1) Cough, asthma. (2) Distension and pain in the chest	0.5–0.8 cun deep perpendicular or horizontal insertion, and avoid deep insertion so as to prevent puncturing the lung
Wuyi	ST 15	In the second intercostal space, 4 cun lateral to the anterior midline of the chest	(1) Cough, asthma. (2) Distension and pain in the chest. (3) Mammary abscess	0.5–0.8 cun deep perpendicular or horizontal insertion, and avoid deep insertion so as to prevent puncturing the lung

(continued)

Table 3.18 (continued)

Points	Code	Location	Indication	Manipulation
Yingchuang	ST 16	In the third intercostal space, 4 cun lateral to the anterior midline of the chest	(1) Cough, asthma. (2) Distension and pain in the chest. (3) Mammary abscess	0.5–0.8 cun deep perpendicular or horizontal insertion, and avoid deep insertion so as to prevent puncturing the lung
Ruzhong	ST 17	In the fourth intercostal space, 4 cun lateral to the anterior midline of the chest, at the center of the nipple	This point serves only as a landmark for locating points on the chest and the abdomen	Acupuncture and moxibustion are prohibited
Rugen	ST 18	In the fifth intercostal space, vertically below the nipple, 4 cun lateral to the anterior midline of the chest	(1) Mastitis, insufficient lactation. (2) Cough, asthma, hiccups. (3) Chest pain	0.5–0.8 cun deep oblique insertion, and avoid deep insertion so as to prevent puncturing the lung
Burong	ST 19	On the upper abdomen, 6 cun above the center of the umbilicus, 2 cun lateral to the anterior midline of the abdomen	Vomiting, stomachache, abdominal distension, and poor appetite	0.5–0.8 cun deep perpendicular insertion Needling is not advisable for people with hepatomegaly or who have recently had a great feed
Chengman	ST 20	On the upper abdomen, 5 cun above the center of the umbilicus, 2 cun lateral to the anterior midline of the abdomen	Stomachache, vomiting, borborygmus, and poor appetite	0.5–0.8 cun deep perpendicular insertion Needling is not advisable for people with hepatomegaly or who have recently had a great feed
Guanmen	ST 22	On the upper abdomen, 3 cun above the center of the umbilicus, 2 cun lateral to the anterior midline of the abdomen	Abdominal pain and distension, borborygmus, diarrhea, and poor appetite	0.8–1.2 cun deep perpendicular insertion
Taiyi	ST 23	On the upper abdomen, 2 cun above the center of the umbilicus, 2 cun lateral to the anterior midline of the abdomen	(1) Abdominal pain and distension. (2) Vexation, psychosis	0.8–1.2 cun deep perpendicular insertion

Table 3.18 (continued)

Points	Code	Location	Indication	Manipulation
Huaroumen	ST 24	On the upper abdomen, 1 cun above the center of the umbilicus, 2 cun lateral to the anterior midline of the abdomen	(1) Abdominal pain, vomiting. (2) Psychosis	0.8–1.2 cun deep perpendicular insertion
Wai ling	ST 26	On the lower abdomen, 1 cun below the center of the umbilicus, 2 cun lateral to the anterior midline of the abdomen	(1) Abdominal pain, hernia. (2) Dysmenorrhea	1.0–1.5 cun deep perpendicular insertion
Daju	ST 27	On the lower abdomen, 2 cun below the center of the umbilicus, 2 cun lateral to the anterior midline of the abdomen	(1) Lower abdominal distension, difficulty in urination. (2) spermatorrhea, premature ejaculation. (3) Hernia	0.8–1.2 cun deep perpendicular insertion
Shuidao	ST 28	On the lower abdomen, 3 cun below the center of the umbilicus, 2 cun lateral to the anterior midline of the abdomen	(1) Lower abdominal distension, difficulty in urination, hernia. (2) Dysmenorrhea	1.0–1.5 cun perpendicular insertion
Qichong	ST 30	On the lower abdomen, 5 cun below the center of the umbilicus, 2 cun lateral to the anterior midline of the abdomen	(1) Abdominal pain, hernia. (2) Irregular menstruation, infertility, impotence, swelling of the vulva	0.8–1.2 cun deep perpendicular insertion
Biguan	ST 31	On the anterior aspect of the thigh in the depression formed by the sartorius, the tensor fasciae latae, and the proximal portion of the rectus femoris	Weakness, numbness, and pain of the lower limbs, pain of the lower back and leg	1.0–1.5 cun deep perpendicular insertion
Yinshi	ST 33	On the anterolateral aspect of the thigh lateral to the rectus femoris tendon, 3 cun superior to the base of the patella	Pain in the knee, atrophy, and paralysis of the legs	0.5–1.0 cun deep perpendicular insertion
Dubi	ST 35	With the knee flexed, on the knee, in the depression lateral to the patella and its ligament	Motor impairment of the lower limbs, numbness and pain in the lower limbs, pain in the knees	Puncture obliquely from the posterior to interior direction by 0.8–1.5 cun
Tiaokou	ST 38	8 cun inferior to Dubi (ST 35), on the line connecting Dubi (ST 35) and Jiexi (ST 41)	(1) Atrophy and paralysis of the legs. (2) Pain in the abdomen and stomach. (3) Pain in the shoulders and arms	1.0–1.5 cun perpendicular insertion

(continued)

Table 3.18 (continued)

Points	Code	Location	Indication	Manipulation
Chongyang (source point)	ST 42	At the highest point of the dorsum of the foot, between the tendons of M. extensor hallucis longus and digitorum longus, where the dorsal artery of the foot pulsates	(1) Stomach pain, abdominal distension. (2) Deviation of the mouth, swollen face, toothache. (3) Swelling and pain in the dorsum of the foot, weakness and numbness of the foot	0.3–0.5 cun deep perpendicular insertion, avoiding needling the artery
Xiangu (stream point)	ST 43	On the dorsum of the foot, between the second and third metatarsal bones in the depression proximal to the second metatarsophalangeal joint	(1) Facial and general edema. (2) Borborygmus, diarrhea. (3) Swelling and pain of the dorsum of the foot	0.3–0.5 cun deep perpendicular insertion

3.4.1.4 Frequently Used Acupoints on Spleen Meridian of Foot Taiyin

This meridian originates from the tip of the big toe, ascends to the front aspect of the medial malleolus, continues going upwards along the posterior side of the lower leg, then it crosses over and goes in front of the liver meridian of foot jueyin, passing through the anterior media aspect of the knee and thigh, it then enters the abdomen and spleen, its pertaining organ, and connects with the stomach. It travels alongside the throat and arrives at the root of the tongue and spreads over the lower surface of the tongue. The abdomen branch of the meridian goes from the stomach through the diaphragm and enters the heart (Fig. 3.28).

1. **Yinbai (SP 1)** Well Point

    Location: On the medial side of the great toe and about 0.1 cun lateral to the corner of the toenail (Fig. 3.29).

    Indications: (1) Gynecological diseases like hypermenorrhea, metrorrhagia, and metrostaxis. (2) Uterine bleeding, menorrhea, blood in the stool and blood in the urine. (3) Abdominal distention. (4) Psychosis, profuse dreaming, and convulsions.

    Manipulation: Insert the needle 0.1 cun into the skin, or insert a three-edged needle to induce bleeding.

2. **Taibai (SP 3)** Stream Point; Source Point

    Location: On the posterior border of the small head of the first metatarsal bone, at the junction of the red and white skin (Fig. 3.30).

    Indications: (1) Stomach pain, abdominal distension, abdominal pain, diarrhea, dysentery, anorexia. (2) Heaviness of the body, pain in joints.

    Manipulation: 0.5–0.8 cun perpendicular insertion.

Fig. 3.28 The course of
spleen meridian of foot
taiyin

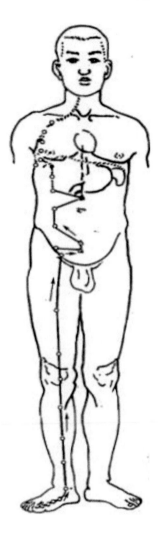

3. **Gongsun (SP 4)** Connecting Point; One of the Eight Confluent Points
   Associating with Chong Vessel
      Location: On the medial border of the foot, anterior to the proximal end of
   the first metatarsal, at the junction of the red and white skin (Fig. 3.30).
      Indications: (1) Stomach pain, vomiting, abdominal distension, abdominal
   pain, diarrhea, dysentery. (2) Epigastric pain, oppression in the chest. (3)
   Insomnia, irritability, somnolence, beriberi.
      Manipulation: 0.5–1.0 cun perpendicular insertions.

Fig. 3.29 Location
of SP 1

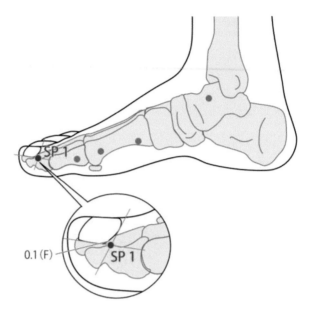

Fig. 3.30 Location of SP
2–SP 5

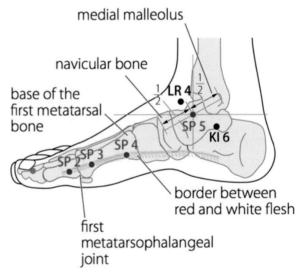

4. **Sanyinjiao (SP 6)**

    Location: 3 cun above the tip of the medial malleolus and on the posterior border of the medial aspect of the tibia (Fig. 3.31).

    Indications: (1) Abdominal pain, abdominal distension, borborygmus, diarrhea. (2) Irregular menstruation, dysmenorrheal, menostasis, leucorrhea, prolapse of the uterus, prolonged labor, infertility, impotence, spermatorrhea. (3) Difficulty in urination, enuresis, edema. (4) Insomnia, dizziness. (5) Atrophy and paralysis of the legs, beriberi.

Fig. 3.31 Location of SP 6–SP 9

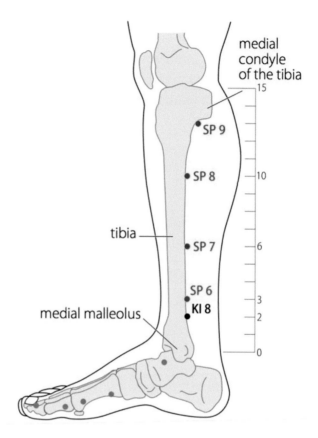

medial condyle of the tibia

SP 9

SP 8

tibia

SP 7

SP 6

KI 8

medial malleolus

Manipulation: 1.0–1.5 cun perpendicular insertion. It is contraindicated for pregnant women.

5. **Diji (SP 8)** Cleft Point

    Location: On the line connecting the tip of the medial malleolus and 3 cun below Yinlingquan (SP 9) (Fig. 3.31).

    Indications: (1) Abdominal distension, abdominal pain, diarrhea. (2) Irregular menstruation, dysmenorrheal, uterine bleeding. (3) Difficulty in urination, edema. (4) Atrophy and paralysis of the legs.

    Manipulation: Puncture perpendicularly by 1.0–1.5 cun.

6. **Yinlingquan (SP 9)** Sea Point

    Location: In the depression inferior to the medial condyle of the tibia (Fig. 3.31).

    Indications: (1) Abdominal distension, diarrhea, jaundice, abdominal pain. (2) Difficulty in urination, edema. (3) Spermatorrhea, pudendal pain. (4) Pain in the knees.

    Manipulation: 1.0–2.0 cun perpendicular insertion.

7. **Xuehai (SP 10)**

    Location: 2 cun superior to the medial end of the base of the patella on the bulge of the vastus medialis muscle (Fig. 3.32).

Fig. 3.32 Location of SP
10–SP12

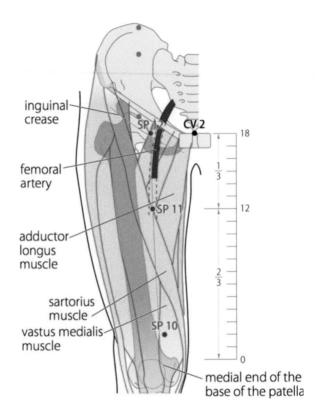

Indications: (1) Irregular menstruation, heavy uterine bleeding, amenorrhea. (2) Urticaria, eczema, erysipelas, abdominal distension, diarrhea, jaundice, abdominal pain, difficulty in micturition, edema. (3) Pain and swelling in the knees.

Manipulation: 1.0–1.2 cun perpendicular insertion.

8. **Daheng (SP 15)**

   Location: 4 cun lateral to the center of the umbilicus (Fig. 3.33).

   Indications: (1) Abdominal pain, diarrhea, and constipation. (2) Hernia.

   Manipulation: 1.0–2.0 cun perpendicular insertion.

9. **Dabao (SP 21)** Major Collateral of the Spleen

   Location: On the midaxillary line, in the sixth intercostal space (Fig. 3.34).

   Indications: (1) Cough, dyspnea. (2) Chest and hypochondriac regions pain. (3) Pain of the whole body, weariness of the four limbs.

   Manipulation: Puncture transversely or obliquely by 0.5–0.8 cun. Deep insertion should be avoided to prevent puncturing the lungs.

10. **Other Points on Spleen Meridian of Foot Taiyin** (Table 3.19).

Fig. 3.33 Location of SP 15, SP 16

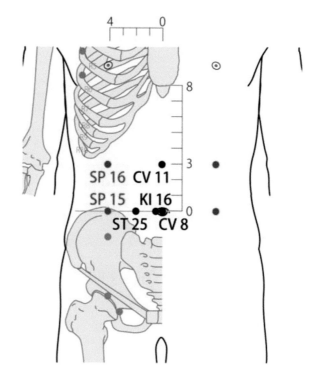

3.4.1.5 Frequently Used Acupoints on Heart Meridian of Hand Shaoyin

It originates from the heart and pertains to the heart system (the tissue where the heart connects other viscera) and connects with the small intestine. The branch that goes upwards through the throat ascends to the head. The straight part of the vessel derived from the heart system runs upwards toward the lungs, runs downwards and emerges from the axilla. It follows along the posterior border of the medial aspect of the forearm and the upper arm and enters the palm. It then travels along the radial side of the little finger and terminates at its tip (Fig. 3.35).

1. **Jiquan (HT 1)**

   Location: At the apex of the axilla, on the pulsation point of the axillary artery (Fig. 3.36).

   Indications: (1) Cardiac pain, palpitations. (2) Hypochondriac and costal pain. (3) Pain in the shoulders and aims, loss of the use of the upper limb. (4) Scrofula.

   Manipulation: Insert the needle perpendicularly by 0.3–0.5 cun deep, avoiding needling the artery.

Fig. 3.34 Location of
SP 21

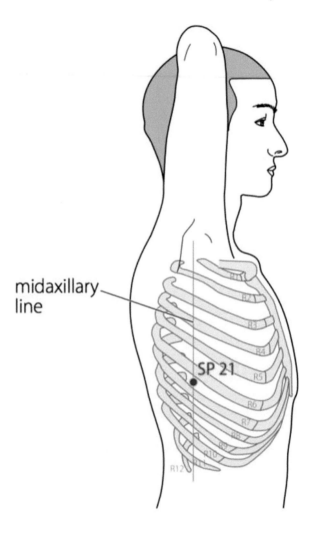

Table 3.19 Other points on spleen meridian of foot taiyin

Points	Code	Location	Indication	Manipulation
Dadu (spring point)	SP 2	In the depression anterior and inferior to the first metatarsophalangeal joint of the big toe, at the junction of the red and the white skin	(1) Abdominal distension, stomach pain, diarrhea, constipation. (2) Febrile disease with absence of sweating	0.5–0.8 cun deep perpendicularly insertion
Shangqiu (river point)	SP 5	In the depression anterior and inferior to the medial malleolus, at the midpoint of the line connecting the tuberosity of the navicular bone and the tip of the medial malleolus	(1) Abdominal distension, borborygmus, diarrhea, constipation, jaundice. (2) Pain in the foot and ankle	0.5–0.8 cun deep perpendicular insertion

Table 3.19 (continued)

Points	Code	Location	Indication	Manipulation
Lougu	SP 7	On the line connecting the tip of the medial malleolus and Yinlingquan (SP 9), 6 cun above the tip of the medial malleolus	(1) Abdominal distention, borborygmus. (2) Seminal emission. (3) Weakness and flaccidity of the lower limbs	1.0–1.5 cun deep perpendicular insertion
Jimen	SP 11	On the medial aspect of the thigh between the sartorius and the adductor longus muscle where the femoral artery pulses, at the junction of the upper 1/3 and lower 2/3 of a line connecting the medial end of the base of the patella and Chongmen (SP 12)	Dysuria, enuresis, swelling, and pain of the groin	0.3–0.5 cun deep perpendicular insertion, avoiding needling the artery
Chongmen	SP 12	At the groin region at the inguinal crease, lateral to the external iliac artery	(1) Abdominal pain, hernia. (2) Uterine bleeding, leukorrhea	0.5–1.0 cun deep perpendicular insertion
Fushe	SP 13	0.7 cun superior and lateral to Chongmen (SP 12), 4 cun lateral to the midline of the abdomen	Abdominal pain, hernia, distension, and masses in the abdomen	0.8–1.2 cun deep perpendicular insertion
Fujie	SP 14	1.3 cun below Daheng (SP 15), 4 cun lateral to the midline of the abdomen	Indications: abdominal pain, diarrhea, and constipation	1.0–1.5 cun deep perpendicular insertion
Fuai	SP 16	3 cun above the center of the umbilicus, 4 cun lateral to the anterior midline of the abdomen	Abdominal pain, diarrhea, dysentery, constipation, and dyspepsia	1.0–1.5 cun deep perpendicular insertion
Shidou	SP 17	In the fifth intercostal space, 6 cun lateral to the anterior midline of the chest	(1) Belching, abdominal distension. (2) Edema. (3) Distension and pain in the chest and hypochondrium	0.5–0.8 cun deep perpendicular insertion, avoiding a deep insertion to prevent needling the lung
Tianxi	SP 18	In the fourth intercostal space, 6 cun lateral to the anterior midline of the chest	(1) Pain in the chest, cough. (2) Acute mastitis, insufficient lactation	0.5–0.8 cun deep perpendicular insertion, avoiding a deep insertion to prevent needling the lung

(continued)

Table 3.19 (continued)

Points	Code	Location	Indication	Manipulation
Xiongxiang	SP 19	In the third intercostal space, 6 cun lateral to the anterior midline of the chest	Distension and pain in the chest and hypochondrium	0.5–0.8 cun deep perpendicular insertion, avoiding a deep insertion to prevent needling the lung
Zhourong	SP 20	In the second intercostal space, 6 cun lateral to the anterior midline	(1) Distension in the chest and hypochondriac regions. (2) Cough, asthma	0.5–0.8 cun deep perpendicular insertion, avoiding a deep insertion to prevent needling the lung

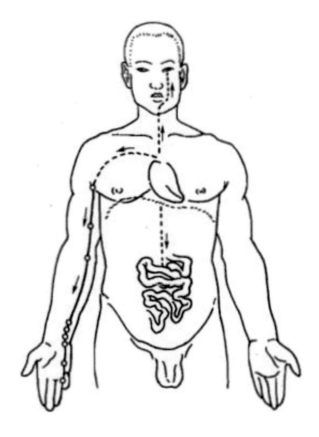

Fig. 3.35 The course of heart meridian of hand shaoyin

Fig. 3.36 Location
of HT 1

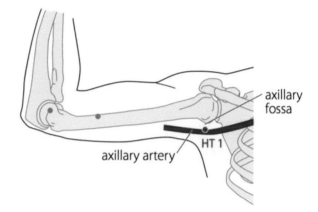

axillary
fossa

HT 1

axillary artery

Fig. 3.37 Location of HT
2, HT 3

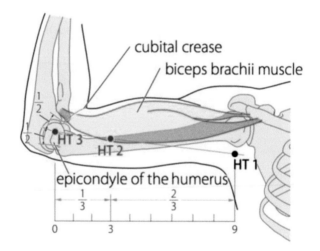

cubital crease

biceps brachii muscle

HT 3

HT 2

HT 1

epicondyle of the humerus

2. **Shaohai (HT 3)** Sea Point

    Location: Anterior to the medial epicondyle of the humerus, level with the cubital crease. With the elbow flexed, at the midpoint of the line connecting the medial end of the cubital crease and the medial epicondyle of the humerus (Fig. 3.37).

    Indications: (1) Cardiac pain. (2) Axillary and hypochondriac pain. (3) Pain of the arm and elbow, paralysis of the upper limbs. (4) Scrofula.

    Manipulation: Insert the needle perpendicularly by 0.5–1.0 cun deep.

3. **Tongli (HT 5)** Connecting Point

    Location: On the palmar aspect of the forearm, 1 cun above the Shenmen (HT 7) point (Fig. 3.38).

    Indications: (1) Sudden loss of voice, stiffness of the tongue, inability to speak. (2) Palpitations. (3) Pain in the wrists and arms.

Fig. 3.38 Location of HT
4–HT 7

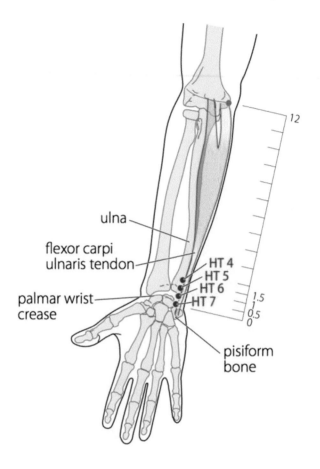

ulna

flexor carpi
ulnaris tendon

palmar wrist
crease

HT 4
HT 5
HT 6
HT 7

pisiform
bone

12

1.5
1
0.5
0

Manipulation: Insert the needle perpendicularly by 0.3–0.5 cun deep. It is not advisable to insert deeply to avoid hurting nerves and vessels.

4. **Yinxi (HT 6)** Cleft Point

Location: On the palmar aspect of the forearm, 0.5 cun above the *Shenmen* (HT 7) point (Fig. 3.38).

Indications: (1) Cardiac pain, fright palpitations. (2) Hematemesis, epistaxis. (3) Steaming heat, night sweats.

Manipulation: Insert the needle perpendicularly by 0.2–0.5 cun deep. It is not advisable to insert deeply to avoid hurting nerves and vessels.

5. **Shenmen (HT 7)** Stream Point; Source Point

Location: On the palmar ulnar end of the transverse crease of the wrist, in the depression on the radial side of the flexor carpi ulnaris tendon (Fig. 3.38).

Indications: (1) Insomnia, forgetfulness, dementia, psychosis, epilepsy. (2) Cardiac pain, palpitations.

Manipulation: Insert the needle perpendicularly by 0.2–0.5 cun deep.

Fig. 3.39 Location of HT
8, HT 9

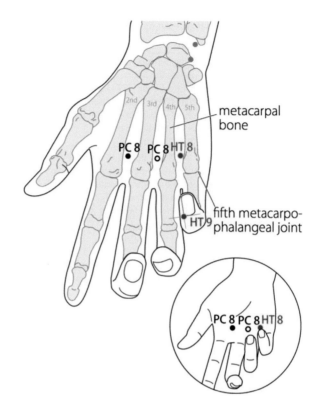

6. **Shaochong (HT 9)** Well Point
     Location: On the radial side of the little finger, approximately 0.1 cun from
   the corner of the nail (Fig. 3.39).
     Indications: (1) Cardiac pain, palpitations. (2) Psychosis, coma. (3) Febrile
   diseases.
     Manipulation: Superficially puncture by 0.1–0.2 cun, or prick to induce
   bleeding.
7. **Other Points on Heart Meridian of Hand Shaoyin** (Table 3.20).

3.4.1.6   Frequently Used Acupoints on Small Intestine Meridian of Hand Taiyang

It originates from the ulnar side of the tip of the little finger, and then runs upwards
along the lateral aspect of the forearm. Then it reaches and emerges at the shoulder
joint and proceeds in a zigzag course along the scapular region, arriving at Dazhui
(GV 14). From here, it descends through the supraclavicular fossa and connects
with the heart, going downwards along the esophagus, passing through the diaphragm to the stomach, and finally ending at the small intestine. A branch from the
supraclavicular fossa ascends along the neck to the head.

Table 3.20 Other points on heart meridian of hand shaoyin

Points	Code	Location	Indication	Manipulation
Qingling	HT 2	On the medial side of the arm and on the line connecting Jiquan (HT1) and Shaohai (HT3), 3 cun above the cubital crease, in the groove medial to the biceps muscle of the arm	(1) Headache, chill. (2) Yellowish eyeballs. (3) Hypochondriac pain, pain in the shoulders and arms	0.5–1.0 cun deep perpendicular insertion
Lingdao (river point)	HT 4	With the elbow flexed, in the center between the medial end of the transverse cubital crease and the medial epicondyle of the humerus	(1) Cardiac pain. (2) Axillary and hypochondriac pain. (3) Pain of the arm and elbow, paralysis of the upper limbs. (4) Scrofula	0.3–0.5 cun deep perpendicular insertion
Shaofu (spring point)	HT 8	On the palm, between the fourth and fifth metacarpal bones, where the tip of the little finger rests when a fist is made	(1) Palpitations, chest pain. (2) Itching and pain of the genitals. (3) Spasmodic pain of the little finger, heat sensations in the palm	0.3–0.5 cun deep perpendicular insertion

A branch from the supraclavicular fossa ascends to cross the neck and cheek to the outer canthus of the eye, and finally turns and enters the ear.

Another branch separates from the previous branch on the cheek and ascends to the zygomatic bone, reaching the side of the nose. It finally terminates at the inner canthus to link with the bladder meridian of foot taiyang (Fig. 3.40).

1. **Shaoze (SI 1)** Well Point

   Location: On the ulnar side of the little finger, approximately 0.1 cun from the corner of the nail (Fig. 3.41).

   Indications: (1) Headache, superficial visual obstruction, sore and swollen throat. (2) Mastitis, insufficient lactation. (3) Coma. (4) Febrile disease.

   Manipulation: Insert the needle superficially by 0.1 cun deep, or prick to induce bleeding. Contraindicate for pregnant women.

2. **Houxi (SI3)** Stream Point; One of the Eight Confluence Points Associating with the Governor Vessel

   Location: On the ulnar side of the hand, when a loose fist is made, proximal to the fifth metacarpophalangeal joint, at the top of the transverse crease, and the junction of the red and white skin (Fig. 3.41).

   Indications: (1) Headache and painful stiff nape of the neck, pain of the lumbar and back region. (2) Red eye, deafness, sore and swollen throat. (3) Night sweats, malaria. (4) Psychosis, epilepsy. (5) Spasm in the fingers, elbows or arms.

   Manipulation: Insert the needle perpendicularly by 0.5–1.0 cun deep.

3. **Wangu (SI 4)** Source Point

   Location: On the ulnar side of the wrist, in the depression between the base of the fifth metacarpal bone and the triquetrum, at the border between the red and white flesh (Fig. 3.42).

Fig. 3.40 The course of
small intestine meridian of
hand taiyang

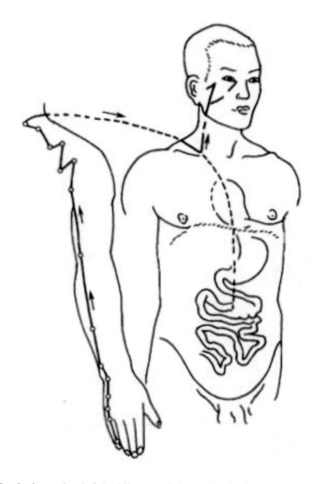

   Indications: (1) Headache and painful stiff nape of the neck, tinnitus, superficial visual obstruction. (2) Jaundice. (3) Diabetes, febrile diseases, malaria. (4)
Pain and spasm in the fingers and wrists.
   Manipulation: Insert the needle perpendicularly by 0.3–0.5 cun deep.
4. **Yanglao (SI 6)** Cleft Point
   Location: On the dorsal ulnar aspect of the forearm, in the depression radial
to the head of the ulnar bone, 1 cun proximal to the dorsal wrist crease (Fig. 3.43).
   Indications: (1) Blurred vision. (2) Numbness and pain in the shoulder, back,
elbow, and arm, stiff neck, acute lumbar pain.
   Manipulation: When the palm of the hand is placed on the chest, insert
obliquely toward the elbow by 0.5–0.8 cun deep.
5. **Zhizheng (SI7)** Connecting Point
   Location: On the dorsal ulnar aspect of the forearm between the medial border of the ulna and the flexor carpi ulnaris, 5 cun proximal to the dorsal wrist
crease (Fig. 3.44).

Fig. 3.41 Location of SI
1–SI 3

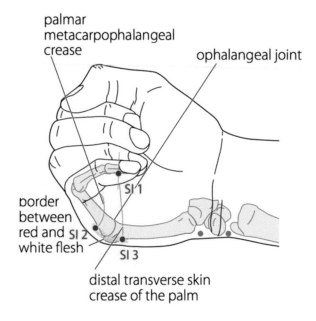

Fig. 3.42 Location of SI
4, SI 5

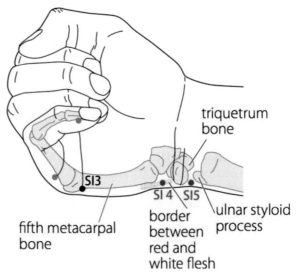

Indications: (1) Headache, stiff neck. (2) Febrile diseases. (3) Psychosis. (4) Aching pain in the elbows and arms.

Manipulation: Insert the needle perpendicularly or obliquely by 0.3–0.8 cun deep.

Fig. 3.43 Location of SI 6

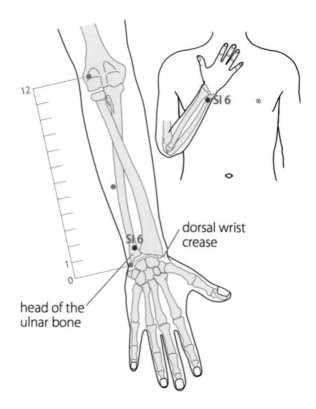

6. **Tianzong (SI 11)**

   Location: In the depression of the center of the subscapular fossa, level with the fourth thoracic vertebra (Fig. 3.45).

   Indications: (1) Scapular pain. (2) Asthma. (3) Mastitis.

   Manipulation: Insert the needle perpendicularly or obliquely by 0.5–1 cun *deep*.

7. **Quanliao (SI 18)**

   Location: On the face, directly below the outer canthus, in the depression below the zygomatic bone (Fig. 3.46).

   Indications: (1) Facial paralysis. (2) Trembling eyelids. (3) Toothache. (4) Swollen lips.

   Manipulation: 0.3–0.5 cun deep perpendicular insertion or 0.5–1.0 cun deep oblique insertion.

8. **Tinggong (SI 19)**

   Location: On the face, anterior to the tragus and posterior to the mandibular condyloid process, in the depression found when the mouth is open (Fig. 3.47).

   Indications: (1) Tinnitus, deafness, epilepsy. (2) Toothache.

   Manipulation: 1.0–1.5 cun deep perpendicular insertion while opening the mouth.

9. **Other Points on Small Intestine Meridian of Hand Taiyang** (Table 3.21).

Fig. 3.44 Location of SI 7, SI 8

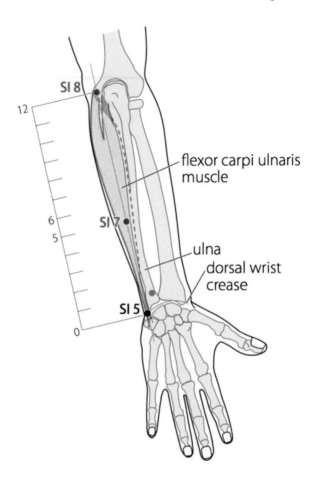

3.4.1.7 Frequently Used Acupoints on Bladder Meridian of Foot Taiyang

The bladder meridian of foot **taiyang** originates from the inner canthus of the eye. It then goes upwards toward the forehead, and connects with the vertex. The straight branch from the vertex enters the brain, and then emerges to descend at the nape of the neck, where the meridian splits into two branches. One of the branches runs downwards along the medial border of the scapular region parallel to the vertebral column, reaching the lumbar region, and then enters the body cavity via the paravertebral muscle to connect with the kidney and bladder. The branch separates into the lumbar region descending via the hip and entering the popliteal fossa of the knee. The branch separates from the nape of the neck and descends along the medial aspect of the scapular region, crosses the hip joint, and then descends along the posteriolateral aspect of the thigh to meet with the previous branch of the meridian in the popliteal fossa. From here, it descends to emerge at the back of the external malleolus, and ends at the lateral side of the small toe (Fig. 3.48).

Fig. 3.45 Location of SI
11, SI 12

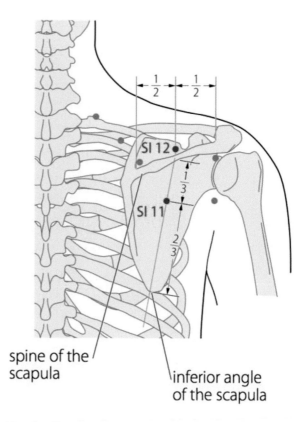

spine of the
scapula

inferior angle
of the scapula

1. **Jingming (BL 1)**

    Location: On the face, in the depression between the superomedial parts of the inner canthus and the medial wall of the orbit (Fig. 3.49).

    Indications: (1) Red and swollen eyes, lacrimation upon exposure to wind, unclear vision, myopia, night blindness, color blindness, blurred vision. (2) Acute lumbar pain. (3) Palpitation and severe palpitation.

    Manipulation: Ordering the patient to close the eye, the doctor slightly pushes the eyeball to the lateral side. Insert the point slowly perpendicularly along the orbital wall for 0.3–0.5 cun. Moxibustion is not applicable. For insertion can easily cause bleeding inside, please use a dry cotton ball to press the puncture site for a moment after withdrawing the needle.

2. **Cuanzu (BL 2)**

    Location: On the face, in the depression of the medial end of the eyebrow, at the frontal notch (Fig. 3.49).

    Indications: (1) Blurred vision, redness, pain and swelling of the eyes, lacrimation, twitching of the eyelid. (2) Headache, pain in the supraorbital region, facial paralysis. (3) Hiccups.

    Manipulation: 0.5–0.8   cun   horizontal   insertion.   Moxibustion   is contraindicated.

Fig. 3.46 Location of SI 18

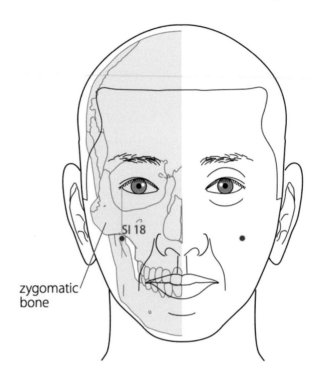

Fig. 3.47 Location of SI 19

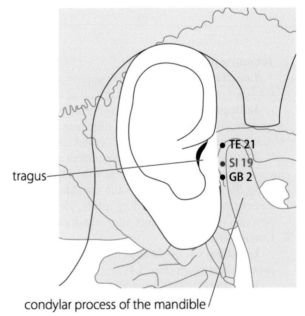

Table 3.21 Other points on small intestine meridian of hand taiyang

Points	Code	Location	Indication	Manipulation
Qiangu (spring point)	SI 2	At the junction of the red and white skin along the ulnar border of the hand, at the ulnar end of the crease of the fifth metacarpophalangeal joint when a loose fist is made	(1) Headache, ophthalmalgia, tinnitus, sore throat. (2) Febriledisease. (3) Acute mastitis	0.3–0.5 cun deep perpendicular insertion
Yanggu (river point)	SI 5	On the ulnar side of the wrist, in the depression between the styloid process of the ulna and the triquetral bone	(1) Headache, dizziness, tinnitus, deafness. (2) Febrile disease. (3) Psychosis, epilepsy. (4) Pain in the wrist	0.3–0.5 cun deep perpendicular insertion
Xiaohai (sea point)	SI 8	With the elbow flexed, in the depression between the olecranon of the ulna and the medial epicondyle of the humerus	(1) Pain in the elbows and arms. (2) Epilepsy	0.3–0.5 cun deep perpendicular insertion
Jianzhen	SI 9	Posterior and inferior to the shoulder joint, 1 cun above the posterior end of the axillary fold with the arm abducted	(1) Numbness and pain in the shoulder and arm. (2) Scrofula	1.0–1.5 cun deep perpendicular insertion
Naoshu	SI 10	On the shoulder, directly above the posterior end of the axillary fold, in the depression inferior to the scapular spine	(1) Pain in the shoulder and arm. (2) Scrofula	0.5–1.2 cun deep perpendicular or oblique insertion
Bingfeng	SI 12	At the scapula region, in the supraspinous fossa superior to the midpoint of the scapular spine	Scapular pain and aching numbness of the upper arm	0.3 cun deep perpendicular or oblique insertion
Quyuan	SI 13	At the scapula region, in the depression superior to the medial end of the scapular spine, midpoint of the line connecting Naoshu (SI 10) and the spinous process of the second thoracic vertebra	Pain in the scapula, back, and neck	0.5–0.8 cun deep perpendicular or oblique insertion
Jianwaishu	SI 14	3 cun lateral to the lower border of the spinous process of the first thoracic vertebrae	Stiffness of nape and back, pain in the shoulders and back	0.5–0.8 cun deep oblique insertion
Jianzhongshu	SI 15	On the back, 2 cun lateral to the lower border of the spinous process of the seventh cervical vertebrae	(1) Cough, asthma. (2) Pain in the shoulders and upper back	0.5–0.8 cun deep oblique insertion

(continued)

Table 3.21 (continued)

Points	Code	Location	Indication	Manipulation
Tianchuang	SI 16	On the lateral aspect of the neck, on the posterior border of the sternocleidomastoideus, posterior to Futu (LI 1 8), and level with the Adam's Apple	(1) Sore and swollen throat, sudden loss of voice, tinnitus, deafness. (2) Pain and stiffness in the nape of the neck	0.5–0.8 cun deep perpendicular insertion
Tianrong	SI 17	Posterior to the mandibular angle in the depression of the anterior border of the stemocleidomastoid muscle	(1) Tinnitus, deafness, sore and swollen throat. (2) Pain and distension in the nape of the neck	0.5–0.8 cun deep perpendicular insertion

Fig. 3.48 The course of bladder meridian of foot taiyang

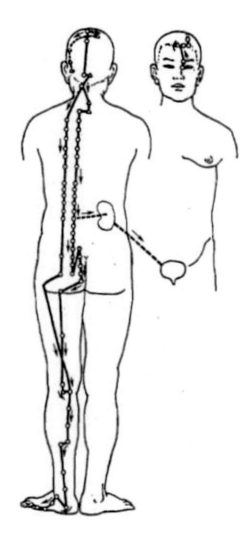

Fig. 3.49 Location of BL 1, BL 2

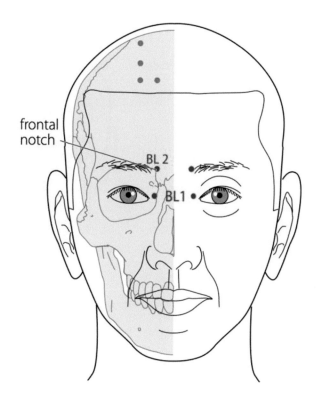

3. **Tianzhu (BL 10)**

   Location: On the nape, in the depression lateral to the trapezius muscle at the level of the superior border of the spinous process of the second cervical vertebra (Fig. 3.50).

   Indications: (1) Headache, dizziness. (2) Blurred vision, nasal congestion. (3) Stiff neck, pain in the upper back and shoulders.

   Manipulation: 0.5–0.8 cun deep perpendicular or oblique insertion, do not puncture deeply upward or inside so as to avoid damaging the medulla.

4. **Fengmen (BL 12)**

   Location: On the back, below the spinous process of the second thoracic vertebrae, 1.5 cun lateral to the posterior midline (Fig. 3.51).

   Indications: (1) Cough due to wind invasion, fever and headache, nasal obstruction, and nose running. (2) Stiffness of nape, pain in the back and shoulders.

   Manipulation: 0.5–0.8 cun deep oblique insertion, deep insertion is not advisable.

5. **Feishu (BL 13)** Back Transport Point of the Lung

   Location: On the back, below the spinous process of the third thoracic vertebra, 1.5 cun lateral to the posterior midline (Fig. 3.51).

   Indications: (1) Cough with asthma, common cold, nasal congestion. (2) High fever, night sweating. (3) Itching of the skin, urticaria.

   Manipulation: 0.5–0.8 cun deep oblique insertion.

Fig. 3.50 Location of BL
9, BL 10

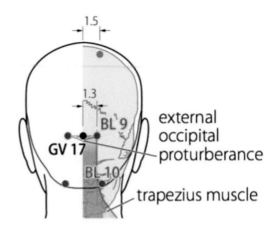

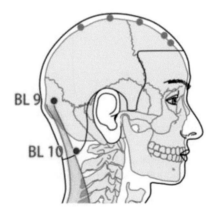

6. **Xinshu (BL 15)** Back Transport Point of the Heart
   Location: On the back, below the spinous process of the fifth thoracic verte-
   brae, 1.5 cun lateral to the posterior midline (Fig. 3.51).
   Indications: (1) Cardiac pain, palpitations, insomnia, forgetfulness, epi-
   lepsy. (2) Cough, hematemesis. (3) Nocturnal emission, night sweats.
   Manipulation: 0.5–0.8 cun deep oblique insertion.
7. **Geshu (BL 17)** One of the Eight Meeting Points (Blood Convergence)
   Location: On the back, below the spinous process of the seventh thoracic
   vertebrae, 1.5 cun lateral to the posterior midline (Fig. 3.51).
   Indications:(1) Stomachache, vomiting, hiccups. (2) Cough with asthma,
   hematemesis, high fever, night sweats. (3) Urticaria.
   Manipulation: 0.5–0.8 cun deep oblique insertion.
8. **Ganshu (BL 18)** Back Transport Point of the Liver

Fig. 3.51 Location of BL
11–BL 24

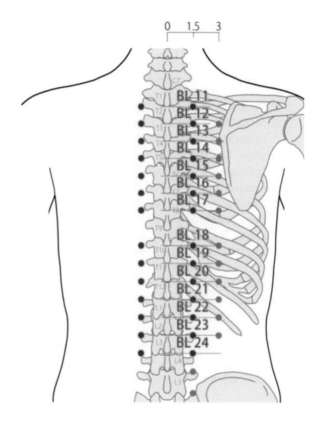

Location: On the back, below the spinous process of the ninth thoracic vertebra, 1.5 cun lateral to the posterior midline (Fig. 3.51).

Indications: (1) Jaundice, hypochondriac pain. (2) Red eyes, blurred vision, night blindness. (3) Hematemesis, epistaxis. (4) Dizziness, depression and psychosis, mania, epilepsy.

Manipulation: 0.5–0.8 cun deep oblique insertion.

9. **Danshu (BL 19)** Back Transport Point of the Gallbladder

Location: On the back, below the spinous process of the tenth thoracic vertebrae, 1.5 cun lateral to the posterior midline (Fig. 3.51).

Indications: (1) Jaundice, bitter taste in mouth, hypochondriac pain. (2) Pulmonary phthisis, high fever.

Manipulation: 0.5–0.8 cun deep oblique insertion.

10. **Pishu (BL 20)** Back Transport Point of the Spleen

Location: On the back, below the spinous process of the 11th thoracic vertebra, 1.5 cun lateral to the posterior midline (Fig. 3.51).

Indications: (1) Abdominal distension, diarrhea, dysentery, hematochezia, anorexia. (2) Edema, jaundice.

Manipulation: 0.5–0.8 cun deep oblique insertion.

11. **Weishu (BL 21)** Back Transport Point of the Stomach

    Location: On the back, below the spinous process of the 12th thoracic vertebrae, 1.5 cun lateral to the posterior midline (Fig. 3.51).

    Indications: (1) Epigastric pain, vomiting, abdominal distension, borborygmus. (2) Chest and hypochondriac pain.

    Manipulation: 0.5–0.8 cun deep oblique insertion.

12. **Shenshu (BL 23)** Back Transport Point of the Kidney

    Location: On the back, below the spinous process of the second lumbar vertebra, 1.5 cun lateral to the posterior midline (Fig. 3.51).

    Indications: (1) Tinnitus, deafness. (2) Seminal emission, impotence, irregular menstruation, morbid leucorrhea, enuresis, difficulty in urination, edema. (3) Lumbar pain. (4) Cough, asthma, asthenic breathing.

    Manipulation: 0.5–1.0 cun deep oblique insertion.

13. **Dachangshu (BL 25)** Back Transport Point of the Large Intestine

    Location: On the back, below the spinous process of the fourth lumbar vertebra, 1.5 cun lateral to the posterior midline (Fig. 3.52).

    Indications: (1) Pain of the lumbar region and lower limbs. (2) Abdominal pain, diarrhea, constipation, dysentery, hemorrhoids.

    Manipulation: 0.5–1.0 cun deep oblique insertion.

14. **Pangguangshu (BL 28)** Back Transport Point of the Bladder

    Location: On the sacrum, level with the second posterior sacral foramen, and 1.5 cun lateral to the median sacral crest (Fig. 3.53).

    Indications: (1) Difficulty in urination, frequent urination, enuresis. (2) Diarrhea, constipation. (3) Stiffness and pain in the lower back.

    Manipulation: 0.8–1.2 cun deep oblique insertion.

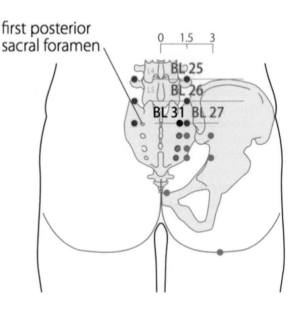

Fig. 3.52 Location of BL 25–BL 27

first posterior sacral foramen

Fig. 3.53 Location of BL 28–BL 30

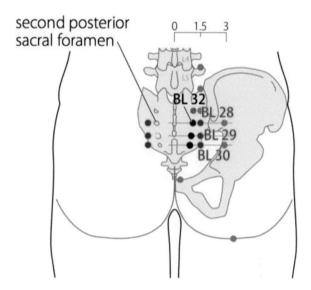

Fig. 3.54 Location of BL 31, BL 32

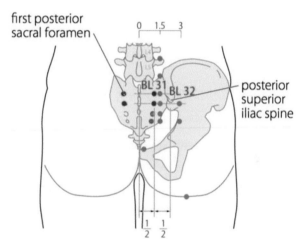

15. **Ciliao (BL 32)**
    Location: On the sacrum, in the second posterior sacral foramen (Fig. 3.54).
    Indications: (1) Irregular menstruation, dysmenorrhea, morbid leucorrhea. (2) Seminal emission. (3) Difficulty in urination. (4) Hernia. (5) Low-back pain, sacral pain, weakness or paralysis in the lower limbs.
    Manipulation: 1.0–1.5 cun deep oblique insertion.
16. **Weiyang (BL 39)** Lower Sea Point of the Triple Energizer
    Location: On the lateral end of the transverse crease of the popliteal fossa, on the medial border of the tendon of the biceps femoris (Fig. 3.55).
    Indications: (1) Abdominal distension, edema, difficulty in urination. (2) Pain and stiffness in the back, spasm of the lower limbs.
    Manipulation: 1.0–1.5 cun deep oblique insertion.

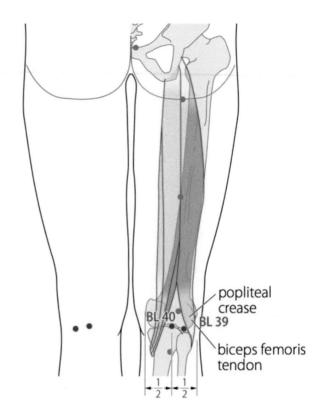

Fig. 3.55 Location of BL 39, BL 40

17. **Weizhong (BL 40)** Sea Point; Lower Sea Point of the Bladder

   Location: On the midpoint of the transverse crease of the popliteal fossa (Fig. 3.55).

   Indications: (1) Lumbar pain, spasm of the popliteal tendons, weakness or paralysis in the lower limbs. (2) Difficulty in urination, enuresis. (3) Acute vomiting and diarrhea, abdominal pain. (4) Erysipelas, urticaria, furuncles.

   Manipulation: 1.0–1.5 cun deep oblique insertion.

18. **Gaohuang (BL 43)**

   Location: On the back, level with the lower border of the spinous process of the fourth thoracic vertebra, 3 cun lateral to the posterior midline (Fig. 3.56).

   Indications: (1) Cough, asthma, pulmonary phthisis. (2) Forgetfulness, seminal, emission, night sweats, consumptive disease. (3) Pain of the shoulder and back.

   Manipulation: 0.5–0.8 cun deep oblique insertion.

19. **Zhishi (BL 52)**

   Location: Level with the lower border of the spinous process of the second lumbar vertebra, 3 cun lateral to the posterior midline (Fig. 3.56).

   Indications: (1) Seminal emission, impotence. (2) Difficulty in urination, edema. (3) Stiffness and pain in the back.

   Manipulation: 0.5–0.8 cun deep oblique insertion.

Fig. 3.56 Location of BL 41–BL 52

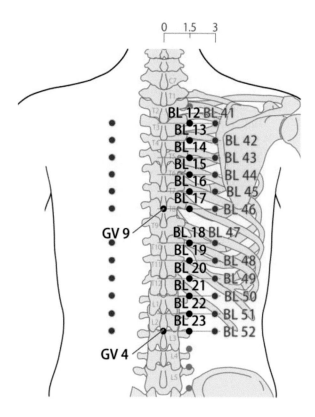

Fig. 3.57 Location of BL 53, BL 54

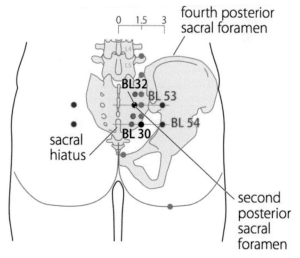

20. Zhibian (BL 54)

Location: Level with the fourth posterior sacral foramen, 3 cun lateral to the median sacral crest (Fig. 3.57).

Indications: (1) Pain in the lumbar areas and legs, atrophy or paralysis in the lower limbs. (2) Hemorrhoids, constipation, difficulty in urination.

Manipulation: 0.5–0.8 cun deep oblique insertion.

21. **Chengshan (BL 57)**

Location: On the posterior aspect of the leg where the calcaneal tendon connects with the two muscle bellies of the gastrocnemius muscle (Fig. 3.58).

Indications: (1) Pain in the lumbar and legs. (2) Hemorrhoids, constipation. (3) Hernia.

Manipulation: 1.0–2.0 cun perpendicular insertion.

22. **Feiyang (BL 58)** Connecting Point

Location: 7 cun directly above Kunlun (BL 60) between the inferior border of the lateral head of the gastrocnemius muscle and the calcaneal tendon (Fig. 3.58).

Fig. 3.58 Location of BL 55–BL 60

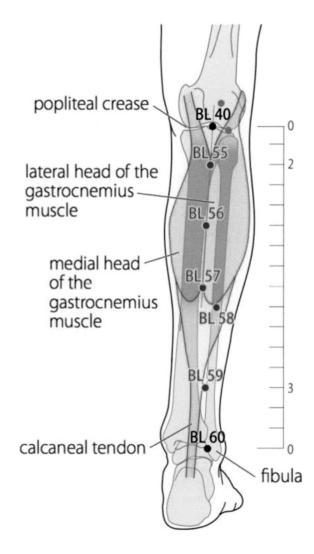

Fig. 3.59 Location of BL
60–BL 62

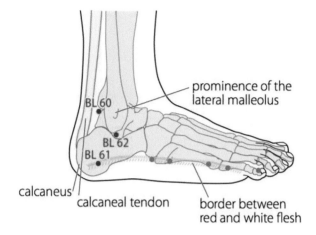

Indications: (1) Pain in the low back and legs. (2) Headache. (3) Dizziness. (4) Hemorrhoids.

Manipulation: 1.0–1.5 cun perpendicular insertion.

23. **Kunlun (BL 60)** River Point

Location: Posterior to the lateral malleolus, in the depression between the tip of the external malleolus and Achilles tendon (Fig. 3.59).

Indications: (1) Headache, stiffness in the nape, spasm of the back and shoulder, dizziness. (2) Low-back pain, heel pain. (3) Epilepsy. (4) Delayed labor.

Manipulation: 0.5–0.8 cun perpendicular insertion. Pregnant woman should not be applied.

24. **Shenmai (BL 62)** One of the Eight Confluence Points Associating with Yang Heel Vessel

Location: On the lateral side of the foot, in the depression directly below the external malleolus (Fig. 3.59).

Indications: (1) Headache, dizziness, stiffness in nape. (2) Epilepsy, mania, insomnia. (3) Pain in the low back and leg.

Manipulation: 0.3–0.5 cun perpendicular insertion.

25. **Shugu (BL 65)** Stream Point

Location: On the lateral side of the foot, posterior to the head of the fifth metatarsal bone, at the junction of the red and white skin (Fig. 3.60).

Indications: (1) Headache, stiff neck, dizziness. (2) Pain in the lumbar area and lower limbs. (3) Psychosis.

Manipulation: 0.3–0.5 cun perpendicular insertion.

26. **Zhiyin (BL 67)** Well Point

Location: On the lateral side of the distal segment of the little toe, 0.1 cun from the corner of the toenail (Fig. 3.61).

Indications: (1) Malposition of fetus, delayed labor. (2) Headache, eyes pain. (3) Nasal obstruction, nosebleed.

Fig. 3.60 Location of BL 63–BL 66

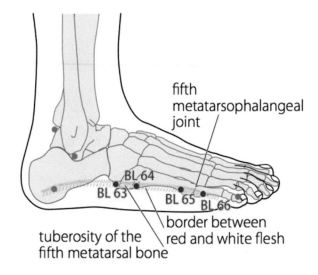

Fig. 3.61 Location of BL 67

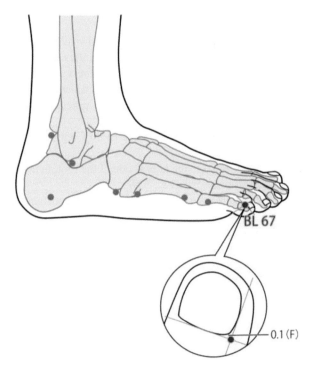

Manipulation: Insert the needle 0.1 cun into the skin, moxibustion is applicable for malposition of fetus.

27. **Other Points on Bladder Meridian of Foot Taiyang** (Table 3.22).

Table 3.22 Other points on bladder meridian of foot taiyang

Points	Code	Location	Indication	Manipulation
Meichong	BL 3	On the scalp, directly above Cuanzu (BL 2), 0.5 cun within the anterior hairline	Headache, dizziness, nasal obstruction, epistaxis	0.3–0.5 cun horizontal insertion
Qucha	BL 4	On the scalp, 0.5 cun within the anterior hairline, 1.5 cun lateral to the midline. At the junction of the medial one-third and lateral 2/3 of the distance from Shenting (GV 24) and Touwei (ST 8)	Headache, dizziness, nasal obstruction, epistaxis	0.5–0.8 cun horizontal insertion
Wuchu	BL 5	On the scalp, 1.0 cun within the anterior hairline, 1.5 cun lateral to the midline	(1) Headache, dizziness, (2) Epilepsy	0.5–0.8 cun horizontal insertion
Chengguang	BL 6	On the scalp, 2.5 cun within the anterior hairline, 1.5 cun lateral to the midline	(1) Headache, dizziness, nasal obstruction. (2) Febrile diseases	0.3–0.5 cun horizontal insertion
Tongtian	BL 7	On the scalp, 4.0 cun within the anterior hairline, 1.5 cun lateral to the midline	(1) Headache, dizziness, nasal obstruction, epistaxis, nasosinusitis. (2) Epilepsy	0.3–0.5 cun horizontal insertion
Luoque	BL 8	On the scalp, 5.5 cun within the anterior hairline, 1.5 cun lateral to the midline	Dizziness, blurred vision, tinnitus	0.3–0.5 cun horizontal insertion
Yuzhen	BL 9	On the posterior aspect of the head, 2.5 cun superior to the posterior hairline, 1.3 cun lateral to the midline and level with the depression on the superior border of the external occipital protuberance	Headache and nape of the neck pain, eye pain, nasal obstruction	0.3–0.5 cun horizontal insertion
Tianzhu	BL 10	On the nape, 1.3 cun lateral to the midpoint of the posterior hairline, and in the depression of the lateral border of the trapezius muscle	Headache, dizziness, stiffness of nape, pain in the back and shoulders, nasal obstruction	0.5–0.8 cun deep perpendicular or oblique insertion. Do not puncture deeply upwards or inside

(continued)

Table 3.22 (continued)

Points	Code	Location	Indication	Manipulation
Dazhu (one of the eight meeting points—bones convergence)	BL 11	On the back, below the spinous process of the first thoracic vertebra, 1.5 cun lateral to the posterior midline	(1) Stiffness of nape, pain in the back and shoulder. (2) Cough	0.5–0.8 cun deep oblique insertion, deep insertion is not advisable
Jueyinshu (back transport point of the pericardium)	BL 14	On the back, level with the lower border of the spinous process of the fourth thoracic vertebra, 1.5 cun lateral to the posterior midline	(1) Cardiac pain, palpitations. (2) Cough, tightness in the chest. (3) Vomiting	0.5–0.8 cun deep oblique insertion
Dushu	BL 16	On the back, level with the lower border of the spinous process of the sixth thoracic vertebra, 1.5 cun lateral to the posterior midline	(1) Cardiac pain, tightness in the chest. (2) Asthma. (3) Stomachache, abdominal distention, hiccups	0.5–0.8 cun deep oblique insertion
Sanjiaoshu (back transport point of the triple energizer)	BL 22	On the back, below the spinous process of the first lumbar vertebra, 1.5 cun lateral to the posterior midline	(1) Edema, difficulty in urination. (2) Abdominal distension, borborygmus, diarrhea, dysentery. (3) Stiffness and pain in the back and lumbar region	0.5–1.0 cun deep oblique insertion
Qihaishu	BL 24	Level with the lower border of the spinous process of the third lumbar vertebra, 1.5 cun lateral to the posterior midline	(1) Lumbar pain. (2) Dysmenorrhea. (3) Abdominal distension, borborygmus, hemorrhoids	0.5–1.0 cun deep perpendicular insertion
Guanyuanshu	BL 26	Level with the lower border of the spinous process of the fifth lumbar vertebra, 1.5 cun lateral to the posterior midline	(1) Pain of the lumbar region and lower limbs. (2) Abdominal distension, diarrhea. (3) Frequent urination or difficulty in urination, enuresis	0.8–1.2 cun deep perpendicular insertion
Xiaochangshu (back transport point of the small intestine)	BL 27	On the sacrum, level with the first posterior sacral foramen, and 1.5 cun lateral to the median sacral crest	(1) Lumbar pain, sacral pain. (2) Lower abdominal pain and distention, diarrhea, dysentery. (3) Seminal emission, morbid leucorrhea. (4) Enuresis, hematuria	0.8–1.2 cun deep oblique insertion

Table 3.22 (continued)

Points	Code	Location	Indication	Manipulation
Zhonglushu	BL 29	Level with the third posterior sacral foramen, 1.5 cun lateral to the medial sacral crest	(1) Diarrhea. (2) Stiffness and pain in the lower back. (3) Hernia	1.0–1.5 cun deep perpendicular insertion
Baihuanshu	BL 30	Level with the fourth posterior sacral foramen, 1.5 cun lateral to the medial sacral crest	(1) Seminal emission, enuresis, morbid leucorrhea, irregular menstruation, hernia. (2) Pain in the lower back	1.0–1.5 cun deep perpendicular insertion
Shangliao	BL 31	In the region of the sacrum, between the posterior-superior iliac spine and the posterior midline, in the first posterior sacral foramen	(1) Irregular menstruation, morbid leucorrhea, prolapsed uterus, seminal emission impotency. (2) Difficulty in urination and defecation. (3) Pain in the lower back	1.0–1.5 cun deep perpendicular insertion
Zhongliao	BL 33	In the region of the sacrum, medial and inferior to Ciliao (BL 32), in the third posterior sacral foramen	(1) Irregular menstruation, morbid leucorrhea, difficulty in urination. (2) Constipation, diarrhea. (3) Lumbosacral pain	1.0–1.5 cun deep perpendicular insertion
Xialiao	BL 34	In the region of the sacrum, medial and inferior to Zhongliao (BL 33), in the fourth posterior sacral foramen	(1) Lower abdominal pain, lumbosacral pain. (2) Difficulty in urination and defecation, morbid leucorrhea	1.0–1.5 cun deep perpendicular insertion
Huiyang	BL 35	In the region of the sacrum, 0.5 cun lateral to the tip of the coccyx	(1) Diarrhea, dysentery, hematochezia, hemorrhoids. (2) Impotency, morbid leucorrhea	1.0–1.5 cun deep perpendicular insertion
Chengfu	BL 36	At the midpoint of the transverse gluteal crease	(1) Pain in the lumbar and legs, weakness or paralysis in the lower limbs. (2) Hemorrhoids	1.0–2.0 cun deep oblique insertion
Yinmen	BL 37	On the line connecting Cheng fu (BL36) and Weizhong (BL40), 6 cun below Cheng fu (BL36)	Pain in the lumbar and legs, weakness or paralysis in the lower limbs	1.0–2.0 cun deep perpendicular insertion

(continued)

Table 3.22 (continued)

Points	Code	Location	Indication	Manipulation
Fuxi	BL 38	On the lateral end of the transverse crease of the popliteal fossa, 1 cun above Weiyang (BL 39) on the medial side of the tendon of the biceps femoris	(1) Pain, numbness, and spasm in the popliteal fossa and knees. (2) Constipation	1.0–1.5 cun deep perpendicular insertion
Fufen	BL 41	On the back, level with the lower border of the spinous process of the second thoracic vertebra, 3 cun lateral to the posterior midline	Stiffness and pain of the neck and back, spasm of the shoulders and back, and numbness of the elbows and arms	0.5–0.8 cun deep oblique insertion
Pohu	BL 42	On the back, level with the lower border of the spinous process of the third thoracic vertebra, 3 cun lateral to the posterior midline	(1) Cough, asthma, pulmonary phthisis. (2) Stiff neck, pain of the shoulders and back	0.5–0.8 cun deep oblique insertion
Shentang	BL 44	On the back, level with the lower border of the spinous process of the fifth thoracic vertebra, 3 cun lateral to the posterior midline	(1) Cardiac pain, palpitations. (2) Cough, asthma, tightness in the chest. (3) Pain in the back	0.5–0.8 cun deep oblique insertion
Yixi	BL 45	On the back, level with the lower border of the spinous process of the sixth thoracic vertebra, 3 cun lateral to the posterior midline	(1) Cough, asthma. (2) Malaria, febrile diseases. (3) Pain of the shoulders and back	0.5–0.8 cun deep oblique insertion
Geguan	BL 46	On the back, level with the lower border of the spinous process of the seventh thoracic vertebra, 3 cun lateral to the posterior midline	(1) Vomiting, hiccups, belching, dysphagia, tightness in the chest. (2) Stiffness and pain of the back	0.5–0.8 cun deep oblique insertion
Hunmen	BL 47	On the back, level with the lower border of the spinous process of the ninth thoracic vertebra, 3 cun lateral to the posterior midline	(1) Distending pain in the chest and hypochondrium, vomiting, diarrhea. (2) Pain in the back	0.5–0.8 cun deep oblique insertion
Yanggang	BL 48	On the back, level with the lower border of the spinous process of the tenth thoracic vertebra, 3 cun lateral to the posterior midline	(1) Borborygmus, abdominal pain, diarrhea. (2) Jaundice, diabetes	0.5–0.8 cun deep oblique insertion

Table 3.22 (continued)

Points	Code	Location	Indication	Manipulation
Yishe	BL 49	On the back, level with the lower border of the spinous process of the 11th thoracic vertebra, 3 cun lateral to the posterior midline	Abdominal distension, borborygmus, diarrhea, and vomiting	0.5–0.8 cun deep oblique insertion
Weicang	BL 50	On the back, level with the lower border of the spinous process of the 12th thoracic vertebra, 3 cun lateral to the posterior midline	(1) Epigastric pain, abdominal distension, indigestion. (2) Edema	0.5–0.8 cun deep oblique insertion
Huangmen	BL 51	Level with the lower border of the spinous process of the first lumbar vertebra, 3 cun lateral to the posterior midline	(1) Abdominal pain, abdominal masses. (2) Constipation	0.5–0.8 cun deep oblique insertion
Baohuang	BL 53	Level with the second posterior sacral foramen, 3 cun lateral to the median sacral crest	(1) Difficulty in urination, swollen vulva. (2) Abdominal distension, constipation. (3) Lumbar vertebral pain	0.5–0.8 cun deep oblique insertion
Heyang	BL 55	On the posterior aspect of the lower leg, 2 cun below Weizhong (BL 40)	Stiffness or pain in the low back, atrophy or paralysis in the lower limbs, hernia, uterine bleeding	1.0–2.0 cun deep perpendicular insertion
Chengjin	BL 56	On the posterior midline of the leg, between Weizhong (BL 40) and Kunlun (BL 60), in the center of the belly of the gastrocnemius muscle, 5 cun below Weizhong (BL 40)	Pain in the low back and legs, hemorrhoids	1.0–1.5 cun perpendicular insertion
Fuyang (cleft point of the yang heel vessel)	BL 59	3 cun directly above Kunlun (BL 60) between the fibula and the calcaneal tendon	Pain in the low back and legs, atrophy or paralysis in the lower limbs, headache	0.8–1.2 cun perpendicular insertion
Pucan	BL 61	On the lateral side of the foot, posterior and inferior to the external malleolus, directly below Kunlun (BL 60), lateral to the calcaneus at the junction of the red and white skin	(1) Atrophy or paralysis in the lower limbs, pain in the heel. (2) Epilepsy	0.3–0.5 cun perpendicular insertion

(continued)

Table 3.22 (continued)

Points	Code	Location	Indication	Manipulation
Jingmen (cleft point)	BL 63	On the dorsum of the foot inferior to the anterior border of the lateral malleolus and posterior to the tuberosity of the fifth metatarsal bone in the depression inferior to the cuboid bone	(1) Headache. (2) Epilepsy, infantile convulsions. (3) Lumbar pain, pain in the lower limbs, pain and swelling in the external malleolus	0.3–0.5 cun perpendicular insertion
Jinggu (source point)	BL 64	On the lateral aspect of the foot, distal to the tuberosity of the fifth metatarsal bone at the border between the red and white flesh	(1) Headache, stiff neck, superficial visual obstruction. (2) Pain in the lumbar and lower limbs. (3) Epilepsy	0.3–0.5 cun perpendicular insertion
Zutonggu (spring point)	BL 66	On the lateral side of the foot, anterior to the fifth metatarsophalangeal joint, at the junction of the red and white skin	(1) Headache, stiff neck, dizziness, epistaxis. (2) Psychosis	0.2–0.3 cun perpendicular insertion

3.4.1.8 Frequently Used Acupoints on Kidney Meridian of Foot Shaoyin

Kidney meridian of foot shaoyin originates from the inferior aspect of the small toe, and proceeds diagonally to the center of the foot sole emerging from the lower border of the navicular tuberosity. It runs posterior to the inner malleolus and enters the heel. It then ascends along the medial aspect of the lower leg and emerges from the medial aspect of popliteal fossa. From the popliteal fossa, it proceeds upwards along the medial and posterior aspect of the thigh and goes toward the vertebral column. It then pertains to the kidney and connects with the bladder. A straight branch from the kidney ascends to enter the lung, and then travels upwards along the throat to reach the root of the tongue. Another branch emerges from the lung to connect with the heart, and depresses into the chest (Fig. 3.62).

1. **Yongquan (KI 1)** Well Point

    Location: On the sole, in the depression which appears on the anterior part of the sole when the foot is in the plantar flexion, at the junction of the anterior third and posterior two-thirds of the line connecting the base of the second and third toes and the heel approximately (Fig. 3.63).

    Indications: (1) Mind diseases like coma, heatstroke, epilepsy, infantile convulsions. (2) Headache, vertigo, dizziness, insomnia. (3) Lung system diseases like swollen pharynx, aphonia. (4) Constipation, dysuria. (5) Up-rushing gas syndrome. (6) Feverish sensation in the sole.

    Manipulation: 0.5–1.0 cun perpendicular insertion, and to avoid hurting plantar deep when inserting the needle. Moxibustion is applicable.

2. **Rangu (KI 2)** Spring Point

Fig. 3.62 The course of
kidney meridian of foot
shaoyin

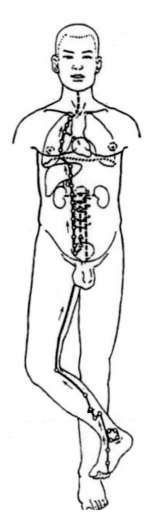

Location: On the medial border of the foot and in the depression below the
tuberosity of the navicular bone, at the junction of the red and white skin
(Fig. 3.64).

Indications: (1) Gynecological diseases like irregular menstruation, morbid
leucorrhea, prolapsed uterus. (2) External genitalia diseases like seminal emission, impotence, and dysuria. (3) Sore and swollen throat, hemoptysis. (4)
Diabetes. (5) Weakness and flaccidity of the lower limbs, pain instep. (6) Tetanus,
lockjaw. (7) Diarrhea.

Manipulation: 0.5–1.0 cun perpendicular insertion.

3. **Taixi (KI 3)** Stream Point; Source Point

Location: Posterior to the medial malleolus, in the depression between the tip
of the medial malleolus and the calcaneal tendon (Fig. 3.64).

Fig. 3.63 Location of KI 1

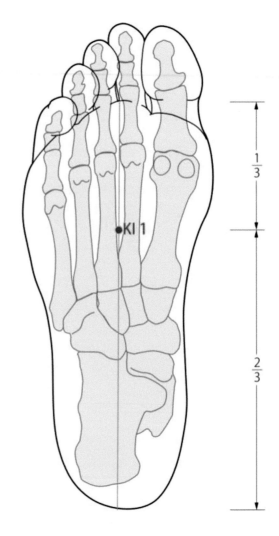

Fig. 3.64 Location of KI
2–KI4

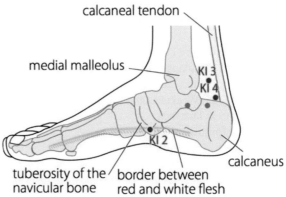

Indications: (1) Headache, dizziness, insomnia, forgetfulness. (2) Sore and swollen throat, toothache, tinnitus, deafness. (3) Cough, asthma, hemoptysis, pain in the chest. (4) Diabetes. (5) Irregular menstruation, seminal emission, impotence, frequent urination. (6) Lumbar pain, cold lower limbs, pain, and swelling in the medial malleolus.

Manipulation: 0.5–1.0 cun perpendicular insertion.

4. **Dazhong (KI 4)** Connecting Point

Location: On the medial side of the foot, posterior and inferior to the medial malleolus, in the depression anterior to the medial side of the attachment of calcaneal tendon (Fig. 3.64).

Indications: (1) Dementia. (2) Retention of urine, enuresis, constipation. (3) Irregular menstruation. (4) Hemoptysis, asthma. (5) Lumbago, pain in the heel.

Manipulation: Puncture perpendicularly by 0.3–0.5 cun.

5. **Zhaohai (KI6)** One of the Eight Confluence Points Associated with Yin Heel Vessel

Location: In the depression below the tip of the medial malleolus (Fig. 3.65).

Indications: (1) Insomnia, epilepsy. (2) Sore and dry throat, red and swollen eyes. (3) Irregular menstruation, dysmenorrheal, morbid leucorrhea, prolapsed uterus. (4) Frequent urination, retention of urine, constipation.

Manipulation:0.5–0.8 cun perpendicular insertion.

6. **Fuliu (KI 7)** River Point

Location: 2 cun directly above *Tai xi* (KI 3), anterior to the achilles tendon (Fig. 3.66).

Indications: (1) Edema, night sweat, febrile diseases with anhidrosis or hyperhidrosis. (2) Abdominal distension, diarrhea, borborygmus. (3) Lumbago, weakness, and flaccidity of the lower limbs.

Manipulation: 0.5–1.0 cun perpendicular insertion.

7. **Other Points on Kidney Meridian of Foot Shaoyin** (Table 3.23).

Fig. 3.65 Location of KI 5, KI 6

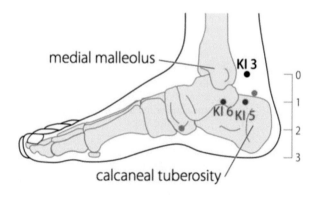

Fig. 3.66 Location of KI
8–KI 10

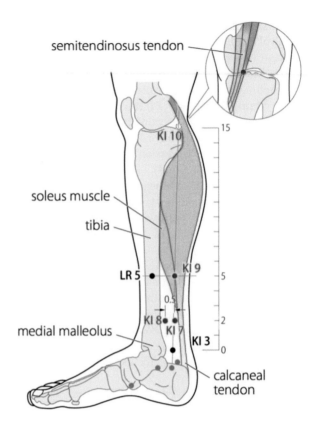

Table 3.23 Other points on kidney meridian of foot shaoyin

Points	Code	Location	Indication	Manipulation
Shuiquan	KI 5	1 cun directly below Taixi (KI 3), in the depression of the medial side of the tuberosity of the calcaneus	Irregular menstruation, dysmenorrhea, prolapsed uterus, difficulty in urination	0.3–0.5 cun deep perpendicular insertion
Jiaoxin	KI 8	On the medial aspect of the lower legs, 2 cun above Taixi (KI 3), 0.5 cun anterior to Fuliu (KI 7), posterior to the medial border of the tibia	(1) Irregular menstruation, uterine bleeding, and prolapsed uterus. (2) Diarrhea, constipation	0.8–1.2 cun deep perpendicular insertion
Zhubin	KI 9	On the line connecting Taixi (KI 3) and Yingu (KI 10), 5 cun above Taixi (KI 3), medial and inferior to the gastrocnemius muscle belly	(1) Psychosis. (2) Hernia. (3) Vomiting. (4) Pain on the medial aspect of the lower legs	1.0–1.5 cun deep perpendicular insertion

Table 3.23 (continued)

Points	Code	Location	Indication	Manipulation
Yingu (sea point)	KI 10	On the posteromedial aspect of the knee lateral to the semitendinosus tendon in the popliteal crease	(1) Psychosis. (2) Impotence, irregular menstruation, uterine bleeding, difficulty in urination. (3) Pain on the medial side of the knees and legs	1.0–1.5 cun deep perpendicular insertion
Henggu	KI 11	On the lower abdomen, 5 cun below the umbilicus, 0.5 cun lateral to the anterior midline	(1) Pain and distension in the lower abdomen, hernia. (2) Seminal emission, impotence, enuresis, difficulty in urination	1.0–1.5 cun deep perpendicular insertion
Dahe	KI 12	4 cun below the center of the umbilicus, 0.5 cun lateral to the anterior midline	(1) Seminal emission, impotence. (2) Prolapsed uterus, morbid leucorrhea, irregular menstruation. (3) Diarrhea and dysentery	1.0–1.5 cun deep perpendicular insertion
Qixue	KI 13	On the lower abdomen, 3 cun below the umbilicus, 0.5 cun lateral to the anterior midline	(1) Irregular menstruation, morbid leucorrhea, infertility, impotence, difficulty in urination. (2) Diarrhea, dysentery	1.0–1.5 cun deep perpendicular insertion
Siman	KI 14	On the lower abdomen, 2 cun below the umbilicus, 0.5 cun lateral to the anterior midline	(1) Irregular menstruation, morbid leucorrhea, seminal emission, enuresis, edema. (2) Abdominal pain, constipation	1.0–1.5 cun deep perpendicular insertion
Zhongzhu	KI 15	In the center of the abdomen, 1 cun below the umbilicus, 0.5 cun lateral to the anterior midline	(1) Irregular menstruation. (2) Abdominal pain, constipation, diarrhea	1.0–1.5 cun deep perpendicular insertion
Huangshu	KI 16	In the center of the abdomen, 0.5 cun lateral to the anterior midline	(1) Abdominal pain and distension, vomiting, diarrhea, constipation. (2) Hernia. (3) Irregular menstruation	1.0–1.5 cun deep perpendicular insertion
Shangqu	KI 17	On the upper abdomen, 2 cun above the umbilicus, 0.5 cun lateral to the anterior midline	Abdominal pain, diarrhea, and constipation	1.0–1.5 cun deep perpendicular insertion
Shi guan	KI 18	On the upper abdomen, 3 cun above the umbilicus, 0.5 cun lateral to the anterior midline	(1) Abdominal pain, vomiting, constipation. (2) Infertility	1.0–1.5 cun deep perpendicular insertion

(continued)

Table 3.23 (continued)

Points	Code	Location	Indication	Manipulation
Yindu	KI 19	On the upper abdomen, 4 cun above the umbilicus, 0.5 cun lateral to the anterior midline	(1) Abdominal pain and distension, borborygmus, constipation. (2) Infertility	1.0–1.5 cun deep perpendicular insertion
Futonggu	KI 20	On the upper abdomen, 5 cun above the umbilicus, 0.5 cun lateral to the anterior midline	Abdominal pain and distension, and vomiting	0.5–1.0 cun deep perpendicular insertion
Youmen	KI 21	On the upper abdomen, 6 cun above the umbilicus, 0.5 cun lateral to the anterior midline	Stomachache, vomiting, abdominal distension, and diarrhea	0.5–1.0 cun deep perpendicular insertion. Do not insert deeply so as to avoid injuring the liver
Bulang	KI 22	On the chest in the fifth intercostal space, 2 cun lateral to the anterior midline	(1) Distension and fullness of the chest and hypochondriac regions, cough, asthma. (2) Vomiting. (3) Mastiffs	0.5–0.8 cun deep horizontal or oblique insertion. Do not insert deeply so as to avoid injuring the heart and lung
Shenfeng	KI 23	On the chest, in the fourth intercostal space, 2 cun lateral to the anterior midline	(1) Cough, asthma, distension and fullness of the chest and hypochondriac regions. (2) Mastitis. (3) Vomiting	0.5–0.8 cun deep horizontal or oblique insertion. Do not insert deeply so as to avoid injuring the heart and lung
Lingxu	KI 24	On the chest, in the third intercostal space, 2 cun lateral to the anterior midline	(1) Cough, asthma, distension and fullness of the chest and hypochondriac regions. (2) Mastitis. (3) Vomiting	0.5–0.8 cun deep horizontal or oblique insertion. Do not insert deeply so as to avoid injuring the heart and lung
Shencang	KI 25	On the chest, in the second intercostal space, 2 cun lateral to the anterior midline	(1) Chest pain, cough, asthma. (2) Vomiting	0.5–0.8 cun deep horizontal or oblique insertion. Do not insert deeply so as to avoid injuring the heart and lung
Yuzhong	KI 26	On the chest, in the first intercostal space, 2 cun lateral to the anterior midline	Cough, asthma, distending pain in the chest and hypochondriac regions	0.5–0.8 cun deep horizontal or oblique insertion. Do not insert deeply so as to avoid injuring the heart and lung
Shufu	KI 27	On the chest, on the lower border of the clavicle, 2 cun lateral to the anterior midline	(1) Cough, asthma, chest pain. (2) Vomiting	0.5–0.8 cun deep horizontal or oblique insertion. Do not insert deeply so as to avoid injuring the heart and lung

3.4.1.9 Frequently Used Acupoints on Pericardium Meridian of Hand Jueyin

It originates from the center of the chest, and pertains to the pericardium. It descends through the diaphragm, passing through the upper, middle, and lower energizer. One branch runs inside the chest to emerge from hypochondrium and runs along the middle of the upper arm, and then it travels along the forearm between the two tendons to enter the palm, passing along the middle finger and ends at its tip. One branch splits from the palm to reach the tip of the ring finger, connecting with the triple energizer meridian of hand shaoyang (Fig. 3.67).

1. **Tianchi (PC 1)**

    Location: On the chest, in the fourth intercostal space, 1 cun lateral to the nipple, 5 cun lateral to the anterior midline (Fig. 3.68).

    Indications: (1) Cough, asthma, pain or distention in the chest. (2) Mastitis. (3) Scrofula.

    Manipulation: Puncture obliquely or transversely by 0.5–0.8 cun. Do not puncture deeply to avoid injuring the lung.

Fig. 3.67 The course of pericardium meridian of hand jueyin

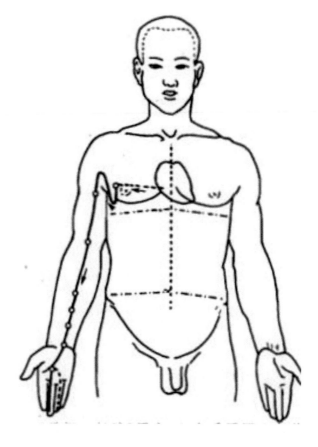

Fig. 3.68 Location of PC
1, PC 2

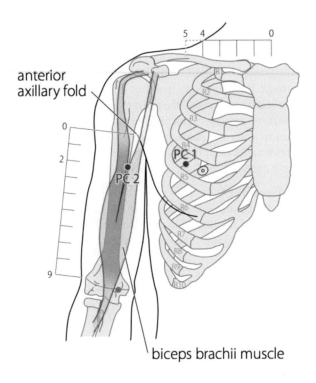

anterior
axillary fold

biceps brachii muscle

2. **Quze (PC 3)** Sea Point
   Location: On the transverse cubital crease, on the ulnar side of the tendon of
   the biceps muscle of the arm (Fig. 3.69).
   Indications: (1) Heart system diseases like cardiodynia, palpitations, etc. (2)
   Stomach diseases like stomachache, hematemesis, vomiting, etc. (3) Sunstroke.
   (4) Pain and cramps in the elbows and arms.
   Manipulation: 1.0–1.5 cun deep perpendicular insertion. Pricking to induce
   bleeding is applicable.
3. **Jianshi (PC 5)** River Point
   Location: On the palmar side of the forearm, 3 cun above the transverse
   crease of the wrist, and between the tendons of the palmaris longus and flexor
   carpi radialis (Fig. 3.69).
   Indications: (1) Heart system diseases like cardiodynia, palpitations, etc. (2)
   Stomach diseases like stomachache, vomiting, etc. (3) Febrile disease, malaria.
   (4) Psychosis, epilepsy. (5) Brachialgia, cramps in the elbow, axillary swelling.
   Manipulation: 0.5–1.0 cun deep perpendicular insertion.
4. **Neiguan (PC 6)** Connecting Point; One of the Eight Confluent Points Associating
   with Yin Link Vessel
   Location: On the palmar side of the forearm, 2 cun above the transverse
   crease of the wrist, and between the tendons of the palmaris longus and flexor
   carpi radialis (Fig. 3.69).

Fig. 3.69 Location of PC 3–PC 7

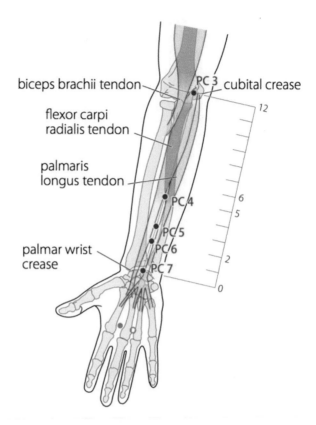

Indications: (1) Heart system diseases like cardiodynia, palpitations, chest pain, oppression in the chest, etc. (2) Stomach diseases like stomachache, vomiting, hiccups, etc. (3) Stroke, dizziness, hemiplegia, migraine. (4) Insomnia, depression, epilepsy, febrile disease. (5) Pain and spasm in the elbows and arms.

Manipulation: 0.5–1.0 cun deep perpendicular insertion.

5. **Daling (PC 7)** Stream Point; Source Point

    Location: In the middle of the transverse crease of the wrist, and between the tendons of the palmaris longus and flexor carpi radialis (Fig. 3.69).

    Indications: (1) Cardiodynia, palpitations, pain and distension in the chest, hypochondriac pain. (2) Stomachache, vomiting, bromopnea. (3) Epilepsy, madness. (4) Pain and spasm in the elbows and arms.

    Manipulation: 0.3–0.5 cun deep perpendicular insertion.

6. **Laogong (PC 8)** Spring Point

    Location: In the middle of the palm, between the second and third metacarpal bones. When the fist is made, the point is just below the tip of the middle finger (Fig. 3.70).

    Indications: (1) Stroke and coma, sunstroke. (2) Cardiodynia, restlessness, epilepsy. (3) Stomatitis, foul breath. (4) Tinea manus.

    Manipulation: 0.3–0.5 cun deep perpendicular insertion.

7. **Zhongchong (PC 9)** Well Point

  Location: In the center of the tip of the middle finger (Fig. 3.70).

  Indications: (1) Stroke and coma, stiff tongue impeding speech, infantile convulsion, sunstroke, syncope. (2) Febrile disease, pain in the hypoglottis.

  Manipulation: 0.1 cun shallow insertion or prick with three-edged needle to induce bleeding.

8. **Other Points on Pericardium Meridian of Hand Jueyin** (Table 3.24).

Fig. 3.70 Location of PC 8, PC 9

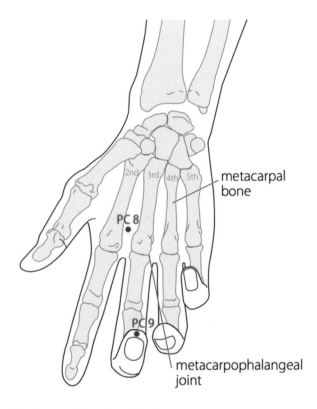

Table 3.24 Other points on pericardium meridian of hand jueyin

Points	Code	Location	Indication	Manipulation
Tianquan	PC 2	On the palmar side of the upper arm, 2 cun below the level of the anterior axillary fold, between the two heads of the biceps brachii muscle	Cardiodynia, cough, distention in the chest, pain in the chest, upper back, and medial side of the upper arms	1.0–1.5 cun deep perpendicular insertion
Ximen (cleft point)	PC 4	On the palmar side of the forearm, 5 cun above the transverse crease of the wrist, and between the tendons of the palmaris longus and flexor carpi radialis	(1) Cardiodynia, palpitations, restlessness, pain in the chest. (2) Hemoptysis, hematemesis, epistaxis. (3) Furunculosis. (4) Epilepsy	0.5–1.0 cun deep perpendicular insertion

3.4.1.10 Frequently Used Acupoints on Triple Energizer Meridian of Hand Shaoyang

It originates from the tips of the ring finger and runs upward between the fourth and fifth metacarpal bones along the dorsum of the hand then continues going upwards between the radius and ulna. It ascends along the lateral aspect of the upper arms to the shoulders and enters the supraclavicular fossa to connect with the pericardium and connects along its pathway with the upper, middle, and lower energizer. One branch separates in the chest region, ascending to emerge from the supraclavicular fossa and rising to the head.

One branch separates in the chest region, ascending to emerge from the supraclavicular fossa and rising along the neck to the posterior border of the ear. It crosses from the superior aspect of the ear to the corner of the forehead, turning downwards the cheek and reaching the inferior aspect of the eye.

Another branch separates behind the ear and enters the ear, and reemerges in front of the ear, crossing the previous branch on the cheek. It then goes to the outer canthus, where it connects with the gallbladder meridian of foot shaoyang (Fig. 3.71).

Fig. 3.71 The course of triple energizer meridian of hand shaoyang

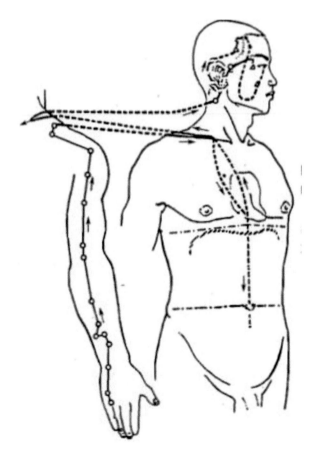

1. **Guɑuchong (TE 1)** Well Point

    Location: On the ulnar side of the distal segment of the fourth finger, 0.1 cun from the corner of the nail.

    Indications: (1) Headache, red eyes, deafness, sore throat, stiff tongue. (2) Febrile diseases, coma, sunstroke (Fig. 3.72).

    Manipulation: Insert the needle shallowly by 0.1 cun deep or prick with three-edged needle to induce bleeding.

2. **Zhongzhu (TE 3)** Stream Point

    Location: On the dorsum of the hand proximal to the fourth metacarpophalangeal joint, in the depression between the fourth and fifth metacarpal bones (Fig. 3.72).

    Indications: (1) Headache, red eyes, tinnitus, deafness, sore throat. (2) Febrile diseases, sunstroke.

    Manipulation: 0.3–0.5 cun deep perpendicular insertion.

3. **Yangchi (TE 4)** Source Point

    Location: At the midpoint of the dorsal crease of the wrist, in the depression on the ulnar side of the tendon of the extensor muscle of the finger (Fig. 3.73).

    Indications: (1) Red and swollen eyes, deafness, sore throat. (2) Diabetes, febrile diseases. (3) Pain in the arms and wrists. (4) Malaria.

    Manipulation: 0.3–0.5 cun deep perpendicularly insertion.

4. **Waiguan (TE 5)** Connecting Point; One of the Eight Confluent Points Associating with Yang Link Vessel

Fig. 3.72 Location of TE 1–TE 3

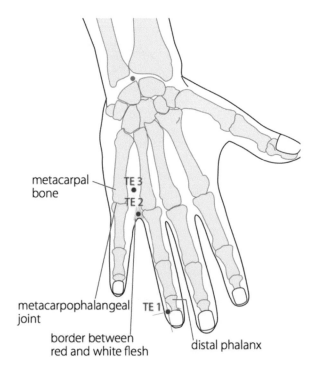

Fig. 3.73 Location of TE 4, TE 5

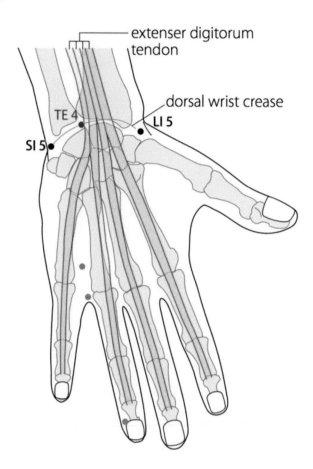

extenser digitorum tendon

dorsal wrist crease

TE 4

LI 5

SI 5

Location: On the dorsal side of the forearm and on the line connecting *Yang chi* (TE 4) and the tip of the olecranon, 2 cun proximal to the dorsal crease of the wrist, between the radius and ulna (Fig. 3.74).

Indications: (1) Febrile disease. (2) Headache, cheek pain, red and swollen eyes, tinnitus, deafness. (3) Scrofula. (4) Hypochondriac pain. (5) Pain, numbness, flaccidity, and muscle atrophy in the upper limbs.

Manipulation: 0.5–1.0 cun deep perpendicular insertion.

5. **Zhigou (TE 6)** River Point

    Location: On the dorsal aspect of the forearm, 3 cun above the transverse crease of the dorsum of the wrist between the ulna and radius (Fig. 3.74).

    Indications: (1) Tinnitus, deafness, sudden loss of voice. (2) Hypochondriac pain. (3) Constipation. (4) Scrofula. (5) Febrile disease.

    Manipulation: 0.5–1.0 cun deep perpendicular insertion.

6. **Jianliao (TE 14)**

    Location: On the shoulder girdle in the depression between the acromial angle and the greater tubercle of the humerus (Fig. 3.75).

Fig. 3.74 Location of TE 5–TE 8

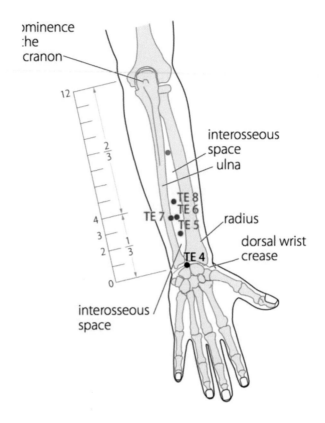

Indications: (1) Pain in the shoulders and arms, heaviness of the shoulder with inability to raise the arm. (2) Pain in the hypochondriac regions.

Manipulation: 1.0–1.5 cun deep perpendicular insertion.

7. **Yifeng (TE 17)**

   Location: Posterior to the ear lobe, in the depression between the mastoid process and the angle of the mandible (Fig. 3.76).

   Indications: (1) Tinnitus, deafness. (2) Deviation of the mouth and eye, locked jaw, toothache. (3) Scrofula.

   Manipulation: 0.5–1.0 cun deep perpendicular insertion.

8. **Ermen (TE 21)**

   Location: In front of the supratragic notch, in the depression of the posterior border of the condylar process of the mandible when the mouth is open (Fig. 3.77).

   Indications: (1) Tinnitus, deafness. (2) Toothache.

   Manipulation: 0.5–1.0 cun deep perpendicular insertion.

Fig. 3.75 Location of TE 14, TE 15

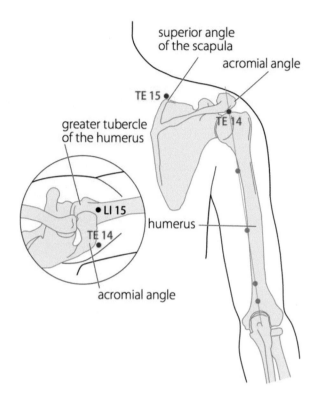

9. **Sizhukong (TE 23)**

   Location: On the face and in the depression of the lateral end of the eyebrow (Fig. 3.78).

   Indications: (1) Psychosis and epilepsy. (2) Redness, swelling, and pain of the eyes, twitching of the eyelids, migraine. (3) Toothache.

   Manipulation: 0.3–0.5 cun deep horizontal insertion.

10. **Other Points on Triple Energizer Meridian of Hand Shaoyang** (Table 3.25).

3.4.1.11   Frequently Used Acupoints on Gallbladder Meridian of Foot Shaoyang

Gallbladder meridian of foot shaoyang originates from the outer canthus, ascends to the corner of the forehead, and then descends to the posterior of the ear. Descending further along the neck to the shoulder, it enters the supraclavicular fossa.

   One branch emerges behind the ear and enters the ear, reemerging in front of the ear, and then reaching the posterior aspect of the outer canthus.

Fig. 3.76 Location of TE 17, TE 18

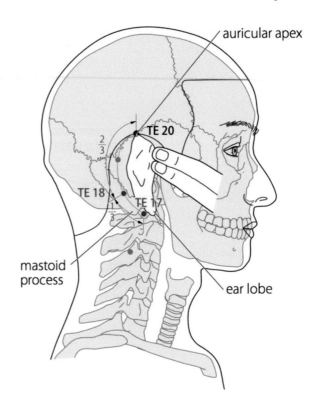

Fig. 3.77 Location of TE 21

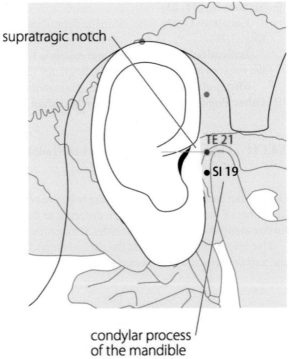

Fig. 3.78 Location of
TE 23

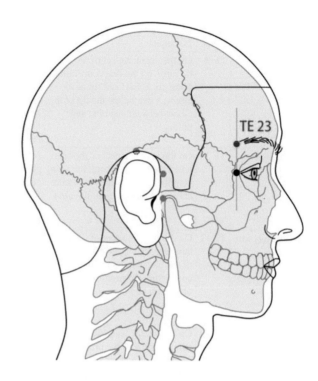

Table 3.25 Other points on triple energizer meridian of hand shaoyang

Points	Code	Location	Indication	Manipulation
Yemen (spring point)	TE 2	On the dorsum of the hand, proximal to the margin of the web between the fourth and fifth fingers, at the junction of the red and white skin	(1) Headache, red eyes, tinnitus, deafness. (2) Malaria. (3) Pain in the upper limbs	0.3–0.5 cun deep perpendicular insertion
Huizong (cleft point)	TE 7	On the dorsal aspect of the forearm, 3 cun above the transverse crease of the dorsum of the wrist, on the ulnar side of Zhi gou (TE 6), and on the radial side of the ulna	(1) Tinnitus, deafness. (2) Epilepsy	0.5–1.0 cun deep perpendicular insertion
Sanyang luo	TE 8	On the dorsal aspect of the forearm, 4 cun above the transverse crease of dorsum of the wrist, between the ulna and radius	(1) Deafness, sudden loss of voice, toothache. (2) Atrophy or paralysis in the upper limbs	0.5–1.0 cun deep perpendicular insertion

(continued)

Table 3.25 (continued)

Points	Code	Location	Indication	Manipulation
Sidu	TE 9	On the dorsal aspect of the forearm, on the line connecting Yang chi (TE 4) and tip of the elbow, 5 cun below the tip of the elbow between the ulna and radius	(1) Numbness and pain of the upper limbs. (2) Deafness, sudden loss of voice, toothache, headache	0.5–1.0 cun deep perpendicular insertion
Tianjing (sea point)	TE 10	On the lateral aspect of the arm, when the elbow is bent, the point is in the depression about 1 cun above the olecranon of the ulna	(1) Migraine, deafness, epilepsy. (2) Scrofula. (3) Pain in the elbows and arms	0.5–1.0 cun deep perpendicular insertion
Qinglengyuan	TE 11	On the lateral aspect of the arm, 2 cun proximal to the prominence of the olecranon on a line connecting the prominence of the olecranon and the acromial angle	(1) Pain in the shoulders and arms, paralysis of the upper limbs. (2) Headache, eye pain	0.5–1.0 cun deep perpendicular insertion
Xiaoluo	TE 12	On the lateral aspect of the arm, 5 cun proximal to the prominence of the olecranon on a line connecting the prominence of the olecranon and the acromial angle	(1) Numbness and pain of the upper limbs. (2) Headache, toothache, stiff neck. (3) Epilepsy	1.0–1.5 cun deep perpendicular insertion
Naohui	TE 13	On the lateral aspect of the arm, 3 cun inferior to the acromial angle, on the posterior and inferior border of the deltoid muscle	(1) Scrofula, goiter. (2) Spasm and pain in the upper limbs	1.0–1.5 cun deep perpendicular insertion
Tianliao	TE 15	In the scapula region, in the depression above the superior angle of the scapula, midpoint of a line connecting Jianjing (GB 21) and Quyuan (SI 13)	(1) Pain in the shoulders and arms. (2) Spasm of the nape of the neck	0.5–0.8 cun deep perpendicular insertion
Tianyou	TE 16	On the side of the neck, directly inferior to the posterior aspect of the mastoid process, at the level of the angle of the mandible, on the posterior border of the sternocleidomastoideus	(1) Headache, stiff neck, dizziness, eye pain, deafness. (2) Scrofula	0.5–1.0 cun deep perpendicular insertion
Chimai	TE 18	On the head, posterior to the ear in the center of the mastoid process, at the junction of the middle and lower third of the curved line along the ear helix connecting Jiaosun (TE 20) and Yifeng (TE 17)	(1) Migraine, tinnitus, deafness. (2) Infantile convulsions	0.3–0.5 cun deep horizontal insertion

Table 3.25 (continued)

Points	Code	Location	Indication	Manipulation
Luxi	TE 19	On the head, at the junction of the upper and middle third of the curved line along the ear helix connecting Jiaosun (TE 20) and Yi feng (TE 17)	(1) Migraine, tinnitus, deafness. (2) Infantile convulsions	0.3–0.5 cun deep horizontal insertion
Jiaosun	TE 20	On the head, on the hairline directly above the ear apex where the ear is folded forward	(1) Migraine, stiff neck. (2) Mumps, toothache. (3) Cataracts, red and swollen eyes	0.5–1.0 cun deep horizontal insertion
Erheliao	TE 22	On the side of the head, on the posterior border of the hairline of the temple, at the level with the root of the ear, posterior to the superficial temporal artery	(1) Migraine, tinnitus. (2) Locked jaw	0.3–0.5 cun deep horizontal or oblique insertion, avoiding needling the artery

Another branch starts from the outer canthus, descends to the Daying (ST5) and ascends to the infraorbital regions, passing near Jiache (ST6) and descending along the neck where it joins the previous branch at the supraclavicular fossa.

These meridians descend from head to the supraclavicular fossa, and meet a branch coming from lateral side of eye. Then it descends to enter the chest to connect with the liver and pertains to the gallbladder. It then travels along inside the hypochondriac region to reach *qi pathway*, curving along the margin of the pubic hair and running transversely into *Huantiao* (GB 30). The straight branch in pelvis descends from the supraclavicular fossa to *Huantiao* (GB 30) to meet the previous branch passing through the axillary region, the lateral side of the chest, and the free ends of the ribs. It continues going down the lateral side of the thigh and knee to descending along the anterior side of fibula to reach the anterior aspect of the lateral malleolus. It then follows the dorsum of the foot to end on the lateral side of the tip of the fourth toe. One branch splits from Zu *linqi* (GB 41) and emerges from the tip of the big toe. Then it comes back to enter the nail and go out of the hairy region to connect with the liver meridian of foot jueyin (Fig. 3.79).

1. **Tongziliao (GB 1)**

    Location: In the depression 0.5 cun lateral to the outer canthus and on the lateral side of the orbital margin (Fig. 3.80).

    Indications: (1) Pain and red eyes, cataracts. (2) Migraine, deviation of the mouth and eye.

    Manipulation: 0.3–0.5 cun deep horizontal insertion.

2. **Tinghui (GB 2)**

    Location: Anterior to the intertragic notch, in the depression posterior to the condyloid process of the mandible when the mouth is open (Fig. 3.81).

Fig. 3.79 The course of
gallbladder meridian of
foot shaoyang

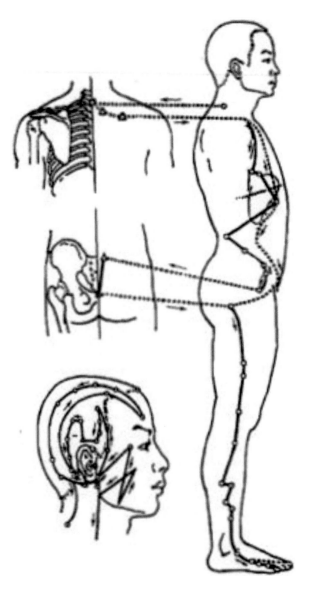

Indications: (1) Tinnitus, deafness. (2) Toothache, deviation of the mouth
and eye.

Manipulation: Puncture perpendicularly by 0.5–0.8 cun.

3. **Yangbai (GB 14)**

Location: On the forehead, directly above the pupil,1 cun above the eyebrows (Fig. 3.82).

Indications:(1) Headache, vertigo. (2) Deviation of the mouth and eye. (3)
Pain in the eyes, blurred vision, trembling eyelids.

Manipulation: 0.5–0.8 cun horizontal insertion.

Fig. 3.80 Location of GB 1

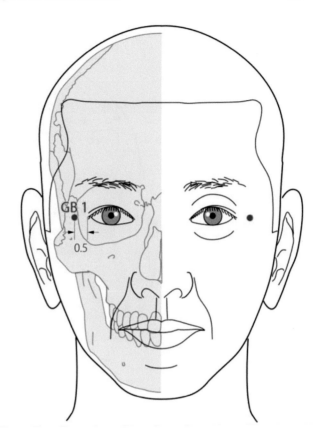

Fig. 3.81 Location of GB 2–GB 4

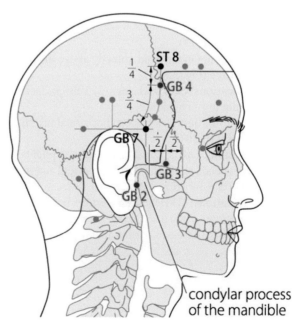

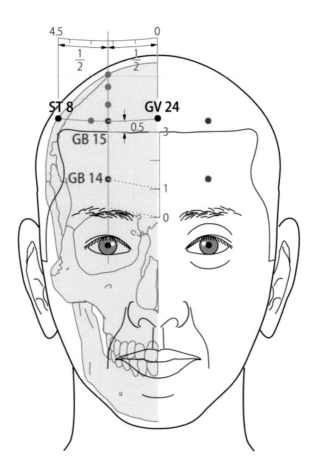

Fig. 3.82 Location of GB 14, GB 15

4. **Toulinqi (GB 15)**

   Location: On the head, directly above the pupil and 0.5 cun above the anterior hairline (Fig. 3.82).

   Indications: (1) Headache. (2) Vertigo, lacrimation. (3) Nasal obstruction. (4) Infantile convulsion.

   Manipulation: 0.5–0.8 cun horizontal insertion.

5. **Fengchi (GB 20)**

   Location: On the nape, below the occipital bone, in the depression between the upper ends of the sternocleidomastoid and trapezius muscles, on the level of Fengfu (GV 16) (Fig. 3.83).

   Indications: (1) Headache, vertigo, red and swollen eyes, tinnitus, deafness. (2) Common cold, nasal congestion, nasosinusitis, mania and epilepsy, apoplexy, febrile diseases, malaria, and goiter. (3) Rigidity and pain in the nape and back.

Fig. 3.83 Location of GB
19, GB 20

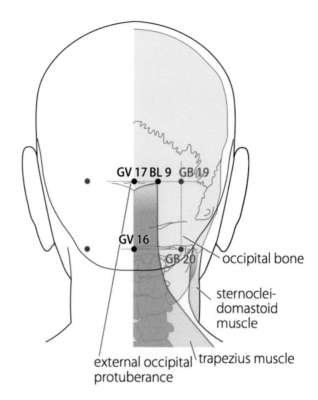

GV 17 BL 9 GB 19

GV 16

GB 20   occipital bone

sternoclei-
domastoid
muscle

external occipital trapezius muscle
protuberance

Manipulation: Puncture with the needle tip slightly pointed downwards, or toward the tip of the nose for 0.8–1.2 cun, or puncture horizontally toward Feng fu (GV 16). The medulla is located in the deep part to insert the needle must strictly grasp the depth and angle.

6. **Jianjing (GB 21)**

   Location: At the midpoint of a line connecting the spinous process of the seventh cervical vertebra and the lateral end of the acromion (Fig. 3.84).

   Indications: (1) Pain in the shoulders and upper back, stiffness and pain in the neck. (2) Mastitis, insufficient lactation. (3) Delayed labor. (4) Scrofula.

   Manipulation: 0.5–0.8 cun *deep* perpendicular insertion. Do not insert the needle too deep. Acupuncture is contraindicated for pregnant women.

7. **Riyue (GB 24)** Alarm Point of the Gallbladder

   Location: Directly below the nipple, 4 cun lateral to the anterior midline, in the seventh intercostal space (Fig. 3.85).

   Indications: (1) Jaundice, pain in the hypochondriac regions. (2) Epigastric pain, vomiting, hiccups.

   Manipulation: 0.5–0.8 cun *deep* perpendicular insertion. Do not insert the needle too deep so as to avoid hurting the inner viscera.

Fig. 3.84 Location of
GB 21

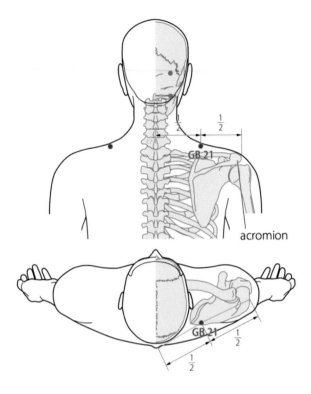

Fig. 3.85 Location of
GB 24

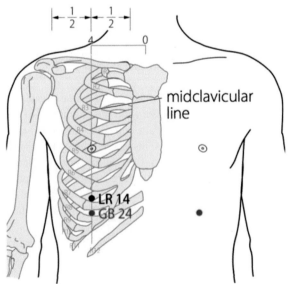

Fig. 3.86 Location of GB
24, GB 25

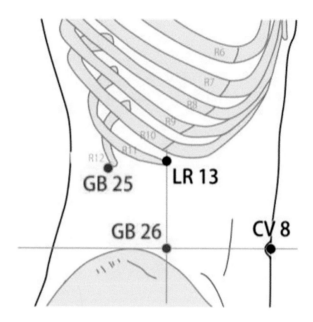

8. **Daimai (GB 26)**

   Location: At the junction of the vertical line of the free end of the 11th rib and the horizontal line of the umbilicus (Fig. 3.86).

   Indications: (1) Irregular menstruation, morbid leucorrhea, amenorrhea, lower abdominal pain. (2) Lumbar pain. (3) Hernia.

   Manipulation: 1.0–1.5 cun *deep* perpendicular insertion.

9. **Huantiao (GB 30)**

   Location: On the lateral side of the thigh, at the junction of the middle third and lateral third of the line connecting the prominence of the great trochanter and the sacral hiatus when the patient is in a lateral recumbent position with the thigh flexed (Fig. 3.87).

   Indications: (1) Pain in the lumbar areas and legs, hemiplegia, and atrophy or paralysis in the lower limbs. (2) Rubella.

   Manipulation: 2.0–3.0 cun perpendicular insertion.

10. **Fengshi (GB 31)**

   Location: On the lateral aspect of the thigh, in the depression posterior to the iliotibial band where the tip of the middle finger touches when one stands with arms extended downward (Fig. 3.88).

   Indications: (1) Hemiplegia, atrophy or paralysis in the lower limbs. (2) Itching of the entire body, beriberi.

   Manipulation: 1.0–1.5 cun perpendicular insertion.

Fig. 3.87 Location of
GB 30

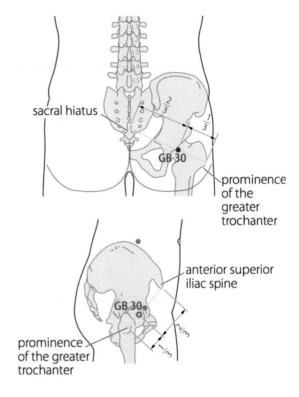

Fig. 3.88 Location of GB
31–GB 33

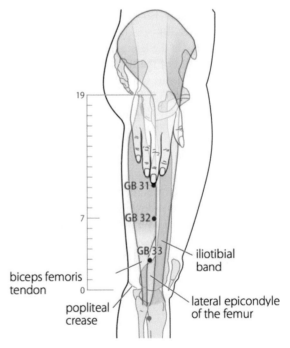

Fig. 3.89 Location of GB 34–GB 39

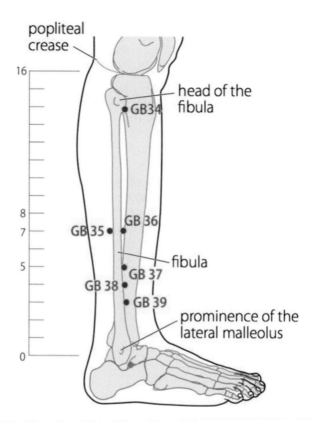

popliteal crease

16

head of the fibula

GB34

8
7
GB 35   GB 36

5
fibula
GB 37
GB 38
GB 39

prominence of the lateral malleolus

0

11. **Yanglingquan (GB 34)** Sea Point; Lower Sea Point of the Gallbladder, One of the Eight Meeting Points (Sinews Convergence)

    Location: On the lateral side of the leg, in the depression anterior and inferior to the head of the fibula (Fig. 3.89).

    Indications: (1) Jaundice, pain in the hypochondriac region, bitter taste in mouth, vomiting. (2) Hemiparalysis, atrophy or paralysis in the lower limbs, beriberi. (3) Infantile convulsion.

    Manipulation: 1.0–1.5 cun perpendicular insertion.

12. **Guangming (GB 37)** Connecting Point

    Location: On the lateral side of the leg, 5 cun above the tip of the external malleolus, on the anterior border of the fibula (Fig. 3.89).

    Indications: (1) Pain in the eyes, night blindness. (2) Atrophy or paralysis in the lower limbs. (3) Distention in the chest.

    Manipulation: 0.5–0.8 cun perpendicular insertion.

13. **Xuanzhong (GB 39)** One of the Eight Meeting Points (Marrow Convergence)

    Location: On the lateral side of the legs, 3 cun above the tip of the external malleolus, on the anterior border of the fibula (Fig. 3.89).

Fig. 3.90 Location of GB 40–GB 42

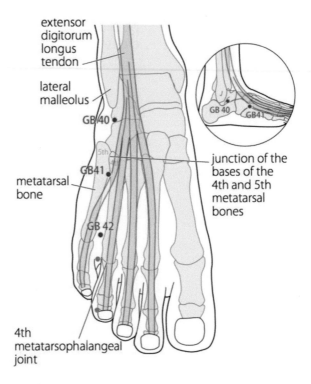

extensor digitorum longus tendon

lateral malleolus

GB 40

GB 40
GB 41

5th

GB 41

metatarsal bone

junction of the bases of the 4th and 5th metatarsal bones

GB 42

4th metatarsophalangeal joint

Indications: (1) Dementia, hemiparalysis. (2) Stiffness in the nape, pain and distention in the hypochondriac region. (3) Atrophy or paralysis in the lower limbs, sore throat, beriberi, hemorrhoid.

Manipulation: 0.5–0.8 cun perpendicular insertion.

14. **Qiuxu (GB 40) Source Point**

Location: Anterior and inferior to the external malleolus, in the depression lateral to the tendon of the long extensor muscle of the toes (Fig. 3.90).

Indications: (1) Red and swollen eyes. (2) Stiffness in neck and nape, pain and distention in the hypochondriac region. (3) Atrophy or paralysis in the lower limbs.

Manipulation: 0.5–0.8 cun perpendicular insertion.

15. **Zulinqi (GB 41) Stream Point; One of the Eight Confluence Points Associated with Belt Vessel**

Location: On the lateral side of the instep of the foot, in the front of the junction of the fourth and fifth metatarsal bones, in the depression lateral to the tendon of the extensor muscle of the small toe (Fig. 3.90).

Indications: (1) Red and swollen eyes, pain in the hypochondriac region, migraine. (2) Irregular menstruation, enuresis, mastitis, malaria, swelling and pain of the dorsum of the feet. (3) Scrofula.

Manipulation: 0.3–0.5 cun perpendicular insertion.

Fig. 3.91 Location of GB
43, GB 44

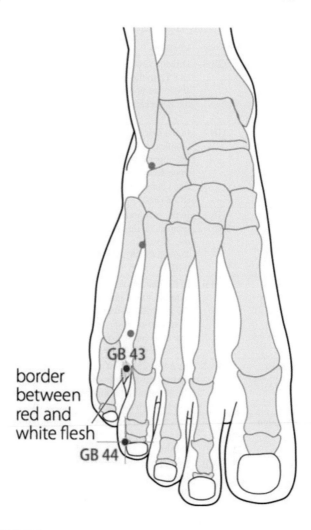

border
between
red and
white flesh

GB 43

GB 44

16. **Zuqiaoyin (GB 44)** Well Point

   Location: On the lateral side of the distal segment of the fourth toe, 0.1 cun from the corner of the toenail (Fig. 3.91).

   Indications: (1) Headache, red and swollen pain, deafness, sore throat, febrile disease, cough, insomnia. (2) Pain in the hypochondriac region. (3) Irregular menstruation.

   Manipulation: Insert the needle 0.1–0.2 cun into the skin, or insert a three-edged needle to induce bleeding.

17. **Other Points on Gallbladder Meridian of Foot Shaoyang** (Table 3.26).

Table 3.26 Other points on gallbladder meridian of foot shaoyang

Points	Code	Location	Indication	Manipulation
Shangguan	GB 3	Directly above Xiaguan (ST 7), in the depression above the upper border of the zygomatic arch	(1) Tinnitus, deafness, toothache, facial pain. (2) Deviation of the mouth and eye, locked jaw	Insert the needle perpendicularly by 0.3–0.5 cun deep
Hanyan	GB 4	In the hair above the temples, at the junction of the upper fourth and lower three-fourths of the curved line connecting Touwei (ST 8) and Qubin (GB 7)	(1) Migraine, vertigo, tinnitus. (2) Toothache	Insert the needle horizontally by 0.5–0.8 cun deep
Xuanlu	GB 5	In the hair above the temples, at the midpoint of the curved line connecting Touwei (ST 8) and Qubin (GB 7)	(1) Migraine, red and swollen eyes. (2) Toothache	Insert the needle horizontally by 0.5–0.8 cun deep
Xuanli	GB 6	In the hair above the temples, at the junction of the upper three-fourths and lower fourth of the curved line connecting Touwei (ST 8) and Qubin (GB 7)	(1) Migraine, red and swollen eyes. (2) Toothache	Insert the needle horizontally by 0.5–0.8 cun deep
Qubin	GB 7	At a crossing point of the vertical posterior border of the temples and horizontal line through the ear apex	(1) Headache. (2) Toothache, swelling and pain in the cheeks and jaw	Insert the needle horizontally by 0.5–0.8 cun deep
Shuaigu	GB 8	1.5 cun from the apex of the ear straight into the hairline	(1) Migraine, dizziness, tinnitus, deafness. (2) Infantile convulsions	Puncture horizontally by 0.5–0.8 cun
Tianchong	GB 9	2 cun from the posterior border of the ear straight into the hairline, 0.5 cun posterior to Shuaigu (GB 8)	(1) Migraine, dizziness, tinnitus, deafness. (2) Goiter. (3) Fright, epilepsy	Insert the needle horizontally by 0.5–1.0 cun deep
Fubai	GB 10	At the junction of the central 1/3 and upper 1/3 of the curved line connecting Tianchong (GB 9) and Wangu (GB 12)	(1) Migraine, tinnitus, deafness. (2) Goiter, scrofula	Insert the needle horizontally by 0.5–0.8 cun deep
Touqiaoyin	GB 11	Posterior and superior to the mastoid process, at the junction of the middle third and lower third of the curved line connecting Tianchong (GB 9) and Wangu (GB 12)	(1) Headache, dizziness, stiffness and pain in the neck. (2) Tinnitus, deafness	Insert the needle horizontally by 0.5–0.8 cun deep

Table 3.26 (continued)

Points	Code	Location	Indication	Manipulation
Wangu	GB 12	In the depression posterior and inferior to the mastoid process	(1) Migraine, tinnitus, deviation of the mouth and eye. (2) Stiffness and pain of the neck. (3) Epilepsy	Puncture horizontally by 0.5–0.8 cun
Benshen	GB 13	0.5 cun above the anterior hairline, 3 cun lateral to Shenting (GV 24)	(1) Headache, dizziness, insomnia, epilepsy. (2) Infantile convulsions, stroke	Insert the needle horizontally by 0.5–0.8 cun deep
Muchuang	GB 16	1.5 cun within the anterior hairline, 2.25 cun lateral to the midline of the head	(1) Headache, dizziness, redness, swelling, and pain of the eyes, infantile convulsions	Insert the needle horizontally by 0.5–0.8 cun deep
Zhengying	GB 17	2.5 cun within the anterior hairline, 2.25 cun lateral to the midline of the head	Headache, dizziness, and epilepsy	Insert the needle horizontally by 0.5–0.8 cun deep
Chengling	GB 18	4 cun within the anterior hairline, 2.25 cun lateral to the midline of the head	Headache, dizziness, disease of the eyes, nasosinusifis and epistaxis	Insert the needle horizontally by 0.5–0.8 cun deep
Naokong	GB 19	On the lateral side of the superior border of the external occipital protuberance, 2.25 cun lateral to the midline of the head	(1) Febrile diseases, headache, stiffness and pain around neck, dizziness, red and swollen eyes. (2) Palpitations, infantile convulsion, epilepsy	Insert the needle horizontally by 0.5–0.8 cun deep
Yuanye	GB 22	On the midaxillary line and in the fourth intercostal space	(1) Pain in the hypochondriac region, swollen axilla, tightness in the chest. (2) Spasm and pain in the upper limbs	Insert the needle horizontally or obliquely by 0.5–0.8 cun deep
Zhejin	GB 23	1 cun anterior to the midaxillary line, in the fourth intercostal space	(1) Pain in the hypochondriac region. (2) Tightness in the chest, asthma. (3) Vomiting, acid regurgitation	Insert the needle horizontally or obliquely by 0.5–0.8 cun deep
Jingmen (alarm point of the kidney)	GB 25	On the inferior free end of the 12th rib	(1) Difficulty in urination, edema. (2) Pain in the hypochondriac region, lumbar pain. (3) Abdominal distension, diarrhea, borborygmus	Insert the needle horizontally by 0.5–1.0 cun deep

(continued)

Table 3.26 (continued)

Points	Code	Location	Indication	Manipulation
Wushu	GB 27	Anterior to the superior iliac spine, level with 3 cun below the umbilicus	(1) Irregular menstruation, morbid leucorrhea, prolapsed uterus, lower abdominal pain. (2) Pain of the lumbar and hip	Insert the needle perpendicularly by 1.0–1.5 cun deep
Weidao	GB 28	Anterior and inferior to the superior iliac spine, 0.5 cun anterior and inferior to Wushu (GB 27)	(1) Irregular menstruation, morbid leucorrhea, prolapsed uterus, lower abdominal pain. (2) Pain of the lumbar and hip	Insert the needle perpendicularly by 1.0–1.5 cun deep
Juliao	GB 29	On the midpoint of the line linking the anteriosuperior iliac spine and the prominence of the greater trochanter	(1) Pain in the lumbar and hip, atrophy or paralysis in the lower limbs. (2) Hernia, lower abdominal pain	Insert the needle perpendicularly by 1.5–2.0 cun deep
Zhongdu	GB 32	On the lateral aspect of the thigh, posterior to the iliotibial band and 7 cun superior to the popliteal crease	Atrophy or paralysis of the lower limbs and hemiplegia	Insert the needle perpendicularly by 1.0–1.5 cun deep
Xiyangguan	GB 33	On the lateral aspect of the knee, in the depression between the biceps femoris tendon and the iliotibial band, posterior and proximal to the lateral epicondyle of the femur	Swelling, pain and spasm in the knees, numbness of the lower legs	Insert the needle perpendicularly by 1.0–1.5 cun deep
Yangjiao (cleft point of yang link vessel)	GB 35	7 cun above the tip of the external malleolus, on the posterior border of the fibula	(1) Distending pain in the chest and hypochondriac region, psychosis, atrophy or paralysis of the lower limbs	Insert the needle perpendicularly by 0.5–0.8 cun deep
Waiqiu (cleft point)	GB 36	7 cun superior to the tip of the external malleolus, on the anterior border of the fibula, level with Yangjiao (GB 35)	(1) Distending pain in the chest and hypochondriac region. (2) Psychosis. (3) Stiffness and pain in the neck. (4) Atrophy or paralysis in the lower limbs	Insert the needle perpendicularly by 1.0–1.5 cun deep

Table 3.26 (continued)

Points	Code	Location	Indication	Manipulation
Yangfu (river point)	GB 38	4 cun superior to the tip of the external malleolus, slightly anterior to the anterior border of the fibula	(1) Migraine, pain in the outer canthus. (2) Pain in the chest and hypochondriac region. (3) Scrofula. (4) Atrophy or paralysis of the lower limbs	Insert the needle perpendicularly by 1.0–1.5 cun deep
Diwuhui	GB 42	On the dorsum of the foot, between the fourth and fifth metatarsal bones, in the depression proximal to the fourth metatarsophalangeal joint	(1) Headache, redness, swelling, and pain of the eye, tinnitus, deafness. (2) Mastiffs. (3) Pain in the hypochondriac region, swelling and pain of the dorsum of the feet	Insert the needle perpendicularly by 0.3–0.5 cun deep
Xiaxi (spring point)	GB 43	Between the fourth and fifth toes, at the junction of the red and white skin, proximal to the margin of the web	(1) Palpitation. (2) Headache, dizziness, tinnitus, deafness, red eye pain. (3) Distending pain in the chest and hypochondriac region, swelling and pain in the dorsum of the feet. (4) Acute mastitis. (5) Febrile diseases	Puncture perpendicularly by 0.3–0.5 cun

3.4.1.12   Frequently Used Points on Liver Meridian of Foot Jueyin

The liver meridian of foot jueyin originates from the dorsal hairy region of the big toe that proceeds upwards along the dorsum of the foot anterior to the medial malleolus. It then travels to the place 8 cun above the medial malleolus where it crosses and runs behind the spleen meridian of foot taiyin and ascends along the medial aspect of the knee. It runs further along the medial aspect of the thigh and enters the pubic region, where it curves around the genitalia. From the genitalia, it goes upwards and enters the lower abdomen, then it pertains to the liver and connects with the gallbladder, it ascends to spread over the hypochondriac region. From here, it runs upwards along the posterior aspect of the throat and goes upwards to the face. The branch splits from the liver, crosses the diaphragm, and proceeds upwards to converge in the chest. It runs upwards along the posterior aspect of the throat, entering the nasopharynx, and connecting with the "eye system." It then proceeds upward and emerges on the forehead and connects with the governor vessel at the vertex (Fig. 3.92).

Fig. 3.92 The course of
liver meridian of foot
jueyin

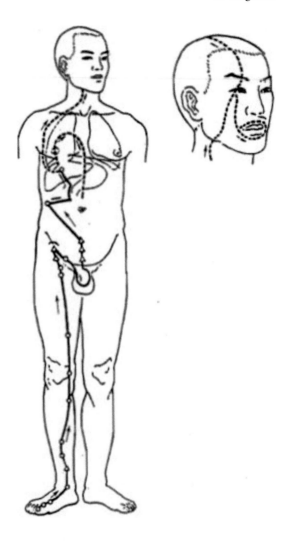

1. **Dadun (LR 1)** Well Point
   Location: On the lateral side of the great toe, approximately 0.1 cun lateral to the corner of the toenail (Fig. 3.93).
   Indications: (1) Hernia, low abdominal pain. (2) Enuresis, dysuria, hematuria. (3) Irregular menstruation, metrorrhagia, contraction of scrotum, colpalgia, prolapsed uterus. (4) Epilepsy, somnolence.
   Manipulation: Insert the needle shallowly by 0.1 cun into the skin, or insert a three-edged needle to induce bleeding.
2. **Xingjian (LR 2)** Spring Point
   Location: On the dorsum of the foot, proximal to the web margin between the first and second toes, at the junction of red and white skin (Fig. 3.93).

Fig. 3.93 Location of LR
1–LR 3

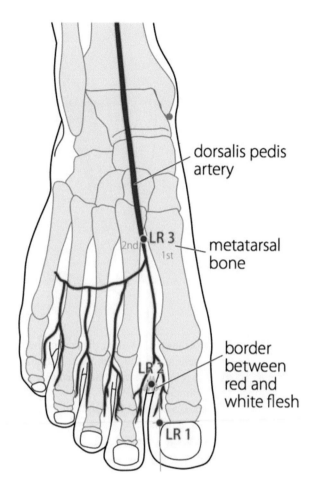

dorsalis pedis
artery

metatarsal
bone

border
between
red and
white flesh

Indications: (1) Dizziness, headache, redness, swelling, and pain in the eyes, deviation of the mouth and eyes, epilepsy, stroke, distending pain in the chest and hypochondriac region. (2) Irregular menstruation, dysmenorrhea, amenorrhea, metrorrhagia, morbid leucorrhea. (3) Colpalgia, hernia, enuresis. (4) Difficulty in urination. (5) Pain in the medial aspect of lower limbs, pain and swelling in the dorsum of foot.

Manipulation: 0.5–0.8 cun perpendicular or oblique upward insertion.

3. **Taichong (LR 3)** Stream Point; Source Point

Location: On the dorsum of the foot, between the first and second metatarsal bones in the depression distal to the junction of the bases of the two bones where the dorsalis pedis artery pulses (Fig. 3.93).

Indications: (1) Vertigo, headache, redness, swelling, and pain in the eyes, tinnitus, angina, deviation of the mouth and eyes, epilepsy, stroke, infantile convulsions. (2) Irregular menstruation, amenorrhea, dysmenorrhea, metrorrha-

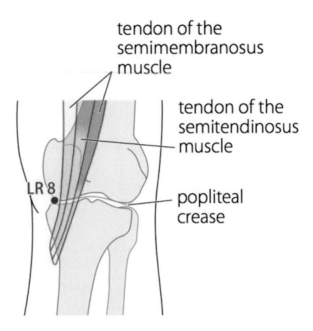

Fig. 3.94 Location of LR 8

tendon of the
semimembranosus
muscle

tendon of the
semitendinosus
muscle

LR 8

popliteal
crease

gia, morbid leucorrhea. (3) Hernia, distending pain in the chest and hypochondriac region, distention in the abdomen, jaundice, vomiting, and hiccup. (4) Enuresis, dysuria. (5) Weakness and flaccidity of the lower limbs, pain and swelling in the dorsum of foot.

    Manipulation: 0.5–0.8 cun perpendicular upwards insertion.

4. **Ququan (LR 8)** Sea Point

    Location: When the knee is flexed, at the medial end of the popliteal crease, in the depression medial to the semitendinosus and semimembranosus tendons (Fig. 3.94).

    Indications: (1) Dysmenorrhea, irregular menstruation, prolapsed uterus, morbid leucorrhea. (2) Seminal emission, impotence, hernia. (3) Difficulty in urination. (4) Weakness and flaccidity of the lower limbs, pain and swelling in the knees.

    Manipulation: 1–1.5 cun perpendicular upwards insertion.

5. **Zhangmen (LR 13)** Alarm Point of the Spleen, One of the Eight Meeting Points (Zang-Viscera Convergence)

    Location: Below the free end of the 11th floating rib (Fig. 3.95).

    Indications: (1) Diarrhea, abdominal distention and pain, vomiting, borborygmus. (2) Pain in the hypochondriac region, jaundice, abdominal mass.

    Manipulation: 0.8–1.0 cun oblique insertion.

6. **Qimen (LR 14)** Alarm Point of the Liver

    Location: Directly below the nipple, at the sixth intercostal space, 4 cun lateral to the anterior midline (Fig. 3.95).

Fig. 3.95 Location of LR
13, LR 14

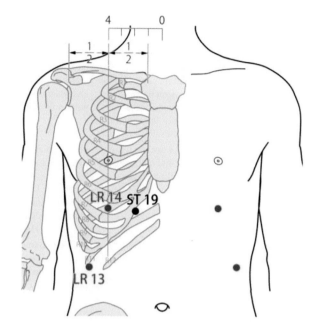

Indications: (1) Distending pain in the chest and hypochondriac region, mastitis, diarrhea, abdominal distention, vomiting, acid regurgitation, hiccup. (2) Up-rushing gas syndrome. (3) Acute mastitis.

Manipulation: 0.5–0.8 cun oblique insertion, do not puncture too deeply in order to prevent hurting the internal viscera.

7. **Other Points on Liver Meridian of Foot Jueyin** (Table 3.27).

3.4.2   Frequently Used Acupoints on the Eight Extra Meridians

3.4.2.1   Frequently Used Acupoints on Governor Vessel

The governor vessel travels backwards along the interior side of the spinal column, reaching Fengfu (GV 16). From there it enters the brain and ascends toward the vertex. From the vertex, it proceeds downwards along the forehead to the columnella of the nose, ends in the upper lip, and connects to Yinjiao (GV 28) (Fig. 3.96).

1. **Changqiang (GV 1)** Connecting Point
   Location: The central point between the tip of the coccyx and the anus below the tip of the coccyx (Fig. 3.97).
   Indications: (1) Hemorrhoids, prolapse of anus, bloody stool, diarrhea, constipation. (2) Psychosis, epilepsy. (3) Lumbago, lower back and coccyx pain.

Table 3.27 Other points on liver meridian of foot jueyin

Points	Code	Location	Indication	Manipulation
Zhongfeng (river point)	LR 4	On the dorsum of foot, 1 cun anterior to the medial malleolus, in the depression on the medial side of the tendon of the anterior tibial muscle	(1) Hernia, seminal emission, difficulty in urination. (2) Pain in the abdomen, swelling and pain in the feet and ankles	0.5–0.8 cun *deep* perpendicular upwards insertion
Ligou	LR 5	5 cun above the tip of the medial malleolus, on the midline of the medial surface of the tibia	(1) Irregular menstruation, morbid leucorrhea, prolapsed uterus. (2) Difficulty in urination, enuresis. (3) Pain in the lumbosacral region. (4) Hernia	Puncture transversely by 0.5–0.8 cun
Zhongdu (cleft point)	LR 6	7 cun above the tip of the medial malleolus, on the midline of the medial surface of the tibia	(1) Hernia, lower abdominal pain. (2) Uterine bleeding, prolonged uterine discharge	0.5–0.8 cun *deep* horizontal insertion
Xiguan	LR 7	Posterior and inferior to the medial condyle of the tibia, 1 cun posterior to Yinlingquan (SP 9)	Swelling and pain of the knees, atrophy or paralysis of the lower limbs	0.5–0.8 cun *deep* horizontal insertion
Yinbao	LR 9	On the medial aspect of the thigh between the gracilis and the sartorius, 4 cun proximal to the base of the patella	(1) Irregular menstruation, difficulty in urination, enuresis. (2) Pain in the lumbosacral region	0.8–1.5 cun *deep* perpendicular insertion
Zuwuli	LR 10	3 cun directly below Qichong (ST 30), inferior to the pubic tubercle	(1) Lower abdominal pain and distension, swelling and pain of the testicles, pruritus vulvae, prolapsed uterus, difficulty in urination. (2) Scrofula	1.0–1.5 cun *deep* perpendicular insertion
Yinlian	LR 11	2 cun directly below Qichong (ST 30), inferior to the pubic tubercle	(1) Lower abdominal pain. (2) Irregular menstruation and morbid leucorrhea	1.0–1.5 cun *deep* perpendicular insertion
Jimai	LR 12	Lateral and inferior to Qichong (ST 30), in the crease of the groin where the femoral artery pulsates, 2.5 cun lateral to the anterior midline	(1) Lower abdominal pain. (2) Phallalgia, prolapsed uterus, and hernia	0.5–0.8 cun *deep* perpendicular insertion, avoiding penetrating the femoral artery

Manipulation: Insert the needle obliquely toward the anterior side of the coccyx by 0.5–1.0 cun deep, deep insertion is not advisable, in order to prevent injuring the rectum.

Fig. 3.96 The course of governor vessel

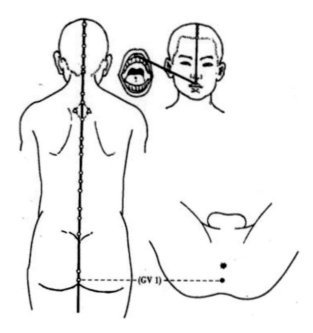

Fig. 3.97 Location of GV 1–GV 3

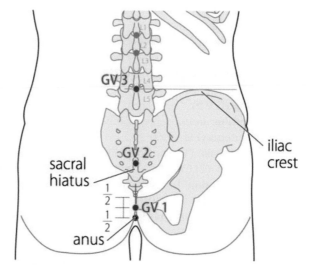

2. **Yaoyangguan (GV 3)**

   Location: On the posterior midline, in the depression below the spinous process of the fourth lumbar vertebra (Fig. 3.97).

   Indications: (1) Lower back pain, atrophy or paralysis in the lower extremities. (2) Irregular menstruation, morbid leucorrhea. (3) Nocturnal emissions, impotence.

   Manipulation: Insert the needle perpendicularly by 0.5–1.0 cun deep, moxibustion is applicable.

Fig. 3.98 Location of GV
4–GV 8

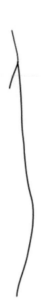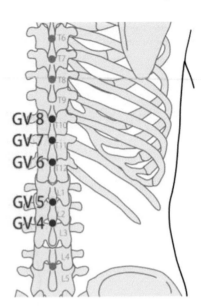

3. **Minmen (GV 4)**

   Location: In the depression below the spinous process of the second lumbar vertebra (Fig. 3.98).

   Indications: (1) Impotence, seminal emission. (2) Irregular menstruation, morbid leucorrhea. (3) Lower back pain. (4) Diarrhea.

   Manipulation: Insert the needle perpendicularly by 0.5–1.0 cun deep, moxibustion is applicable.

4. **Zhiyang (GV 9)**

   Location: In the depression below the spinous process of the seventh thoracic vertebra (Fig. 3.99).

   Indications: (1) Jaundice, distension and fullness in chest and hypochondriac region. (2) Cough, asthma. (3) Stiffness of the spine, pain in the back.

   Manipulation: Insert the needle obliquely upwards by 0.5–1.0 cun deep.

5. **Dazhui (GV 14)**

   Location: On the posterior midline, in the depression below the seventh cervical vertebra (Fig. 3.99).

   Indications: (1) Febrile diseases, malaria, headache, cough, asthma. (2) Epilepsy. (3) Night sweating. (4) Pain in the back and shoulder, stiffness of the lumbar spine. (5) Rubella.

   Manipulation: 0.5–1.0 cun perpendicular insertion.

6. **Yamen (GV 15)**

   Location: On the nape at the posterior midline, in the depression superior to the spinous process of the second cervical vertebra (Fig. 3.100).

   Indications: (1) Sudden aphonia, inability to speak due to stiffness of the tongue. (2) Mania, epilepsy. (3) Headache, stiffness in the neck.

Fig. 3.99 Location of GV
9–GV 14

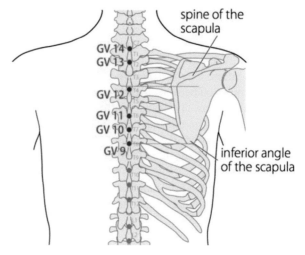

Fig. 3.100 Location of
GV 15, GV 16

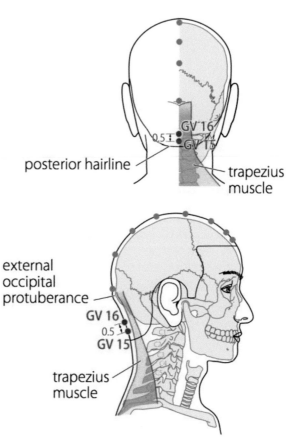

Manipulation: 0.5–1.0 cun perpendicular or oblique insertion downwards. Do not puncture too deep perpendicularly or obliquely upwards to prevent from pricking the medulla. Pay attention to the angle and depth of insertion.

7. **Fcngfu (GV 16)**

    Location: On the nape directly below the external occipital protuberance in the depression between the trapeziuses (Fig. 3.100).

    Indications: (1) Headache, stiffness in the neck, dizziness, swollen and pain throat. (2) Apoplexy with aphasia, mania and epilepsy, hemiplegia.

    Manipulation: 0.5–1.0 cun perpendicular or oblique insertion downwards. Do not puncture deeply to prevent from pricking the medulla.

8. **Baihui (GV 20)**

    Location: On the head, 5 cun directly above the midpoint of the anterior hairline, at the midpoint of the line connecting the apexes of both ears (Fig. 3.101).

Fig. 3.101 Location of GV 20

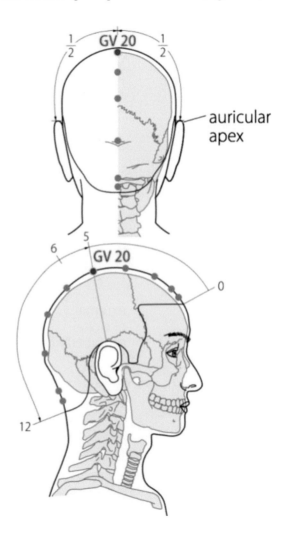

Indications: (1) Headache, dizziness, swollen and painful throat. (2) Hemiplegia, apoplexy with aphasia, mania and epilepsy, insomnia, forgetfulness. (3) Prolapsed anus, prolonged diarrhea, prolapse of uterus.

Manipulation: 0.5–0.8 cun horizontal insertion, moxibustion is applicable.

9. **Shangxing (GV 23)**

Location: On the head, 1 cun directly above the midpoint of the anterior hairline (Fig. 3.102).

Indications: (1) Headache, painful eyes, nasosinusitis, nosebleed. (2) Malaria, febrile diseases. (3) Mania and epilepsy.

Manipulation: 0.5–0.8 cun horizontal insertion.

10. **Shenting (GV 24)**

Location: 0.5 cun directly above the midpoint of the anterior hairline (Fig. 3.102).

Fig. 3.102 Location of
GV 23–GV 25

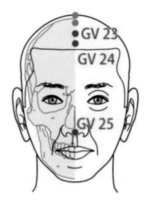

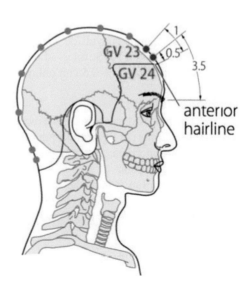

Fig. 3.103 Location of
GV 26, GV 27

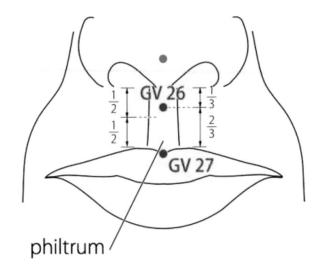

Indications: (1) Headache, vertigo, nasosinusitis, nosebleed, conjunctival congestion, corneal opacity. (2) Insomnia. (3) Psychosis.

Manipulation: 0.5–0.8 cun horizontal insertion.

11. **Suliao (GV 25)**

Location: At the tip of the nose (Fig. 3.102).

Indications: (1) Nasosinusitis, nosebleed. (2) Unconsciousness, apnea, convulsions

Manipulation: 0.5–0.8 cun horizontal insertion, or pricking to induce bleeding with a three-edged needle.

12. **Shuigou (GV 26)**

Location: On the face, at the junction of the upper third and middle third of the philtrum (Fig. 3.103).

Indications: (1) Coma, syncope. (2) Epilepsy, mania and epilepsy, facial paralysis, infantile convulsion. (3) Swollen lips and face, rhinobyon, epistaxis, dentalgia, trismus. (4) Stiffness of the lumbar spine.

Manipulation: 0.3–0.5 cun oblique upwards insertion, or press and knead with fingers.

13. **Yintang (GV 29)**

Location: Midway between the medial ends of the two eyebrows (Fig. 3.104).

Indications: (1) Dementia, epilepsy, insomnia, forgetful. (2) Headache, vertigo. (3) Rhinorrhea, epistaxis. (4) Infantile convulsions, postpartum anemic fainting, eclampsia.

Manipulation: Pinch the local skin, 0.3–0.5 cun horizontal downwards insertion or prick to induce bleeding with three edges needle.

14. **Other Points on Governor Vessel** (Table 3.28).

Fig. 3.104 Location of GV 29

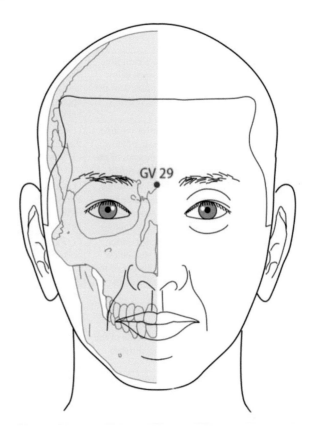

Table 3.28 Other points on governor vessel

Points	Code	Location	Indication	Manipulation
Yaoshu	GV 2	On the posterior midline, in the sacrococcygeal hiatus	(1) Dysentery, prolapsed anus, constipation, irregular menstruation. (2) Lumbago, atrophy or paralysis in the lower extremities. (3) Epilepsy	0.5–1.0 cun deep oblique insertion
Xuanshu	GV 5	On the posterior midline, in the depression below the spinous process of the first lumbar vertebrae	(1) Stiffness and pain of the lumbar region. (2) Abdominal pain, diarrhea	0.5–1.0 cun deep oblique insertion
Jizhong	GV 6	On the posterior midline, in the depression below the spinous process of the 11th thoracic vertebrae	(1) Diarrhea, jaundice, prolapsed anus, hemorrhoids, infantile malnutritional stagnation. (2) Epilepsy. (3) Stiffness and pain of the lumbar region	0.5–1.0 cun deep oblique upwards insertion

(continued)

Table 3.28 (continued)

Points	Code	Location	Indication	Manipulation
Zhongshu	GV 7	On the posterior midline, in the depression below the spinous process of the tenth thoracic vertebra	(1) Jaundice. (2) Vomiting, distension of the abdomen, stomach pain, poor appetite. (3) Lumbar and back pain	0.5–1.0 cun deep oblique upwards insertion
Jinsuo	GV 8	On the posterior midline, in the depression below the spinous process of the ninth thoracic vertebra	(1) Epilepsy. (2) Vomiting, flaccidity of limbs, spasms. (3) Stomach pain	0.5–1.0 cun deep oblique upwards insertion
Lingtai	GV 10	On the posterior midline, in the depression below the spinous process of the sixth thoracic vertebra	(1) Cough, asthma. (2) Furunculosis. (3) Stiffness of the spine, pain in the back	0.5–1.0 cun deep oblique upwards insertion
Shendao	GV 11	On the posterior midline, in the depression below the spinous process of the fifth thoracic vertebra	(1) Palpitation, angina, pectoris, amnesia. (2) Cough and asthma. (3) Stiffness of the spine, pain in the back	0.5–1.0 cun deep oblique upwards insertion
Shenzhu	GV 12	On the posterior midline, in the depression below the spinous process of the third thoracic vertebra	(1) Cough, asthma, fever, headache. (2) Stiffness of the spine, pain in the back. (3) Back carbuncles. (4) Epilepsy, convulsions	Insert the needle obliquely upwards by 0.5–1.0 cun deep
Taodao	GV 13	On the posterior midline, in the depression below the spinous process of the first thoracic vertebra	(1) Cough and asthma. (2) Headache. (3) Fever, tidal fever, malaria. (4) Mania. (5) Stiffness of the spine, pain in the back	0.5–1.0 cun deep oblique upwards insertion
Naohu	GV 17	2.5 cun directly above the midpoint of the posterior hairline, 1.5 cun above Fengfu (GV 16), in the depression on the upper border of the external occipital protuberance	(1) Headache, stiff neck, vertigo. (2) Aphonia. (3) Epilepsy	0.5–0.8 cun deep oblique insertion
Qiangjian	GV 18	4 cun directly above the midpoint of the posterior hairline, 1.5 cun above Naohu (GV 17) and on the midpoint of the line joining Fengfu (GV 16) and Baihui (GV 20)	(1) Headache, stiff neck, vertigo. (2) Psychosis	0.5–0.8 cun deep oblique insertion
Houding	GV 19	5.5 cun directly above the midpoint of the posterior hairline, 1.5 cun above Qiangjian (GV 18) or 1.5 cun below Baihui (GV 20)	(1) Headache, stiff neck, vertigo. (2) Psychosis, epilepsy	0.5–0.8 cun deep oblique insertion

Table 3.26 (continued)

Points	Code	Location	Indication	Manipulation
Qianding	GV 21	3.5 cun directly above the midpoint of the anterior hairline, 1.5 cun above Baihui (GV 20)	(1) Headache, vertigo. (2) Nasosinusitis. (3) Psychosis, epilepsy	0.3–0.5 cun deep oblique insertion
Xinhui	GV 22	2 cun directly above the midpoint of the anterior hairline, 1.5 cun above Qianding (GV 21)	(1) Headache, vertigo. (2) Nasosinusitis. (3) Psychosis, epilepsy	0.3–0.5 cun deep oblique insertion
Duiduan	GV 27	On the midline, at the junction of the margin of the upper lip and the philtrum	(1) Unconsciousness, syncope, psychosis. (2) Facial distortion, swollen, painful gums, nosebleed	0.2–0.3 cun deep oblique upwards insertion
Yinjiao	GV 28	In the superior frenulum, at the junction of the upper lip and the gums	(1) Facial distortion, swelling and pain of the gums, halitosis, nosebleed nasal obstruction. (2) Psychosis	0.2–0.3 cun deep oblique superior insertion or prick to induce bleeding

3.4.2.2   Frequently Used Acupoints on Conception Vessel

The conception vessel arises inside of the lower abdomen, passing through some points such as Guanyuan (CV 4), and reaches the throat. It ascends further to curve around the lips, passing through the maxillary part and entering the infraorbital region.

1. **Zhongji (CV 3)** Alarm Point of the Bladder

   Location: On the anterior midline, 4 cun below the umbilicus (Fig. 3.105).

   Indications: (1) Dysuria, enuresis. (2) Seminal emission, impotence. (3) Irregular menstruation, morbid leucorrhea, and infertility, metrorrhagia and metrostaxis, prolapse of the uterus, pruritus vulvae.

   Manipulation: Insert the needle perpendicularly by 0.5–1.0 cun deep after urination. The point is contraindicated in pregnant women.

2. **Guanyuan (CV 4)** Alarm Point of the Small Intestine

   Location: On the anterior midline, 3 cun below the umbilicus (Fig. 3.105).

   Indications: (1) Asthenic disease, exhaustion syndrome. (2) Abdominal pain, hernia. (3) Diarrhea, dysentery, rectocele, hemafecia. (4) The five kinds of stranguria, dysuria, hematuria, urodialysis, and enuresis. (5) Seminal emission, impotence, premature ejaculation. (6) Irregular menstruation, dysmenorrheal, morbid leucorrhea, and infertility. (7) Commonly used moxibustion point for promoting health.

   Manipulation: Insert the needle perpendicularly by 0.5–1.0 cun deep after urination. Moxibustion is applicable. This point is contraindicated in pregnant women.

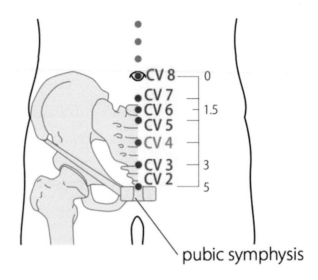

pubic symphysis

3. **Qihai (CV 6)**

   Location: On the anterior midline, 1.5 cun below the umbilicus (Fig. 3.105).

   Indications: (1) Exhaustion syndrome. (2) Abdominal pain, diarrhea, constipation, indigestion, dysentery. (3) Dysuria, enuresis. (4) Irregular menstruation, dysmenorrheal, morbid leucorrhea. (5) Seminal emission, impotence, premature ejaculation. (6) Commonly used moxibustion point for promoting health.

   Manipulation: Insert the needle perpendicularly by 1.0–1.5 cun deep. Moxibustion is applicable. The point is contraindicated in pregnant women.

4. **Shenque (CV 8)**

   Location: In the center of the umbilicus (Fig. 3.105).

   Indications: (1) Asthenic disease, exhaustion syndrome. (2) Abdominal distension, abdominal pain, constipation, diarrhea. (3) Edema, dysuria. (4) Commonly used moxibustion point for promoting health.

   Manipulation: Acupuncture is prohibited and moxibustion is applicable.

5. **Xiawan (CV l0)**

   Location: On the anterior midline, 2 cun above the umbilicus (Fig. 3.106).

   Indications: (1) Abdominal distension, abdominal pain, diarrhea, vomiting, indigestion. (2) Abdominal masses.

   Manipulation: Insert the needle perpendicularly by 1.0–1.5 cun deep.

6. **Zhongwan (CV 12)** Alarm Point of the Stomach, One of the Eight Meeting Points (Fu-Viscera Convergence)

   Location: On the anterior midline, 4 cun above the umbilicus, or midway between the umbilicus and the xiphisternal symphysis (Fig. 3.106).

   Indications: (1) Stomachache, vomiting, acid regurgitation, hiccup, poor appetite, abdominal distension, diarrhea. (2) Jaundice. (3) Psychosis, epilepsy.

   Manipulation: Insert the needle perpendicularly by 1.0–1.5 cun deep.

Fig. 3.106 Location of
CV 9–CV 16

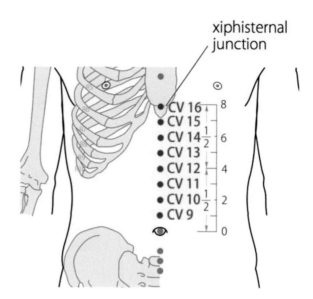

Fig. 3.107 Location of
CV 17–CV 20

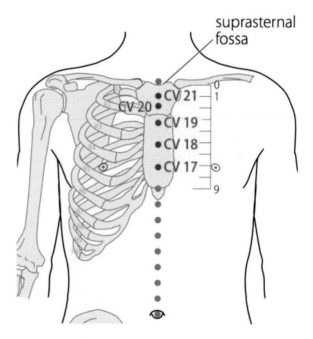

7. **Danzhong (CV 17)** Alarm Point of the Pericardium, One of the Eight Meeting
   Points (Qi Convergence)
   Location: On the anterior midline, level with the fourth intercostal space or
   at the midpoint between the nipples (Fig. 3.107).

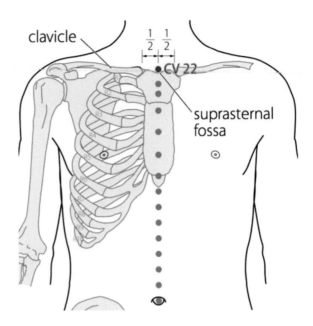

Fig. 3.108 Location of CV 22

Indications: (1) Oppression in the chest, shortness of breath, pain in the chest, palpitations, cough, asthma, vomiting, cardiac spasms. (2) Lack of lactation, acute mastitis, nodules of breast.

Manipulation: Insert the needle horizontally by 0.3–0.5 cun deep.

8. **Tiantu (CV 22)**

    Location: On the anterior midline, at the center of the suprasternal fossa (Fig. 3.108).

    Indications: (1) Cough, asthma, chest pain, swollen and painful throat, apoplexy with aphasia. (2) Goiter, globus hystericus, dysphagia.

    Manipulation: 0.2 cun deep perpendicular insertion at first. Then turn the needle tip downwards and insert it along the posterior side of the sternum closely and slowly by 0.5–1 cun deep. Moxibustion is applicable.

9. **Lianquan (CV 23)**

    Location: On the neck and on the anterior midline, above the laryngeal protuberance, on the midpoint above the upper border of the hyoid bone (Fig. 3.109).

    Indications: Swollen sublingual region, increased salivation, aphasia with stiff tongue, sudden loss of voice, dysphagia, difficulty in swallowing.

    Manipulation: 0.5–0.8 cun deep oblique insertion toward the root of tongue.

10. **Chengjiang (CV 24)**

    Location: On the face, in the depression at the midpoint of the mentolabial sulcus (Fig. 3.110).

    Indications: (1) Facial paralysis, swollen gums, salivation. (2) Sudden loss of voice. (3) Epilepsy

    Manipulation: 0.3–0.5 cun deep oblique insertion.

11. **Other Points on Conception Vessel** (Table 3.29).

Fig. 3.109 Location of CV 23

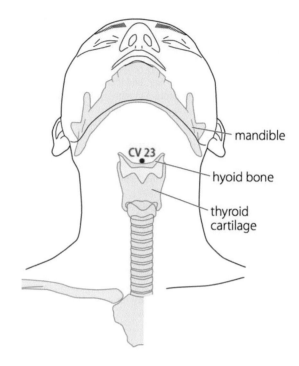

mandible

CV 23

hyoid bone

thyroid cartilage

Fig. 3.110 Location of CV 24

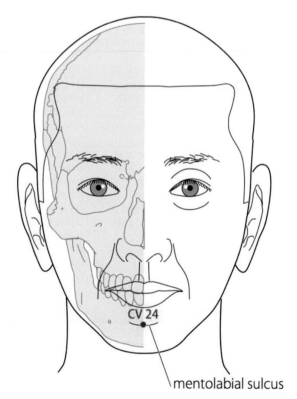

CV 24

mentolabial sulcus

Table 3.29 Other points on conception vessel

Points	Code	Location	Indication	Manipulation
Huiyin	CV 1	On the perineum, midway between the anus and the scrotum in men, and the anus and the posterior labial commissure in women	(1) Irregular menstruation, difficulty in urination, nocturnal emissions, vaginal pain, pruritus vulva. (2) Asphyxiation from drowning, unconsciousness, psychosis	Insert the needle perpendicularly by 0.5–1.0 cun deep. The point is contraindicated in pregnant women
Qugu	CV 2	On the anterior midline, 5 cun below the umbilicus, in the depression on the midpoint of the upper border of the pubis symphysis	Difficulty in urination, enuresis, irregular menstruation, dysmenorrhea, morbid leucorrhea, nocturnal emissions, impotence, and eczema of the scrotum	Insert the needle perpendicularly by 0.5–1.0 cun deep. The point is contraindicated in pregnant women
Shimen (alarm point of the triple energizer)	CV 5	On the anterior midline, 2 cun below the umbilicus	(1) Abdominal distension, edema, diarrhea. (2) Nocturnal emissions, impotence, uterine bleeding, morbid leucorrhea, difficulty in urination	Insert the needle perpendicularly by 0.5–1.0 cun deep. The point is contraindicated in pregnant women
Yinjiao	CV 7	On the anterior midline, 1 cun below the umbilicus	(1) Abdominal pain. (2) Edema. (3) Irregular menstruation, morbid leucorrhea, hernia	Insert the needle perpendicularly by 0.5–1.0 cun deep. The point is contraindicated in pregnant women
Shuifen	CV 9	On the anterior midline, 1 cun above the umbilicus	(1) Edema, difficulty in urination. (2) Abdominal pain, abdominal distension, diarrhea, regurgitation	Insert the needle perpendicularly by 0.5–1.0 cun deep
Jianli	CV 11	On the anterior midline, 3 cun above the umbilicus	(1) Stomachache, abdominal distension, poor appetite, vomiting. (2) Edema	Insert the needle perpendicularly by 1.0–1.5 cun deep
Shangwan	CV 13	On the anterior midline, 5 cun above the umbilicus	(1) Abdominal distension, stomach pain, vomiting, acid regurgitation, hiccups, poor appetite. (2) Epilepsy	Insert the needle horizontally by 1.0–1.5 cun deep
Juque (alarm point of the heart)	CV 14	On the anterior midline, 6 cun above the umbilicus, or 2 cun below the xiphisternal symphysis	(1) Chest pain, palpitation. (2) Psychosis, epilepsy. (3) Stomach pain, vomiting, acid regurgitation	Insert the needle obliquely downwards by 0.5–1.0 cun deep, avoiding a deep insertion so as to avoid damaging the liver

Table 3.29 (continued)

Points	Code	Location	Indication	Manipulation
Jiuwei (connecting point)	CV 15	On the anterior midline, 7 cun above the umbilicus, or 1 cun below the xiphisternal symphysis	(1) Oppression in the chest, pain in the chest, palpitation. (2) Psychosis, epilepsy. (3) Abdominal distension, hiccups, vomiting	Insert the needle obliquely downwards by 0.5–1.0 cun deep
Zhongting	CV 16	On the anterior midline, level with the fifth intercostal space, on the center of the xiphisternal symphysis	(1) Oppression in the chest, cardiac pain. (2) Vomiting, infantile milk regurgitation	0.2–0.3 cun deep oblique insertion
Yutang	CV 18	On the anterior midline, level with the third intercostal space	(1) Oppression in the chest, pain in the chest. (2) Cough, asthma. (3) Vomiting	0.3–0.5 cun deep oblique insertion
Zigong	CV 19	On the anterior midline, level with the second intercostal space	(1) Cough, asthma. (2) Oppression in the chest, pain in the chest	0.3–0.5 cun deep oblique insertion
Huagai	CV 20	On the anterior midline, level with the first intercostal space, at the midpoint of the sternal angle	(1) Cough, asthma. (2) Distension and pain in the chest and hypochondriac region	0.3–0.5 cun deep oblique insertion
Xuanji	CV 21	On the anterior midline, on the center of the manubrium of the sternum	(1) Cough, asthma, pain in the chest. (2) Swelling and pain in the throat. (3) Dyspeptic disease	0.3–0.5 cun deep oblique insertion

3.4.2.3   The Course of the Chong Vessel

It starts inside of the lower abdomen and emerges from the perineum. It runs upwards along the inside part of the spinal column where its superficial branch passes through the region of Qichong (ST 30) and communicates with the kidney meridian, traveling along both sides of the abdomen. It goes up to the throat and curves around the lips (Fig. 3.111).

3.4.2.4   The Course of the Belt Vessel

It starts below the hypochondriac region and runs obliquely downwards Daimai (GB 26), Wushu (GB 27), and Weidao (GB 28). It then runs transversely around the waist like a belt (Fig. 3.112).

Fig. 3.111 The course of
chong vessel

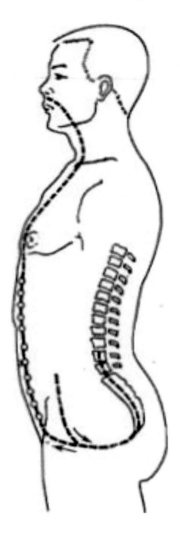

3.4.2.5   The Course of the Yin Link Vessel

It starts from the medial aspect of the lower leg, ascends along the medial aspect of
the thigh to the abdomen to communicate with the spleen meridian. It then runs
along the chest, and communicates with the conception vessel at the neck
(Fig. 3.113).

Fig. 3.112 The course of
belt vessel

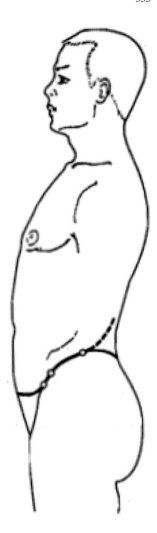

3.4.2.6   The Course of the Yang Link Vessel

It starts from the lateral aspect of the heel, and runs upwards along the external malleolus, ascending along the gallbladder meridian, passing through the hip region,
and running upwards along the posterior aspect of the hypochondriac region and
posterior aspect of the axilla to the shoulder, and then to the forehead. It then turns
backwards the back of the neck to communicate with the governor vessel
(Fig. 3.114).

Fig. 3.113 The course of
yin link vessel

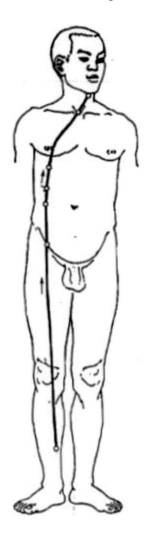

3.4.2.7   The Course of the Yin Heel Vessel

It starts from the posterior aspect of the navicular bone, goes up to the upper portion
of the medial malleolus, and runs straight up along the posterior border of the medial
aspect of the thigh to the external genitalia. It then travels upwards along the chest
to the supraclavicular fossa and runs upwards laterally to the region in front of
Renying (ST 9) along the zygomatic arch to reach the inner canthus and communicate with both the bladder meridian and the yang heel vessel (Fig. 3.115).

Fig. 3.114 The course of
yang link vessel

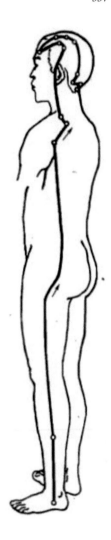

3.4.2.8   The Course of the Yang Heel Vessel

It starts from the lateral side of the heel, runs upwards along the external malleolus, and passes the posterior border of the fibula, going up along the lateral side of the thigh and posterior side of the hypochondriac region to the posterior axillary fold. It travels to the shoulder and ascends along the neck to the corner of the mouth, entering the inner canthus to communicate with the yin heel vessel. Finally, it runs up along the bladder meridian to the forehead, where it meets the gallbladder meridian at Fengchi (GB 20) (Fig. 3.116).

Fig. 3.115 The course of
yin heel vessel

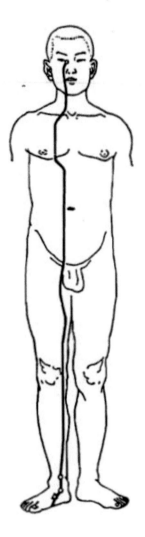

3.4.3   Extra Points

3.4.3.1   Extra Points of Head and Neck (EX-HN)

1. **Sishencong (EX-HN 1)**

   Location: This name refers to four points located on the vertex, 1 cun posterior, anterior, and lateral to Baihui (GV 20) (Fig. 3.117).

   Indications: (1) Vertigo, headache. (2) Forgetfulness, insomnia, epilepsy,
   mania. (3) Paralysis.

   Manipulation: 0.5–0.8 cun horizontal insertion or pricking with a three-
   edged needle to induce bleeding.

Fig. 3.116 The course of
yang heel vessel

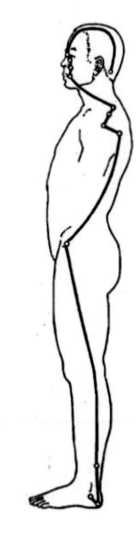

Fig. 3.117 Location of
EX-HN 1

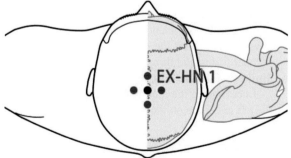

Fig. 3.118 Location of
EX-HN 5

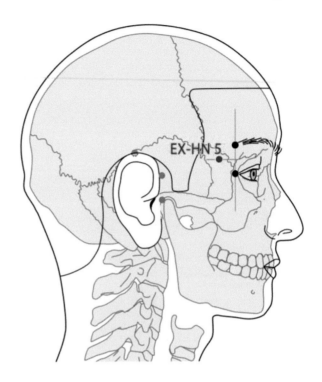

2. **Taiyang (EX-HN 5)**

   Location: In the position about one fingerbreadth posterior to the midpoint between the lateral end of the eyebrow and the outer canthus (Fig. 3.118).

   Indications: (1) Red and swollen eyes. (2) Headache, dizziness. (3) Facial paralysis, wry face and eyes, toothache.

   Manipulation: 0.3–0.5 cun perpendicular or oblique insertion or prick to induce bleeding with three edges needle. Moxibustion is applicable.

3. **Qiuhou (EX-HN 7)**

   Location: In the junction of the lateral 1/4 and medial 3/4 of the infraorbital margin (Fig. 3.119).

   Indications: (1) Eye diseases.

   Manipulation: Gently push the eye ball upward, insert the needle slightly downwards toward the optic foramen along the orbital margin for 0.5–1.5 cun without lifting and thrusting.

4. **Jinjin (EX-HN 12), Yuye (EX-HN 13)**

   Location: In the mouth, on the two veins under the lingual frenum, Jinjin on the left and Yuye on the right (Fig. 3.120).

Fig. 3.119 Location of
EX-HN 7

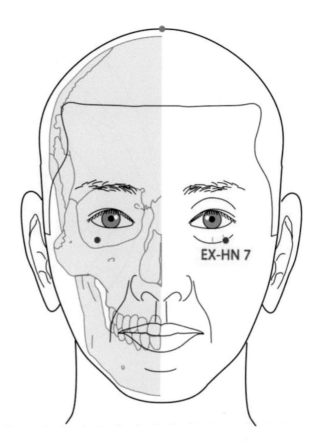

Indications: (1) Swollen tongue, stiff tongue, ulcers in the mouth, aphasia. (2) Vomiting, diarrhea, diabetes.

Manipulation: Prick to induce bleeding.

5. **Qianzheng (EX-HN)**

   Location: 0.5–1.0 cun anterior to the earlobe (Fig. 3.121).

   Indications: Facial paralysis, and ulcers in the mouth.

   Manipulation: 0.5–0.8 cun *forward* oblique insertion.

6. **Yiming (EX-HN 14)**

   Location: On the neck, 1 cun posterior to Yifeng (TE 17) (Fig. 3.122).

   Indications: (1) Vertigo, headache, insomnia. (2) Diseases of eyes, tinnitus.

   Manipulation: 0.5–1.0 cun perpendicular insertion, moxibustion is applicable.

Fig. 3.120 Location of
EX-HN 12, EX-HN 13

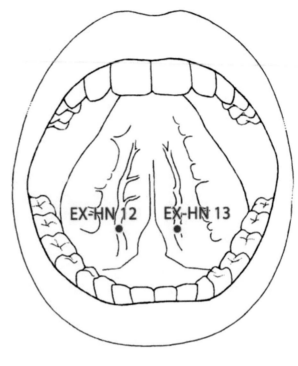

Fig. 3.121 Location of
EX-HN 5, Qianzheng

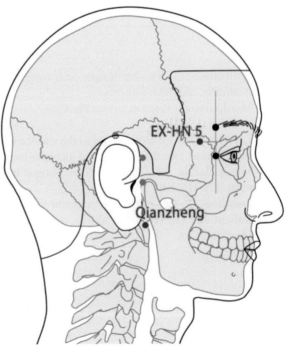

Fig. 3.122 Location of
EX-HN 14

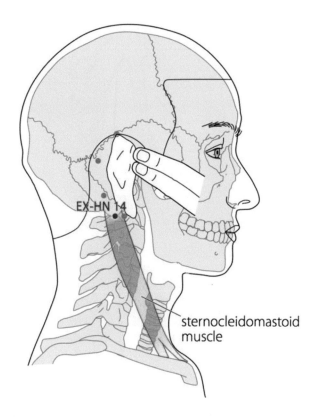

sternocleidomastoid
muscle

3.4.3.2 Extra Points of Chest and Abdomen (EX-CA)

1. **Zigong (EX-CA 1)**
   Location: 4 cun below the center of umbilicus, 3 cun lateral to Zhongji (CV 3) (Fig. 3.123).
   Indications: (1) Irregular menstruation, uterine bleeding, dysmenorrheal, prolapsed uterus, infertility, hernia.
   Manipulation: 0.8–1.2 cun perpendicular insertion.
2. **Sanjiaojiu (EX-CA 2)**
   Location: On the hypogastric region, making an equilateral triangle with the length of patient's corner of the mouth, the angulus parietalis is on the umbilicus, the bottom margin should be horizontal and the two base angles are the points (Fig. 3.123).
   Indications: (1) Abdominal pain, hernia.
   Manipulation: Moxibustion with 5–7 moxa cone.

Fig. 3.123 Location of
EX-CA 1, EX-CA 2

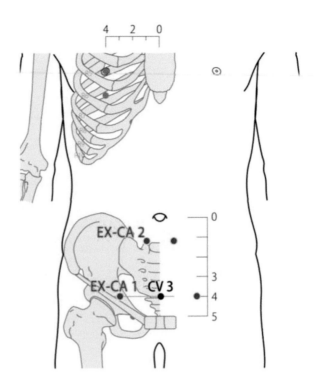

3.4.3.3 Extra Points of Back (EX-B)

1. **Dingchuan (EX-B 1)**
   Location: Below the spinous process of the seventh cervical vertebra, 0.5 cun lateral to the posterior midline (Fig. 3.124).
   Indications: (1) Asthma, cough. (2) Rigidity and pain in the shoulder and back, stiff neck.
   Manipulation: 0.5–0.8 cun perpendicular insertion.
2. **Jiaji (EX-B 2)**
   Location: 0.5 cun lateral to the lower border of each spinous process from the first thoracic vertebrae to the fifth lumbar vertebrae. There are 17 points on each side, 34 points in total (Fig. 3.125).
   Indications: There are many **Indications**. The Jiaji *(EX-B 2)* points on the upper back are indicated for disorders of the heart, lung, and upper limbs, while those on the lower back are indicated for disorders of the spleen and stomach, and those on the lumbar region are indicated for disorders of the lumbar region and lower abdomen, and lower limbs.
   Manipulation: 0.3–0.5 cun perpendicular or oblique insertion. The plum-blossom needling technique can be utilized.

Fig. 3.124 Location of
EX-CA 1

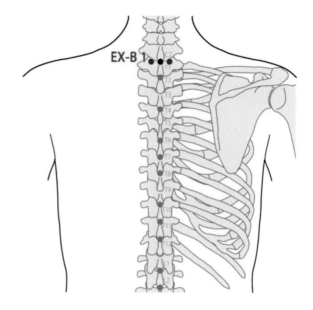

Fig. 3.125 Location of
EX-B 2

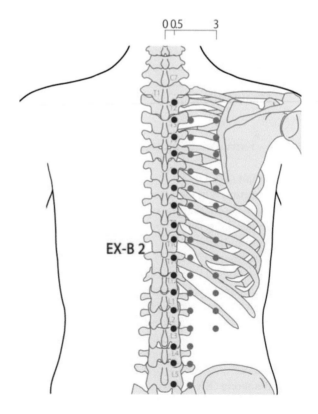

Fig. 3.126 Location of
EX-B 7

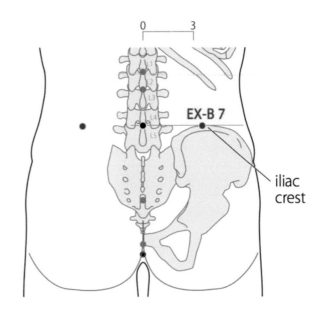

3. **Yaoyan (EX-B 7)**

   Location: In the depressed region, 3.5 cun lateral to the lower border of the spinous process of the fourth lumbar vertebra (Fig. 3.126).

   Indications: (1) Lumbago. (2) Morbid leucorrhea, irregular menstruation. (3) Consumptive diseases.

   Manipulation: 1.0–1.5 cun perpendicular insertion.

3.4.3.4 Extra Points of Upper Extremities (EX-UE)

1. **Jianqian (EX-UE 1)**

   Location: On the anterior area of the shoulder, the point is on the midpoint between the anterior end of the axillary fold and Jianyu (LI 15) point (Fig. 3.127).

   Indications: Acute lumbar muscle sprain.

   Manipulation: 1.0–1.5 cun perpendicular insertion.

2. **Yaotongdian (EX-UE 7)**

   Location: On the dorsum of the hand, between the second and third, fourth and fifth metacarpal bones respectively, at the middle points from the line through the metacarpal-phalangeal joints to the transverse crease of the wrist. There are two points on each hand, four points in total (Fig. 3.128).

   Indications: Acute lumbar muscle sprain.

   Manipulation: Acupuncture obliquely 0.5~0.8 cun *toward the center of the palm*.

3. **Wailaogong (EX-UE 8)**

   Location: On the dorsum of the hand, between the second and third metacarpal bones, 0.5 cun posterior to the metacarpal-phalangeal joint (Fig. 3.128).

Fig. 3.127 Location of
EX-UE 1

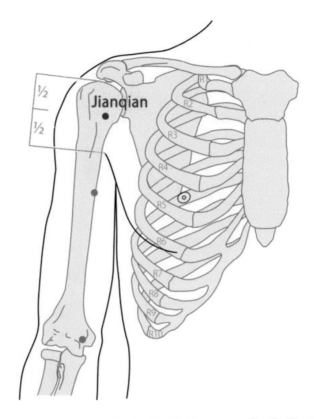

Indications: (1) Stiff neck, swelling and redness in the back of the hands, numbness of the fingers. (2) Umbilical tetanus.

Manipulation: 0.5–0.8 cun perpendicular insertion.

4. **Baxie (EX-UE 9)**

Location: Hand slightly flexed, on the dorsum of hands, in the fingerweb between each finger, eight points on the dorsum of left and right hands (Fig. 3.128).

Indications: (1) Swelling and pain on the dorsum of the hand, numbness and spasmodic pain in the interphalangeal joints. (2) Vexation, fever. (3) Eye pain. (4) Venomous snake bite.

Manipulation: 0.5–0.8 cun oblique insertion, or prick to induce bleeding.

5. **Sifeng (EX-UE 10)**

Location: On the palmar side of the index, middle, ring, and little fingers at the center of the proximal interphalangeal joints (Fig. 3.129).

Indications: (1) Infantile malnutrition and pertussis, infantile diarrhea. (2) Pertussis and asthma.

Manipulation: Prick 0.1–0.2 cun deep until yellowish mucus comes out.

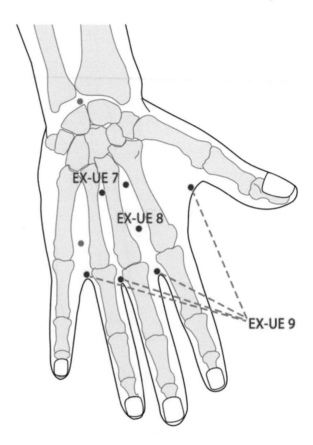

Fig. 3.128 Location of EX-UE 7–EX-UE 9

6. **Shixuan (EX-UE 11)**

   Location: At the tips of the ten fingers, about 0.1 cun distal to the nails, ten points on left and right fingers in total (Fig. 3.130).

   Indications: (1) Coma, infantile syncope. (2) Epilepsy. (3) High fever, sore throat, numbness of the fingers.

   Manipulation: Insert shallowly about 0.1 cun into the skin, or insert a three-edged needle to induce bleeding.

3.4.3.5 Extra Points of Lower Extremities (EX-LE)

1. **Heding (EX-LE 2)**

   Location: On the upper part of the knee, in the depressed region above the midpoint of the base of the patella (Fig. 3.131).

   Indications: (1) Knee pain, weakness of the leg and foot, paralysis of lower extremities, beriberi.

   Manipulation: 0.8–1.0 cun perpendicular insertion.

Fig. 3.129 Location of
EX-UE 10

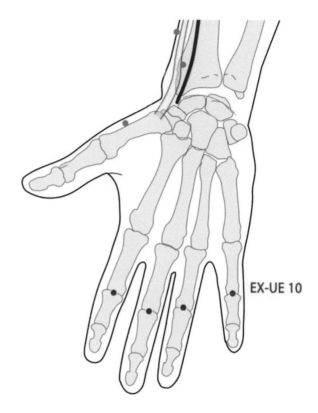

EX-UE 10

2. **Baichongwo (EX-LE 3)**

 Location: When the knee is flexed, the point is on the medial side of the thigh, 3 cun above the medial side of the patella,1 cun above the point Xuehai (SP 10) (Fig. 3.132).

 Indications: (1) Ascariasis. (2) Itching of the skin, eczema, rubella, skin ulcers on the lower part of the body.

 Manipulation: 1.5–2.0 cun perpendicular insertion.

3. **Neixiyan (EX-LE 4)**

 Location: In the depressed region, medial side of ligament patellae when the knee is flexed. The medial side is called Neixiyan (EX-LE 4) (Fig. 3.131).

 Indications: (1) Pain in the knee and lower limbs. (2) Beriberi.

 Manipulation: 0.5–1.0 cun oblique insertion.

4. **Dannang (EX-LE 6)**

 Location: On the lateral aspect of the lower leg, 2 cun directly below the head of the fibula (Fig. 3.133).

 Indications: (1) Pain in the hypochondriac region, cholelithiasis, acute and chronic cholecystitis, biliary ascariasis, jaundice. (2) Pain and weakness of the lower limbs.

 Manipulation: 1.0–2.0 cun perpendicular insertion.

Fig. 3.130 Location of
EX-UE 11

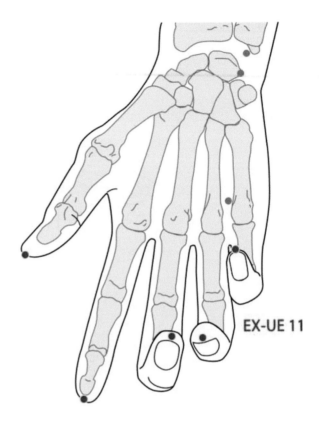

EX-UE 11

5. **Lanwei (EX-LE 7)**

   Location: On the superior anterior aspect of the lower leg, 5 cun below Dubi (ST35), one-fingerbreadth from the anterior crest of the tibia (Fig. 3.134).

   Indications: (1) Acute or chronic appendicitis, stomachache. (2) Poor appetite.(3) Weakness and pain of the lower limbs.

   Manipulation: 1.5–2.0 cun perpendicular insertion.

6. **Bafeng (EX-LE 10)**

   Location: On the dorsum of the foot, between the web of the toes, proximal to the web margin, four points on one side, eight points in total (Fig. 3.135).

   Indications: (1) Pain and swelling on the dorsum of the foot. (2) Venomous snake bite. (3) Beriberi.

   Manipulation: Insert the needle obliquely, 0.5–0.8 cun deep, or prick to induce bleeding.

7. **Other Extra Point** (Table 3.30).

Fig. 3.131 Location of
EX-LE 2, EX-LE 4

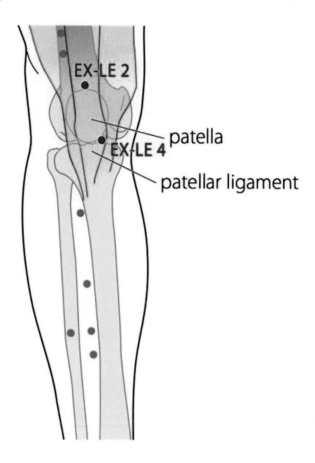

Fig. 3.132 Location of
EX-LE 3

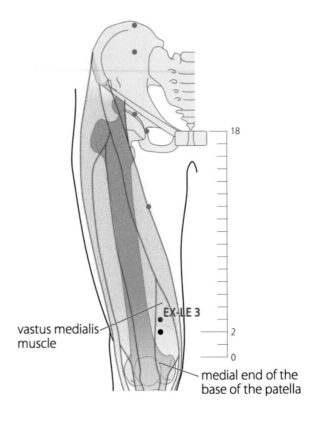

Fig. 3.133 Location of
EX-LE 6

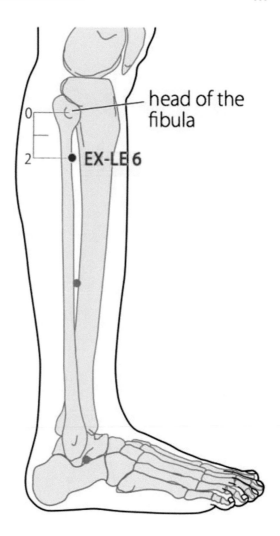

head of the
fibula

0

2 • EX-LE 6

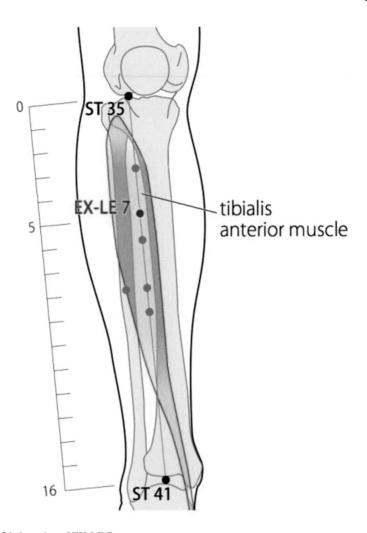

Fig. 3.134 Location of EX-LE 7

Fig. 3.135 Location of
EX-LE 10

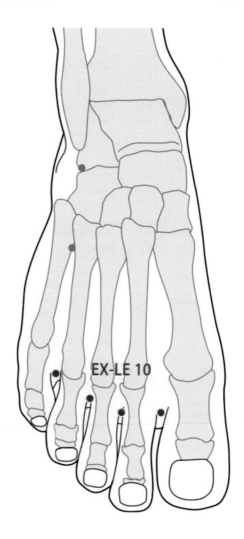

Table 3.30 Other extra point

Point	Code	Location	Indication
Dangyang	EX-HN 2	On the head directly above the pupil, 1 cun superior to the anterior hairline	Headache, vertigo, insomnia, forgetfulness, epilepsy
Yuyao	EX-HN 4	At the center of the eyebrow in the depression directly above the pupil when the eyes are looking straight ahead	Twitching of the eyelid, deviation of the mouth and eye, ptosis of the eyelid, red and painful eyes, trigeminal neuralgia
Erjian	EX-HN 6	On the top region of the ear, fold the ear forward, the point is at the apex of the ear	(1) Swollen and painful eyes, hordeolum. (2) Swelling and pain in the throat. (3) Headache, vertigo
Shangyingxiang	EX-HN 8	On the region of the face, at the junction of the cartilage of the ala nasi and the nasal concha, near the upper end of the nasolabial groove	Nasal obstruction, sinusitis, soreness and furuncles in the nasal region
Neiyingxiang	EX-HN 9	Inside of the nostrils, on the mucosal membrane at the junction of the cartilage of the ala nasi and the nasal concha	(1) Diseases of the nose, inflammation of the throat, swelling and pain in the eyes. (2) Febrile disease, sunstroke. (3) Vertigo
Juquan	EX-HN 10	In the mouth cavity at the midpoint of the center line of the tongue	Cough, asthma, aphasia after cerebrovascular events
Haiquan	EX-HN 11	In the mouth at the midpoint of the lingual frenulum	Aphtha, sore tongue, vomiting, diarrhea, hyperpyrexia, unconsciousness, pharyngitis, aphasia after cerebrovascular events, diabetes
Jingbailao	EX-HN 15	On the neck 2 cun directly superior to the seventh cervical spinous process and 1 cun lateral to the posterior midline	Bronchitis, bronchial asthma, phthisis, cervical spondylosis
Anmian	EX-HN 18	On the neck, on the midpoint between Yifeng (TE 17) and Fengchi (GB 20)	(1) Vertigo, headache, insomnia. (2) Madness
Weiwanxiashu	EX-B 3	1.5 cun lateral to the lower border of the spinous process of the eighth thoracic vertebra	(1) Stomachache, pain in the chest and hypochondriac region, abdominal pain. (2) Diabetes, dry throat
Pigen	EX-B 4	In the lumbar region level with the inferior border of the spinous process of the first lumbar vertebra, 3.5 cun lateral to the posterior midline	Gastrospasm, gastritis, gastrectasia, hepatitis, hepatosplenomegaly, hernia, nephroptosis, lumbar muscle strain

Table 3.30 (continued)

Point	Code	Location	Indication
Xiajishu	EX-B 5	In the lumbar region on the posterior midline and below the spinous process of the third lumbar vertebra	Nephritis, enuresis, enteritis, lumbar muscle strain
Yao yi	EX-B 6	In the lumbar region level with the inferior border of the spinous process of the fourth lumbar vertebra, 3 cun lateral to the posterior midline	Lumbar soft tissue injury, low-back pain, profuse uterine bleeding, spinal myospasm
Shiqizhui	EX-B 8	In the lumbosacral region on the posterior midline in the depression below the spinous process of the fifth lumbar vertebra	Irregular menstruation, dysmenorrhea, functional uterine bleeding, hemorrhoids, sciatica, poliomyelitis syndrome, lumbosacral pain
Yao qi	EX-B 9	In the sacral region 2 cun above the apex of the coccyx in the depression of the sacral horn	Epilepsy, insomnia, headache, constipation
Zhoujian	EX-UE 1	Behind the elbow on the tip of the olecranon process of the ulna	Scrofula, carbuncles, sores
Erbai	EX-UE 2	On the palmar side of the forearm, 4 cun proximal to the transverse crease of the wrist, on both sides of the flexor carpi radialis tendon. Each side has one point; each arm has two points	(1) Hemorrhoids, Constipation, prolapse of the rectum. (2) Pain in the chest and hypochondriac region, pain in the forearm
Zhongquan	EX-UE 3	On the dorsal transverse wrist crease in the depression on the radial side of the extensor digitorum tendon	Bronchitis, bronchial asthma, gastritis, enteritis
Zhongkui	EX-UE 4	The midpoint of the proximal interphalangeal joint of the dorsum of the middle finger	Acute gastritis, cardiac obstruction
Dagukong	EX-UE 5	Midpoint of the interphalangeal joint of the dorsum of the thumb	Conjunctivitis, keratitis, cataract, nasal hemorrhage, acute gastroenteritis
Xiaogukong	EX-UE 6	Midpoint of the proximal interphalangeal joint of the dorsum of the little finger	Eye disorders, pharyngitis, metacarpophalangeal joint pain
Kuangu	EX-LE 1	On the anterior region of the both thighs 1.5 cun lateral to Liang qiu (ST 34); 2 points on each side	Arthritis
Neihuaijian	EX-LE 8	At the prominence of the medial malleolus	Toothache, gastrocnemius spasms
Waihuaijian	EX-LE 9	At the prominence of the lateral malleolus	Toothache, gastrocnemius spasms

(continued)

Table 3.30 (continued)

Point	Code	Location	Indication
Duyin	EX-LE 11	On the sole of the foot, at the midpoint of the plantar surface of the distal interphalangeal joint of the second toe	Angina pectoris, irregular menstruation
Qiduan	EX-LE 12	At the center of the tip of the each of the ten toes 0.1 cun distal to the nails; ten points in total	Cerebrovascular accident, numb toe

3.5 Acupuncture and Moxibustion Techniques

Acupuncture and moxibustion therapy, which regulate internal functions through outside stimuli, are unique therapy approachs and indispensable components of TCM. The acupuncture treatment is the insertion of different fine needles on the body's surface according to a certain acupoint, to stimulate certain parts of the body and use various methods to evoke the meridians and collaterals as well as the qi of human body, in order to adjust physiological functioning of the body so to cure diseases. Moxibustion is the burning of moxa on or near a person's skin as a counterirritant. For a long time, acupuncture and moxibustion treatment are often combined together in clinical practice application; therefore, we collectively referred to them as acupuncture-moxibustion therapy.

Acupuncture treatment includes either the administration of manual, mechanical, thermal, electrical stimulation of acupuncture needles, the use of laser acupuncture, and magnetic therapy, etc. Most commonly used acupuncture needles are filiform needle, skin needle, three-edged needle, intradermal needle, fire needle, etc.

3.5.1 Filiform Needle Therapy

According to ancient Chinese medical records and archaeological findings, the primitive Chinese people used bian stone, the earliest acupuncture instrument, to treat diseases. Afterward, with the further development of the society, bone needles and bamboo needles replaced stone ones. Then the development and improvement of metal casting techniques brought about metal medical needles. Such as bronze, iron, gold, and silver ones. Nine types of needles are described in *Miraculous Pivot*, namely, filiform needle, shear needle, round-pointed needle, spoon needle, lance needle, round-sharp needle, stiletto needle, long needle, and big needle. At present, filiform needles are widely used.

3.5.1.1   Structure and Specification of Filiform Needles

The filiform needles are usually used in clinical treatment. Most of them are made of stainless steel. The filiform needle may be divided into five parts (Fig. 3.136):

1. Tail: the part at the end of the handle.
2. Handle: the part that the fingers hold. It is wrapped with fine copper or aluminum wire.
3. Body: the part between the handle and the tip.
4. Root: the connecting section between the body and the handle.
5. Tip: the sharp end of the needle.

As the main tool, the filiform needles should be kept and maintained with great care to avoid damage. The needles should be carefully checked before use. If it is bent, the shaft eroded, or the tip hooked or blunt, the needle is defective and should be discarded.

The length of a filiform needle is also shown as "cun" (Table 3.31). The filiform needles vary in length and diameter (Table 3.32). Clinically the needles ranging from gauges 28 to 32 in diameter and from 1 to 3 cun in length are frequently used in clinical treatment.

Points over bony areas, such as the scalp, face, ears, and distal limbs require the shortest needles. Those over the thorax, abdomen, and lightly muscled areas require medium length needles and those over heavily muscled areas, such as the lumbar area, the hindquarter (buttock and thigh) area, and the heavy muscles of the shoulder area require the longest needles.

Fig. 3.136 Structure of filiform needles

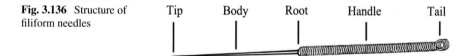

Tip   Body   Root   Handle   Tail

Table 3.31 Length of different filiform needles

Cun	0.5	1.0	1.5	2.0	2.5	3.0	3.5	4	4.5	5
mm	15	25	40	50	65	75	90	100	115	125

Table 3.32 Diameter of different filiform needles

Gauge	26	28	30	32	34
Dia (mm)	0.45	0.38	0.32	0.28	0.22

3.5.1.2   Practicing Needling Skills

A filiform needle is slim and soft. Strong and skillful hand manipulation is required to make efficient acupuncture. Beginners must practice the basic manipulation technique. Paper or cotton pads should be used for practice. The method helps to gain personal experience of needling sensation in clinical practice.

Paper pad practice: Fold some soft paper into a pad (8 × 5 × 2 cm), bind it with gauze thread. Hold the pad with left hand. Hold the needle-handle with the right thumb, index finger, and middle finger similar to holding a brush. Insert needle into packet, rotate in and out clockwise and counterclockwise (Fig. 3.137).

Cotton pad practice: Make cotton ball 5–6 cm diameter wrapped in gauze. Hold the ball with left hand and needle-handle with right hand. Insert needle into ball and practice rotating, lifting, thrusting procedure (Fig. 3.138).

3.5.1.3   Preparation Prior to Treatment

1. Explanation

    In order to get good acupuncture results, the patients' cooperation is needed. Some first visiting patients may be afraid of needling. The acupuncturist should explain to the patients in order to make them relax.

2. Selection and check of the instruments

    The suitable needle, long or short, thick or thin, should be selected according to the patient's age, sex, body type, constitution, disease diagnosis, the depth and

Fig. 3.137 Paper pad practice

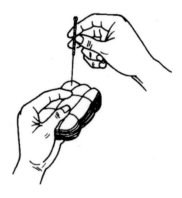

Fig. 3.138 Cotton pad practice

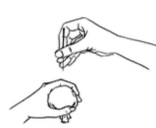

shallowness of the site, and the different acupoints. Generally, for a large or strong male whose disease is deep inside, we choose a large, long filiform needle. We choose slim, short filiform needles for opposite characteristics. Needles should be carefully inspected before use. Prepare needles with different sizes, trays, forceps, and some 75% alcohol cotton balls. If the needle body is bent or eroded, or the needle tip is barbed, too sharp or too dull, the needle should be discarded. This will help prevent hurting the patient or breaking the needle.

3. Sterilization

(a) Needle sterilization: Sterilized needles, which should be used only once, are recommended. The needles for repeated use should be sterilized with autoclave; boiling sterilization or medical sterilization with 75% alcohol.

(b) Disinfection of the region selected for needling: The area selected for needling must be sterilized with a 75% alcohol cotton ball. The selected area is sterilized from the center to the sides. After sterilization, measures should be taken to avoid recontamination.

(c) Disinfection of the acupuncturist's fingers: Before needling, the acupuncturist should wash his or her hands with soapsuds or sterilize with 75% alcohol cotton balls.

4. Selection of the patient's postures

Appropriate posture of the patient is important for correct location of acupoints, prolonged retention of the needle and prevention of bending and breaking the needle as well as fainting during acupuncture. Before needling, the patient is advised to relax himself or herself, keep a comfortable and natural posture so as to maintain the position for a longer time.

(a) Lying posture is most frequently used, especially for the aged, the patients with poor constitution or serious diseases or nervousness. Therefore lying position is significant in preventing fatigue or fainting.

- Supine posture: Suitable for needling the acupoints on the head and face, chest and abdominal regions, and the limbs (Fig. 3.139).
- Lateral recumbent posture: Suitable for needling the acupoints on the posterior region of the head, neck, back, and the lateral side of the limbs (Fig. 3.140).

Fig. 3.139 Supine posture

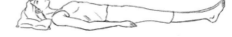

Fig. 3.140 Lateral recumbent posture

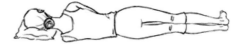

- Pronation posture: Suitable for needling the acupoints located on the posterior region of the head, neck, back, lumbar and buttock regions, and the posterior region of the lower limbs. Sitting position (Fig. 3.141).

(b) Sitting position is suitable for needling the acupoints located on the head, neck, upper extremities or the back of the patient whose illness is mild.

- Sitting in pronation posture: Applicable to the acupoints located on the posterior region of the head, neck, and back (Fig. 3.142).
- Sitting in supination posture: Applicable to the acupoints located on the head and face as well as the upper chest region (Fig. 3.143).
- Sitting in flexion posture: Applicable to the acupoints located on the head, neck, and back (Fig. 3.144).

Fig. 3.141 Pronation posture

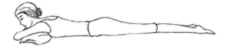

Fig. 3.142 Sitting in pronation posture

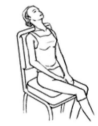

Fig. 3.143 Sitting in supination posture

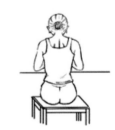

Fig. 3.144 Sitting in flexion posture

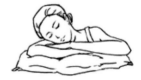

3.5.1.4   Needle Methods

The left hand, known as the pressing hand, presses against the area close to the point to be punctured to fix the skin. The touching and pressing with the pressing hand assist on the accurate location of acupoint. In case of inserting with a long needle, the left hand helps to stabilize the body of the needle. The needle usually should be held with the right hand known as the puncturing hand. The thumb and the index finger of the puncturing hand hold the body of the needle, like holding a writing brush (Fig. 3.145). The tip of the needle is punctured rapidly into the point with a certain finger force, then the needle is rotated to a deep layer.

Different needle inserting methods are employed according to length of the needle and location of the point. In the clinic, the common methods of insertion are as follows:

1. Insertion of the needle with single hand
    Hold the needle with the thumb and index finger of the right hand, the third finger touching the body of the needle, then insert the needle into the acupoint. This method is suitable for puncturing with short needles.
2. Insertion of the needle with both hand

    (a) Fingernail-pressing needle insertion
        Press the area close to the acupoint with the nail of the thumb or the index finger of the left hand, then hold the needle with the right hand and keep the needle tip closely against the nail of the left hand, insert the needle into the acupoint. This method is suitable for puncturing with short needles (Fig. 3.146).
    (b) Hand-holding insertion
        Hold a sterilized dry cotton ball round the needle tip with the thumb and index fingers of the left hand, leaving 0.2–0.3 cm of its tip exposed, and hold

Fig. 3.145 Posture of holding the needle

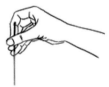

Fig. 3.146 Fingernail-pressing needle insertion

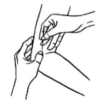

the needle with the thumb and index finger of the right hand. Then insert the needle into the acupoint with the right hand. This method is suitable for puncturing with long needles (Fig. 3.147).

(c) Skin spreading needle insertion

Stretch the skin where the point is located with the thumb and index finger of the left hand, hold the needle with the right hand, and insert it into the acupoint between the two fingers. This method is suitable for the points located on the abdomen where the skin is loose (Fig. 3.148).

(d) Pinching needle insertion

Lift and pinch the skin up around the acupoint with the thumb and index finger of the left hand, insert the needle into the acupoint with the right hand. This method is suitable for puncturing the points on the face, where muscle and skin are thin (Fig. 3.149).

3. Needle insertion with tube

The guide tube is a hollow tube, made of plastic or stainless steel, about 10–13 mm shorter than the needle. The guide is placed firmly on the point and held with one hand. The needle is inserted into the tube and the needle-handle,

Fig. 3.147 Hand-holding insertion

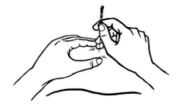

Fig. 3.148 Skin spreading needle insertion

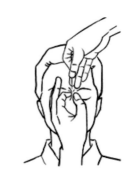

Fig. 3.149 Pinching needle insertion

protruding from the guide, is tapped firmly with the finger of the free hand to drive the needle 10–13 mm deep. The guide is then removed and the needle is advanced to the correct depth. This method is suitable for beginners.

3.5.1.5   Manipulations

Needle manipulation may induce needling effect, for which several methods can be used. Correct manipulations are prerequisite to better therapeutic effects. Manipulations can be divided into two tapes: primary manipulation techniques and supplementary manipulation techniques.

1. Primary manipulation techniques

    (a) Lifting and thrusting

    Lifting and thrusting manipulation is conducted by lifting perpendicularly from the deep layer to the superficial layer, then thrusting the needle from the superficial layer to the deep layer after the needle is inserted to a certain depth, which is repeatedly performed as required. Generally, lifting and thrusting in a large degree and high frequency may induce a strong stimulation, and in a small degree and low frequency lead to a weak stimulation (Fig. 3.150).

    (b) Twirling or rotating

    After the needle is inserted to the desired depth, the needle is twirled and rotated clockwise and counterclockwise continuously with the thumb, index, and middle fingers of the right hand. Generally, the needle is rotated with amplitude from 180 to 360. Rotating clockwise or counterclockwise alone may twine the muscle fibers and produce pain and difficulty in further manipulation.

    Twirling-rotating and lifting-thrusting are the two basic manipulations and can be used individually or in combination. The amplitude of twirling and the scope of lifting-thrusting as well as the frequency and duration of manipulation depend upon the patient's constitution, pathological conditions, and the acupoints to be needled (Fig. 3.151).

Fig. 3.150 Lifting and thrusting

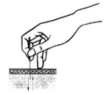

Fig. 3.151 Twirling or rotating

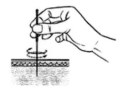

2. Supplementary manipulation techniques

   During the process of acupuncture, no matter what manipulation it is, the arrival of qi must be achieved. When there is no needling reaction, or the arrival of qi is not apparent after needle is inserted, manipulations for promoting the qi should be conducted. In clinic, following six kinds of supplementary manipulation techniques are commonly applied.

   (a) Massage along meridian

   Slightly massage the skin along the course of the meridian. The action of this method is to facilitate movement of qi through target meridian and strengthen its sensation at the point. This method is used in patients whose needling sensation is delayed.

   (b) Flying method

   Twirl the needle for several times, and then separate the thumb and the index finger from it (the movement of the fingers looks like the birds wing waving) until the needling sensation is strengthened.

   (c) Handle-scraping method

   The thumb (the index finger or the middle finger) of the right hand is placed on the tail end to keep the needle body steady, then scrape the handle with the nail of the index finger (the middle finger or the thumb) of the right hand upward or downward. The function of this method is to strengthen the needing sensation and promote the dispersion of the sensation (Fig. 3.152).

   (d) Handle-flicking method

   Flick the handle of the needle lightly, causing it to tremble for the enhancement of the stimulation. This is reinforcing method. This method is used for patients with retarded qi sensation due to qi deficiency (Fig. 3.153).

   (e) Handle-waggling method

   Hold the handle of the needle and shake the needle as the movement of a scull. This is an auxiliary method for reducing. "Before withdrawing the needle, shake the needle to drive pathogenic factors out." Shaking is combined with lifting at the withdrawal of the needle in perpendicular insertion.

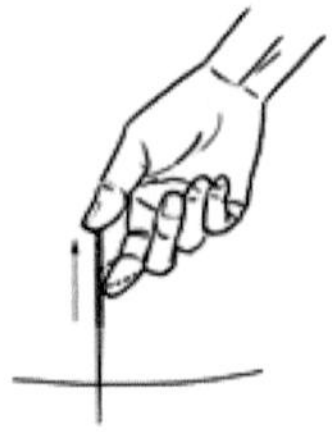

Fig. 3.152 Handle-scraping method

Fig. 3.153 Handle-flicking method

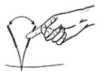

When the needle is obliquely or transversely inserted, shake the needle by moving the handle left and right, but the needle body inside the point is kept at the same place. It is used to push the needling sensation in certain direction.

(f) Trembling method

Hold the needle with the fingers of the right hand and apply lift-thrust or twirl movement in a rapid frequency but small amplitude to cause vibration. It is for promoting the arrival of qi or strengthening the needling sensation.

3.5.1.6 Arrival of Qi

After the needle is inserted, physicians will look for the appearance of needling sensation. TCM calls this de qi literally, the "arrival of qi." The sensation of "arrival of qi" is perceived by both patients and practitioners. The patient may feel a dull ache, heaviness, distention, tingling, or electrical sensation either around the needle or traveling up or down the affected meridian. Meanwhile, the practitioner may experience tightness and dragging around the needle similar to a fish taking the bite. This needling sensation varies greatly from person to person.

The needling sensation is influenced by many factors, such as the constitution of a patient, severity of the illness, location of the acupoints and the needling techniques. In general, if the needling sensation occurs easily and the qi can travel to stimulate the lesion, the therapeutic effect will be better; if qi is difficult to secure, then the effect is not so good. For individuals who get this sensation slowly or faintly, the physician will further manipulate to adjust the position, direction, and depth of the needle; this includes techniques like lifting and thrusting the needle into place, twirling the needle in a specific manner, plucking or scraping the handle of the needle, and also pressing the skin up and down along the course of the meridian with the fingers.

Techniques are carefully chosen based on the condition of the patient and the location of the acupoints. Common factors to determine the needling techniques include: those with strong bodies or the more muscular regions may be inserted deeper and can accept more vigorous techniques; while the elderly, small children and those with weakened bodies, and for those regions with a thin skin layer should have shallower needle insertions and be stimulated more gently.

3.5.1.7 Reinforcing and Reducing Manipulations of the Filiform Needle

Reinforcing manipulation refers to the method which is able to invigorate the body resistance and strengthen the weakened physiological functions. Reducing manipulation refers to the method which is able to eliminate the pathogenic factors and harmonizes the hyperactive physiological functions. Reinforcing manipulation should be selected for deficiency syndrome and reducing manipulation should be selected first for excess syndrome.

1. Twirling reinforcement and reduction

      The reinforcing and reducing of this kind can be differentiated by the ampli-
   tude and speed used. Be careful not to rotate and twirl to one direction, otherwise
   lead to the stuck needle.

   (a) The reinforcing manipulation

            When the needle is inserted to a certain depth and the qi arrives, rotating
         the needle gently and slowly with small amplitude and lower frequency for
         relatively a short period using the thumb to twirl the needle forward and the
         index finger to twirl it backward is called reinforcing.

   (b) The reducing manipulation

            When the needle is inserted to a certain depth and the qi arrives, rotating
         the needle forcefully with a larger amplitude and higher frequency for rela-
         tively a long period using the thumb to twirl. When the needle is inserted to
         a certain depth and the qi arrives, rotating the needle gently and slowly with
         small amplitude and lower frequency for relatively a short period using the
         thumb to twirl the needle forward and the index finger to twirl it backward
         is called reducing.

2. Lifting-thrusting reinforcement and reduction

      The reinforcing and reducing of this kind can be differentiated by the force
   and speed used.

   (a) The reinforcing manipulation

            After the needle is inserted to a given depth and the needling sensation
         appears, the reinforcing method is performed by briefly thrusting the needle
         forcefully and rapidly and lifting it gently and slowly.

   (b) The reducing manipulation

            After the needle is inserted to a given depth and the needling sensation
         appears, the reducing method is performed by lifting the needle forcefully
         and rapidly, thrusting the needle gently and slowly.

3. Rapid-slow reinforcement and reduction

      The reinforcing and reducing of this kind can be differentiated by the speed
   of insertion and withdrawal of the needle.

   (a) The reinforcing manipulation

            During manipulations, the reinforcing method is performed by inserting
         the needle to a given depth slowly and lifting it rapidly beneath the skin.

   (b) The reducing manipulation

            During manipulations, the reducing method is performed by inserting the
         needle rapidly to a given depth swiftly and lifting it slowly beneath the skin.

4. Directional reinforcement and reduction

      It is the main leading principles of reinforcing and reducing manipulation in
   acupuncture.

   (a) The reinforcing manipulation

            During manipulations, the reinforcing method is conducted by guiding
         the needle tip along the direction of the course of the meridian. The puncture

is applied by running along the flowing direction of the meridian qi, to reinforce and benefit the healthy qi, so as to strengthen the hypoactive condition.
  (b) The reducing manipulation
       During manipulations, the reducing method is conducted by making the
    needle tip against the direction of the course of the meridian. The puncture
    is applied by running against the flowing direction of the meridian qi, to
    reduce and eliminate the pathogenic qi, so as to weaken the hyperactive
    condition.
5. Respiratory reinforcement and reduction
    During manipulations, told the patient to breathe deeply and slowly.
  Respiration can be cooperate by other reinforcing-reducing manipulation for
  making the blood-qi moving smoothly.

  (a) The reinforcing manipulation
       The reinforcing is achieved by inserting the needle when the patient
    breathes out and withdraw it when the patient breathes in.
  (b) The reducing manipulation
       The reducing is achieved by inserting the needle when the patient breathes
    in and withdraw it when the patient breathes out.
6. Open-close reinforcement and reduction

  (a) The reinforcing manipulation
       When withdrawing of the needle, pressing the needling hole quickly to
    close it is known as the reinforcing. The purpose of this method is to prevent
    the health qi from escaping.
  (b) The reducing manipulation
       When withdrawing the needle, shaking the needle to enlarge the needled
    hole without pressing is known as the reducing. The purpose of this method
    is to allow the pathogenic factor going out.
7. Neutral reinforcement and reduction
    This method is used to treat diseases atypical to deficiency or excess in nature.
  Lift, thrust, and rotate the needle evenly and gently at moderate speed to cause a
  mild sensation, withdraw the needle at moderate speed as well.

3.5.1.8 Angle and Depth of Insertion

The angle and depth of insertion depend on the location of points, the therapeutic
purpose, condition, constitution, and body type of a patient. Correct angle and depth
help to induce the needling sensation, bring about desired therapeutic results, and
guarantee safety.

1. Angle
    The angle of insertion refers to the angle between the needle and the skin
  surface when the needle is inserted into the skin. It varies according to the location of the acupoint and the aim of the needling. There are three kinds of angles:
  perpendicular, oblique, and transverse (Fig. 3.154).

Fig. 3.154 Angle of
insertion

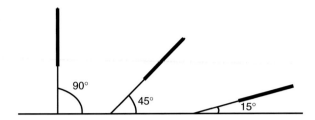

(a) Perpendicular insertion: The needle is inserted perpendicularly, forming an
    angle of 90° with the skin surface. Most points on the body can be punctured
    in this way.
(b) Oblique insertion
    The needle is inserted obliquely, forming an angle of approximately 45°
    with the skin surface. It is commonly used in areas with few muscles or
    areas with important viscera underneath. Points on the chest and back are
    often needled in this way.
(c) Transverse insertion
    Also known as subcutaneous or transverse insertion, the needle is inserted
    horizontally, forming an angle of 15–25° with the skin. It is commonly used
    in areas with thin muscle mass, such as the head or sternum.

2. Depth
   The depth is related to the conditions of each acupoint and related to patient's
   physique, age, state of illness. The principle for depth is to induce better needling sensation but not to hurt any important viscera. Generally, insert shallowly
   in areas like head, face, chest, and back, and deeply in areas like limbs, hips, and
   abdomen. For the elderly often suffering from qi and blood deficiency, infants
   with delicate constitution, areas such as head and face and certain back region,
   shallow needle insertions are advisable. For the young and middle-aged with
   musculature or fatty shape, or for the points on the four extremities, buttocks,
   and abdomen, deep insertion is employed. Oblique and horizontal insertion
   should be shallow, but perpendicular insertion can be very deep.

3.5.1.9 Retaining and Withdrawing the Needle

1. Retaining
   Retaining means to hold the needle in place after it is inserted to a given depth
   below the skin and manipulated. The purpose of it is to prolong the needling
   sensation and for further manipulation. For common diseases, the needles can be
   withdrawn or be retained for 10–20 min; but for some special diseases, such as
   chronic, intractable, painful, spastic cases, or for patients with a slow and weak
   needling sensation, the time for retaining the needle may be prolonged more
   than 20 min. Meanwhile, manipulations may be given at intervals in order to
   strengthen the therapeutic effects.

2. Withdrawing

For the withdrawal of the needle, press the skin around the point with the thumb and index finger of the pressing hand, rotate the needle gently and lift it slowly to the subcutaneous level, then withdraw it quickly and press the punctured point with a sterilized dry cotton ball for a while to prevent bleeding. The practitioner should make sure that all the needles are withdrawn. Be sure not to leave any needle on the body.

3.5.1.10 Management and Prevention of Accident

1. Fainting in acupuncture

   (a) Cause of fainting in acupuncture

   This is often due to nervous tension, delicate constitution, hunger, fatigue, inappropriate position or fierce needling manipulation.

   (b) Manifestations of fainting in acupuncture

   During acupuncture treatment, there may appear palpitation, dizziness, vertigo, nausea, cold sweating, pallor, and weak pulse. In severe cases, there may be cold limbs, drop of blood pressure, incontinence of urine and stool, loss of consciousness, etc.

   (c) Management of fainting in acupuncture

   When fainting appears, stop needling immediately and withdraw all needles. Then make the patient lie flat, offer some warm or sweet water. Symptoms will disappear after a short rest. In severe cases, in addition to above management, press hard with fingernail or needle Shuigou (GV 26), Hegu (LI 4), Neiguan (PC 6), and Zusanli (ST 36), or apply moxibustion to Baihui (GV 20), Qihai (CV 6), Guanyuan (CV 4), and Yongquan (KI 1). The patient will usually respond rapidly to these measures, but if the symptoms persist, emergency medical assistance will be necessary.

   (d) Prevention of fainting in acupuncture

   The needling procedure and the sensations it may cause should be carefully explained before starting. For those about to receive acupuncture for the first time, treatment in a lying position with gentle manipulation is preferred. Needles should not be retained for long time. The complexion should be closely watched and the pulse frequently checked to detect any untoward reactions as early as possible. If there appear some prodromal symptoms such as pallor, sweating or dizziness, management should be taken promptly.

2. Stuck needle

   (a) Cause of stuck needle

   It may result from nervousness, muscle spasm, rotation of the needle with too wide an amplitude, rotation in only one direction causing muscle fibers to tangle around the needle, or from change of position of the patient after the insertion of the needles.

  (b) Manifestations of stuck needle

      After insertion, one may find it difficult or impossible to rotate, lift, and thrust, or even to withdraw the needle.

  (c) Management of stuck needle

      The patient should be asked to relax. If the cause is excessive rotation in one direction, the condition will be relieved when the needle is rotated in the opposite direction. If stuck needle is caused by spasm of muscles temporarily, leave needle in place for a while, then withdraw it by rotating, massaging the muscle near the point, or by inserting another needle nearby to transfer patient's attention and to ease muscle tension. If stuck needle is caused by changed position, resume the original position, then withdraw the needle.

  (d) Prevention of stuck needle

      Sensitive and nervous patients should be encouraged to release tensions. Avoid muscle tension during needle insertion. Patient's posture should keep unchanged during the retention of the needles. Fierce needling manipulation should not be applied. Avoid puncturing the muscular tendon during insertion. Do not twirl needle with excessive amplitude or only in one direction.

3. Bent needle

  (a) Cause of bent needle

      This may arise from unskillful or fierce manipulation, or the needle striking on the hard tissue, a sudden change of the patient's posture, or from an improper management of the stuck needle.

  (b) Manifestations of bent needle

      It is difficult to lift, thrust, rotate, and withdraw the needle, and the patient feels painful.

  (c) Management of bent needle

      When the needle is bent, do not lift, thrust or rotate the needle. The needle should be removed slowly and withdrawn by following the course of bending. If bent needle is caused by change of patient's posture, help the patient to resume the original position to relax local muscles and then remove the needle. Never withdraw the needle with force, otherwise, the needle may be broken inside the body.

  (d) Prevention of bent needle

      Perfect insertion and even manipulation should be applied. Prior to treatment, the patient should have a comfortable position and do not change position when needles are retained. The needling place should not be impacted or pressed by an external force.

4. Broken needle

  (a) Cause of broken needle

      This may result from the poor quality of the needle, erosion between the shaft and the handle, strong muscle spasm or sudden movement of the patient, incorrect withdrawal of a stuck or bent needle, or prolonged use of galvanic current.

(b) Manifestations of broken needle

The needle body is broken during manipulation and the broken part is below the skin surface or a little bit out of the skin surface.

(c) Management of broken needle

If a needle breaks, the patient should be told to keep calm and not to move, so as to prevent the broken part of the needle from going deeper into the tissues. If a part of the broken needle is still above the skin, remove it with forceps. If it is at the same level as the skin, press around the site gently until the broken end is exposed, and then remove it with forceps. If it is completely under the skin, ask the patient to resume his/her previous position and the end of the needle shaft will often be exposed. If this is unsuccessful, surgical intervention will be needed.

(d) Prevention of broken needle

Needles should be of high-quality material, preferably stainless steel. All needles should be regularly inspected. Twisted, rusty or imperfect needles should be discarded. During insertion, a needle becomes bent, and it should be withdrawn and replaced by another. Too much force should not be used when manipulating needles, particularly during lifting and thrusting. The junction between the handle and the shaft is the part that is apt to break. Therefore, in inserting the needle, one-quarter to one-third of the shaft should always be kept above the skin.

5. Hematoma

(a) Cause of hematoma

This may due to injury of blood vessels during insertion, or from absent pressing of the point after needle withdrawal.

(b) Manifestations of hematoma

Local swelling, distension and pain after the withdrawal of the needle. The skin of the local place is blue and purplish.

(c) Management of hematoma

Generally, mild hematoma may disappear by itself. If the local swelling, distension, and pain are serious, apply cold compression locally to stop bleeding, hot compression can be applied to promote resolution of the blood stasis, after bleeding completely ceased. Hematoma will disappear by itself. If local swelling and pain are serious, light massage or warming moxibustion will help disperse the hematoma.

(d) Prevention of hematoma

Avoid injuring the blood vessels and points are pressed with sterilized cotton ball as soon as the needle is withdrawn.

3.5.1.11   Precautions of Acupuncture

It is advisable to delay giving acupuncture treatment to the patient who are very nervous, or overfatigued. Acupuncture may induce labor and, therefore, unless needed for other therapeutic purposes, it should not be performed in pregnancy. Acupuncture is contraindicated for puncture points on the lower abdomen and lumbosacral region during women with menstruation. Acupoints on the fontanel is not closed. Acupoints on the areas with infection, ulcer, scar or tumor should not be needled. Needling should be avoided in patients with bleeding and clotting disorders, or who are on anticoagulant therapy or taking drugs with an anticoagulant effect. Acupoints on the ocular area, neck, or close to the vital viscera or large blood vessels should be carefully needled.

3.5.2   Moxibustion Therapy

According to Internal Classic, the coldness hidden in the body would bring illness which could be expelled through moxibustion. Moxibustion is a therapy that utilizes cauterization or heating with ignited flammable material (moxa wool or other materials) applied to certain areas on the body.

The material mainly used for moxibustion is moxa. Moxa, the leaf of Aiye, is a perennial, herbaceous plant. Due to its special aroma, bitter and pungent flavor, and warm nature, as well as its flammability and moderate heat, moxa is an ideal option of moxibustion. After being dried in the sun, moxa leaves would be pounded and purified. It is thus processed into mugwort wool for clinical use. The reason for using old, dry moxa wool instead of fresh new wool, is that the latter contains so much volatile oil that when burned it gives off too much heat.

3.5.2.1   Actions of Moxibustion

1. Warming meridian and dispersing coldness
   Moxibustion can warm and dredge the meridians, promote circulation of qi and blood, expel cold and dampness. Clinically, it is applied for all diseases caused by cold obstruction, blood stagnation, and blockages of the meridians, such as cold-damp arthralgia, dysmenorrhea, amenorrhea, stomachache, and epigastric pain.
2. Supporting yang to rescue collapse
   Moxibustion can help bring the body into balance and strengthen the Original qi. It has active regulating functions of improving and rectifying the disturbance and dysfunction of certain viscera in the body. It has been widely applied to many serious diseases due to insufficiency, sinking or depletion of yang qi, such as enuresis, rectocele, prolapse of the genitalia, menorrhagia, leukorrhea, and chronic diarrhea.

3. Remove blood stasis and dissipate masses.

Moxibustion can help ensure a consistent flow of qi and blood, remove blood stasis and dissipate pathological accumulation. In the clinical setting, it is commonly used to treat diseases related to qi and blood stagnation, such as the early stages of acute mastitis, scrofula, and goiter.

4. Disease prevention and health maintenance and strengthening the body resistance

Moxibustion on Zusanli (ST 36) or other acupoints, has the function of preventing diseases and maintaining health. It was called healthy moxibustion, which means maintaining the habit by doing moxibustion even though one enjoys good health. This method can invigorate healthy qi and strengthen the immunity to keep one full of vitality and increase longevity.

3.5.2.2 Classifications of Moxibustion

There are many kinds of commonly used moxibustion (Table 3.33).

1. Moxibustion with moxa wool

In the clinic, the common methods of moxibustion with moxa wool are as follows: moxibustion with moxa cone, moxibustion with moxa stick, and moxibustion with warmed needles.

(a) Moxibustion with moxa cone

To make a moxa cone, roll mugwort fluff into the shape of a cone. The moxa cones vary in size from as small as a grain of wheat to the size of a

Table 3.33 The classification of moxibustion

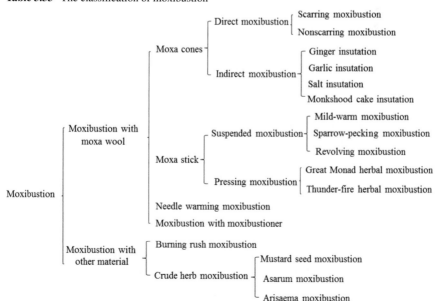

core of a date. During the treatment with moxibustion, one moxa cone used at one point is called zhuang. Moxibustion with moxa cone is subdivided into direct moxibustion and indirect moxibustion, depending on whether there is something between the moxa cone and the skin.

• Direct moxibustion

The ignited moxa is applied to selected acupoints either directly or indirectly. A moxa cone placed directly on the point and ignited is called direct moxibustion. It is subdivided into scarring moxibustion, and no scarring moxibustion. Direct moxibustion means that the moxa cone is placed directly on the acupoint and ignited. This type of moxibustion is either scarring or nonscarring according to the degree of burning over the skin (Fig. 3.155).

– Scarring moxibustion: Prior to moxibustion, some garlic juice can be applied to the site in order to increase the adhesion of the moxa cone to the skin, then put the moxa cone on the point and ignite it until it completely burns out and then remove the ash. Repeat the procedure for about 5–10 zhuang. This will cause a local blister, festering, and scarring on the skin after healing. It is often used to treat certain chronic diseases, such as asthma and pulmonary tuberculosis.
– Nonscarring moxibustion: Apply a small amount of Vaseline to the area around the point. Place a moxa cone on the point and ignite. When 2/5 of a moxa cone is burnt, or when the patient feels a burning pain, the cone is replaced by a new one. The moxibustion continues until the local skin becomes reddish but without blisters. Usually each acupoint can be moxibusted for 3–7 zhuang without suppuration and scar formation. It is often used to treat asthenia-cold syndrome.

• Indirect moxibustion (also known as moxibustion with material insulation)

The ignited moxa cone is insulated from the skin by the materials of ginger, salt, garlic, and Fuzi cake, in order not to contact on the skin directly and avoid burning the skin (Fig. 3.156). Moxibustion with ginger: Fresh ginger is cut into slices, about 2–3 cm wide and 0.2–0.3 cm thick. Punch several holes on it with needle and place it on the acupoints selected. The moxa cone is then placed on top of the ginger slice where it

Fig. 3.155 Direct moxibustion

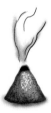

Fig. 3.156 Indirect
moxibustion

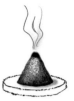

is ignited and burned. Repeat it for several times until the local skin turns reddish but without blisters formed. Indications: vomiting, abdominal pain, diarrhea due to cold, and arthralgia syndrome due to wind-cold.

Moxibustion with garlic: Garlic cloves are cut into slices, each about 0.2–0.3 cm thick, then holes are punched into them. Then place a moxa cone on the garlic and ignite the moxa cone until the patient feels pain. Then remove the cone and place for another one. Repeat it for several times. Indications: early stage of carbuncle and phlegmon.

Moxibustion with salt: Fill the navel with salt, place a large moxa cone on the top of salt and then ignite it. Replace the burning moxa. This method has the function to restore yang from collapse. Indications: abdominal pain, diarrhea due to pathogenic cold, and flaccid-type wind-stroke.

Moxibustion with Fuzi cake: Mix Fuzi with wine and shape it like a coin, then punch several holes on it with needle for ventilation. Indications: yang deficiency syndrome like impotence, premature ejaculation, bed-wetting, and chronic carbuncle.

(b) Moxibustion with moxa stick

To make a moxa roll, place some mugwort fluff into a sheet of paper and roll it up into a tight stick. Apply a burning moxa stick with a certain distance apart over the selected point. Moxibustion with moxa stick can be performed in two ways: suspended moxibustion and pressing moxibustion.

- Suspended moxibustion

  This method is done by holding the moxa stick over the acupoint/area during the treatment. Note: The end of the moxa stick should not make contact with the skin. It is subdivided into mild-warming, sparrow-pecking, and revolving moxibustion.

  Mild moxibustion: Ignite a moxa stick at its one end and place it 2–3 cm away over the site to bring a mild warmth to the local place, but not burning, for some 15 min until the skin becomes slightly red. It is suitable for all the syndromes indicated by moxibustion (Fig. 3.157).

  Sparrow-pecking moxibustion: In this method, the ignited moxa stick is moved up and down over the point like a bird pecking or moving left and right, or circularly. It is indicated for numbness and pain of the limbs (Fig. 3.158).

  Circling moxibustion: When using this method, though the end of the moxa stick is kept 2 or 3 cm above the skin, it is moved back and forth or circularly.

Fig. 3.157 Mild
moxibustion

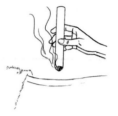

Fig. 3.158 Sparrow-
pecking moxibustion

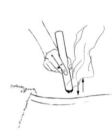

Fig. 3.159 Warming
needle moxibustion

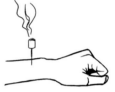

- Pressing moxibustion

    This method of moxibustion is done by pressing the burning end of a
    moxa stick, partitioned off by several layers of cloth or cotton paper, on
    the acupoints to allow the heat to penetrate the skin and muscle. After the
    fire is extinguished, it should be ignited again and repeated. Taiyi miracu-
    lous moxa stick and thunder-fire miraculous moxa stick are com-
    monly used.

(c) Warming needle moxibustion

    Warming needle moxibustion is a combination of acupuncture and moxi-
    bustion, and is used for conditions in which both retaining of the needle and
    moxibustion are needed. During the manipulation, after the arrival of qi and
    with the needle retained in the point, affix a small section of moxa stick
    (about 2 cm long) on the needle's handle, ignite the moxa stick from its bot-
    tom till it burns out. When the moxa stick burns out, remove the ash, and
    take out the needle. This method has the function of warming the meridians
    and promoting the flow of qi and blood so as to treat bi syndrome caused by
    cold-damp and paralysis (Fig. 3.159).

(d) Moxibustion with moxa burner

    The moxa burner is a special instrument used for moxibustion. There are
    two kinds: the box and the canister. During the manipulation, put some

moxa wool, either alone or together with the special ingredients previously mentioned, into the box or canister. Ignite the argyi wool and make sure its lid is properly secured. Then, place it on the acupoints or affected area of the body to be treated. The desired effect is to make the local skin warm and flushed. This method of doing moxibustion is especially useful for children and other individuals who are afraid of being burnt by an open flame.

3.5.2.3 Precautions of Moxibustion

1. Order of moxibustion

   Generally, it starts from the upper part of the body, then to the low part, first the back, second the abdomen; first the head, then the four limbs. Clinically, it may be applied freely in accordance with the pathological state.
2. Reinforcement and reduction with moxibustion

   For reinforcement, do not assist combustion by blowing, let the moxa burn naturally till it burns out; for reduction, while the moxa is burning, blow air to it time after time to make the combustion vigorous. This method is recorded in the book *Miraculous Pivot*.
3. Moxibustion contraindications

   (a) In principle, excess heat syndrome or the syndrome of yin deficiency with heat signs is contraindicated to moxibustion.
   (b) Direct moxibustion is prohibited to perform on face and head, and the place close to the large blood vessels.
   (c) The abdomen and lumbosacral region are not allowed to use moxibustion in pregnancy.
   (d) Precautions should be taken with patients suffering from skin allergies or ulcers.

3.5.2.4 Cupping Therapy

Cupping is a therapy in which a jar is attached to the skin to induce local congestion and blood stasis through the negative pressure created by consuming the air inside the cup with fire or other methods.

Cupping therapy, also known as "jar suction therapy" or the "horn method" in ancient China, was recorded as early as in *Formulas for Fifty-two Diseases*, a silk book unearthed in Emperor Ma's tomb during the *Han* dynasty. Discussions can be found in the TCM literature of other dynasties. Cupping was primarily used to drain stagnant blood and pus from carbuncles and ulcers during surgery. However, with medical progress, not only have the materials and methods of cupping therapy improved, but the scope of its indications has also greatly increased. Clinically, it is often employed in conjunction with acupuncture and moxibustion.

3.5.2.5 Types of Cups

Cups are made from a wide variety of materials, among which three types are most common used: bamboo cup, glass cup, pottery cup, and suction cup (Fig. 3.160).

1. Bamboo cup

    A section of firm bamboo, 3–6 cm in diameter and 6–9 cm in length, is cut to form a short cylinder. One end is used as the base; the other as the opening at the top. The rim of the cup should be made smooth with a piece of sandpaper. The bamboo jar is light, economical, and not easy to break; but it cracks easily from shrinkage if left to dry for long.

2. Glass cup

    The glass cup is transparent, therefore, the skin in the cup can be visualized to help control the appropriate treatment time. However, one disadvantage of glass cups is that they can be easily broken. These cups are shaped like a ball with smooth, open mouth.

3. Suction cup

    Presently, suction cups, for the most part, are made of plastic. Each cup has a fitting on the crown where a suctioning device is attached to remove the air. Through suction, the skin is drawn into the cup by creating a vacuum in the cup placed on the skin over the targeted area. Suction cups are convenient, break-resistant, safe, and the suction force can be easily regulated with very simple adjustments. However, one disadvantage of suction cups is that it cannot provide warm effect.

3.5.2.6 Cup-Sucking Methods

1. Fire cupping method

    A cup is attached to the skin surface through the negative pressure created by an ignited material inside the cup to consume the air. Following are the five methods: fire twinkling method, fire throwing method, alcohol firing method, cotton firing method, and firing method for cup laid on treatment location.

    (a) Flash-fire cupping

        Ignite a 95% alcohol soaked cotton ball held with a clamp, put it inside the cup, quickly turn it around in one to three circles and take it out immedi-

Fig. 3.160 Bamboo cup, glass cup, and pottery cup

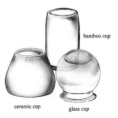

ately, then press the cup on the selected area; the cup will be attached itself to the skin. This is a safe and the most common used method. However, caution should be taken to avoid scalds or burns by overheating the mouth of the cup.

(b) Fire-insertion cupping

A 95% alcohol-soaked cotton ball is ignited and placed into the cup. After a short time, the cup is rapidly placed firmly against the skin on the selected area. Since there is burning material inside the cup which is apt to drop down and burn the skin, it is often applied for the lateral side of the body. The quantity of alcohol should be moderate and avoid of dripping to burn the skin.

(c) Alcohol-dropping cupping

Put one to three drops of alcohol into a cup (only a small amount should be used, to prevent it from dripping out of the cup and burning the skin), turn the cup to distribute the alcohol evenly on the surface of the walls. Promptly place the cup on the area to be treated after igniting the alcohol for a few seconds.

(d) Cotton-burning cupping

Stick an appropriate-sized alcohol-soaked, cotton ball on the inner wall of the cup; ignite the cotton ball and quickly place the cup on the area to be treated. With this method, the cotton ball should not be soaked with too much alcohol, otherwise the skin would be burned when the burning alcohol drops down.

2. Water-boiled cupping

With this method, the negative pressure is created when boiling water draws the air out of the cup so that it can attach to the skin. Generally, a bamboo cup is chosen to put in the boiling water or herbal liquid for several minutes; then the cup is grasped with clamped, with the mouth facing downwards. The cup is immediately placed on the selected location and attached to the body surface.

3. Suction cupping

A suction cup is placed firmly on the chosen area, where a device is used to withdraw the air. When a sufficient amount of negative pressure is produced, the cup will attach itself to the skin. The negative pressure can be adjusted according to the quantity of air withdrawn, to regulate the suction force.

3.5.2.7 Cupping Methods

1. Retaining cupping

This could also be called the cup-waiting method, as it involves attaching the cup to the skin and retaining it on the selected location for 10–15 min before removal. In clinical practice, a single-cup or multicup retaining can be used.

2. Sliding cupping

A lubricant, such as Vaseline or oil, should be applied to the skin over the treatment, the cup then is sucked to the skin. Hold the cup with hand and slide it across the skin until the skin becomes congested, or even blood stagnation is seen. It is suitable for treatment of a large, thickly muscled area, such as the back, the lumbus, the buttocks, and the thigh.

3. Flash cupping

    This method is applied by rapidly placing and removing the cup repeatedly over the same place until the skin becomes hyperemic. It is suitable for treating local numbness of the skin or diseases of deficiency with impairment of viscera functions.

4. Pricking and cupping

    After disinfecting the treatment area, prick the points with a three-edged needle to cause bleeding, or tap with plum-blossom needle, then apply cupping. Retain the cup on the area for 10–15 min. It enhances blood circulation and relieves swelling and pain by removing the blood stasis. It is indicated for erysipelas, sprains, and acute mastitis.

5. Cupping with retaining of needle

    Sometimes referred to as needle cupping for short, this method is done by applying a cup over the center of the site where a needle has been inserted. The cup is removed when the skin turns rosy, congested, and blood stagnation appears. This method combines cupping with acupuncture.

6. Medicated cupping

    There are actually two methods involved here. One is to boil a bamboo cup in an herbal decoction for 10–15 min and place it on the affected area; the other is to put the herbal decoction in the suction cup and apply it to the affected location. The prescription is made according to the illness, for example, herbal medicine with the properties of dispelling wind and promoting blood circulation, such as Qianghuo, Duhuo, Danggui. Honghua, Mahuang, Aiye, Chuanjiao, Mugua, Chuanwu, and Caowu, can be selected for treating wind-cold-dampness syndrome.

3.5.2.8 Effects and Indications of Cupping

Cupping therapy has the action of warming the meridians, promoting qi and blood circulation, relieving blood stagnation, alleviating pain and swelling, and dispelling dampness and cold. It is commonly applied for wind-cold-dampness impediment disease; acute strains and sprains, soft tissue sprains and contusions, common colds, headaches, facial paralysis, hemiplegia, cough, stomach pains, diarrhea, abdominal pain, the early stages of abscesses, and dysmenorrheal.

3.5.2.9 Removal of Cup and Precautions

1. Removal of cup

    Generally, the cup is retained in the location for 10–15 min, then it should be removed. Hold the cup with the one hand and press the skin by the edge of the jar, break the seal created by the suction, let the air come into the cup, and release cup. If the strength of suction is too strong, the cup should not be pulled forcibly, to avoid injuring the skin.

2. Precautions

(a) Generally, select areas with abundant muscle mass, and ensure the patients are comfortably positioned. Sites with hair, joints, and depressions are not suitable for cupping therapy since it is difficult to achieve a seal and the jar may fall off. Flash cupping should be used on areas that are difficult for cups to stick.

(b) The size of the cups must be chosen according to the cupping location. The mouth of the jar must be round and smooth, without chips or cracks. Otherwise the skin may be injured.

(c) Precautions should be taken to avoid scalding the skin. It is normal if small blisters appear on the skin after cupping therapy. It is not necessary to treat them. Prolonged retention and overheating of the mouth of the cup may cause blisters to arise. If the local blood stasis is severe, it is inadvisable to apply more cupping therapy to the same area. In the event that this occurs, small blisters should be covered with sterile gauze to avoid scraping; bigger ones should be punctured with a sterile syringe, followed by the application of a sterile dressing to prevent infection. If there is purple or even black agglomeration left, the warm towel can be used; or we can press the local area, in order to promote the blood circulation, and relieve the symptom.

(d) It is not advisable to apply cupping therapy to a patient with skin ulcers, skin sensitivity, or edema, as well as on the precordium and places supplied with large blood vessels. It is also contraindicated for those who have high fevers accompanied by convulsions, and on the abdominal and sacral regions of pregnant women.

3.5.3   Other Acupuncture-Related Therapies

3.5.3.1   Three-Edged Needle Therapy

The three-edged needle is used for bleeding. Presently made of stainless steel, being 2 cun long, is a thick, round-handled needle with a triangular head and a sharp tip (Fig. 3.161).

Fig. 3.161 Three-edged needle

1. Manipulations
   (a) Point-pricking method
      Hold the handle of the three-edged needle with the right thumb and index finger, prick the selected sterilized acupoint or local reactive spot quickly and induce bleeding, withdraw the needle immediately. Then squeeze and press the area to cause bleeding for several drops. Finally, press the punctured acupoint by a sterilized dry ball to stop bleeding. For instance, pricking Shaoshang (LU 11) to treat sore throat, pricking Taiyang (EX-HN 5) or apex of the auricle to treat acute conjunctivitis, and pricking Weizhong (BL40) to treat lumbago due to stagnation of blood.
   (b) Collateral-Pricking method
      Sterilize the skin, prick the selected superficial vein to let a little blood, then press the punctured hole with a sterilized dry cotton ball to stop bleeding. For instance, pricking the superficial vein at the popliteal space and the medial side of the elbow for sun stoke.
   (c) Scattered needling method
      Prick around a small area or a reddened swelling, then press the skin or apply cupping to let the stagnated blood escape to alleviate swelling and pain. It is indicated for intractable tinea, carbuncles, erysipelas, sprain, and contusion, etc.
   (d) Piercing method
      Press and fix the local skin by the left hand, prick the sterilized acupoint or local reactive spot with a three-edged needle to let blood or fluid, or further prick 0.5 cm deep to break the white subcutaneous fibrous tissue and induce bleeding, afterwards, cover the punctured site with a clean dressing. For multiple folliculitis, try to find the red spots at the both sides of the vertebra, and then prick them with a three-edged needle till bleeding.
2. Effects and indications
   The three-edged needling has the function of dispelling blood stasis, eliminating heat, removing toxin, dispersing swelling to alleviate pain, and assisting resuscitation. It is advisable to treat syndromes such as acute heat syndromes especially fever, emergency condition of coma, heatstroke, convulsion and syncope, sore throat, carbuncles, hemorrhoids, intractable Bi syndrome, local hyperemia, swelling, numbness, paralysis, etc.
3. Precautions
   Aseptic operation is applied to avoid infection. The pricking should be slight, superficial, and rapid. The bleeding should not be excessive. Avoid injuring the deep large arteries. It is not advisable to be applied for those who are weak, pregnant, and those susceptible to bleeding.

3.5.3.2 Dermal Needle Therapy

The dermal needle is also known as the plum-blossom needle, 7-star needle, and temple-guard needle, which is made of 5, 7, and 18 stainless steel needles inlaid onto the end of a handle. The 7-star needle is composed of 7 short stainless steel needles attached vertically to a handle 5–6 in. long. The plum-blossom needle is composed of five stainless steel needles in a bundle. The temple-guard needle is composed of 18 stainless steel needles in a bundle (Fig. 3.162).

1. Manipulations

    After routine sterilization, hold the handle of the needle with the index finger and tap vertically on the skin with a gentle and flexible movement of the wrist. The area to be tapped may be along the course of the meridians, or on the points selected, or on the affected area, or along the both sides of the spinal column. The intensity of tapping may be light, moderate or heavy in accordance with the constitution, the age, the pathological state, and the location of the patient.

    (a) Light tapping: Light tapping is applied with slight force, and shorter time of contact of the needles with the skin until the skin becomes congested without bleeding spots. It is applied for the kids, the women, the weak, and the elderly, or for areas on the head and face with thin muscles.
    (b) Moderate tapping: The force exerted in the moderate tapping is between that of the light and heavy tapings. Moderate tapping is required to cause congestion and with slight pain, but no bleeding, suitable for the majority of the patients, ordinary diseases, and general locations.
    (c) Heavy tapping: Heavy tapping is conducted by exerting a relatively strong force and longer time of contact of the needles with the skin until the skin becomes congested with bloody spots, associated with a little pain. It is applied for patients with the strong, the excess syndrome, or for areas with thick muscles.

2. Effects and indications

    The dermal needling is used to prick the skin superficially by tapping to promote the smooth flow of qi in the meridians and regulate the functions of the zang-fu viscera. It is particularly suitable to treat disorders of the nervous system and skin disease such as headache, dizziness and vertigo, insomnia, hypertension, myopia, alopecia, neurodermatitis, as well as general disorders—painful joints and paralysis, gastrointestinal disease, gynecological disease, etc.

Fig. 3.162 Dermal needle

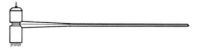

3. Precautions

First, check the needles carefully before needling. The tips of the needle should be sharp, smooth, and free from any hooks. When tapping, the tips of the needles should strike the skin at a right angle to the surface to reduce pain. Sterilize the needles and the location of treatment should be disinfected. After heavy tapping, the local skin surface should be sterilized to prevent infection. Tapping should be avoided to apply to the location of trauma and ulcers.

3.5.3.3 Intradermal Needle Therapy

The intradermal needle is a kind of short needle made of stainless steel, used for embedding in the skin or subcutaneously. It can exert the continuous stimulation produced by the implanted needle. There are two types: the thumbtack-type and grain-like type, the former is about 0.3 cm long with a head like a thumbtack. Theater is about 1 cm long with a head like a grain of wheat.

1. Manipulations

The thumbtack-type needle is generally applied to the ear region, while the grain-like needle is applied to points or tender spots on various parts of the body. Embed the sterilized needle into the point, leaving its handle lying flat on the skin surface, and fixing it with a piece of adhesive tape.
2. Effects and indications

The intradermal needle is mostly used to treat some chronic or painful diseases which need long-time retaining of the needle, such as headache, stomachache, asthma, insomnia, enuresis, abnormal menstruation, dysmenorrhea, etc.
3. Precautions

The points selected for embedding should be located in an area of the body where the needle can be fixed relatively easily. Avoid embedding the intradermal needle around the joints to prevent pain on motion. During the embedding, if pain is experienced, the needle should be removed and embedded again; do not select too many points for embedding for each treatment, 2–3 points selection is recommended. The duration of implantation depends on the pathological conditions in different seasons. In summer, the retaining of needle should not be for more than 2 days. In autumn or winter, retain the needles for 2–7 days. During the embedding period, keep the area around the needle clean to prevent infection. The intradermal needle is not suitable for ulcer, inflammation, and hard masses with unclear reasons.

3.5.3.4 Skin Scraping

Skin scraping, also known as Gua Sha, is based on the skin theory of traditional Chinese medicine: by using a smooth-edged tools such as jade, ox horn, a ceramic Chinese soup spoon, or a coin, scraping and rubbing repeatedly the relevant parts of

Fig. 3.163 Skin scraping

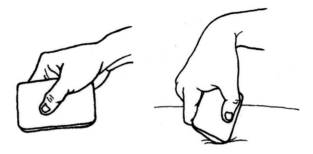

the skin, to dredge the meridian, and activate blood circulation to dissipate blood stasis. Gua means to scrape or rub. Sha is the term used to describe blood stasis in the subcutaneous tissue before and after it is raised as petechiae (Fig. 3.163).

1. Manipulations

    Skin is typically lubricated with massage oil. The smooth edge of skin scraping tool is placed against the skin surface, pressed down firmly, and then moved down the muscles or along the pathway of the meridians, with each stroke being about 4–6 in. long. The intensity of scraping may be light, moderate or heavy in accordance with the constitution, the age, the pathological state, and the location of the patient. The places to be scraped may be along the course of meridian, or on the points selected, or on the affected locations, especially at the both sides of the vertebra.

2. Effects and indications

    Skin scraping has the function of dredging the meridian, improving the circulation, removing toxin, promoting metabolism, strengthening the body resistance, and maintaining healthy. Skin scraping is mostly used to treat soft tissue pain, stiffness, fever, headache, insomnia, cough, vomiting, diarrhea, heatstroke, and health care, etc.

3. Precautions

    It is not advisable to apply skin scraping therapy to patients with skin ulcers, allergies. It is also contraindicated for those susceptible to bleeding, and on the abdominal and sacral regions of pregnant women. During skin scraping therapy, keep the room warm, avoid the wind blowing directly. After the treatment, drink a cup of warm boiling water (preferably add a bit sugar and salt in the water), and rest for 15–20 min. The next scraping therapy should be applied until the bruise (Sha) caused by the scraping has disappeared, so the interval between 2 treatments should be 3–7 days.

3.5.3.5 Electroacupuncture

Electroacupuncture is a form of acupuncture by which the needle is attached to a trace pulse current after it is inserted to the selected acupoint for the purpose of producing synthetic effect of electric and needling stimulation. It substitutes for prolonged hand maneuvering, otherwise, it is easier to control the frequency of the stimulus and the amount of stimulus than with hand manipulation of the needles.

1. Electroacupuncture device

   Electroacupuncture device is an electric pulse generator and the low-frequency impulse current is generated by an oscillator. The device is equipped with host, electrode wire, electrode plates, and electrode clip, etc. With special rotary knob to adjust wave form, time, frequency, and output strength, it is easy to be operated.

2. Manipulation

   Insert the needle on the selected acupoints, after the needling sensation is obtained and reinforcing or reducing needling manipulation is conducted, set the output potentiometer of the electroacupuncture device to "0," connect the two wires of the output respectively to the handles of the two needles switch on the power supply, select the desired wave pattern and frequency, gradually increase the output current until the patient gets a tolerable soreness and numbness sensation. Duration of standard treatment with electroacupuncture is usually 10–20 min, usually no more than 30 min. When the treatment is over, turn the potential to "0" and switch off the electroacupuncture device, disconnect the wires from the needles, and withdraw the needles. The negative electrode is attached to what is considered the main point, while the positive electrode is attached to a secondary point attach to an electroacupuncture device in the case of a direct current. However, in the case of alternating current, the two electrodes in any pair are equivalent, so there is no strict distinction between positive and negative electrode.

   Electroacupuncture uses the same points as acupuncture, and operates on a similar principle. In general, 1–3 pair of points are selected from the same side of the body or limbs. Generally, and avoid to apply electrostimulation at high intensities in the head or across the midline of the body.

3. Stimulating parameters

   (a) The actions of electropulse

   The low-frequency pulsation of the stimulator would stimulate the point via the inserted filiform needle so as to affect the physiological function of the body, relieve the muscular spasm and pain, induce sedation, and promote the blood circulation. As the pulsation varies in frequency and wave pattern, the actions of the pulses may be different. The high-frequency pulse 50–100 s^{-1} is known as dense wave, the low-frequency pulse 2–5 s^{-1} termed as rarefaction wave.

   (b) Undulate wave forms, amplitude of waves

   - Undulate wave forms
     Dense wave: high-frequency wave (>30 Hz, 50–100 pulse)
     It may reduce the nerve irritability, produce inhibition on sensory never and motor nerve, commonly used for acupuncture analgesia, sedation and pain relief, relaxation of muscles, and vessels spasm, etc.

Sparse wave: low-frequency wave (<30 Hz, or 2–5 pulse/s)

It is comparatively strong and can cause contraction of the muscles and enhance the tension of muscle and ligaments, commonly used for flaccidity, atrophy and the impairment of muscle, joint, ligament, and tendons.

Irregular wave: alternately dense and sparse wave

This is a kind of wave, which spontaneously alternates appearance of low and high waves within time of 1.5 s. It has a better excitation effect during treatment, can promote metabolism and blood circulation, improve tissue nutrition, and eliminate inflammatory edema. It is commonly used for sprain and contusion, periarthritis, facial paralysis, etc.

Intermittent wave: rhythmically interrupted electric dense wave for 1.5 s each phase.

As a regular intermittent rarefaction wave, it can increase the excitation of muscular tissue and produce good stimulation to the muscle and make it contract perfectly, especially for striated muscle. It is commonly used for muscular weakness and atrophy, paralysis, etc.

Serrated wave (saw-tooth wave)

This is an undulated wave in which impulse amplitude undulates automatically in a serrated form 16–20 times or 20–25 times a minute, which is close to human's respiration, therefore also known as respiratory wave. It is used for rescuing a person with respiratory failure by making artificial electrorespiration through stimulation of the phrenic nerve.

- Amplitude of waves: The difference between the maximum and minimum voltage and current, the intensity of electroacupuncture mainly depends on the amplitude of the wave (0–20 V, or 1–2 mA). In the clinic practice, the intensity can be selected according to the tolerance of the patient.

4. Effects and indications

The indications of electroacupuncture is quite similar to that of traditional acupuncture, particularly for manic-depressive psychosis, neurasthenia, neuralgia, sequelae of cerebrovascular accident, sequelae of poliomyelitis, muscular flaccidity, gastrointestinal diseases, arthralgia syndrome, painful joints as well as acupuncture analgesia.

5. Precautions

(a) Check the electric stimulator to make sure that its output is normal before each treatment. Turn the output to 0 before treatment.

(b) Adjust the flow of the electric current from small to large gradually, so as not to cause a sudden strong muscular contraction or pain to the patient.

(c) In treating patient with serious heart disease, take care to prevent the current going through the heart. It is generally recommended to avoid placing electrodes on patient with pacemaker.

(d) Do not apply electroacupuncture on the lower abdomen or lower back, and sacrum regions of pregnant women. For the elderly, people with weak constitution, drunk, overhungry, overeating or overstrain, electroacupuncture should be used with caution.

(e) A filiform needle, which has been burned during the process of moxibustion and has lost the capability of conduction due to the oxidation of its handle, is not suitable for electric needling use.

3.5.3.6 Scalp Acupuncture

Scalp acupuncture refers to the acupuncture technique that targets functional zones on the scalp. The needling points are scalp areas corresponding to the functional areas of the cerebral cortex, the nomenclature of the areas (lines) are in accordance with the functional area of the cerebral cortex.

Scalp acupuncture is based on ancient fundamental theories of Chinese medicine and modern knowledge of western biomedicine. In the 1970s, scalp acupuncture was developed as a complete acupuncture system. Three major contributors to the development of this system, *Jiao Shunfa, Fang Yunpeng*, and *Tang Songyan*, each proposed different diagrams and groupings of scalp acupuncture points. A standard of nomenclature for acupuncture points has been published (adopted in 1984 and reconfirmed in 1989), indicating 14 therapeutic lines or zones based on a combination of the thoughts of the different schools of scalp acupuncture. In our book, the name and location of scalp therapeutic lines are based on the 1989 edition.

1. The locations and indications of the stimulating areas

    (a) MS 1 Middle line of forehead
        Location: On the front of the forehead, draw a straight line from Shenting (GV 24), the length of the line will be 1 cun (Fig. 3.164).
        Application: Headache, dizziness, epilepsy, redness, swelling, and pain of the eyes.
    (b) MS 2 Lateral line 1 of forehead (thoracic region)
        Location: On the front of the forehead, draw a straight line from Meichong (BL 3), the length of the line will be 1 cun (Fig. 3.164).
        Application: Allergic asthma, bronchitis, angina, rheumatic heart disease (palpitation, edema, short of breath, oliguria), tachycardia.
    (c) MS 3 Lateral line 2 of forehead (gastric region, liver, and gallbladder region)
        Location: On the front of the forehead, draw a straight line from Toulinqi (GB 15), the length of the line will be 1 cun (Fig. 3.164).
        Application: Acute chronic gastritis, gastric ulcer, duodenal ulcer.
    (d) MS 4 Lateral line 3 of forehead (reproductive region, intestine region)
        Location: On the front of the forehead, draw a straight line from the point (0.75 cun lateral to Touwei (ST 8)), the length of the line will be 1 cun (Fig. 3.164).

Fig. 3.164 Lines of the forehead

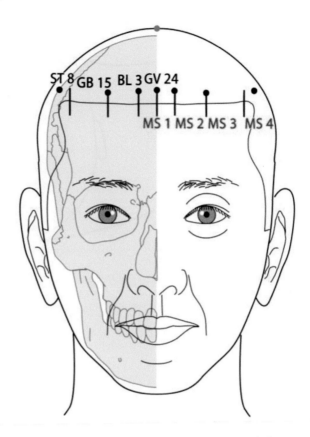

Application: Dysfunctional uterine bleeding, combine with both foot motor sensory area to treat acute cystitis (frequent urination, urgent urination) or diabetes (thirst, profuse urination, polydipsia, impotence, prolapse of uterus, spermatorrhea), especially relieve the lower abdomen pain.

(e) MS 5 Middle line of vertex

Location: On the top of the head, draw a straight line from Baihui (GV 20) to Qianding (GV 21) (Fig. 3.165).

Application: Headache, vertigo, stroke, aphasia, syncope, mental disorder, epilepsy.

(f) MS 6 Anterior oblique line of vertex-temporal (motor region)

Location: Draw an oblique line from Qianshencong (EX-HN1) to Xuanli (GB 6), then divide into five segments (Fig. 3.166).

Application: Superior 1/5 segment will treat the contralateral lower limbs paralysis. Middle 2/5 segment, treat the contralateral upper limbs paralysis. Inferior 2/5 segment (the first speech area), for the contralateral facial paralysis, motor aphasia, salivation, dysphonia.

Fig. 3.165 Middle line of vertex

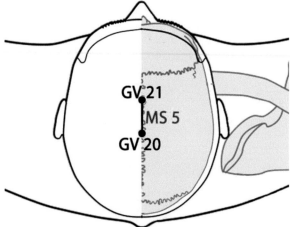

Fig. 3.166 Anterior oblique line of vertex-temporal and posterior oblique line of vertex-temporal

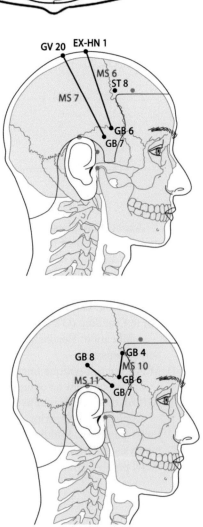

(g) MS 7 Posterior oblique line of vertex-temporal (sensory region)
       Location: Draw an oblique line from Baihui (GV 20) to Qubin (GB 7),
       then divide into five segments (Fig. 3.166).
       Application: Superior 1/5 segment will treat the contralateral waist and
       legs pain, numbness, paresthesia, stiff neck, tinnitus. Middle 2/5 segment,
       treat the contralateral upper limbs pain, numbness, paresthesia. Inferior 2/5
       segment (the first speech area), for the contralateral facial pain, numbness,
       and so on.
(h) MS 8 Lateral line 1 of vertex
       Location: On the front of the head, draw a straight line from Chengguang
       (BL 6), the length of the line will be 1.5 cun (Fig. 3.167).
       Application: Headache, vertigo, tinnitus, blur vision.
(i) MS 9 Lateral line 2 of vertex
       Location: On the front of the head, draw a straight line from Zhengying
       (GB 17), the length of the line will be 1.5 cun (Fig. 3.167).
       Application: Headache, vertigo, migraine.
(j) MS 10 Anterior temporal line
       Location: Draw a straight line from Hanyan (GB 4) to Xuanli (GB 6)
       (Fig. 3.167).
       Application: Headache, migraine, tinnitus, epilepsy.
(k) MS 11 Posterior temporal line
       Location: Draw a straight line from Shuaigu (GB 8) to Qubin (GB 7)
       (Fig. 3.167).
       Application: Headache, migraine, vertigo, febrile convulsion.
(l) MS 12 Upper middle line of occiput
       Location: Draw a straight line from Qiangjian (GV 18) to Naohu (GV
       17) (Fig. 3.168).
       Application: Headache, dizziness, vertigo, stiff neck, mental disorder,
       epilepsy.

Fig. 3.167 Lines of the temporal

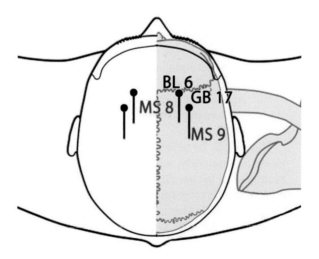

Fig. 3.168 Lines of the occiput

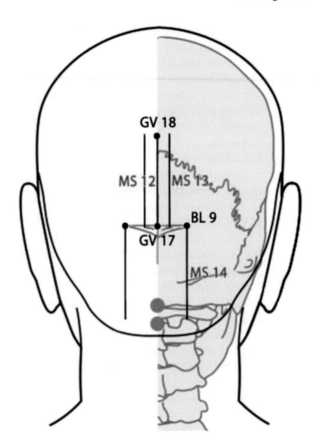

(m) MS 13 Upper lateral line of occiput (optic area)
    Location: At the posterior of head, 0.5 cun lateral beside, draw a straight line parallel to upper middle line of occiput (Fig. 3.168).
    Application: Cortex vision impairment, cataract.
(n) MS 14 Lower lateral line of occiput (balance area)
    Location: At the posterior of head, below the external occipital protuberance, draw a straight line from Yuzhen (BL 9), the length of the line will be 2 cun (Fig. 3.168).
    Application: Headache, stiff neck, vertigo, balance disorder caused by cerebellum impairment.
2. Manipulation
    Patient may be treated with a sitting position or lying position. Disinfect the local place routinely, select a 1.5 cun or 2 cun long filiform needle No. 28–30, swiftly insert the needle subcutaneously, in 30 angle to the scalp, when the needle reaches the subgaleal layer and the practitioner feels the insertion resistance becomes weak, further insert the needle by twirling method, which parallels with the scalp until it goes to the periosteum, the depth of insertion varies with the

areas, generally 0.5–1.5 cun. After the needle being inserted to the required depth, conduct manipulation.

In scalp acupuncture, the needle is manipulated only by twirling method, no lifting or thrusting of the needle. The depth of insertion keeps constant, and the needle is twirled in a frequency of 130–200 times per minute, it is first manipulated for 2–3 min and the needle is retained for 5–10 min, then the needle is withdrawn. For hemiplegia, during the manipulation and retention of the needle, the patient is encouraged to exercise the affected limbs so as to raise the therapeutic effect. (In severe case, passive movement of the limbs of the patient is conducted.)

Electrostimulation can be connected to the needles in the main areas to replace the hand manipulation. It is in a mode of high frequency and weak stimulation (Fig. 3.169).

3. Indications

It is mainly indicated for cerebral disorders, such as hemiplegia, numbness, aphasia, dizziness and vertigo, tinnitus, chorea, etc. It is also applied for headache, low-back and leg pain, nocturia, trigeminal neuralgia, scapulohumeral periarthritis, and other diseases of nervous system.

4. Precautions

Generally, scalp acupuncture is a strong stimulation, fainting therefore should be avoided. The practitioner should keep a close eye on the complexion of the patient and the intensity of the stimulation should be appropriately controlled. Wind stroke due to cerebral hemorrhage with coma, fever, high blood pressure, etc. in the acute stage is not suggested to treat by scalp acupuncture. The treatment may be applied until the pathological state is stable. Patients with acute inflammation, high fever, and heart failure should be dealt with great care if scalp acupuncture is used.

Fig. 3.169 Manipulation of the scalp acupuncture

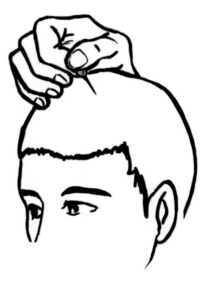

3.5.3.7 Auricular Acupuncture

Auricular acupuncture is one of the acupuncture therapies used to prevent and treat diseases by stimulating certain points in the auricle with needles or other tools.

1. The history of auricular acupuncture

    Auricular acupuncture has been utilized in the treatment of diseases for thousands of years. In the moxibustion classic of 11 Yin and Yang Meridians for Moxibustion excavated from Western Han dynasty mausoleum, it was first recorded as Ear meridian, which was connected with upper limbs, eyes, cheeks, and laryngopharynx. In the classic TCM literature of Internal Classic, which was compiled in around 500 BC, the correlation between the auricle and the body had been described; each of the six yang meridians has a connection to the ear. Yang meridians connect in pairs to yin meridians. Therefore even yin viscera have contact with the ear. In the literature of Miraculous Pivot, it described, "for the deaf who can't hear, needle the center of the ear." It is also recorded in Essential Prescriptions Worth a Thousand Gold for Emergencies that needling point "center" is an appropriate treatment for jaundice, diseases due to cold, summer heat or epidemic, pathogenic factors. In other classic medical literary texts, there are descriptions of stimulating the ears and certain auricular areas with needles, moxibustion, massage, and herbal suppositories to treat and prevent diseases; as well as inspecting and palpating the auricles to assist in disease diagnoses. Modern auriculotherapy got its start in 1957 when a French neurologist named Dr. Paul Nogier, developed the map of reflex points on the ear, based upon the concept of an Inverted Fetus arrangement. Since 1982, the World Health Organization (WHO) has worked to try to bring about a standardization of international acupuncture terminology in naming meridians and acupuncture points. In 1992, the Chinese national standard of nomenclature and location of auricular points was published, and it was revised in 2008. In our book, auricular points are based on the 2008 revised edition.

2. The Relationship between the ear, meridians, and zang-fu viscera

    (a) Relationship between the ear and meridians

    The meridians of the hand taiyang, hand shaoyang, foot shaoyang, and the collateral of the hand yangming enter the ear. The meridians of foot yangming and foot taiyang travel to the front of the ear and above the ear, respectively. The divergent meridian of the hand jueyin comes out from the back of the ear. The vessels of the yang heel and yin heel go to the back of the ear. The six yin meridians connect to the ear by means of their divergent meridians that separate, enter, resurface, and finally join their interior-exterior related yang meridians respectively.

    (b) Relationship between the ear and zang-fu viscera

    The ear has close relation with zang-fu viscera as well. According to records in *Classic of Difficult Issues*, the ear links to the five zang-viscera physiologically. In *Li Zheng An Mo Yao Shu* (*The Extensive Techniques of Massage*), the back of the ear is divided into five parts that correspond to the five zang-viscera respectively.

Fig. 3.170 The anatomy
of the auricle

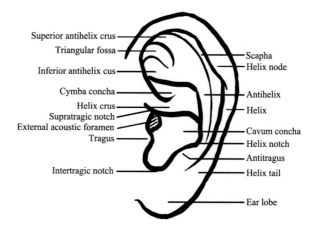

Superior antihelix crus
Triangular fossa
Inferior antihelix cus
Cymba concha
Helix crus
Supratragic notch
External acoustic foramen
Tragus
Intertragic notch

Scapha
Helix node
Antihelix
Helix
Cavum concha
Helix notch
Antitragus
Helix tail
Ear lobe

3. The anatomy of the auricle

(a) Helix and antihelix (Fig. 3.170)

Helix: Curling edge of the lateral border of the auricle.

Helix crus: Transverse edge of the helix reaching backward into the ear cavity.

Antihelix: Medial aspect of the helix, on the elevated edge parallel to the helix. Its upper portion branches out into the superior antihelix crus and the inferior antihelix crus.

(b) Earlobe, tragus, and antitragus

Earlobe: Lowest part of the auricle without cartilage.

Tragus: Curved flap in front of the auricle.

Antitragus: Small tubercle opposite to the tragus and superior to the ear lobe.

(c) Triangular fossa, cymba concha, cavum concha

Triangular fossa: Triangular depression between the two crura of the antihelix.

Cymba concha: Olive cavum between the helix crus and the inferior antihelix crus.

Cavum concha: Cavum inferior to the helix crus.

(d) Scapha, helix tubercle

Scapha: Narrow curved depression between the helix and the antihelix.

Helix tubercle: Small tubercle at the posterior-superior aspect of the helix.

(e) Supratragic notch, intertragic notch, helix notch

Supratragic notch: Depression between the upper border of the tragus and the helix crus.

Intertragic notch: Depression between the tragus and antitragus.

Helix notch: Shallow depression between antitragus and antihelix.

4. The concept and distribution of auricular points

Auricular points are the specific areas distributed over the ear. One of the most popular representations is a picture of a little child huddled up in the fetal position in the form of the external ear. The distribution of auricular points is as follows: Points related to the portion of the head are located on the ear lobe. Points related to the upper limbs are located on the scapha. Points related to the trunk and lower limbs are located on the body of the antihelix and superior and inferior antihelix crus. Points related to the viscera in the abdomen are located on the cymba concha. Points related to the viscera in the chest are located on the cavum concha. Points related to the digestive tract are distributed around the helix crus (Fig. 3.171).

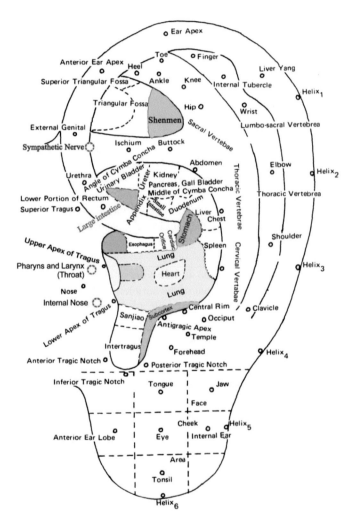

Fig. 3.171 The distribution of auricular points

5. Auricular Points

  (a) Auricular points of helix zone

    • Ear Center; (HX 1)
        Location: On the helix crus
        Indications: Hiccup, skin rash, neurodermatitis, enuresis in children, hemoptysis
    • Rectum; (HX 2)
        Location: At the end of the helix approximate to the superior tragic-notch, at the level with point large intestine.
        Indications: Constipation, diarrhea, prolapse of the rectum, hemorrhoids.
    • Urethra; (HX 3)
        Location: At the level with point bladder, superior to point urethra.
        Indications: Frequent micturition, urgent and painful urination, retention of urine.
    • External genitals; (HX 4)
        Location: At the level with point sympathetic, superior to point urethra.
        Indications: Orchitis, epididymitis, pruritus vulvae.
    • Anus; (HX 5)
        Location: At the level with the lower border of the superior antihelix crus.
        Indications: Hemorrhoids, anal fissure.
    • Ear Apex(Erjian); (HX 6, 7i)
        Location: At the tip of the helix, at the level with the upper border of the superior antihelix crus.
        Indications: Fever, hypertension, acute conjunctivitis
    • Node; (HX 8)
        Location: On the helix tubercle.
        Indications: Dizziness, headache.
    • Helix 1–6; (HX 9–12)
        Location: Region from lower border of auricular tubercle to midpoint of lower border of lobule is divided into five equal parts.
        Indications: Tonsillitis, infection of the upper respiratory tract, fever.

  (b) Auricular points of Scapha

    • Finger; (SF 1)
        Location: Scapha is divided into five equal parts, from the upper part to the lower part. The first part.
        Indications: Finger numbness and pain, paronychia.

- Wind steam; (SF 1, 2i)
    Location: The area between point finger and point wrist.
    Indications: Urticaria, cutaneous pruritus, allergic rhinitis.
- Wrist; (SF 2)
    Location: The second part.
    Indications: Wrist pain.
- Elbow; (SF 3)
    Location: The third part.
    Indications: Elbow pain, external humeral epicondylitis.
- Shoulder; (SF 4, 5)
    Location: The fourth part.
    Indications: Shoulder pain, shoulder peripheral arthritis.
- Clavicle; (SF 6)
    Location: The fifth part.
    Indications: Peripheral arthritis of the shoulder.

(c) Auricular points of antihelix

- Heel; (AH 1)
    Location: At superior and anterior angle of superior antihelix crus, approximate to the upper part of triangular fossa.
    Indications: Heel pain.
- Toe; (AH 2)
    Location: At superior and posterior angle of superior antihelix crus, approximate to ear apex.
    Indications: Paronychia, pain of the toe.
- Ankle; (AH 3)
    Location: Midway between point Heel and point Knee.
    Indications: Ankle sprain.
- Knee; (AH 4)
    Location: At the middle 1/3 at superior antihelix crus.
    Indications: Swelling and pain of the knee joint.
- Hip; (AH 5)
    Location: At the interior 1/3 of the superior antihelix crus.
    Indications: Pain of the hip joint, sciatica.
- Sciatic nerve; (AH 6)
    Location: At anterior 2/3 of the inferior antihelix crus.
    Indications: Sciatica.
- Sympathetic; (AH 6a)
    Location: At the border between the terminal of the inferior antihelix crus and helix.
    Indications: Gastrointestinal colic, biliary colic, angina pectoris, urinary stone, automatic nervous system function disorder.
- Gluteus; (AH 7)
    Location: At the posterior 1/3 of the inferior antihelix crus.
    Indications: Pain of the lumbosacral region, sciatica.

- Abdomen; (AH 8)

    Location: On the border of cavum conchae of Lumbosacral Vertebrae.

    Indications: Abdominal pain and distention, diarrhea.

- Lumbosacral vertebrae; (AH 9)

    Location: A curved line from helixtragic notch to the branching area of superior and inferior antihelix crus can be divided into five equal parts. The lower 1/5 is cervical vertebrae, the middle 2/5 is thoracic vertebrae, the upper 2/5 is lumbosacral vertebrae.

    Indications: Pain in the lumbosacral region.

- Chest; (AH 10)

    Location: On the border of cavum conchae of thoracic vertebrae.

    Indications: Pain in the thoracic and hypochondriac regions, fullness sensation in the chest.

- Thoracic Vertebrae; (AH 11)

    Location: Vertebrae, the upper 2/5 is lumbosacral vertebrae.

    Indications: Pain in the chest and back.

- Neck; (AH 12)

    Location: On the border of cavum conchae of thoracic vertebrae.

    Indications: Stiff neck, swelling and pain of the neck.

- Cervical vertebrae; (AH 13)

    Location: A curved line from helixtragic notch to the branching area of superior and inferior antihelix crus can be divided into five equal parts. The lower 1/5 is cervical vertebrae, the middle 2/5 is thoracic vertebrae, and the upper 2/5 is lumbosacral vertebrae.

    Indications: Neck pain.

(d) Auricular points of triangular fossa

- Superior triangular fossa; (TF 1)

    Location: Superior to the anterior 1/3 of triangular fossa.

    Indications: Hypertension.

- Internal genitals; (TF 2)

    Location: Inferior to anterior 1/3 of triangular fossa.

    Indications: dysmenorrhea, irregular menstruation, dysfunctional uterine bleeding, profuse leukorrhea, nocturnal emission, premature ejaculation.

- Middle triangular fossa; (TF 3)

    Location: Middle 1/3 of the triangular fossa.

    Indications: Asthma.

- Shenmen; (TF 4)

    Location: Superior to the posterior 1/3 of triangular fossa.

    Indications: Insomnia, dream-disturbed sleep, pain.

- Pelvis; (TF 5)

    Location: Inferior to the posterior 1/3 of triangular fossa.

    Indications: Pelvic inflammation.

(e) Auricular points of tragus

- Upper tragus; (TG 1)
    Location: Upper half of the external aspect of the tragus.
    Indications: Pharyngitis, rhinitis.
- Lower tragus; (TG 2)
    Location: Lower half of the external aspect of the tragus.
    Indications: Rhinitis.
- External ear; (TG 1u)
    Location: Supra tragus notch close to the helix.
    Indications: Inflammation of the external auditory canal, otitis media, tinnitus.
- Apex of tragus; (TG 1p)
    Location: At the tip of the upper protuberance on the border of the tragus.
    Indications: Fever, toothache.
- External nose; (TG 1, 2i)
    Location: At the anterior to center of lateral aspect of tragus.
    Indications: Nasal obstruction, rhinitis.
- Adrenal gland; (TG 2p)
    Location: At the top of the lower protuberance on the border of the tragus.
    Indications: Hypotension, allergic diseases
- Pharynx and Larynx; (TG 3)
    Location: At the upper half of the medial aspect of the tragus
    Indications: Hoarseness, pharyngolaryngitis, tonsillitis.
- Internal nose; (TG 4)
    Location: At the lower half of the medial aspect of the tragus.
    Indications: Rhinitis, paranasal sinusitis, epistaxis.
- Anterior intertragal notch; (TG 2l)
    Location: Anterior to intertragus, notch, the lowest point of the tragus.
    Indications: Stomatitis, pharyngitis.

(f) Auricular points of Antitragus

- Forehead; (AT 1)
    Location: At the anterior inferior corner of the lateral aspect of the antitragus.
    Indications: Headache, dizziness, insomnia, dream-disturbed sleep.
- Posterior intertragal notch; (AT 1l)
    Location: Posterior to intertragus notch, anterior and inferior part of antitragus.
    Indications: Frontal sinusitis.
- Temple; (AT 2)
    Location: At the midpoint of the lateral aspect of the antitragus.
    Indications: Migraine.

- Occiput; (AT 3)
    Location: At the posterior superior corner of the lateral aspect of the antitragus.
    Indications: Headache, dizziness, asthma, epilepsy.
- Subcortex; (AT 4)
    Location: On the medial aspect of the antitragus.
    Indications: Pain, neurasthenia.
- Apex of antitragus; (AT 1, 2, 4i)
    Location: At the top of the antitragus.
    Indications: Asthma, mumps, cutaneous pruritus
- Central rim (brain); (AT 2, 3, 4i)
    Location: Midway between the antitragic apex and helixtragic notch.
    Indications: Enuresis, internal auditory vertigo.
- Brain stem; (AT 3, 4i)
    Location: Helixtragus notch.
    Indications: Occipital headache, dizziness, temporary myopia.

(g) Auricular points of Conchae

- Mouth; (CO 1)
    Location: Anterior 1/3 of inferior part of helix crus.
    Indications: Facial paralysis, stomatitis, gallbladder stone, cholecystitis, withdrawal syndrome.
- Esophagus; (CO 2)
    Location: Middle 1/3 of inferior part of helix crus.
    Indications: Esophagitis, esophagus spasm.
- Cardia; (CO 3)
    Location: Posterior 1/3 of inferior part of helix crus.
    Indications: Cardio spasm, nervous vomiting.
- Stomach; (CO 4)
    Location: Area where the helix crus terminates.
    Indications: Gastro spasm, gastritis, gastric ulcer.
- Duodenum; (CO 5)
    Location: At the posterior part of the superior aspect of the helix crus.
    Indications: Duodenal ulcer, pylorospasm.
- Small intestine; (CO 6)
    Location: At the middle part of the superior aspect of the helix crus.
    Indications: Indigestion, abdominal pain.
- Large intestine; (CO 7)
    Location: At the posterior part of the superior aspect of the helix crus.
    Indications: Diarrhea, constipation, cough, acne.
- Appendix; (CO 6, 7i)
    Location: Midway between small intestine and large intestine.
    Indications: Simple appendicitis, diarrhea.
- Angle of superior concha; (CO 8)
    Location: At the anterior superior angle of cymba conchae.
    Indications: Prostatitis, urethritis.

- Bladder; (CO 9)
  Location: Between kidney and angle of superior concha.
  Indications: Cystitis, retention of urine, enuresis.
- Kidney; (CO 10)
  Location: On the lower border of the inferior antihelix crus directly above small intestine.
  Indications: Lumbago, tinnitus, insomnia, dizziness, enuresis, irregular menses.
- Ureter; (CO 9,10i)
  Location: Between kidney and bladder.
  Indications: Colic pain of the ureter calculus.
- Pancreas and gallbladder; (CO 11)
  Location: Between liver and point kidney.
  Indications: Pancreatitis, cholecystitis, cholelithiasis.
- Liver; (CO 12)
  Location: the posterior and interior border of the cymba conchae.
  Indications: Hypochondriac pain, dizziness, irregular menstruation.
- Center of superior concha; (CO 6, 10i)
  Location: In the middle of the cymba conchae.
  Indications: Abdominal pain, abdominal distention.
- Spleen; (CO 13)
  Location: At the posterior and superior aspect of the cavum conchae.
  Indications: Abdominal distention, diarrhea, loss of appetite.
- Heart; (CO 13)
  Location: In the center of the cavum conchae.
  Indications: Palpitation, angina pectoris, neurasthenia.
- Trachea; (CO 16)
  Location: Between the orifice of the external auditory meatus and point heart.
  Indications: Cough, asthma.
- Triple energizer; (CO 17)
  Location: Posteral-inferior part of the orifice of the external auditory meatus and CO(18).
  Indications: Constipation, abdominal distention, stomachache.
- Lung; (CO 14)
  Location: Around the center of the cavum conchae.
  Indications: Cough, asthma, skin diseases.
- Endocrine; (CO 18)
  Location: At the base of cavum conchae in the intertragic notch.
  Indications: Dysmenorrhea, irregular menstruation, acne.

(h) Auricular points of Lobe

On the area from the lower border of the cartilage of the intertragic notch to the lower border of the ear lobe, draw three horizontal lines by which the area is horizontally and equally divided, then draw two vertical lines by which the area is vertically and equally divided, thus the area is divided into nine equal sections. These sections are numbered from the anterior section posterior and from the upper section downward.

- Tooth; (LO 1)
    Location: Anterior-superior part of the ear lobule.
    Indications: Toothache, hypotension, periodontitis.
- Tongue; (LO 2)
    Location: Superomedian part.
    Indications: Glossitis, stomatitis.
- Jaw; (LO 3)
    Location: Posterior-superior part of the earlobe.
    Indications: Toothache, submandibular arthritis.
- Anterior ear lobe; (LO 4)
    Location: Anterior medial part of the earlobe.
    Indications: Toothache, neurasthenia.
- Eye; (LO 5)
    Location: Center part of the earlobe.
    Indications: Acute conjunctivitis, pseudomyopia
- Internal ear; (LO 6)
    Location: Posterior medial part of the earlobe.
    Indications: Tinnitus, impaired hearing, internal auditory vertigo.
- Cheek; (LO 5,6i)
    Location: Between (LO 5) and LO(6).
    Indications: Facial paralysis, trigeminal neuralgia, acne.
- Tonsil; (LO 7,8,9)
    Location: Inferior part of the earlobe.
    Indications: Acute tonsillitis, pharyngitis.

(i) Auricular points of Posterior Surface

- Heart of posterior surface; (P 1)
    Location: Superior part of the posterior auricle.
    Indications: Coronary heart disease, insomnia, dreaminess.
- Lung of posterior surface; (P 2)
    Location: Medial to the central part of the posterior auricle.
    Indications: Asthma, neurodermatitis.
- Spleen of posterior surface; (P 3)
    Location: Central part of the posterior auricle.
    Indications: Stomachache, indigestion, anorexia.
- Liver of posterior surface; (P 4)
    Location: Lateral to the central part of the posterior auricle.
    Indications: Cholelithiasis, cholecystitis, hypochondriac pain.
- Kidney of posterior surface; (P 5)
    Location: Inferior part of the posterior auricle.
    Indications: Headache, dizziness, neurosis.

- Groove of posterior surface; (P 6)
  Location: Through the backside of superior antihelix crus and inferior antihelix crus, in the depression as a "Y" form.
  Indications: Hypertension, neurodermatitis.

(j) Auricular points of Ear Root

- Upper ear root; (R 1)
  Location: At the upper border of the auricular root.
  Indications: Hypertension.
- Root of ear vagus; (R 2)
  Location: At the junction of retro auricle and mastoid, level with helix crus.
  Indications: Cholecystitis, cholelithiasis, biliary ascariasis.
- Lower Ear Root; (R 3)
  Location: At the lower border of the auricular root.
  Indications: Hypotension.

6. Clinical application of auricular acupuncture

(a) Principles for selecting auricular points

- Based on the position of the disease or affected area of the body
  The whole body can be mapped on the ear; therefore, every part of an viscera or tissue has a corresponding point on the viscera or tissue's corresponding ear area.
  E.g., Select the stomach (CO 4) for the treatment of gastritis.
- According to TCM theory
  The auricular points corresponding to the five zang and six fu viscera are especially significant in TCM. E.g., Choose the kidney (CO 10) for alopecia. Choose the lung (CO 7) and large intestine (CO 14) for skin diseases.
- According to knowledge of modern medicine
  E.g., Choose Shenmen (TF 4) and Subcortex (AT 4) for painful conditions and inflammation. Choose the large intestine (CO 7) for toothache.
- According to clinical experience
  E.g., Select external genital (HX 4) for pain in the lower back and legs. Choose Ear apex (HX 6,7i) for bloodletting and for red, swollen, and painful eyes.

(b) Exploration of auricular points

- Inspection
  Auricular inspection is to check for abnormal changes on the ear in order to diagnose diseases or disorders. The most commonly seen positive changes include deformities, discoloration, pimples, desquamation, nodules, congestion, blister, and so on. Red color of ear indicates heat. Pale color of ear indicates deficiency. Bluish-black color of ear indicates

cold stagnation. Pale purple color of ear indicates qi stagnation. Reddish purple color of ear indicates blood stagnation. Excess moisture on the ear indicates dampness. Pimples on the ear indicates damp heat. Dry flaky skin means blood or yin deficiency.

- Detection of the tender spot

    This method searches for the tender spots on the ears with a probe, the head of an acupuncture needle-handle, or the end of a matchstick by pressing and moving on the surface of the ear gently and smoothly.

- Measurement of electrical resistance

    This technique detects decreased electrical resistance in points with an electrical detector that has an indicator lamp or special sound.

(c) Effects and indications of auricular acupuncture

Auricular acupuncture therapy has the action of assistant diagnosis. When there is an illness in the body, especially the organic disease, it may manifest on the ear as positive reactions. There may be tenderness, deformities, discoloration, and disturbance in the skin's electrical properties. We can establish the diagnosis according to these reactions combined with symptoms, signs, and medical history. It is commonly applied for acute and chronic pain, addictions, neurological, gynecological, allergic, endocrinal and metabolic disorders, inflammatory conditions, beauty therapy, antiaging, and disease prevention.

(d) Manipulation of auricular acupuncture

After diagnosis and point prescription are made, detect the tender spots on the area where the ear points are selected. If marked tenderness is not located, give the treatment with auricular points' therapy. After the selected points are located, strict skin disinfection is necessary. Beside disinfect the needles and fingers of acupuncturist, the auricular points should be swabbed with 2% iodine first and then with 75% alcohol as routine asepsis. If disinfection is not strict, it is easy to lead to auricular perichondritis due to infection. The manipulation techniques are as follows:

- The filiform needle methods

    Filiform needles that are 0.5 cun in length or special thumbtack needle are selected for auricular acupuncture. To begin with the procedure, stabilize the ear with the left hand and insert the needle with right hand, then penetrate the cartilage but do not penetrate through the ear. During the needle retention, the needles should be rotated intermittently. Filiform needles are allowed to be retained for 20–30 min. However, they may be prolonged by 1–2 h or even longer for chronic conditions. After the needle has been removed, press the punctured hole with a dry clean cotton ball for 20 s. Once a week treatment, ten times for one course of treatment. For the thumbtack-type intradermal needle insertion, the needle should be fastened to the ear with a piece of adhesive tape and kept in place for 2–3 days. There will be local pain or heat sensation in most of the patients after the needle insertion.

- Electrotherapy

  This method is used to treat diseases of the nervous system, spasm and pain in zang and fu-viscera, asthma, etc.
- Needle-embedding therapy

  After the thumbtack needle is embedded, ask the patient to press it three times a day by himself; retain the needle on the point for 3–5 days.
- Auricular-seed-pressing therapy

  It is a simple stimulating method by tapping small seed-shape herb on the auricular point. This method is safe, painless, and has fewer side effects. It will not cause auricular perichondritis. It is suitable for the elderly people and children or the patient who is afraid of acupuncture. The material, such as rape seed, a mung beam, radish seed, a seed of Vaccaria segetalis, magnetic bead, etc., can be used.

  The points may also be treated with the ear-pressing method. Magnetic beads or Vaccaria segetalis are fastened to the ear with a piece of adhesive tape on the auricular points and kept in place for 3–5 days. The patient is asked to press the selected points 2–4 times a day.

(e) Precautions

Filiform needling on auricular areas may produce strong pain, so explanation is necessary before treatment in order to obtain cooperation from patients. Strict antisepsis to avoid infection. Needling fainting should also be prevented from happening during auricular acupuncture. Prompt intervention is needed if this happens.

For needle-embedding therapy, auricular-seed-pressing therapy, use hypoallergenic adhesive tape for people with adhesive allergies. Do not rub in a sideways or circular motion while pressing the taped auricular points. If it will influence the sleep, only one side points can be used.

(f) Contraindications

Auricular acupuncture should be contraindicated for pregnant women or women with a history of abortion. This therapy is not advisable for patients with frostbite, inflammation, or infection of the ear, and patients with severe diseases or bad anemia. In the treatment of severe heart disease or severe hypertension, strong stimulation should be avoided.

3.6 General Introduction on Acupuncture Treatment

3.6.1 The Function of Acupuncture Treatment

The acupuncture treatment has various effectively curing functions to different diseases, such as tranquilizing effect to insomnia, analgesic effect to pain, antitussive effect to cough, etc. But in brief, the functions of acupuncture treatment are worked out by regulating yin and yang, strengthening body resistance and dispelling pathogenic factors, and dredging meridians and collaterals.

3.6.1.1   Regulating Yin and Yang

As we know, normal physiological states depend on the balance between yin and yang, while diseases mainly result from excess or deficiency of yin or yang. In the fifth chapter of *Miraculous Pivot*, it is said that "how to regulate yin and yang is most important in acupuncture treatment." So that regulation of yin and yang can be recognized as the fundamental effect of clinical acupuncture treatment. Regulation of yin and yang by acupuncture is closely related with point prescription and needling manipulations depending on the different conditions of imbalance of yin and yang. For example, drowsiness due to yin excess and yang deficiency; while insomnia due to yang excess and yin deficiency. Both Zhaohai (KI 6) of yin heel vessel and Shenmai (BL 62) of yang heel vessel could be selected for acupuncture treatment. But different manipulations would be used as for drowsiness reinforcement method is used at Shenmai (BL 62) to strengthen deficient yang and reduction method at Zhaohai (KI 6) to reduce excessive yin, meanwhile for insomnia reinforcement method is used at Zhaohai (KI 6) to tonify deficient yin and reduction method at Shenmai (BL 62) to reduce excessive yang. With these different methods, both drowsiness and insomnia can be treated.

3.6.1.2   Strengthening the Body Resistance and Dispelling Pathogenic Factors

According to the theories of Traditional Chinese Medicine, the occurrence, development process, and outcome of the disease are really the process of struggle between healthy and pathogenic qi in human body. The insufficiency of healthy qi indicates the weakness of body resistance, so the body tends to be attacked by pathogenic qi and cannot dispel the pathogenic factors easily. Another crucial function of acupuncture or moxibustion treatment is strengthening the body resistance and dispelling the pathogenic factors. For example, pricking for bleeding method can be used for dispelling the excessive heat on excessive heat syndrome; reinforcement method like needling and moxibustion can be used for restoring yang qi and helping yang qi warm the body on asthenia cold syndrome; while reinforcement and reduction methods can be used simultaneously on the syndrome complicated with both asthenia and sthenia.

3.6.1.3   Dredging Meridians and Collaterals

Physiologically speaking, meridians and collaterals can connect exterior and interior, zang-fu viscera and outside limbs; promote qi and blood circulation. If there are some blocks in meridians, the qi and blood circulation will be stagnated and clinically manifested as pain, numbness, nodule, swelling, bruising, and other symptoms. However, the appropriate acupoints and needling methods could solve all problems above casily. The basic and direct function of acupuncture is helping to clear the blocked point in the meridians and collaterals in human's body and effectively recover the original functions like connection among viscera and limbs and circulation of qi and blood. Meanwhile, meridians, collaterals, and acupoints are also the gateway for exogenous pathogenic qi to infect into and be driven out from the body. So strengthening the body resistance and dispelling pathogenic factors function of acupuncture treatment is also achieved by dredging meridians and collaterals.

In conclusion, the functions of acupuncture treatment are bidirectional benign effects for human body by dredging qi and blood of meridians and collaterals, and regulating yin and yang. The functions are closely related with the conditions of human body, the methods of acupuncture, and the selection of acupoints.

3.6.2 Principles of Acupuncture Treatment

3.6.2.1 Tonifying the Deficiency and Reducing the Excess

Tonifying the deficiency and reducing the excess is not only the most important function but also the basic principle of acupuncture.

Deficiency indicates insufficient of healthy qi, including qi or blood deficiency and qi sinking; while excess indicates superabundance of pathogenic factors, including stagnation of qi, blood, and phlegm. The deficiency of qi or/and excess of pathogenic factors results in the entire process of diseases. So the basic principle of acupuncture treatment is tonifying the deficiency and reducing the excess, also referring as strengthening the body resistance and dispelling the pathogenic factors.

According to this principle, to tonify the deficiency, reinforcing methods especially moxibustion can be used at Pishu (BL 20) and Zusanli (ST 36) for spleen qi deficiency, Shenshu (BL 23) and Taixi (KI 3) for Kidney qi deficiency, Qihai (CV 6) and Guanyuan (CV 4) for primordial qi deficiency, and Baihui (GV 20) for qi sinking. To reduce the excess, reducing methods such as needling, pricking for bleeding can be used at Taichong (LR 3) for qi stagnation, Fenglong (ST 40) for phlegm, etc.

3.6.2.2 Clearing the Heat and Warming the Cold

Heat and cold are the key guidelines of the diseases nature and manifested in most process of diseases. Clearing the heat and warming the cold is the acupuncture treatment principle directing against heat syndromes and cold syndromes.

Many kinds of heat syndromes could be treated by the method of clearing heat. For exterior or interior heat syndromes manifested as sunstroke, sore throat, and fever, needles must be inserted shallowly and pulled out fast, or pricking for bleeding can also be used. For cold syndromes caused by exogenous cold invasion or endogenous yang deficiency, the method of warming cold is applicable. Moxibustion can be used to treat the exogenous cold in meridians; while the excess cold congealing in viscera, needles must be inserted deeply and retained with the manipulation of heat-producing needling.

3.6.2.3 Concentrating on the Fundamental Contradiction of Diseases

The fundamental and incidental contradictions of diseases are relative to each other, but referring to different meanings. The incidental is generally the phenomenon and the secondary aspect, the fundamental causes generally the nature and the primary aspect of a disease. According to different conditions of human body, the genuine qi is fundamental, and the pathogenic factors are incidental; the cause is fundamental, and the symptoms are incidental; the primary disease is fundamental, while the consequent disease is incidental.

Generally speaking, the key principle of acupuncture treatment is concentrating on the fundamental contradiction of diseases. As it is much more effective to solve the fundamental causes than to relieve the symptoms. Mostly when the fundamental contradiction is solved, the incidental contradiction would also be dispelled. Such as for deficiency cold syndromes, nourishing yang will bring out the relieving of cold.

While in emergency, the acute incidental contradiction must be relieved before the fundamental one, so as to save life or relieve emergent condition. For example, severe constipation and dysuria resulted by aeipathias should be treated with the points helping defecation and urinate, to relieve the acute symptoms firstly. After the relief of severe conditions, the points for the primary cause or original disease are selected to treat the disease and prevent the acute constipation and dysuria.

3.6.2.4 Selecting Treatment According to the Climatic, Geographical, and Individual Conditions

This principle is one of the applications of the "holism of human beings and nature." As the continuous changes of the environment, such as season, weather, and living conditions will affect the human body directly or indirectly. While people with different constitutions will have different manifestation to the same pathogenic factors. All above these factors resulting in the corresponding physiological or pathological reaction, should be considered while treating diseases with acupuncture treatment.

1. Temporal factors

    Not only season and climate, day and night, but rhythmic circulation of qi and blood in the meridians, and the regularities of occurrence or aggravation can be considered as temporal factors. For example, midnight-noon ebb-low acupuncture therapy indicating the point selection by midday-midnight flowing of qi-blood, is recognized as one of the Chronomedicine.

2. Geographical environment

Different areas have different natural conditions, such as climate, cultural customs, and habits. For instance, in cold northern China, moxibustion is frequently used with more moxa cones, but in hot and humid southern China, moxibustion is used fewer.

3. Individual conditions

The same disease has various syndromes and manifestations in different person according to the age, gender, and constitution. For women, acupoints belonging to chong vessel and conception vessel would be used more frequently, and pregnancy is a very important factor for acupuncture treatment selection. While the manipulations of needling on patients in weak constitution should also be lighter than those with strong constitutions.

3.6.3 Selection of Acupoints

Based on the theory of meridians and collaterals, successful acupuncture treatment depends on proper prescription of acupoints. The key principles are selecting according to the symptoms, the causes of the diseases, the functions of the related meridians, and the natures of the points.

3.6.3.1 Principles of Acupoints Selection

Adjacent or local acupoints are commonly selected to treat the diseases, such as Dicang (ST 4) and Yingxiang (LI 20) for facial paralysis, Zhongwan (CV 12) and Shangwan (CV 13) for stomachache. While distal acuponts especially below the elbows and knees are also selected to treat diseases according to the symptoms or the distributions of the meridians, such as Hegu (LI 4) can be selected for facial paralysis according to the distributions of the meridians, while for ache according to the special analgesia on the symptom.

In addition, the application of the specific acupoints is another important principle of acupoints selection. Such as the eight meeting points are mentioned to the eight specific points where the vital energy of the zang-viscera, fu-viscera, qi, blood, sinews, pulse, vessels, bones, and marrow gather. In clinical application, all diseases of the zang-viscera, fu-viscera, qi, blood, sinews, pulse, vessels, bones, and marrow can be treated by the respective meeting points.

3.6.3.2 Combination of Acupoints

1. Combination of the exterior-interior acupoints

This combining method is based on the exterior-interior relationship of the yin meridians and yang meridians according to the differentiations of zang-fu and meridians. The acupoints of the exterior-interior related meridians can be selected at the same time to strengthen the effect. For example, for low-back pain of kidney deficiency, Taixi (KI 3) of kidney meridian of foot Shaoyin can be selected combining with Kunlun (BL 60) and Weizhong (BL 64) of the bladder meridian of foot taiyang. Additionally, the combination of the source points and the connecting points in specific points is a concrete application of this method in clinic.

2. Combination of the anterior-posterior acupoints

   This combining method is based on the theory of the thoracic-abdominal region (anterior) belonging to Yin, and the lumbodorsal region (posterior) belonging to Yang. Thus, the selection of the points on the anterior and posterior regions makes up a prescription for the diseases of zang-fu and trunk. For example, anterior Zhongwan (CV 12) and posterior Weishu (BL 21) are selected for stomachache.

3. The Combination of the distal-local acupoints

   This combining method is based on the local and distal curative effect of all acupoints. Usually, the adjacent or local acupoints will be selected combining with the distal acuponts especially on the same meridians or the exterior-interior related meridians. For example, Dicang (ST 4) and Yingxiang (LI 20) are selected as the local acupoints combining with Hegu (LI 4) as distal acuponits for facial paralysis.

4. The combination of the left-right acupoints

   The combining method is based on the theory that the symmetrical distribution of the meridians and collaterals, therefore the points on both sides can be selected to strengthen the coordinating effects on the diseases of zang-fu. For example, Hegu (LI 4) on the right side can be selected to treat facial paralysis on the left side according to the distribution of the large intestine meridian of hand yangming, while Zusanli (ST 36) on both side can be selected to strengthen the effects for stomachache.

3.6.4 Selection of Acupuncture and Moxibustion Technique

Successful acupuncture treatment depends on not only the proper acupoints selections with correct combinations, but also suitable selection of acupuncture and moxibustion manipulations.

3.6.4.1 Selection of Methods

The acupuncture and moxibustion therapy include various methods, as filiform acupuncture, electroacupuncture, moxibustion, cupping, pricking for bleeding, pyropuncture, auriculotherapy, etc. These methods can be chosen independently or in combination with each other according to the conditions of the diseases. For example, moxibustion will also be used based on filiform acupuncture to treat deficiency cold syndrome.

3.6.4.2 Selection of Manipulations

After methods are selected, the manipulations must be confirmed. Such as filiform acupuncture, for acute excessive syndrome, reducing manipulation should be used; while for chronic-deficient syndrome, reinforcing manipulation is more suitable. The duration and frequency of needling also depend on the conditions and reactions of the patients.

3.6.4.3 Selection of Treatment Timing

Treatment timing is another influencing factor to the effect of acupuncture. Generally speaking, for the diseases with obvious time regularity of attack or aggravation, acupuncture therapy should be used before the attack or aggravation. For example, acupuncture could be used at 3–7 days before menstruation to treating dysmenorrhea. Additionally, midnight-noon ebb-low acupuncture and eight methods of sacred tortoise are specific applications of treatment timing selection.

3.7 Summary

Acupuncture and moxibustion mainly include theory of meridian and acupoint, operation techniques, and clinical application of acupuncture and moxibustion.

Acupuncture and moxibustion emphasize clinical practice. It is an effective way to learn this subject by practicing locating the acupoints and various manipulation techniques, forming clinical thinking mode of acupuncture and moxibustion gradually in clinical training.

Questions
1. What are meridians and collaterals? What are acupoints?
2. What are regularities of the 12 meridians?
3. What are special points? What are the categories of special points?
4. How does an acupoint be located according to proportional bone measurement?
5. What are the courses of the 12 meridians, governor vessel, and conception vessel?
6. What is arrival of qi? Discuss the phenomena of arrival of qi.

7. How do you operate reinforcing and reducing manipulations of the filiform needle?
8. What are classifications of moxibustion?
9. What are precautions of moxibustion and cupping therapy?
10. What are the principles of acupuncture and moxibustion treatment?

Chapter 4
Other Therapies

Naiqi Li, Hua Sui, and Yong Huang

Objectives

To master the concepts and the characteristics of traditional Chinese tuina, dietary therapy, qigong, and Tai Chi.

To know the historical developments of those therapies and basic methods.

Guideline

This chapter includes four sections. The first part is traditional Chinese tuina; the second part is dietary therapy; the third part is qigong; and the last part is Tai Chi. From each section, we can learn the history, basic theory, the specific content or manipulation, and cautions of those four therapies.

4.1 Introduction

The other therapies of TCM are plentiful, which include traditional Chinese tuina massage, dietary therapy, qigong, and Tai Chi. They use different ways to treat and prevent diseases according to different theory and methods. Some therapies, such as massage and dietary therapy, have a full theory to guide the practice. Nowadays, the qigong and Tai Chi are usually taken as physical exercises to prevent diseases. Due to the non-invasive, non-pharmaceutical features, now the other therapies of TCM are getting more and more attention in the world.

N. Li
Southern Medical University, Guangzhou, China

H. Sui
Dalian Medical University, Dalian, China

Y. Huang (✉)
School of Traditional Chinese Medicine, Southern Medical University, Guangzhou, China

© Zhengzhou University Press 2024   417
Y. Huang, L. Zhu (eds.), *Textbook of Traditional Chinese Medicine*,
https://doi.org/10.1007/978-981-99-5299-1_4

4.2   Traditional Chinese Tuina

4.2.1   General Introduction to Massage

Massage is based on TCM theory, using body parts to perform manipulations on human in order to take precaution of disease and alleviate pain from illness. The earliest record of massage dates back to 3000 years ago, and the long history has enriched its connotation which makes it one of the most important medical therapies in TCM. In modern TCM, massage is generally classified into adult massage and infantile massage. Adult massage also includes a unique classification namely Spinal manipulation. With its characteristic theory and special manipulations, massage is used to treat many kinds of illness in a natural and mostly harmless way. Moreover, basic exercises for massage practice (massage gong method) are an essential part of massage practicing which requires long time hard training for students of massage and will certainly determine the curative effect. Due to the wide spreading of TCM, massage is now studied by more and more people all around the world.

4.2.1.1   History of Massage

Massage was created by ancient Chinese during labor activity and struggles with cruel nature. Human inevitably got injured when fighting with beasts or defending themselves in ancient times. The Chinese ancestors instinctively pressed the injured part of their body and by accident found it relieving pain. After years and years of practice, they summed up the primitive experiences and developed it into a mature medical mode nowadays we call massage.

Massage has a very long history. The earliest reference to massage dates back to the culture of Yin Ruin (about 3000 years ago) according to the archeological studies in recent years. Massage was early recorded in the inscriptions on bones or tortoise shells of the *Shang* dynasty. This reveals the fact that massage had been widely used to treat illness since this period of time.

1. *Qin* and *Han* dynasties.

   The dynasties of Qin and Han are considered to be an important stage in the history of massage. According to *Han Shu* (*History of the Han Dynasty*), there was a monograph about massage—*Huang Di Qi Bo An Mo Shi Juan* (*Ten Volumes on Massage Therapies Developed by Yellow Emperor and Qi Bo*) that was the first medical book, not only in Chinese history but also in the history of the world, specially discussed massage therapy. However, this book was unfortunately lost due to various reasons. *Internal Classic* is the earliest existing medical book of TCM. It was published in the same period with the former book and contained a great amount of ancient literature about massage. *Internal Classic* pointed out that massage was originated in the central area of ancient China and the book clearly put forward the positive effects of treating illness with massage. It also covers a dozen of massage manipulations such as pushing, pressing, rubbing, nailing, flicking, stretching, searching, stroking, shaking, bending, stepping, and pulling. Because the manipulation of pressing (An) and rubbing (Mo) was used together at that time, so massage was once called Anmo. In *Han* dynasty, an extraordinary doctor named *Zhang Zhongjing* wrote a book—*Synopsis of Prescriptions of the Golden Chamber*. In his work, for the first time, ointment rubbing manipulation was adopted and suggested as a way for disease prevention. Also, in his great piece of work he recorded a massage method used for saving people in danger after trying to commit a suicide by hanging. Another famous doctor named *Hua Tuo* created a conduction exercise imitating five kinds of animals called five mimic-animal exercise, which is still practiced by people today to improve health. Therefore, *Qin* and *Han* dynasties are the first peak in the development process of massage.

2. *Sui* and *Tang* Dynasties.

The *Sui* and *Tang* dynasties were a flourishing period in massage history. In *Sui* dynasty, the Imperial Hospital set up a position for specialists of Anmo (at this time massage it was called Anmo). Later, The *Emperor Taizong* of *Tang* developed the Imperial Hospital and set up the Anmo department, dividing Anmo manipulators into four levels from high to low, namely Anmo Doctor, Anmo technician, Anmo worker, and Anmo student. The Anmo Doctor will teach Anmo student to practice Anmo with the assistance of Anmo technician and Anmo worker. In addition, self-massage (one performing massage to himself/herself) was highly advocated and put into an important position of people's daily life. Self-massage was both recorded in *Ge Hong*'s *Handbook of Prescriptions for Emergencies* and *Sun simiao*'s *Essential Prescriptions Worth a Thousand Gold for Emergencies*. The widespread use of self-massage reveals that patients are more self-helping in fighting with illness. Also, the ointments used in rubbing manipulation were improved by *Sun Simiao* and its application was enlarged, for example, using it to prevent or treat infantile diseases. It was also in this period of time that massage was for the first time introduced to Korea, Japan, India, Arabian, and European countries.

3. *Song Jin* and *Yuan* dynasties.

In *Song Jin* and *Yuan* Dynasties, massage was mostly used in orthopedics and infantile which contributed to the classification between the spinal manipulation in adult massage and infantile massage. With the development of massage in this time, study of manipulation became more valued by erudite for massage. The work *Sheng Ji Zong Lu* (*General Records of Holy Universal Relief*) devoted a special chapter and gave the summary and induction about massage. The book turns out to be the earliest and most complete special record of massage. However, massage department was canceled in medical organizations of government in this time. But the position of erudite for massage still exists.

4. *Ming* and *Qing* dynasties.

   Ming and *Qing* dynasties were another flourishing period in massage history. In this time, the number of monographs about infantile massage sharply increased. In 1601, the first special monograph about infantile massage was born------*The Canon of Anmo for Children*. Then, several monographs were gradually published and until this time infantile massage formally became an independent system. In addition, massage department was back in the Imperial Hospital in *Ming* dynasty but canceled again later. Although there was no department of massage in *Qing*'s Imperial Hospital, massage was still commonly and widely used in official occasion and among the civilians due to its remarkable curative effects. It was right in this period of time that the name massage was first introduced and later replaced Anmo for the name of this subject.

5. Modern times.

   Massage has come into a brand new stage for integrated development with its golden opportunity, especially since the founding of the People's Republic of China. Firstly, more and more ancient literatures about massage were unearthed and have been carefully studied and published. Secondly, main schools of massage began to form and got the chance to be propagated. There are several present main schools of massage with great influence namely qi-concentrated single-finger pushing manipulation massage, *Ding*'s rolling manipulation massage, internal exercise massage, etc. Thirdly, education system and scientific studies about massage have developed significantly; also, there continually occurs spirited innovations which keep enriching the content of this both ancient and dynamic subject.

4.2.1.2   Theory of Massage

Massage theory is based on TCM theories. Several important TCM theories that are highly related to massage will be introduced below.

1. Pathogenesis of defense-qi-nurtient-blood (wei qi ying xue) theory

   TCM thinks human's physiological activity is greatly based on qi and blood. Qi and blood are needed to nourish from zang-fu viscera, bones and muscle, collateral, meridian to fur, and skin. So it is very important for massage to take qi and blood into account when treating diseases. The conception of qi refers to two aspects: one is the refined nutritive substance that builds up human body and maintains human living activities. Another one is the physiological function or power of zang-fu viscera. The most essential qi in human body is the original qi, and its existence relies on innate essence and acquired essence. The function of original qi is to regulate qi movement. There are other two important kinds of qi. One is defense qi and the other is nutrient qi. Defense qi moves outside vessels, protecting human body from pathogenic qi of six climatic influences. Nutrient qi moves inside vessels, nourishing human body. Nutrient qi can also generate blood and flow with blood, so it is also known as nutrient blood. Blood flows in vessels and carries nutrient substance to all parts of human body. Qi and blood are tightly connected. Qi is able to generate blood, impel blood, and control blood while blood is the foundation of qi. Blood carries qi all the way through the vessels, and blood also nourishes qi. Because of the high activity of qi, qi must rely on blood to stay regular. Disease can be divided into four levels (defense, qi, nutrient, blood) according to the level of illness from mildness to seriousness. Massage therapy uses this theory to instruct different treatments or manipulations for different level of illness.

2. Meridian and collateral theory

As we know from the previous chapter that specially discusses meridian and collateral, there are fourteen meridians and lots of branches distributing in human body carrying qi and blood. Meridian and collateral also connect the zang-fu viscera and body extremities to communicate internal parts and external parts of the body. As the ancient literature says about meridian and collateral "No blockage, no pain," only if we keep the meridian and collateral unblocked, are we able to do with the pain of our body. Once blockages are in meridian and collateral, qi and blood stop flowing regularly, which leads to the loss of nutrients and weakness of skin, muscles, tendons, vessels, and joints. The effect of massage is to propel the circulation of qi and blood, adjust yin and yang, and nourish tendons and joints. All these effects happen through the meridian and collateral by performing manipulations on the meridian and collateral or on the projected superficial portion of the body corresponding to a certain zang-fu viscera inside. Moreover, massage manipulations will cause stimulation on an acupoint or even the whole meridian and collateral system which improve physiological functions of viscera, tissues, and organs throughout the passing meridian and collateral.

3. Tendons along twelve meridians

Tendons along twelve meridians are subsidiary part of the twelve meridians. It is the gathering and distributing of qi from twelve meridians to limbs and body. The function of the tendons along twelve meridians is connecting limbs and body, restraining bones, managing joint movements, and maintaining natural body position. Tendons along twelve meridians are huge balanced biological structure of soft tissue. The word "jin" in Chinese means strong fibrous tissue that contains and generates power and force for body movement. Different from the twelve meridians, the twelve musculature start at the tendons along the bladder meridian of foot taiyang. In other words, the twelve musculature start at limbs, gather in joints, distribute in chest and back, and finally connect all parts of body. Therefore, tendons along twelve meridians generally run centripetally. Pathological changes of the tendons along twelve meridians system usually appear as spasm, stiffness, and convulsion. Massage can prevent and treat this kind of diseases by acting on the tendons along twelve meridians system.

4. Muscle and bones theory

A series of diseases will happen due to certain abnormal changes of anatomical position with soft tissues (mostly muscle) and bones. Massage manipulation is used to correct these abnormal changes and deal with dislocation of joints as well as soft tissues. In TCM, the famous saying "Tendons are out of line, bones are out of place" describes the pathogenesis of this kind of diseases. When a part of soft tissue of our body like muscle or tendon is in injury, a pain will be felt and then act on related body part through reflexion of nerves to alarm us that there is an injury. This kind of injuries can happen due to some anatomical changes such as dislocation and subluxation. However, the pain is a protective action for human body which is to reduce body movements and avoid a second injury. In massage theory, we adopt traction and countertraction, rotating and pulling or flicking-poking manipulation to repair joint dislocation, joint subluxation, return the sprained soft tissue to normal position, and put slipped tendons in order. The effect of this kind of manipulations is instant and remarkable. It can eliminate spasm of muscle, alleviate pain, and promote the recovery of the injured soft tissues or joints. Furthermore, diseases that are commonly seen on patients in massage department such as cervical spondylosis, periarthritis of shoulder, and lumbar disk herniation can be well treated with massage manipulation.

5. Pediatrics of TCM

In pediatrics of TCM, there are special diagnostics and treatment for children. For example, younger children can easily caught by exogenous contraction and have problem in digesting milk. In TCM, children are considered to be immature in yin-yang and zang-fu viscera. Generally, for children, heart and liver viscera are in excess while lung, spleen, and kidney viscera are in deficiency. This characteristic leads to a high occurrence of lung diseases caused by wind pathogen. Children can also be easily harmed by dryness pathogen and summer heat pathogen which result in lung and stomach yin deficiency. Moreover, children's diseases are likely to become heat diseases due to their constitution of pure yang. Pestilent qi is another common factor that always threatens children's health. It is a kind of strongly infectious pathogenic factor bringing serious and fast-developing syndromes.

There are several things we should pay attention to when treating pediatric diseases with massage therapy. First of all, the timing to start treatment should be as early as possible. Because of the pure yin and yang constitution, diseases develop rapidly in pediatrics. The earlier the treatment begins, the less possibly the illness is going to develop. Therefore, accurate and on time treatment is the guarantee of effect. Secondly, principles of pediatric massage are gentle, mild, and moderate. We should be cautious when choosing treatment in order to protect the young and weak healthy qi of child. Moreover, we should attach importance to taking care of spleen-stomach zang-fu viscera (always in deficiency) while avoid abuse of treating deficiency with reinforcement. Last but not the least, always remember to treat the earlier coming syndromes first, and then, the latter coming ones. Especially when treating exogenous contractions, controlling the former syndrome is important for ceasing the development of illness.

4.2.1.3 Categories

Before we begin, we should understand that there is the difference between massage in traditional Chinese medicine and the commonly seen massage. Firstly, massage is instructed by traditional Chinese medicine theory which includes yin-yang theory, meridian and collateral theory, zang-fu viscera theory, five elements theory, and so on. General massage does not have a basic theory instruction. Secondly, the slaying of massage in Western country refers to manipulations with no joint movement and adjustment. A number of manipulations in massage need to have joint movement and aim at adjusting irregular joint location. Thirdly, massage is a non-medical behavior for relaxation and leisure. On the opposite, performing massage is a medical behavior that happens in medical setting like hospital and clinics. Massage therapy is used to treat certain diseases which have clear and accurate diagnosis. For practitioner, massage practitioner must have a license of doctor. Massage is often practiced by people with no practitioner's license. In a word, there are differences between massage in traditional Chinese medicine and the commonly seen massage. In ancient times, massage was not classified into adult massage and infantile massage. In modern times, scholars put forward the conception of adult massage in order to make it different from the well-developed infantile massage. After a history of more than 3000 years, massage is now generally divided into adult massage, infantile massage, and a special kind named spinal manipulation.

4.2.1.4 Massage Manipulation

Manipulation is an important way to treat disease in traditional massage. It refers to the standard techniques performed with performer's hand or other part of the body to exert a stimulating effect on the body part to the patient for medical purpose. The promising quality of manipulation with correct clinical differentiation is the key to a good therapeutic effect. The performers are required to perform a manipulation continuously, forcefully, evenly, softly, and thoroughly. "Continuously" means performer should keep the manipulation for a certain period of time according to the requirement. "Forcefully" means performers should have a certain force and be able to adapt different patients and different situations. "Evenly" means the force and frequency of the manipulation should be the same during the whole time. "Softly" means the force of manipulation should be well controlled and be gentle but not superficial, and heavy but not retained. The change of movements should be natural and fluent. "Thoroughly" means the manipulation should reach deep down to the affected part of the patient's body on the basis of achieving the four previous key points.

Students can practice massage manipulations on sand bag or rice bag first and
then on human body. The sand bag or rice bag is squared and about 8 cun (about
3.3 cm) in length and 5 cun in width. The training and practice of fingers, wrist, and
arms are the key point of practicing massage manipulations.

Massage manipulations can be classified by movements into pushing manipulation, pressing manipulation, and pulling manipulation, classified by targeted body
parts into soft issue manipulation and joint manipulation, classified by schools
which we've introduced in the previous paragraph, classified by difficulties and
divided into simple manipulation and complex manipulation. In this book, we adopt
the first classification to introduce massage manipulation.

4.2.2   Adult Massage

Adult massage is used to take precaution of adult diseases as well as treating diseases. Compared with infantile massage, manipulation in adult massage has a
greater range with heavier strength. Adult massage manipulation is generally
divided into categories of pushing rolling manipulations, scrubbing manipulations,
squeezing-pressing manipulations, tapping manipulations, vibrating manipulations,
and mobilizing manipulations.

4.2.2.1   Basic Exercises for Massage Practice

The basic exercises for massage practice are a series of training designed for erudite
for massage; it is also called massage gong fa. Gong means function and ability; fa
means method of specialized training. Therefore, basic exercises for manipulation
practice refer to a process for massage practitioner to improve their body and adapt
the ability of practicing massage through long-term repeated and diligent practice
and training of specific exercises. Traditional massage attaches great importance to
basic exercises and considers it as the guarantee of clinical curative effect. There is
also a saying of "the more effort, the more effect" which indicates the great connection between basic exercises and curative effect. To be an erudite for massage, a
basic exercise of the specific training is not only a kind of medical technology that
needs to master but also a compulsory training for his professional technique.

Generally, basic exercises for massage practice include Tai Chi, Shaolin internal
cultivation exercise, and Sinew-transforming exercise, etc. The functions of basic
exercises for massage practice are as follows: first, enhance the health status of
practitioner and fully develop strength, endurance, sensibility, and flexibility which
give the practitioner the ability in persistent, continuous manipulation of massage.
Second, the structure and function of manipulating part of human body will be
improved though basic exercises practice. Third, concentrate on practicing basic
exercises can improve the coordination of organisms used in massage manipulation.
Last, practicing basic exercise can cultivate the beneficial qi which makes erudite

for massage stay healthy and have a high efficiency of work. It is the guarantee of manipulation quality and curative effort. Furthermore, practicing basic exercises of massage can strengthen muscles, bones, ligaments and joint, promote blood circulation, and improve respiratory system, nerve system, and digestion system according to recent research.

Some basic exercises for massage practice are not only for erudite for massage but also practiced by patients. Patients can practice basic exercises under the instruction of erudite for massage to improve their health status, accelerating the recovery.

4.2.2.2 Adult Massage Manipulations

Adult massage manipulations mainly include 6 categories: pushing rolling manipulations, scrubbing manipulations, squeezing-pressing manipulations, tapping manipulations, vibrating manipulations, and mobilizing manipulations. The five key points of performing adult massage manipulations especially on soft tissue are "continuously, forcefully, evenly, softly and thoroughly."

1. Category of pushing rolling manipulations.

    Continuously and regularly swaying the forearm to exert force on part of body is the basic operation for category of pushing rolling manipulations, including Qi-concentrated single-finger pushing manipulation, and rolling manipulation with the ulnar side of the palm and kneading manipulation.

    (a) Qi-concentrated single-finger pushing manipulation.

    Pushing with the tip of the thumb or the whorled surface of the thumb on the region to be treated by swaying your forearm to lead your finger is called Qi-concentrated single-finger pushing manipulation. It is the typical manipulation of the qi-concentrated single-finger pushing manipulation school.

    - Direction for performing manipulations.

      Clench a hollow fist with suspended and flexed wrist and palm, then stretch the thumb straight naturally to cover your fist hole. Push the targeted region with the tip or the whorl surface of the thumb. Lower the shoulder, drop the elbow, and suspend the wrist. Sway the forearm to lead the wrist swing inward and outward while flexing and extending the thumb joint to reach a frequency of 120 to 160 times per minute. The thumb should go heavily and come lightly continuously and alternately (Fig. 4.1).

      The key point of performing this manipulation is lowering shoulders, dropping elbow, suspending wrist, exert force to thumb, emptying palm, and pushing forcefully and moving slowly.
    - Medical application.

      The characteristics of this manipulation are that the targeted region is small but the applied force is great and thorough, and the stimulation is regular and mild. This manipulation is commonly used on all the merid-

Fig. 4.1 Qi-concentrated
single-finger pushing
manipulation

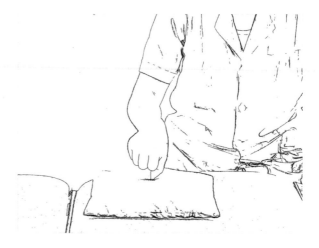

ians and collaterals and acupoints all over the body. In departments of
internal medicine, gynecology, traumatology, five sense organs, and
pediatrics, it is used to treat common diseases such as headache, dizziness, insomnia, hypertension, stagnation of the liver qi, arthralgia-
syndrome, and especially diseases of gastrointestinal alimentary system.
(b) Rolling manipulation with the ulnar side of the palm.

Rolling manipulation with the ulnar side of the palm refers to using the
ulnar side of the palm to press the affected region. Sway the forearm to drive
the wrist to extend and flex and roll on the target region. It is the typical
manipulation of the rolling manipulation school (*Ding*'s rolling
manipulation).

- Direction for performing manipulations.

    The performer straightens the thumb naturally and makes a hollow
    fist. The little finger and the ring finger flex naturally and the flexed angle
    of the other two fingers reduces gradually to make the palm round along
    the palm surface. Press the target region with the dorsal palm of the hand
    near the lateral side of the little finger. Sway the forearm to extend and
    flex the wrist in a wide range and rotate the forearm as well. Roll the
    ulnar side of the hand of the target region continuously in a frequency
    about 120 times per minute (Fig. 4.2).

    The key points of performing this manipulation are lowering shoul-
    ders and dropping elbow with the wrist joint flexed naturally. Keep a
    hollow fist. Fix on the target region with the dorsal part of your palm near
    the little finger. The stimulation should be done lightly and heavily alter-
    nately, rolling forward three times heavier than rolling back.
- Medical application.

    Rolling manipulation has a large area of stimulation with strong effect,
    evident deepness and thoroughness, is one of the most commonly used

Fig. 4.2 Rolling
manipulation

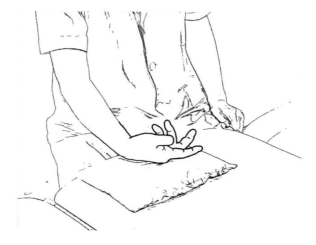

manipulations in clinical work, especially suitable for the lumbodorsal region, lumbo-buttock region, and thick muscle regions of the limbs. It is good for treating the diseases in motor system and nerve system.

(c) Kneading manipulation.

Fix on targeted body surface with certain part of your hand and knead in circles to rotate slowly and softly the subcutaneous tissues is called kneading manipulation. According to different touching areas, it can be divided into palm-base kneading manipulation, major thenar kneading manipulation, finger kneading manipulation, and forearm kneading manipulation.

- Direction for performing manipulations.

     The key points of kneading manipulation are quite similar. The key points are lowering your shoulders. Fix on the targeted body surface with certain part of your hand. Bring the subcutaneous tissue to move when performing this manipulation. Avoid rubbing or slipping between the treated part and the body surface. The wrist is relaxed in major thenar kneading manipulation but should keep tight in palm-base kneading manipulation and finger kneading manipulation.

- Medical application.

     The effect of kneading manipulation is light, soft, and slow but deep and thorough. Warm effect can be delivered to the deep of tissue by the internal rubbing caused by kneading. Major thenar kneading manipulation is suitable for swelling or aching parts of the limbs caused by acute sprain and contusion. Palm-base kneading manipulation is commonly used on the well-developed muscular regions of the limbs, lumbodorsal region, and buttock region. Finger kneading manipulation is used for pointing acupoints or meridians and collateral all over the body. Forearm kneading manipulation is good at treating deep tissue problem.

2. Category of Scrubbing Manipulations.

Use the tip of finger or palm to touch the targeted region and precede rhythmic and circular movements. This is called scrubbing manipulations.

(d) Circular rubbing manipulations.

Using the palm or the finger to make a circular rubbing movement on surface of human body is called circular rubbing manipulations. It is mainly divided into finger circular rubbing manipulation (zhi mo method) and palm circular rubbing manipulation (zhang mo method).

- Direction for performing manipulations.

Finger circular rubbing manipulation: use your fingertip as the touching area with the fingers juxtaposed, the palm straightened naturally, and the wrist joint flexed slightly. Use the elbow joint as a pivot, and move the forearm to rub with the palm side of the fingers circularly on the target region. It can be clockwise or counterclockwise with a frequency of 100 to 120 times per minute.

Palm circular rubbing manipulation: press on the body surface with the fingers juxtaposed. Straighten your palm naturally and the wrist joint slightly tight. Consider the elbow as a pivot, move the forearm to rub circularly with the palm on the target region. It can be clockwise or counterclockwise with a frequency of 100 to 120 times per minute.

- Medical application.

Rubbing manipulation is mainly applied to treating problems on the chest, hypochondrium, and the epigastric region. It has an effect of relieving the depressed liver and regulating the circulation of qi, warming the middle energizer, and regulating the stomach. It is also good at treating diseases in digest system.

(e) Pushing manipulation.

Using the touching part to make a one-way pushing in a straight line is called pushing manipulation. It can be divided into linear pushing with the finger, linear pushing with the palm and linear pushing with the elbow. We take linear pushing with the palm as an example to introduce. The following direction is for linear pushing with the palm. Linear pushing with the palm is the most commonly used pushing manipulation in clinical work.

- Direction for performing manipulations.

Use the palm or palm base as the touching part. Stretch the elbow to make a linear pushing. Use both palms to perform in the same time can also be called separating pushing manipulation.

- Medical application.

This manipulation can exert both "warmth and force." Therefore, it has a good effect on warming and dredging the meridians and collaterals, promoting blood circulation and qi, warming the yang, etc. It is suitable for thoracodorsal region and lumbo-abdominal region. It is commonly used to treat oppressed feeling in the chest, diseases in the upper energizer, diseases in digestive system for example throw up, nausea and stomachache, depression of the liver qi, lumbago, deficiency of the kidney, etc.

(f) Scrubbing manipulation.

Exert force on the target region with the major thenar to perform straight to-and-fro rubbing movement. Make the warm effect penetrate into the deep layer of tissue. This is called scrubbing manipulation. It can be divided into to-and-fro rubbing manipulation with palm, to-and-fro rubbing manipulation with finger, to-and-fro rubbing manipulation with minor thenar, and to-and-fro rubbing manipulation with major thenar.

- Direction for performing manipulations.

   Keep your wrist in tense. Put the touching part on the body surface and make a little pressing. Use shoulder joint and elbow joint to combine a bend and stretch movement. Make the touching part move evenly to-and-fro in a straight line (Fig. 4.3).
- Medical application.

   This manipulation has a strong rubbing force with a large range of movement. So it has evident warming effect and the function of removing obstruction. It is suitable for all parts of the body. It can warm the body and dispel dampness pathogen. It is good at treating cold manifestation syndrome. Be careful not to rub for a long time in case the surface skin will be injured.

3. Category of Squeezing-Pressing Manipulations.

Using finger, palm, or other parts of body to press vertically or squeezing oppositely is called squeezing-pressing manipulations. It can be divided into vertical press and opposite squeeze. Pressing manipulation and grasping manipulation are two typical manipulations for this category.

Fig. 4.3 Scrubbing manipulation with the palm

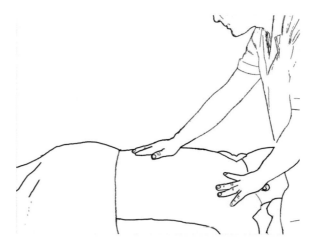

(g) Pressing manipulation.

Press a certain acupoint or part of the body surface with finger, palm, or elbow. Then, exert force gradually is called pressing manipulation.

- Direction for performing manipulations.

Vertically press the target region with the touching part, press gradually from lightly to heavily. When using pressing with palm, you should lean your body to strengthen the force on your palm. Performing this manipulation should make patients cooperate with breath like press with exhale and leave with inhale (Fig. 4.4).

- Medical application.

This manipulation has small and concentrated acting area, and the acting layer is deep with evident stabbing pain effect, and it is applied to indurate tissue of muscles or between bones or tenderness points. It is good at relieving pains.

(h) Grasping manipulation.

Exert force symmetrically with the thumb and the other four fingers to lift, pinch, or clip the extremities or the skin. Such a manipulation is called grasping manipulation. It can be divided into three fingers grasping manipulation and five fingers grasping manipulation.

- Direction for performing manipulations.

Relax the wrist joint and clip the operated part tightly with the thumb, index finger, and middle finger or with the thumb and the whorl surface of the other four fingers. Lift the skin and repeat the performance of kneading and pinching continuously and alternatively in a form of forceful and gentle way.

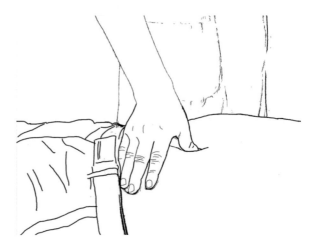

Fig. 4.4 Pressing manipulation with the thumb

- Medical application.

    This manipulation is deep and heavy but has a mild stimulation. It is commonly suitable for the cord soft tissues such as the muscles and tendons of the neck, shoulder, back, lateral abdomen, upper and lower limbs, etc. It is good at inducing resuscitation and restoring consciousness, expelling pathogenic wind and cold, relaxing muscles and tendons to promote blood circulation, relieving spasm, and pain, etc.

4. Category of Tapping Manipulations.

    Using hand or tools to tap the body face in a rhythm is called tapping manipulations. It mainly includes patting manipulation and knocking manipulation. The most commonly used tool in this manipulation is mulberry stick.

(i) Patting manipulation (pai method).

    Pat on the body surface rhythmically with an empty palm is called patting manipulation.

- Direction for performing manipulations.

    Coalesce the fingers and slightly flex the metacarpophalangeal joint so as to form an empty palm. Then, pat the operated part rhythmically in a frequency of 100 to 120 times per minutes.

- Medical application.

    This manipulation is mainly used on the shoulder and back, lumbosacral portion, and the thigh. Light patting can also be used on thoracic-abdominal region and the head. It is used to treat various kinds of diseases such as arthralgia due to pathogenic wind-dampness, stiffness, and pain in the chest and dizziness, etc.

(j) Knocking manipulation.

    Hit the operated part rhythmically with the palm base, the minor thenar, the back of a fist, the fingertip, or a mulberry stick. This is called knocking manipulation.

- Direction for performing manipulations.

    Steadily use finger, palm, or mulberry stick to knock on the targeted region. When using hand to perform, relax your wrist and keep a hollow fist or slightly bent fingers. Before performing, the patient should be noticed previously.

- Medical application.

    Fist-back-knocking manipulation is mainly used on Dazhu (GV 14) and the lumbosacral portion. Palm-knocking manipulation is for the Baihui (GV 20). It is good at activating the flow of blood and qi in the meridians and collateral.

5. Category of Vibrating Manipulations.

Continuously stimulating the targeted region with a rhythmic high frequency is called vibrating manipulations. It generally includes shaking manipulation and vibrating manipulation.

(k) Shaking manipulation.

Hold the distal end of the patient's target extremities with one hand or both hands to shake constantly up and down or from the left to the right. This is called shaking manipulation.

   • Direction for performing manipulations.

   Hold the distal end of the patient's targeted extremities. Lift the treated extremity to a certain angle. While pulling with slight force shake constantly in small amplitude to cause the parenchyma of the target region to shake and transmit to the proximal end of the extremity.

   • Medical application.

   This manipulation is mainly applied to extremities and mostly after twisting manipulation with both palms as a combination and reinforcement. It is commonly used in the lumbar area to treat lumbar intervertebral disk protrusion with shaking both two lower limbs simultaneously. It can enlarge the space inside the lumbar vertebrae to help reduce projecting nucleus pulpous, relax adhesion between the projection and nerve roots to remit or release its pressure upon nerve roots. It has a great effect on relieving pain for lumbar intervertebral disk protrusion.

(l) Vibrating manipulation.

Using finger or palm to make a vertical rapid vibrating movement is called vibrating manipulation. It generally includes vibrating with the palm and vibrating with the finger.

   • Direction for performing manipulations.

   Drop the elbow and put the tip of the middle finger or the palm on the targeted region. Exert force statically with the forearm and hand, and contract the muscle alternatively to direct the vibration produced by arm to the body in a frequency of 300 to 400 times per minute (Fig. 4.5).

   • Medical application.

   This manipulation is suitable for all the acupoints on the body, especially to the craniofacial region and the thoracic-abdominal region. It is good at relaxing anxious feeling.

6. Category of Mobilizing Manipulations.

Make the joint passively move and generate sliding, separation, twisting, bending, and stretching. Such manipulation is called mobilizing manipulations. It generally includes rotating manipulation and pulling-stretching manipulation

(m) Rotating manipulation.

A passive movement performed within the range of joint or semi-joint is called rotating manipulation. It is one of the common manipulations of mas-

Fig. 4.5 Vibrating
manipulation with finger

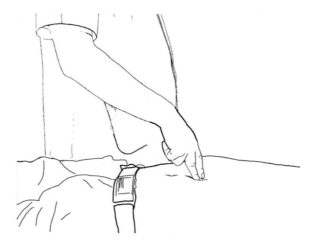

sage and performed with different methods when applied to different parts. It generally includes rotating of the neck, rotating of the shoulder, rotating of the elbow, rotating of the wrist, rotating of the lumbar, rotating of the hip, rotating of the knee, and rotating of the ankle.

- Direction for performing manipulations.

    There are many kinds of rotating manipulation based on different parts, but there is still something in common. Movements of rotating manipulation should be moderate and mild with steady force. The frequency of the rotation should be slow and even, especially at the beginning. The amplitude of the rotation should be gradually increased and adjusted according to individual conditions. Generally, the joint should be kept within the limitation of normal physical movement. Rotating manipulation should not be done violently or violate the movement of normal physical activity. Rotating manipulation is forbidden to be used to treat patients with fracture or dislocation of joint.
- Medical application.

    This manipulation is suitable for joints all over the body. It has the effect of lubricating joints, releasing adhesion, relaxing muscles and tendons, relieving spasm, and strengthening and renewing articular moving ability.

(n) Pulling-stretching manipulation.

    Fix one end of a joint or an extremity, pull and extend the other end with constant force to enlarge the joint space. Such a manipulation is called pulling-stretching manipulation. It can be applied to different joints in many regions such as neck, shoulder, elbow, wrist, fingers, waist, hip, knee, and ankle.

- Direction for performing manipulation.

    According to different regions, the patient should take different positions to adjust. This manipulation should make it stable and gentle with the strength intensified gradually. When the traction reaches a certain degree, it should be kept steady for a while. The angle of the traction should be well adjusted and the pulling should be done around the longitudinal axis of the extremity.

- Medical application.

  This manipulation can be applied to joints of cervical vertebrae, lumbar vertebrae, and extremities, with the effect of restoring and treating injured soft tissues, reducing dislocation of joints, enlarging joint spaces, remitting nerve compression, and relaxing adhesion.

7. Comprehensive manipulations and special manipulations.

   Comprehensive manipulations are a series of manipulations composed by more than one of the six basic manipulations. Special manipulations are a series of manipulations that cannot be classified into the six basic manipulations but used commonly in clinical work.

   (o) Grasping-kneading manipulation.

   Grasping-kneading manipulation is a combination with grasping manipulation and kneading manipulation.

   - Direction for performing manipulations.

     The methods for performing this manipulation are similar to performing grasping manipulation. Grasping-kneading manipulation uses grasp as main manipulation and knead as assistance. Also, the thumb and other fingers need to knead in rotation.

   - Medical application.

     This manipulation has advantages in both grasping manipulation and kneading manipulation. It is mainly applied to extremities and neck region. It is generally used to treat neck pain, cervical spondylosis, and periarthritis of shoulder, etc.

   (p) Thumb-pushing and circular rubbing manipulation (tui mo method).

   The thumb performing qi-concentrated single-finger pushing manipulation while the other four fingers performing finger-rubbing manipulation are called thumb-pushing and circular rubbing manipulation. It is often applied on the chest, abdomen, and back.

   - Direction for performing manipulations.

     Exert force with the side of the thumb; swing the forearm to perform Qi-concentrated single-finger pushing manipulation. At the same time, the other four fingers straighten and coalesce to perform rubbing manipulation.

   - Medical application.

     This manipulation is mainly used in chest, abdomen, lumbosacral region, and shoulder. It is good at treating distension and pain in abdomen, digestive system problem, genital system problem, and periarthritis of shoulder, etc.

(q) Sweeping manipulation (sao san method).

Using the radial side of the thumb and other fingertips quickly sweeping from the head of temporal to the back of ear forward and backward is called sweeping manipulation.

- Direction for performing manipulations.

    The doctor gently supports the patient's head with one hand and touches the patient's temporal region with the radial side of the thumb and the tips of the other fingers of the other hand, then moves the hand along an arc route from the temporal region to the occipital region (along the running route of the gallbladder meridian) from the anterior-superior to the posterior-inferior.

- Medical application.

    Sweeping manipulation is performed with even force, mainly used for operation on the head. It has the effect of calming the liver to suppress hyperhepatic yang, dispelling wind, and dispelling pathogenic cold, tranquilizing and inducing resuscitation, relaxing tendons, and relieving pain. Headache, vertigo, hypertension, insomnia, poor memories are often treated with this technique.

(r) Pinching of the two sides of spine.

Continuously pinching the skin of spine from top to bottom is called the pinching of the two sides of spine. It is a special manipulation first used in adult but lately mainly used in infantile.

- Direction for performing manipulations.

    The operator may first push the skin with the tip of thumb and then use the index finger or other finger to pinch up the skin. Then grasp and lift the skin up with the three fingers simultaneously. Do the lifting and pinching operation with both hands alternately and move forward. Or use the radial aspect of the middle knuckle of the flexed index finger to support the skin, the thumb to press forward. Then grasp and lift the skin forcefully with the two fingers and move forward while both hands are alternately doing the manipulation.

- Medical application.

    The technique has the effect of promoting digestion to eliminate stagnation, strengthening the spleen-stomach, regulating the spleen-stomach to dissipate dampness, relaxing tendon, and removing obstruction and promote qi circulation to activate blood. Epigastria distension and fullness, indigestion, anorexia, and chronic diarrhea can be treated with the manipulation.

4.2.2.3 Cautions

Massage is a safe, effective, and generally side effect-free therapy. However, there may have some accidents like dizziness, pain, bruise, and fracture when manipulations are used in a wrong way. In case these situations would happen, we should have emergency response plan and be careful when performing massage.

Massage manipulations have several contraindications. First, people should not be treated with massage after sports or in a condition of tiredness or weakness. Second, people should not be treated with hunger or too fullness and within an hour after a meal. Third, abdomen and lumbosacral region of pregnant women should not be treated while other parts can be treated with light strength, but some acupoints that can possibly cause abortion must be avoided. Fourth, drunk people should not be treated with massage. Finally, patients with fracture, spinal cord injury, body part with cancer, infectious disease, and serious should be forbidden from massage.

4.2.3 Infantile Massage

Infantile massage is a series of massage manipulation designed for infants though the long-term practices. It comes from the summary of infantile characteristics, physiological characteristics, pathological characteristics, and special acupoints. Also, it is well known for its great curative effect on infantile diseases. In infantile massage, a number of acupoints are different from adult and some of them are special designed for infantile. In manipulation aspects, infantile massage manipulation attaches great importance to softness, steadiness, smoothness, correctness, and painlessness. Furthermore, many manipulations in infantile massage require the external use of medical medium. There are eight general manipulations in infantile massage, namely pressing, rubbing, pinching, circularly pushing, kneading, pushing, nipping, and pounding. Although some of those manipulations have the same name as in adult massage, their performing may be quite different.

4.2.3.1 Acupoints of Infantile Massage

Acupoints of infantile massage have several characteristics: First, most of acupoints of infantile massage are not located on the fourteen meridians but located in hand. It is called hundreds of channels and vessels of child gathering in the hand. Secondly, the form of acupoint of infantile massage is classified into point form, line form, and cover form. Thirdly, most of the infantile acupoints are combined with specific manipulation and tend to specific effect.

1. Erhougaogu (prominent bone behind the ear).
   Location: In the depression inferior to the mastoid process behind the eye and superior to the posterior hairline.

Manipulation: Kneading the point with the tip of the thumbs or middle fingers. Repeat 30 to 50 times.

Indication: Headache, dysphoria, and common cold.

2. Tianmen.

Location: The line from the midpoint between the two eyebrows to the anterior hairline.

Manipulation: Push the point straight upward with the pads of both thumbs alternately, known as opening Tianmen. Repeat 30 to 50 times.

Indication: Headache, cold, vertigo, night cry, and insomnia.

3. Kangong.

Location: The transverse line from the medial end to the lateral end of the eyebrow.

Manipulation: Push the points respectively from the medial ends of the eyebrow to the lateral ends with both thumbs.

Indication: Exogenous fever, redness and pain of eyes, convulsion, and myopia.

4. Tianzhu.

Location: The line from the midpoint of the posterior hairline to Dazhui (GV14).

Manipulation: Pushing the point straight downward with the pads of the thumb or the index and middle fingers. Repeat 100 to 500 times.

Indication: Nausea, vomiting, cold, fever, sore throat, and stiff nape.

5. Spleen Meridian.

Location: On the radial border of the thumb and from the tip to the root.

Manipulation: Flex the thumb of the child patient and then push along the radial border of the thumb toward the wrist. This is called reinforcing spleen meridian. Pushing the opposite direction is called clearing spleen meridian. Repeat 100 to 500 times.

Indication: Diarrhea, constipation, abdominal distension, dysentery, anorexia, and jaundice due to damp heat.

6. Stomach meridian.

Location: At the junction of red and white skin of the greater thenar.

Manipulation: Pushing from the root to the palmar root is considered as a reinforcing method, called reinforcing stomach meridian. Pushing the opposite direction is called clearing stomach meridian. Repeat 100 to 500 times.

Indication: Nausea, vomiting, belching, no appetite, abdominal distension, halitosis, and constipation.

7. Liver meridian.

Location: The whorl surface of the distal interphalangeal joint of the index finger.

Manipulation: Pushing from fingertip to the root is considered as a reinforcing manipulation, called reinforcing liver meridian. Pushing the opposite direction is called clearing liver meridian. Repeat 100 to 500 times.

Indication: Conjunctive congestion, bitter taste in the mouth, dry throat, convulsion, restlessness, and feverish sensation over five centers.

8. Heart meridian.

Location: The whorl surface of the distal interphalangeal joint of the middle finger.

Manipulation: Pushing from fingertip to the root is considered as a reinforcing manipulation, called reinforcing heart meridian. Pushing the opposite direction is called clearing heart meridian. Repeat 100 to 500 times.

Indication: Orolingual ulceration, short and hot urination, coma due to high fever, and feverish sensation over the palms and soles.

9. Lung meridian.

Location: The whorl surface of the distal interphalangeal joint of the ring finger.

Manipulation: Pushing from fingertip to the root is considered as a reinforcing manipulation, called reinforcing lung meridian. Pushing the opposite direction is called clearing lung meridian. Repeat 100 to 500 times.

Indication: Cold, cough, panting, wheezy phlegm, spontaneous sweating, night sweat, pale face, prolapse of the rectum, enuresis, and constipation.

10. Kidney meridian.

Location: The ungual whorl surface of the distal part of the small finger.

Manipulation: Pushing from fingertip to the tip is considered as a reinforcing manipulation, called reinforcing kidney meridian. Pushing the opposite direction is called clearing kidney meridian. Repeat 100 to 500 times.

Indication: Congenital defect, weakness due to lingering illness, diarrhea, enuresis, cough, panting, redness of the eye, and painful urination.

11. Four transverse creases.

Location: On the surface of palm, at the midpoint of the transverse creases of the first interphalangeal joints of the index, middle, ring, and little fingers.

Manipulation: Pressing and kneading the point with the nail of the thumb is called nipping Shengwen. Repeat 100 to 300 times.

Indication: Indigestion, abdominal distention, abdominal pain, disharmony of qi and blood, panting and fissure on the lip.

12. Large intestine.

Location: On the radial border of the index finger, from the fingertip to the margin between the index finger and the thumb.

Manipulation: Pushing from the fingertip to the wed margin is considered as a reinforcing method, known as reinforcing large intestine. Pushing to the opposite direction is considered as a clearing method, known as clearing large intestine. Repeat the manipulation 100 to 300 times.

Indication: Diarrhea, dysentery, constipation, and abdominal pain.

13. Small intestine.

Location: On the ulnar side of the little finger and the line from the fingertip to the root.

Manipulation: Pushing from the fingertip to its root is considered as a reinforcing method known as reinforcing small intestine. Pushing to the opposite direction is considered as a clearing method, known as clearing small intestine. Repeat the manipulation 100 to 300 times.

Indication: Hot and difficult urination, watery diarrhea, boils in the mouth, and tidal fever in the afternoon.

14. Shending.

Location: On the tip of the small finger.

Manipulation: Pressing and kneading the point with the tip of the thumb or index finger are called kneading Shending. Repeat the manipulation 100 to 500 times.

Indication: Spontaneous perspiration, night sweating, and metopism in child.

15. Small palmar transverse crease.

Location: On the surface of palm, at the root of the little finger, on the ulnar end of transverse crease.

Manipulation: Pressing and kneading the point with the tip of the thumb or middle finger is called kneading small palmar transverse crease. Repeat the manipulation 100 to 500 times.

Indication: Orolingual ulcer, salivation, pneumonia, phlegm retention, and panting.

16. Small transverse crease.

Location: On the surface of palm, the transverse crease of metacarpal interphalangeal joints of the index, middle, ring, and little finger.

Manipulation: Nipping the crease with the nail of the thumb is called small intestine; pushing the crease with the side of the thumb is called pushing small transverse crease. Nipping the crease of each finger for five times or pushing 100 to 300 times.

Indication: lip ulcer, boils in the mouth, abdominal distention, fever, and restlessness.

17. Major thenar.

Location: On the surface of the greater thenar.

Manipulation: Kneading the point with the fingertip is called kneading major thenar. Pushing from finger root to the transverse crease of the wrist is called pushing manipulation from Banmen to Hengwen and the opposite direction is called pushing manipulation from Hengwen to Banmen. Repeat the kneading manipulation 30 to 50 times or pushing manipulation 100 to 300 times.

Indication: anorexia, indigestion, vomiting, diarrhea, abdominal distension, panting, and belching.

18. Small center of sky.

Location: In the depression of the junction between the major thenar and the minor thenar eminences.

Manipulation: Kneading the point with the tip of the middle finger is called kneading small center of sky.

Indication: Spasm, night crying, hot and difficult urination, conjunctival congestion with pain, orolingual ulcers, and strabismus.

19. Triple pass.

Location: On the radial aspect of the forearm and the line between Yangchi (TE 4) and Quchi (LI11).

Manipulation: Pushing from the transverse crease of the wrist to that of the elbow with the index finger pulp and middle finger pulp is called pushing Sanguan. Repeat the manipulation 100 to 300 times.

Indication: Abdominal pain, diarrhea, aversion to cold, lassitude of limb, weakness due to illness, wind cold, and all other deficiency and cold syndrome.

20. Tianheshui.

Location: Along the mid-line of forearm from convergent tendon to Hongchi (middle of transverse cubital crease).

Manipulation: Pushing from the transverse crease of the wrist to that of the elbow is called clearing Tianheshui. Repeat the manipulation 100 to 300 times.

Indication: All heat symptoms, such as exogenous fever, tidal fever, internal heat, restlessness, thirst, orolingual ulcers, cough, wheezing phlegm, and sore throat

21. Liufu.

Location: On the ulnar aspect of the forearm and the line between the ulnar side of palmar transverse striation at wrist and the transverse crease of the elbow.

Manipulation: Pushing from the transverse crease of the elbow to that of the wrist with the tip of the thumb, or tips of the index and middle fingers is called pushing Liufu. Repeat 100 to 300 times.

Indication: High fever, polydipsia, convulsion, sore throat, and constipation.

22. Ershanmen.

Location: On the dorsum of the hand and in the depression on both sides of the root of the middle finger.

Manipulation: Pinching the point with the nail of the thumb is called pinching Ershanmen. Repeat 5 times.

Indication: Cold, fever, diaphoresis, and asthmatic breathing.

23. Shangma.

Location: On the dorsum of the hand and in the depressions proximal to the metacarpophalangeal joint of the ring and little fingers.

Manipulation: Kneading the point with the tip of the thumb is called kneading Shangma. Nipping it with the nail of the thumb is called nipping Shangma. Repeat the nipping manipulation 3 to 5 times or kneading manipulation 100 to 300 times.

Indication: Hot and difficult urination, abdominal pain, enuresis, indigestion, asthma, and toothache.

24. Yiwofeng.

Location: On the dorsum of the hand and on the midpoint of the transverse crease of the wrist.

Manipulation: Kneading the point with the tip of a finger is called kneading Yiwofeng. Repeat the manipulation 100 to 300 times.

Indication: Abdominal pain, borborygmus, wind cold, acute and chronic convulsion, and difficult joint movement.

25. Rupang.

Location: 0. 2 cun lateral to the breast.

Manipulation: Kneading the point with the tip of the middle finger. Repeat the manipulation 20 to 50 times.

Indication: Chest oppression, wheezing, cough, and vomiting.

26. Dantian.

Location: On the lower abdomen, 2 or 3 cun below the umbilicus.

Manipulation: Kneading or rubbing the point respectively is called kneading Dantian or rubbing Dantian. Knead Dantian 50 to 100 times or rub it for 5 min.

Indication: Enuresis and abdominal pain.

27. Dujiao.

Location: 2cun below the umbilicus and 2 cun lateral to Shimen (CV5).

Manipulation: Grasping with the thumb, index, and middle finger is called grasping Dujiao and pressing with the tip of the middle finger is called pressing Dujiao. Repeat the manipulation 3 to 5 times.

Indication: Abdominal pain and diarrhea.

28. Qijiegu.

Location: On the spine, the part from the fourth lumbar vertebra to the end of the coccyx, or Changqiang (GV1).

Manipulation: Pushing the spine upward with the radial side of the thumb or the pads of the index and middle fingers is called pushing Qijiegu upward. Pushing in the opposite direction is called pushing Qijiegu downward. Repeat 100 to 300 times.

Indication: Diarrhea, constipation, and fever.

29. Guiwei.

Location: At the end of the coccyx.

Manipulation: Kneading the point with the tip of the thumb or the middle finger is called kneading Guiwei. Repeat 100 to 300 times.

Indication: Constipation, diarrhea, and enuresis.

4.2.3.2   Basic Manipulations of Infantile Massage

1. Pressing manipulation.

Pressing a certain part or point with the fingers or palm steadily is called pressing manipulation. It is divided into finger pressing and palm pressing manipulation.

2. Rubbing manipulation.

Fix the palm surface or the pad of the thumb, index, or middle figure on a certain part or point, using the wrist together with the forearm to make clockwise or counterclockwise movements.

3. Pinching manipulation.

Holding the limbs or grasping the skin with the pads of the thumb, index, and middle finger, squeezing with opposite force, pinching, and releasing repeatedly.

4. Circularly pushing manipulation.

Circularly pushing manipulation is performed by pushing on certain points in an arc rotational way with the whoil surface of the thumb or middle finger.

5. Kneading manipulation.

Kneading manipulation is performed by fixing the thenar or whorl surface of the middle finger or thumb on a certain part or point and making circular movements. Kneading manipulation can be further classified according to different operating methods into middle finger kneading manipulation, thumb kneading manipulation, and thenar kneading manipulation.

6. Pushing manipulation.

Exert force on the targeted region or certain acupoint by pushing straight forward or making rotational movements on the point with the pad of the thumb or the pads of the index and middle fingers is called pushing manipulation. It can be divided into straight pushing manipulation, rotational pushing manipulation, and separative-pushing manipulation and combined pushing manipulation.

7. Nipping manipulation.

Nipping manipulation is done by hitting a point or area with the nail of the thumb.

8. Pounding manipulation.

Pounding manipulation is performed by striking certain acupoint with the tip of the middle finger or the interphalangeal joints of the flexed index and middle fingers.

4.2.3.3   Indications and Contraindications

Infantile massage is suitable for children under 6 years old, especially suitable for infant under 3 years old. Indications for infantile massage are quite a lot, and some of them we have mentioned above in acupoints. Infantile massage is also commonly used for disease prevention and health care for children.

Although infantile massage is safe and widely used, there are several contraindications should be noticed. Contraindication for infantile massage is similar to adult massage. Skin injury, infectious disease, bleeding tendency, cancer and tuberculosis, serious organism disease should be forbidden to treat with infantile massage.

4.2.3.4   Cautions

Certain perspectives should be noticed when performing infantile massage:

1. The environment of clinic should be quiet, clean, and with appropriate temperature. Wind and sharp light should be avoided. Stop unauthorized people from moving around. Keep the children warm after treatment and cold food or drink is forbidden.
2. Keep the performer's hand clean and decorations are not allowed. Performers should be kind, patient, and careful. The hand should be kept warm when the weather is cold.

3. The time of treatment should be considered according to the age, the illness and the manipulation as well. Generally, infantile massage treatment should be kept within 20 min and only once a day. Acute diseases like high fever can be treated twice a day.
4. Acupoints in upper limbs are generally treated for only one side. Other parts can be both sides.
5. Remember to use medical medium while performing infantile massage.
6. For convulsions, be careful for the asphyxia and let the child take a side lying position then find related department for help.
7. Infantile massage should be performed an hour after the child had meal.
8. Sterilize before treating every child in case mutual infection.

4.2.4 Spinal Manipulations

Spinal manipulations are also known as the pulling manipulation of spine. It can be generally divided into cervical rotational and local manipulation, thoracic resetting manipulation, and lumbar resetting manipulation. Spinal manipulations are widely used in all segments of spine. It has the effect of smoothing the joints and resetting subluxation.

4.2.4.1 Manipulations

1. Cervical rotational and local manipulation.

   (a) Oblique pulling of the cervical vertebra.
       Manipulation: The patient has a sitting position with the head slight antexion, and the neck should be relaxed. The operator stands behind the patient, holding patient's head at the occiput with one hand, and the chin with the other. Two hands coordinate to rotate patient's head slowly (rotate patient's head to left side if the disorder is on the left side and vice versa.). When the head is turned to certain amplitude and the operator feels resistance on hand, stop rotation for a moment, then do a quick and controlled twisting movement (amplitude increased about 3–5 degree), and cracking sound is often heard at the moment.
   (b) Positioning rotating-pulling of the cervical vertebra.
       Manipulation: The patient is to take a sitting position. Operator steps aside and stands behind the patient. Use the inner side of elbow to hang the patient's jaw, and the palm holds the back head while the other hand's thumb presses against the spinous process of the targeted vertebrae. Use the former arm to lead the neck to make an antexion movement in a certain degree to open the inner space of cervical vertebrae. Slowly rotate the head to the

dislocated direction until there is a resistance. Stop rotation for a moment, then do a quick and controlled twisting movement (amplitude increased about 3–5°); cracking sound is often heard at this time.

2. Thoracic resetting manipulation

(c) Positioning rotating-pulling of the thoracic vertebrae.

Manipulation: The patient is to take a sitting position, and the assistant fixes the patient's leg (normal side of the treating part) to make the pelvis stable. The operator stands behind and uses the thumb of one hand to press on the subluxation vertebrae spinous process. The other hand traverses through the patient's axilla and hold on his neck. Ask the patient to lean forward until the space of thoracic vertebrae is open. Coordinate with two hands to twist the spine to the resistant degree. Stop rotation for a moment, then do a quick and controlled twisting movement (amplitude increased about 3 to 5°). In the same time, use the thumb to push on the spinous process from the injured side to the normal side in order to reset subluxation. Cracking sound is often heard at this time.

(d) Antagonistic reduction of thoracic vertebrae.

Manipulation: The patient is asked to have a sitting position and put his hands behind the occiput; the body slightly leans forward. The operator stands behind the operator, puts his knee against the diseased area, extends his arms by passing patient's armpits to hold patient's forearms at posterior aspects. Ask patient to have a few bending forward and extending backward movements. Then, the operator pulls patient's arm backward and upward when his knee tries to push the diseased vertebra forward and downward. Hands and knee coordinate to make thoracic vertebrae move.

3. Lumbar resetting manipulation

(e) Positioning rotating-pulling of the lumbar vertebrae in sitting position.

Manipulation: The patient is to take a sitting position, and the assistant fixes the patient's leg (normal side of the treating part) to make the pelvis stable or let the patient bestraddle on the treatment desk. The operator sitting behind, use the thumb of one hand to press against on the spinous process of the dislocated vertebrae. The other hand traverses through the patient's axilla and then hold on his neck. Ask the patient to lean forward until the space of lumbar vertebrae is open. Coordinate with two hands to twist the spine to the resistant degree. Stop rotation for a moment, then do a quick and controlled twisting movement (amplitude increased about 3 to 5°). In the same time, use the thumb to push on the spinous process from the affected side to the normal side in order to reset subluxation. Cracking sound is often heard at this time.

(f) Oblique pulling of the lumbar vertebrae (yao zhui xie ban method)

Manipulation: The patient is to have a lateral recumbent position—lie on one side with hip and knee flexed. The operator stands by facing the patient, puts one hand over the front of patient's shoulder, the other hand or forearm over patient's hip. Two hands push coordinately and slowly to opposite direction. Make a controlled sudden twisting movement with increased amplitude when lumbar vertebrae are rotated to an extremity (when there is resistance.). It implies a successful manipulation if cracking sound is heard.

(g) Backward stretching and pulling of the lumbar vertebrae (yao zhui hou shen ban method)

Manipulation: The patient is asked to take a prone position. The operator stands beside on the affected side of body. Use the part of pisiform bone on the palm base to press on the subluxation spinous process of the lumbar vertebrae. Use the other hand to hold the far end of the opposite leg and then pull upwards until the resistant area. Enlarge the rear protraction amplitude of lumbar vertebrae for 3 to 5°. At the same time, use the palm base to press and push on the spinous process.

4.2.4.2 Indications and Contraindications

Indications: Cervical spinal manipulations are suitable for subluxation of cervical vertebrae. Antagonistic reduction of thoracic vertebrae is suitable for the subluxation of the fourth to tenth thoracic vertebrae and the reset of costovertebral joint. Positioning rotating-pulling of the thoracic vertebrae is suitable for dislocation reset under the eighth thoracic vertebrae. Oblique pulling of the lumbar vertebrae and positioning rotating-pulling of the lumbar vertebrae in sitting position are suitable for all segments of lumbar vertebrae. Backward stretching and pulling of the lumbar vertebrae is suitable for lower lumbar vertebrae reset.

Cervical spinal manipulations are used to treat diverse kind of cervical spondylosis. Thoracic spinal manipulations are used to treat subluxation of thoracic vertebrae and internal problem due to subluxation. Lumbar spinal manipulations are used to treat protrusion of lumbar intervertebral disk and posterior joint derangement of lumbar vertebrae.

Contraindications: First, for spine injures of unknown reason with symptoms of spinal cord injuries, spinal manipulation is not allowed to use. Second, for the aged people with serious hyperostosis or rarefaction of bone, spinal manipulation is not allowed. Third, patients with tuberculosis and tumor of bones are forbidden to receive spinal manipulations. Fourth, be careful with spinal canal stenosis when spinal manipulation is needed.

4.2.4.3 Cautions

1. Spinal manipulation performers should know well of anatomy and must master the structure and characteristics of spinal joint as well as the physiological degree of mobility.
2. Control your strength when performing spinal manipulation and violent force is not allowed. Pursuit of cracking sound is not suggested in spinal manipulation. Operators should train for a long time before practicing on human body.

3. Every single manipulation should be controlled in the physiological degree of mobility, otherwise spinal cord, cauda, and nerve root may be injured. Such points should be noticed especially in cervical manipulation and thoracic manipulation.
4. Pay attention to the reaction of patient while performing spinal manipulation. Once the patient has very uncomfortable feelings, stop the manipulation immediately and find the reason.

4.3 Dietary Therapy

4.3.1 Introduction to Dietary Therapy

Dietary therapy has long been a common approach to health among Chinese people. A number of ancient Chinese medical books displayed an early Chinese interest in healing effect of food. The earliest extant Chinese dietary text is a chapter of *Sun Simiao*'s *Essential Prescriptions Worth a Thousand Gold for Emergencies*, which was completed in the 650 s during the *Tang* dynasty. *Sun* presented current knowledge about food so that people would first turn to food rather than drugs when suffering from an ailment.

4.3.1.1 Concept of Traditional Chinese Dietary Therapy

Dietary therapy also called food therapy or nutrition therapy is a method of treating diseases with diet. Traditional Chinese dietary therapy is a subject under the guidance of the theory of Traditional Chinese Medicine to study diet treatment of diseases. It is an important part of TCM clinical medicine.

4.3.1.2 Brief History of TCM Dietary Therapy

In Chinese medicine, food is classified according to its energetic effects rather than according to its component parts. Certain foods are viewed as warming and nourishing while others are seen as cooling and eliminating; some foods are useful for building qi while others have blood, yang or yin building proprieties.

In ancient times, people found that many foods were both nutritious and able to treat diseases. This kind of food is classified as drugs, so-called Medicine and food homology. *Internal Classic* laid a theoretical foundation for the development of dietotherapy and pointed out that excessive diet or partial food could lead to disease. The five flavors of food have a certain effect on human pathophysiology. *Internal classics* has recorded 13 prescriptions, of which 6 are dietotherapy prescriptions. The application of dietotherapy is not only extensive in *Handbook of Prescriptions for Emergency*, but also records a lot of contents with high scientific value. In *Collective Commentaries on the Classic of Materia Medica*, there are 195 kinds of food medicine, including grain, vegetable, fruit, and animal medicines.

The TCM dietetics of the Tang Dynasty made great progress. A special chapter on food therapy in *Essential Prescriptions Worth a Thousand Gold for Emergencies* emphasizes the importance of diet therapy. *Compendium of Materia Medica* of *Li Shizhen* also contributed a lot to the diet therapy. Many methods and drugs for dietotherapy were collected. In modern times, on the basis of the accumulated experience, dietotherapy has been further developed, and now it has become an independent subject in TCM.

4.3.2 Main Tenets of TCM Dietary Therapy

4.3.2.1 Characteristic of Dietary Therapy

1. Holism.

    Holism is the guiding ideology of the theoretical system of TCM. Holism means unity, integrity, and interconnection. As one of the most essential characteristics of TCM, holism is applied throughout the theory system, including physiology, pathology, diagnostics, syndrome differentiation, and treatment. It offers important guidance to dietary therapy too.

    Diet is an important factor in overall coordination. Diet has an important impact on the integrity of the human body. The nutrients in the diet are absorbed to generate qi, blood, and body fluids. A reasonable diet is an important factor in the coordination of the human body and nature. Diet is the most closely related factor in human contact with nature. Phagoiatreusiology presents the time, local diet view, used to adjust the relationship between man and nature. For example, when the weather is cool, we should avoid eating cold food; when the climate is warm, we avoid eating warm food.

2. Choose diet based on constitution and syndrome differentiation.

    First, select different foods according to different constitutions. According to the information collected by four ways of looking, listening, questioning, and feeling the pulse, yin, yang, qi, blood conditions are analyzed to make judgment of constitution. Choose different foods to keep health according to the constitution.

    Second, choose diet based on syndrome differentiation. Syndrome differentiation is the precondition and basis of food therapy. Dietotherapy is one of the means and methods of treating disease. In the diet treatment, first of all pay attention to the syndrome differentiation and then the right choice of food selection. For example, when people catch a cold, which may be caused by cold wind or heat wind, we need to choose hot or cold pungent drugs for the treatment depending on syndrome differentiation.

3. Pay attention to regulating the spleen-stomach function.

One of the major features of TCM dietary therapy is to regulate the function of the spleen-stomach. Dietary activity is one of the important manifestations of human life activities and is the guarantee of healthy and long life. The place of food digestion and absorption is the spleen-stomach. Digestion and absorption depend on the healthy function of the spleen-stomach. Only when the spleen-stomach function is strong, can the food be transformed into nutriment and transported to nourish the whole body and viscera. Improper diet is harmful for the spleen-stomach function, and various kinds of diseases may appear.

4.3.2.2 Methods of Dietary Therapy

Food, maintaining different functions to be selected by cooking and processing can change to different TCM therapies, such as sweating therapy, purgation therapy, harmonizing therapy, warming therapy, clearing therapy, resolving therapy, tonifying therapy, and so on. (Table 4.1).

Table 4.1 Methods of dietary therapy and representative foods

Methods	Specific methods	Functions	Representative foods
Diaphoresis method	Relieving superficies syndrome with pungent and warm natured drugs	Dispelling cold for relieving superficies syndrome, ventilating lung qi for arresting cough	Fresh ginger, bulbus allii fistulosi, pepper fruit, purple perilla
	Resolving superficies syndrome with pungent and cool natured drugs	Clearing lung-heat for relieving superficies syndrome, arresting cough	Peppermint, kudzu vine root, chrysanthemum flower, mulberry leaf
Eliminating phlegm and relieving cough method	Ventilating lung qi for dissipating phlegm	Ventilating lung qi, eliminating cold-phlegm and heat-phlegm	Radish seed, perilla fruit, white mustard seed
	Arresting cough and relieving asthma	Ventilating lung qi and eliminating phlegm to relieve asthma, benefiting qi and moistening lung	Pear, loquat, radish seed, bitter apricot seed, tendrilleaf fritillary bulb
Heat clearing therapy	Clearing heat-fire	Clearing heat-fire, relieving restlessness, promoting the production of body fluid, quenching thirst	Reed rhizome, watermelon pericarp, lotus plumule, lotus leaf, luffa, henon bamboo leaf
	Clearing heat and removing toxicity	Clearing away the heat-evil and expelling superficial evils	Heart leaf houttuynia herb, olive, wild chrysanthemum flower, purslane herb, mung bean, mung bean, honeysuckle bud, and flower

Table 4.1 (continued)

Methods	Specific methods	Functions	Representative foods
Regulating qi flowing method	Dispersing stagnated liver qi and regulating qi flowing	Dispersing stagnated liver qi for relieving qi stagnation, regulating qi flowing to to remove stagnation from spleen-stomach	Finger citron, tangerine pericarp, rose flower, lychee seed, nutgrass galingale rhizome
	Invigorating the stomach and activating qi flowing	Regulating qi flowing for strengthening spleen, drying the wetness-evil and eliminating phlegm	Tangerine pericarp, poria Cocos, finger citron, wax gourd seed, pinellia tuber
Benefiting qi and strengthening spleen method	Benefiting qi	Benefiting lung qi and spleen qi, strengthening function of zang-fu	Chinese date, honey, chicken meat, ginseng
	Strengthening spleen	Strengthening spleen to remove dampness, benefiting qi to cure prolapse syndrome	Lotus seed, coix seed, mud eel, large head atractylodes rhizome, ginseng, milkvetch root, peanut, longan aril, pseudo-ginseng
Tonifying blood and nourishing yin method	Tonifying blood	Promoting production of blood, supplementing blood shortage, nourishing heart and liver	Carrot, peanut, spinach, Chinese date, rice field eel, longan aril, chicken meat, pig liver, mutton, milkvetch root, ginseng, Chinese angelica
	Nourishing yin	Nourishing yin-fluid, nourishing tendon and bones	Mulberry fruit, black soybean, turtle carapace, oyster meat, yolk, debark peony root, barbary wolfberry fruit
Replenishing kidney essence method		Replenishing kidney essence	Sesame, black soybean, barbary wolfberry fruit, mulberry fruit, walnut meat, chestnut, desert living cistanche, epimedium herb, holothuroids, sea cucumber, pilose antler, pig bone marrow
Benefiting yin and promoting fluid production method	Benefiting stomach to promote the production of body fluid	Benefiting stomach yin, promoting the production of body fluid	Pear, sugar cane, Chinese water chestnut, lotus rhizome, sesame, honey, dwarf lilyturf tuber, dendrobium
	Moistening dryness to promote the production of body fluid	Moistening lung dryness, promoting the production of body fluid	Pear, lily bulb, lotus rhizome, Chinese water chestnut, loquat, honey, coastal glehnia root, dwarf lilyturf tuber, tremella

4.3.2.3 The Properties and Flavors of Food

1. The four properties.

   Foods and herbs are divided according to four properties of being hot, warm, cool, and cold. These categories describe the way the food makes the body react and what kind of sensations are generated. Hot foods generate warmth in the body, whereas cold foods make the body feel cold.

   If we know the constitution of our body, we can choose to eat the foods that compensate for our weaknesses. If one often feels cold and experiences pain in cold weather, he may limit foods with a cold property and increase the intake of warming foods. Another technique would be using warm foods to neutralize the cold in foods so as not to aggravate one's condition.

   More specifically, hot food generates heat and warms the internal organs; warm food disperses cold and helps to restore Yang qi; cool food reduces heat; and cold food creates cold, cool the organs, lowers fire, and detoxifies. It is important to avoid hot foods when there are signs of heat like infections and inflammation. Redness is often a sign of excess heat in the body. Likewise, it is important to avoid cold foods when a person often feels cold or has cold hands and feet because the yang of the body is deficient.

   The four properties are meant to be a guideline. Here are a few foods which are absolute. Hot foods include chili, ginger, hot spices, most alcohol (not beer), rich, or fatty foods. Warm foods include high protein and high fat foods such as most meats, chocolate, coffee, curry, and monosodium glutamate because they speed up metabolism. Many artificial flavors and preservatives have this affect. Cool foods are usually fleshy and watery like watermelon or foods that have been boiled for a long time in water. Neutral foods are those neither warming nor cooling and include most grains

2. The five flavors.

   The five classic flavors correspond to the 5 element theory and include sweet, pungent, salty, sour, and bitter. Neutral has also been added to flavors to account for foods with less effect and not fit in other categories. The flavors tell what action the food has on the body and what organ the food has an effect on (Table 4.2).

4.3.2.4 Eating with the Seasons

Life cultivation in accordance with seasonal conditions refers to regulating one's mind, living conditions, and diet at opportune times throughout the year in order to achieve and maintain good health, prevent diseases, and prolong life. These opportune times are determined according to the principles and features of the climatic variations and the waxing and waning of yin and yang during the year. The name "life cultivation" suggests that life itself is not something to be taken for granted but something like a farmer's crop that needs to be tilled, sowed, nourished, and cultivated.

TCM holds that humans, as a part of nature, exist between the heaven and the earth and are closely related to nature. Conversely, the climatic variations in nature may influence the human body directly or indirectly, causing corresponding

Table 4.2 The five flavors of food with examples

Flavors	Organs	Functions	Avoid	Overuse
Sweet	Spleen and stomach	Warms, tonifies, supplements deficiency, and relaxes	Avoid if you are suffering from too much flesh (overweight)	Weakens the function of the heart causing difficult breathing and distention of the chest. Too much sweet also injures the flesh
Pungent	Lung and large intestine	Induces sweating and promotes energy circulation	Avoid if the lungs are dry or if the qi (energy) or blood is weak because pungent is dispersing	Can result in muscles and pulse to become weak and injure the spirit. It can also injure the skin and body hair
Salty	Kidney and bladder	Softens hardness and masses and descends. It is useful in hardened muscles or glands and to lubricate and disperse any hardness	Avoid if you are suffering from blood diseases or if the heart is struggling. Salt has a cold energy and should also be avoided when the yang (heat) of the body is weak (feels cold, edema)	Can result in the pulse to become sluggish from congestion of the qi (energy) and the complexion loses its vitality. The bones may weaken and the function of the heart will be suppressed, low spirits and poor coloring will occur from injury of the blood
Sour	Liver and gallbladder	Astringent, absorbent, and astringent (constricting). It is good for diarrhea and excess perspiration, but it can obstruct	Avoid if muscles and tendons are tense or tight	Injures the muscles, making the flesh contract, drying the lips, and allowing the liver to produce too much fluids which injure the spleen
Bitter	Heart and small intestine	Drying and hardening, purging. In general, bitter reduces body heat, dries up the body fluids and can cause diarrhea if it is purging. It also activates the liver function	Avoid in bone disease or if the bones are old or crumbling	Injures the spirit, dries up the skin and makes the body hair fall out. Too much bitter weakens the spleen's function to transform fluids

physiological or pathological changes. Humans live in the natural environment and all the vital activities should conform to the objective principles of the seasonal waxing and waning and transformations of yin and yang. Only in this way may one enjoy good health and longevity. On the contrary, if one does not conform to the seasonal changes and violates the natural principles one's health will suffer, giving rise to disease. Throughout history, those considered sages in the art of life cultivation have insisted on the need to regulate one's daily life including one's mental activities, diet, and overall life style in accordance with the seasons. In order for normal physiological functions to occur, there must be a harmonious balance between the internal and external environments (Table 4.3).

Table 4.3 Cultivating yang in spring and summer, nourishing yin in autumn and winter

Season	Five Element	Color Favor Organ	Food Recommended	Food/Herb Restricted
Spring	Wood (germination)	Blue Sour Liver	Garlic, chive, leaf mustard, onion, lily bulb, lotus seed, radish, perillia leaf, black fungus, white fungus, mushroom, American ginseng, chrysanthemum flower, cassia seed, polygonum, Chinese yam, bamboo shoot, fish	Cucumber, winter gourd, eggplant, green bean sprout mutton, quail, ginseng. Cinnamon, fennel seeds, hot pepper, wine
Summer	Fire (growth)	Red Bitter Heart	Mung bean, mung bean sprout, pear, winter melon, bitter melon, cucumber, tomato, mint, lotus root, honeysuckle flower, lotus leaf, watermelon, grape, pineapple, coconut, mulberry fruit, lemon, strawberry, lemon, persimmon, dark plum	Longan, lichee, chive, onion, hot pepper, cinnamon, wine, ginseng, mutton, dog meat
Autumn	Metal (reaping)	White Pungent Lung	Glehnia, lily bulb, chestnut, lotus seed, Chinese red date, walnut, peanut, white fungus, pear, ginseng, wolfberry, kelp, astragalus, euryale seed, tomato, honey, sesame	Winter melon, cucumber, bitter melon, watermelon, mung bean, hot pepper, cinnamon, mung bean sprout, fennel seeds, honeysuckle flower, chrysanthemum flower, mutton
Winter	Water (storage)	Black Salty Kidney	Walnut, lotus seeds, lily bulb, longan, lichee, onion, cinnamon, wine, ginseng, sesame, walnut, peanut, black fungus, beef, mutton, codonopsis	Raw and cold vegetables and fruits, watermelon, mung bean, mung bean sprout, honeysuckle flower chrysanthemum flower, American ginseng, banana, persimmon, shrimp, crab

4.3.2.5 Taboo of Dietotherapy

Different foods have their own characteristics. Therefore, in the prevention and control of disease, according to the principle of dialectic, we should choose the food with significant nutrition and efficacy. If the application is not appropriate or abused, it is not only useless for the treatment of disease, but also may have a negative effect.

Food taboo is that in some cases, some food cannot be eaten; otherwise, it will cause disease, or aggravate the disease. For example, some special foods such as persimmons and crabs can't be used together. In addition, pregnant women should also ensure not to eat too hot and pungent food. Postpartum women cannot eat cold food. In addition, we should adapt to the changes in the four seasons to choose the right food based on dietary taboos of four seasons.

4.3.3   TCM Constitution Dietary Therapy

The constitution of each person is influenced by congenital and acquired factors, and this varies from person to person. In the other words, the body's metabolism, functioning of organs and organ structure all combine to determine the susceptibility to pathogenic factors. Either for health cultivation or disease treatment, Traditional Chinese Medicine must be used in accordance with each individual's body constitution. What are the body constitutions of modern people? Professor *Wang Qi* of Beijing University of Chinese Medicine has led a research group studying Traditional Chinese Constitutional Medicine. Human constitution can be classified into 9 basic constitutional types. Certain constitutional types can lead to certain diseases. Imbalanced constitutions can be regulated and rebalanced to health.

4.3.3.1   Yang Deficiency Constitution Dietary Therapy

Yang deficiency manifestation: Fair skinned and large body size, flaccid muscles, pale white complexion, pale lips, aversion to cold with cold limbs, tiredness and weakness, shortness of breath, weak pulse, abdominal cold pain, pale and fat tongue, low body temperature.

Dietary method: Foods which are warm and sweet in nature to warm and tonify spleen yang and kidney yang.

Disease tendency: Phlegm retention, edema, diarrhea, impotence.

Recommended food: Cinnamon, zanthoxylum, clove, shrimp, walnut meat, dog meat, mutton, leek, venison, bullwhip, dog whip, chili, monopterus albus, wheat, sorghum, onion, garlic, chicken, sea cucumber, cherry, Chinese dates, longan, ginger, and fennel.

Food to avoid: Cold, raw, bitter or greasy food such as cucumber, lotus root, watermelon, crabs, bitter melon, mung bean, green tea.

4.3.3.2   Yin Deficiency Constitution Dietary Therapy

Yin deficiency manifestation: Emaciated, flushed cheeks or feverish face, feverish sensation in the palm and soles, dry mouth and throat, dry skin, skin easily wrinkles, dry and irritating sensation in the eyes, blurred vision, dizziness, poor sleep, constipation, spermatorrhea, night sweats, early menstruation.

Dietary method: Nourishing yin and clearing heat, use foods with sweet and cold nature.

Disease tendency: Easily get dry cough, dry syndrome, seminal emission, premature ejaculation, amenorrhea, and metrorrhagia.

Recommended food: Honey, tofu, pig, bird's nest, pine nuts, sesame, black beans, black sesame, ophiopogon root, mulberry, bananas, pears, tomatoes, duck's egg, lean pork, duck meat, turtle, mung beans, winter melon, and lily bulb.

Food to avoid: Warm and dry foods such as mutton, chive, onion, hot pepper, garlic, and sunflower seeds.

4.3.3.3   Qi Deficiency Constitution Dietary Therapy

Qi deficiency manifestation: Shortness of breath, no desire to speak, fatigue, dispiritedness, sweating, weak and soundless voice, palpitations, dizziness, tinnitus, poor appetite, abdominal distension, diarrhea, pale tongue with white coating, white, weak pulse.

Dietary method: Take foods that have the effects of invigorating spleen and replenishing qi, and both tonifying heart and kidney. Avoid cold, greasy, strong flavor of food.

Disease tendency: Common cold, flu, visceroptosis, consumptive diseases.

Food recommended: Rice, glutinous rice, millet, barley, buckwheat, chestnut, peanut, letinous edodes, brown sugar, yellow croaker, perch, rice, chicken, yellow croaker fish, shitake mushroom, Chinese red date, Chinese yam, honey.

Food to avoid: Bin Lang (betel nut), water spinach, radish.

4.3.3.4   Blood Deficiency Constitution Dietary Therapy

Blood deficiency manifestation: Pale or sallow complexion, palpitation, insomnia, dizziness, numbness, menstruation, pale inside of eyelid, thin and weak pulse.

Dietary method: Eat more ferric food, and high-quality protein. Fasting greasy.

Disease tendency: Anemia, forgetfulness, insomnia.

Food recommended: Sheep liver, litchi, longan pulp, brown sugar, mulberry, carrots, beef liver, rabbit liver, chicken liver, brown sugar, grape, Chinese date, black chicken, gelatin, medlar, schisandra, black fungus, sesame, animal blood.

Food to avoid: Chili, dog meat.

4.3.3.5   Phlegm-Dampness Constitution Dietary Therapy

Phlegm-dampness manifestation: Obese, large and flaccid abdomen, oily facial skin, pale yellow dull complexion, swollen face and eyes, excessive sticky sweating, chest oppression, lots of sputum, the tongue is greasy.

Dietary method: Tonifying spleen, remove dampness, reduce phlegm, dieresis, reduce weight, quitting smoking and drinking abstinence. Light diet with bland taste.

Disease tendency: Diabetes, stoke, coronary disease, high blood pressure, high cholesterol.

Food Recommended: Coix seed, small red bean, hyacinth dolichos bean, lotus leaf, carp, winter melon, dried purple seaweed, bamboo shoot, onion, garlic.

Food to avoid: Sweet, sticky, greasy, nourishing foods such as fried foods, lard, white fungus, sesame, walnut, chestnut, watermelon, peach, pear, banana.

4.3.3.6 Blood Stasis Constitution Dietary Therapy

Blood Stasis manifestation: Mostly skinny, dark dull complexion, dark purplish skin rashes, dark skin color, dark circles, dark or dull nose, dry flakey skin, thready, and uneven pulse.

Dietary method: Activating blood and removing stasis, dredging meridians and collaterals. Foods have effects of invigorating spleen, promoting qi circulation, promoting blood circulation.

Disease tendency: Hemorrhage, stroke, coronary disease.

Food recommended: Black soybeans, dried orange peel, soybean, hawthorn, black fungus, oyster mushroom, onion, leek, fennel, shitake mushroom, eggplant, mango, rose, papaya, brown sugar, wine.

Food to avoid: Foods that are cold, cool, warm and dry, greasy and blood astringing are contraindicated, such as ebony, balsam pear, persimmon, plum, guava, and groundnut kernels. Foods rich in fat and cholesterol such egg yolk, shrimp, and cheese should be avoided as well.

4.3.3.7 Qi Stagnation Constitution Dietary Therapy

Qi Stagnation manifestation: Mostly skinny, unhappy facial expression, emotional disturbance (stressed, anxious, depressed, etc.), often sigh and hiccup, fullness, and distention in the chest and hypochondrium.

Dietary method: Food that has the effects of regulating qi to alleviate mental depression and recuperating spleen-stomach with bland and cold nature.

Disease tendency: Depression syndrome, hysteria, insomnia.

Food recommended: Buckwheat, sorghum, sword bean, mushroom, orange, radish, onion, balsam pear, towel gourd, chrysanthemum, and rose.

Food to avoid: Astringing and sour foods such as pumpkin, guava, wax berry, pickle, star fruit, strawberry, plum, and lemon.

4.3.3.8 Dampness-Heat Constitution Dietary Therapy

Dampness-heat constitution manifestation: Obese, large and flaccid abdomen, oily facial skin, swollen face and eyes, excessive sticky sweating, chest oppression, lots of sputum, bad breath, bad temper, irascibility, the tongue is greasy and red.

Dietary method: Heat clearing and humidification. Fasting greasy.

Disease tendency: Furuncle, jaundice, fever.

Food recommended: Coix seed, lotus seed, red bean, mung bean, carp, melon, lettuce, gourd, bitter gourd, cucumber, watermelon, cabbage, celery, cabbage, lotus root, water spinach, and duck.

Food to avoid: Quitting smoking and drinking abstinence.

4.4 Qigong

4.4.1 General Introduction of Qigong

Qigong is one of the essence of Chinese traditional culture and a treasure of the Chinese nation. In the field of medicine, qigong therapy is an important part of Traditional Chinese Medicine. It has been developed for thousands of years. Qigong is still used in clinical practice, and in recent years, modern medicine and science have paid more and more attention to it.

4.4.1.1 Concept of Qigong

Traditional Chinese medicine qigong (TCM qigong) is a discipline that combines TCM with qigong studies. So the concept of qigong include "of traditional Chinese medicine" and "qigong."

Now the most accepted concept of qigong is "qigong is an exercise skill which has function of 'three in one': coordinating body, breath, and mind." This concept includes four levels of meaning. The first level is the content of qigong practice: coordinating body, breath, and mind. Second, the purposes of these three practices are to integrate these three contents together. Third, according to the position of qigong practice in modern disciplinary classification, it is both physical and mental exercise, relating to both physiological and psychological factors. Fourth, the knowledge category of qigong belongs to a kind of skilled knowledge.

4.4.1.2 Brief History of TCM Qigong

Qigong can be traced back to the dawn of written history, or over 2000–3000 years ago. The art of qigong took cohesive shape and became recognized during the rule of the *Yellow Emperor*. Since then, numerous branches of qigong have emerged, distinguished by their goals and practice methods. By the mid-twentieth century, most schools of qigong fell into five major branches: Medical, Taoist, Buddhist, Confucian, and Martial Arts.

From the 1950s, the word "qigong" has been widely used. The period of 1949–1965 was the first qigong climax, and qigong therapy was collated, explored, and promoted. In 1954, *Liu Guizhen* established the name "qigong" to refer to the system of life-preserving practices, developed on the basis of physical and breathing exercise and traditions. Since 1979, qigong has been rapidly restored and developed and got its second climax in China. At this stage, a large number of qigong exercises emerged, qigong entered the field of modern scientific research, foreign exchanges are also very active, and more and more foreign countries begin to know qigong. Qigong development has become more and more standardized since 2000. In contemporary China, the emphasis of qigong practice has shifted away from traditional philosophy, spiritual attainment, and folklore, to health benefits, traditional medicine and martial arts applications, and a scientific perspective. Qigong is now practiced by millions of people worldwide, primarily for its health benefits.

4.4.2 Major Schools of Qigong

In the long history of development, qigong has gradually absorbed the theoretical perspectives and methods which are beneficial to the physical and mental health of human beings in different periods and different disciplines and gradually formed different academic schools among which Medical, Taoist, Buddhist, Confucian, and Martial Arts qigong are the most major schools.

Medical qigong is one of the fastest growing, popular and the most abundant schools in these five. Originated in the *Internal Classic,* its history is more than 2000 years. *Internal Classic* involves theory, operation, application, etc., about qigong, concise, and comprehensive, laid the foundation for the development of medical qigong. Medical qigong has three important characteristics. First, it is guided by the TCM theory, including operation, application, and researches all aspects. Second, the law of medical qigong is clear, the operation is standard, the popularization is widespread, and the influence is great. The most representative medical qigong includes five mimic-animal exercise, six healing sounds, and eight-sectioned exercise. Third, choose the practice method from other schools like Medical, Taoist, Buddhist, Confucian, and Martial Arts according to specific clinical needs.

Taoist qigong can be traced back to the *pre-Qin* period. Daoist qigong are claimed to provide a way to achieve longevity and spiritual enlightenment as well as a closer connection with the natural world. The main characteristic is the emphasis on both the life and body. The school incorporates various ancient sects, beliefs, and philosophies. Its key concept is "Tao," and it emphasizes living and acting naturally, without premeditation. Taoist practice is the art of "inner alchemy," and it trains the body and the mind simultaneously. The mental training includes the "Tao in mind," a method of practice that facilitates stillness of the mind, or the qigong state. The most representative Taoist qigong is Zhoutian Gong (Fig. 4.6).

The Buddhist and the Taoist schools of qigong share many elements. In order to adjust heart in Buddhist qigong, breathing exercises are emphasized and keeping static is normal, in which a representative exercise is meditation.

Fig. 4.6 Xiao Zhoutian
microcosmic orbit

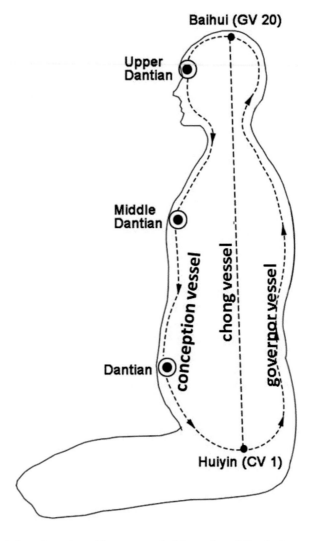

The Confucian branch is based on the ethics-centered philosophy of Confucius. Its goal is to regulate the mind, purge one's emotions, cultivate ethical values, heighten one's creative abilities, and seek perfection for the sake of society. The practitioner seeks peace and tranquility. The name of the Martial Arts (or boxing) school is self-explanatory. Its purpose is to strengthen the body and the spirit so that the practitioner can defeat enemies and defend himself. Martial arts practice enables instant, yet composed reactions in any situation. Self-regulation and healing are also emphasized. After all, a warrior must be in shape and able to recover fast. However, in terms of healing methodology, the Martial Arts school differs significantly from the other schools. It includes a few styles of wushu-qigong. Among them are the well-known hard qigong and the less-known soft qigong.

4.4.3   Modern Research

The modern research of qigong is based on qigong research methodology. It describes and verifies qigong's function by applying modern science (including modern medicine) and experimental research methods, discusses the principle of qigong's action, and establishes the modern qigong scientific theory. The modern scientific research of qigong began in the middle of the twentieth century. In general, the modern research on qigong is still in its infancy, and there is no major breakthrough at present. Although clinical research examining health effects of qigong is increasing, there are still a limited number of studies meet accepted medical and scientific standards of randomized controlled trials (RCTs). Clinical research concerning qigong has been conducted for a wide range of medical conditions, including bone density, cardiopulmonary effects, physical function, related risk factors, quality of life, immune function, inflammation, hypertension, pain, Parkinson's disease, and cancer.

4.4.4   Different Qigong Exercises

4.4.4.1   Five Mimic-Animal Exercise

Five mimic-animal exercise is a set of qigong exercises mainly characterized by imitating animals' actions and expressions in order to prevent and cure illness and to prolong life, developed during the *Han* dynasty (202 BC-220 AD). *Huatuo* is believed to be the author of this qigong sequence.

Created nearly 2000 years ago, it is the pioneer of modern five animal exercises. It is an effective method of physical and breathing exercise for health preservation. A complete discussion of five mimic-animal exercise was found in *Yang Sheng Yan Ming Lu* (*Extracts on Nourishing Spiritual Nature and Prolonging Bodily Life*) written by *Tao Hongjing*. The five animals in the exercises are tiger, deer, bear, monkey, and crane. According to TCM theory of five elements, each animal has two exercises corresponding to zang-fu viscera. It is a bionic exercise. Regular exercising of five mimic-animal exercise can dredge the main and collateral meridians, regulate qi and blood, nourish the viscera and strengthen muscle and bones, sooth joint activities, and thus achieve the purpose of disease prevention and life prolonging.

The bear's movement is slow and stable while the bird is light and flexible. The tiger is violent and powerful while the deer is relaxed and limber, and the monkey, active, agile, and alert. Qi circulation is the most stable in the bear's movements while in the bird (often described as a crane) movements, qi moves gently up, down, and around the body. The five animals can also be performed in accordance with the seasons (Fig. 4.7).

1. Bear Exercise.
   Bear relates to the earth element, the season of late summer and therefore the spleen-stomach. The spleen's emotion is thinking and is the central organ in the

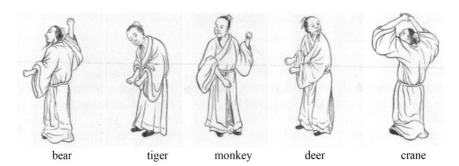

bear   tiger   monkey   deer   crane

Fig. 4.7 Five mimic-animal exercise

production of qi and blood from the food and drink we ingest. The spleen's transformation and transportation of food qi is paramount in the process of digestion
which is the basis for the formation of qi and blood. The spleen is where the idea
is said to reside and is responsible for applied thinking and the generating of
ideas, memorizing, and concentration. This animal is cumbersome and its awk-
ward traits are expressed in each movement. It starts off with circular abdominal
massage to aid digestion by warming and supporting spleen yang, using the
entire upper torso to move the hands. The arms are then poised to open and
stretch the armpit activating the spleen's close relationship with heart and liver
(heart is the mother of spleen and liver stores blood) by stretching the flanks. The
palms are empty to open as the hip is raised to shift the leg forward while keeping the knee straight. The swinging torso and heavy step activates kidney yang
to support spleen yang in heating and "cooking" food.

So in general this method can disperse the liver qi, strengthen spleen-stomach,
tonify liver and kidney, and benefit the movement function of limbs. It is very
useful for spleen deficiency, chronic gastritis, hypertension, gastric ulcer, constipation, gastroptosis, kidney deficiency, and low back pain.

2. Tiger exercise.

Tiger relates to the wood element, the season of spring, and therefore the liver
and gall bladder. The liver's emotion is anger and has many important functions
including storing blood, ensuring the smooth movement of qi in the body and
housing the ethereal soul. Liver blood nourishes the sinews, therefore allowing
physical exercise. The liver is often compared to an army general because it is
responsible for the smooth flow of qi, essential to all physiological processes of
every organ and part of the body. The emphasis of this exercise is grasping and
stretching. By reaching up to bring down Heaven and reaching down to draw up
Earth, grasping is encouraged, which relates to sinews and therefore the liver.
Rolling through the spine stimulates both yin and yang of conception vessel and
governor vessel meridians activating the microcosmic orbit. This is then completed with a slow "stalking" forward bend and sudden shout (release of anger)
as the Tiger catches its prey with vigor while standing on one leg, to stretch the

sinews while activating the well points at the tips of the fingers, incorporating another important wood trait-balance.

This practice has double effects for shape and qi improvement. Strengthening the muscles and enhancing the qi of body at the same time, the human spirit and bone marrow having reinforced training, can regulate the central nervous system with a significant effect on the prevention and treatment of neurasthenia and old chronic bronchitis and other diseases.

3. Monkey exercise.

Monkey relates to the fire element, the season of summer, and therefore the heart and small intestine. The heart is considered the most important and therefore the "emperor" of the internal organs. It relates to the emotion joy and its main function is to govern and circulate blood in the vessels to nourish tissues and house the spirit. Spirit is used to indicate the entire sphere of mental and spiritual aspects of a human being and therefore encompasses inferior soul, will, idea and inferior spirit. Similar to the heart, the monkey is forever moving like the flickering of a flame. With the first exercise, suddenly lifting the hands with hook palms up toward the chest, the shoulders toward the ears and balancing on the toes with the monkey looking to the side squeeze the heart and pumps blood as you release down again. The second part calms spirit by clearing the mind (moving the branch) to grasp the peach. Grasping in this exercise relates to the liver's ability to hold and store blood, while the lifting of the back heel activates the kidneys also supporting the heart. The peach is then brought into view, but it is too heavy and the situation must be supported as the monkey enjoys his find and soon to be "treat."

It has the function of tonifying the kidney, running qi and blood, lubricating the joints, regulating the nervous system of the whole body, and enhancing the coordination of the body. It also has a certain effect on neurasthenia, diarrhea, constipation, and senile osteoarthropathy.

4. Deer exercise.

Deer relates to the water element, the season of winter and therefore the kidney and bladder. The kidney emotion is fear and is often referred to as the "root of life" as they store essence. Essence determines basic constitution and is derived from parents and established at conception. The kidneys are the foundation of yin and yang in the body and therefore every other organ and govern birth, growth, reproduction, and development. They also produce marrow and control bones and the life gate, while housing will. By twisting the torso, the energy of one kidney is opened while the other is closed creating a pump to regulate chong vessel and therefore primordial qi. Fire (heart) and water (kidney) must connect energetically to maintain health. The hand gesture replicating horns calms spirit and connects with the heart by keeping the middle fingers in touch with the palms via the pericardium and triple energizers meridians. The eyes are the window to spirit and are smiling and joyous as we turn to look at the back heel and medial malleolus (kidney meridian), also connecting fire.

This movement can fully extend and exercise the spine, stretch muscles, and regulate the meridian. Enhancing visceral, massaging stomach, and promoting gastrointestinal peristalsis will have good curative effects on chronic diarrhea, constipation, prostate disease, cardiovascular disease, old chronic bronchitis, and other diseases.

5. Crane Exercise.

Crane relates to the metal element and the season of autumn and therefore the lung and large intestine. The lung emotion is sadness and lung governs qi and respiration, while being in charge of inhalation and the regulation of water passages. They are the intermediary organs between man and his environment, likened to a prime minister in charge of qi regulation particularly in the blood vessels to assist the heart in controlling blood circulation. The lung houses inferior spirit which is the most physical and material part of the human soul governing sensations and emotions. The activation of the microcosmic orbit is again featured by firstly working the spine in a concave fashion. The shoulders are raised and squeezed into the neck to squeeze the heart and pump blood while the arms are brought up to mimic a beak and the tailbone is thrust out. The arms are brought back along with one leg to mimic gliding. The second part of the exercise regulates the ascending (liver blood) and descending (lung qi) function of qi in the lung. The ultimate yin and yang expressed by breathing in (kidney) and breathing out (lung) connects these two organs to regulate blood and assist the heart. The rhythm created by the up and down movement of the body, the opening and closing of the arms (lung and large intestine meridians) and the in and out breath helps us adapt to the rhythmical changes of the seasons. The final stretch upwards on one leg stretches the flanks and therefore the liver and gall bladder meridians to balance with the lung. The lung is said to be spoilt being the last organ to start working just after birth and are therefore fragile and sensitive to change, explaining why gentle exercise is preferred.

This action can smooth liver qi and nourish liver blood and regulate the heart and lung, spleen-stomach function. It has a certain effect on hypertension, diabetes, depression, anxiety, cholecystitis, and other diseases.

4.4.4.2   The Six Healing Sounds

The six healing sounds is one of the common forms of Chinese qigong and involves the coordination of movement and breathing patterns with specific sounds. The six healing sounds is based on the yin and yang and five elements theory, in accordance with the attributes of the five zang viscera according to the spring, summer, autumn, and winter seasons, corresponding to the notes of the ancient pentatonic scale (gong, shang, jue, zhi, yu). With breathing, thinking, and limb guidance, to guide the yin of earth to rise, respire the yang of sky to decline, spit out the dirty air of organ, and inhale the clear air of nature, with the qi of body to make the zang and fu viscera and whole body healthy.

SI (belong to lung and metal), CHUI (belong to kidney and water), XU (belong to liver and wood), HE (belong to heart and fire), HU (belong to spleen and earth), XI (belong to triple energizers).

The term The six healing sounds first appears in a book called *On Caring for the Health of the Mind and Prolonging the Life Span* written by *Tao Hongjing* of the *Southern and Northern* dynasties. A leading figure of the Maoshan School of Taoism, *Tao* was renowned for his profound knowledge of TCM. "One has only one way for inhalation but six for exhalation," he wrote in the book.

The sounds of six healing sounds:

XU (pronounced like "shoe" with the lips rounded)—"deep sigh" or "hiss"— Level the liver qi. It can be used to treat eye diseases. Practicing this skill is effective for diseases related to liver fire, liver deficiency, liver swelling, in appetence, indigestion, and dry eyes, dizziness, and other symptoms.

HE (pronounced like "her")—"yawn" or "laughing sound"—Supplement the heart qi. It is used for the treatment of palpitation, angina, insomnia, forgetfulness, excessive sweating, erosion of the tongue, and other diseases.

HU (pronounced like "who")—"to sigh," "to exhale," or "to call"—Cultivate (or shore up) the spleen/pancreas qi. This method is used to treat spleen deficiency, diarrhea, abdominal distension, skin edema, muscle atrophy, indigestion, loss of appetite, hematochezia, menstrual disease, limb fatigue.

XI (pronounced like "she" with tongue high, and well forward, in the mouth)— "mirthful"—Regulate the triple burner qi. This method is suitable for cold, fever, cough, shortness of breath, shortness of breath, and less frequency of urine.

CHUI (pronounced "chway" or "chwee," depending on locale)—"to blow out," "to blast," or "to puff"—Supplement the kidney qi. This method is suitable for waist and leg weakness, eye soreness, forgetfulness, hectic fever, dizziness and tinnitus, spermatorrhea, impotence and premature ejaculation, tooth mobility, and hair loss.

SI (pronounced like "sir")—"to rest"—Supplement the lung qi. It is beneficial to treat tinnitus, vertigo, swollen and sore throat, chest and abdominal distention, unsmooth urine.

All syllables are pronounced on a level tone the so-called first tone (regardless of the dictionary pronunciation of each word); typically, all but the fifth sound are sustained—the fifth sound may be sustained, or pronounced quickly and forcefully.

4.4.4.3 Muscle and Tendon Changing Qigong

Muscle and tendon changing qigong is a manual containing a series of exercises, coordinated with breathing, is said to enhance physical health dramatically when practiced consistently. According to legend, the muscle and tendon changing qigong was invented by Bodhidharma. While some consider these exercises as a form of qigong, it is a relatively intense form of exercise that aims at strengthening the muscles and tendons, so promoting strength and flexibility, speed and stamina, balance and coordination of the body.

The basic purpose of muscle and tendon changing qigong is to turn flaccid and frail sinews and tendons into strong and sturdy ones. The movements of muscle and tendon changing qigong are vigorous and gentle. Their performance calls for a unity of will and strength, using one's will to direct the exertion of muscular strength. It is coordinated with breathing. Better muscles and tendons mean better health and shape, more resistance, flexibility, and endurance. It is obtained as follows:

1. Postures influence the static and nervous structure of the body;
2. Stretching muscles and sinews affect organs, joints, meridians and qi;
3. Torsion affects metabolism and jing production;
4. Breathing produces more and better refined qi;
5. Active working gives back balance and strength to body and mind (brain, nervous system and spirit).

The Exercises Illustrated:

1. Ready position.
   Start with feet together and arms and hands hang naturally by the sides. Step the left foot out so the feet are under the hips. The head is upright. The neck moves back as it touching a collar. The tongue tip is rises up to touch the palate. Loosen the shoulders and let the elbows drop.
2. Wei tuo presenting the pestle 1.
   Stand straight, with the half foot width apart. Throw out the chest, and tighten the abdomen. Hold the head erect, and look straight ahead. Keep the mouth closed, and let the tongue rest on the palate. Cup both hands in front of the chest with the eyes half-closed, inhale deeply through the nose, and exhale through the mouth 3 times. Turn the hands into yin palms (facing the ground) and slowly lift them up to shoulder level. Turn the hand into yin-yang palms (palms face each other) and bring them together in front of the chest. The two Shaoshang (LU 11) acupoints gently touch each other and the fingers point upward. The shoulders relax and the elbows drop. Breathe in Dantian so that qi gathers there.
3. Carrying a demon vanquishing pole across the shoulders.
   Turn the hands into yin palms (palms facing the ground), as you extend the arms out to the sides at the level of the shoulders. Simultaneously lift the heels and stand on tiptoe. Concentrate the heart-mind and look straight ahead with the chin gently drawn in and the back straight. Breathe naturally and concentrate the mind on Laogong (PC 8), in the center of the palm, and on the toes. As you fill inhale and fill Dantian, concentrate on Laogong (PC8). As you exhale, concentrate on the toes.
4. Uphold the heavenly gate in the palms.
   From the previous exercise, inhale and move the hands upward in an arc as you turn the palms upward to become yang palms (palms face upward). The arms form and arch the fingers of the two hands point toward each other just above the Tianmen (2 cun superior to the font hairline) acu-point as if holding the heavenly gate. Lift the heels and stand on tiptoe, moving the heels slightly

outward so as to close Huiyin (CV 1), while opening the Huiyang (BL 35). Gently clench the teeth (tongue tip still touching palate). Use inward vision to gaze through Tianmen at the space between the hands.

Make fists and let the arms follow the same arc they rose along to reach the position from exercise two: yin palms with arms extended out to the sides at the level of the shoulders. Simultaneously exhale and guide qi to Dantian. Repeat the exercise several times.

5. Plucking a star and exchanging a star cluster.

   From the previous exercise, slowly lift the right hand until it is just above and in front of the forehead for a distance of a fist. Simultaneously the left hand forms a fist and put it on the left lower side of the back. Focus your gaze on the right Laogong (PC 8).

6. Pulling nine cows by their tails.

   Following the previous form, take a big step forward with the right foot to form a left bow step, bending the right leg and straightening the left one. Clench the right fist and raise it toward the upper right, with the elbow bent and the thumb facing the waist, as if lifting a huge weight. Clench the left fist in front of the chest, and bend the left elbow. Then cross the fists in front of the lower abdomen and change to the right bow step. Repeat on the other side. Finally, cross the fists again in front of the lower abdomen.

7. Displaying paw-style palms like a white crane spreading its wings.

   Following the previous form, open the fists with palms outward and draw the arms back to the sides of chest, and legs back together. Raise the arms at the front to shoulder level. Stretch the arms forward, with the eyes focused on the hands. Straighten the legs, and apply the toes to the ground. Breathe 10 times as in the previous positions. Then clench the fists and bend the elbows. Draw the fists to the sides of the waist. Repeat 7 times.

8. Nine ghosts drawing swords.

   Following the previous form, raise your right hand upwards, over the head, to encircle the head with it. The palm is attached to the occipital bone, with the forefinger, middle finger, and ring finger, holding and gently pulling the ear tip of the left ear. The shoulder and elbow joints are at one height, and the right axilla is open. Place the left hand behind the back between two shoulder blades, and the left axilla is shut. Repeat on the opposite side of the body. Do 6–7 sets of this movement.

9. Three plates falling on the floor.

   Adopt the horse-riding stance, with the feet apart. Turn the toes slightly in, and the knees out. The knees should make approximately a right angle with the hip joints. Raise the hands to the level of the ears and then move them downwards with the palms down, until they hang loosely by the thighs. Strain both hands with eyes wide open. Do 3–5 sets of this movement—starting from half-squat and ending with a full squat.

10. Black dragon displaying its claws.

    Following the previous form, take back the left leg and be as wide as the shoulder. Lift the right hand to the side of the chest. Clench the fist, and turn the upper

body to the left. Open the right fist, stretch the right hand with the palm up toward
the front left, and stare at the right palm. Then turn the right palm down, and lower
the right arm without bending the elbow. Bend the waist with the movement of the
right hand. Move the right arm across the knees, and stretch it out and to the front.
Straighten the waist, drawing the right fist to the right side of the chest. Turn the
upper body to the right, and repeat the above movements on the other side. Finally,
return the body to an erect position, with the fists clenched at the sides.

11. Tiger springing on its prey.

    Take a big step forward with the right foot to form a right bow step, pressing
the toes to the ground. Lean the upper body forward, with the fingers apart and
slightly bent. Raise both hands with the palms up level with the top of the head.
Move the hands down across the ears to the front of the body and then lower
them to the ground in front of the extended right foot. Press the ground with the
fingers spread and the arms straight. Raise the head, and look forward like a
tiger about to pounce on its prey. Return the body to the erect position. Repeat
the above movements on the other side. Finally, stand straight.

12. Bowing down in salutation.

    Stand with the toes pointing outwards and the heels a fist's width apart.
Clasp the back of the head with both hands, with the palms covering the ears.
Use fingers to snare the back of your head. Bend at the waist and straighten the
knees. Touch the knees with the head. Return to the erect position with the
hands still clasping the back of the head. Do 3–5 sets of this movement.

13. Swinging the tail.

    Move the hands, with the fingers interlaced, to the top of the head. Turn the
palms up and stretch the arms upwards. Then reverse the palms and move them
downwards along the chest. Straighten the knees, and bend the waist, pressing
the palms on the toes. Hold the head up and look straight ahead. Then turn the
head to look to the right then look to the right. Do not raise the heels. However,
if you are unable to touch your toes, move the heels up and down in coordination with the breath. Finally, return to the erect position, stretch the arms forward horizontally with the fingers interlaced and palms forward.

14. Closing from.

    The two hands stand up and the two heels are slightly raised. Two palms out,
and draw an arc outward to the sides of the body, then take the hand back to the
armpit, the palm down. At the same time, the heel fell to the ground and the feet
were raised. Repeat 7 times.

4.4.4.4 Eight-Sectioned Exercise

Eight-sectioned exercise is one of the most common forms of Chinese qigong used
as exercise. Variously translated as eight-sectioned exercise, eight-section brocade,
eight silken movements or eight silk weaving, the name generally refers to how the
eight individual movements of the form characterize and impart a silken quality
(like that of a piece of brocade) to the body and its energy. The "Ba Duan Jin" is
primarily designated as a form of medical qigong, meant to improve health. This is

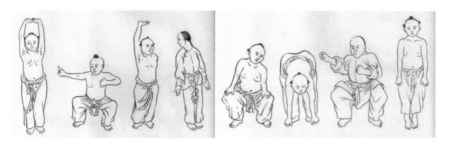

Fig. 4.8 Movements of eight-sectioned exercise

in contrast to religious or martial forms of qigong. The eight-sectioned exercise includes standing exercise and sitting exercise (Fig. 4.8).

Standing Exercise:

1. Both hands carry heaven to regulate the triple burner.

     This move is said to stimulate the triple energizers meridian. It consists of an upward movement of the hands, which are loosely joined and travel up the center of the body.
2. Draw the bow left and right as if to shoot a vulture.
3. While in a lower horse stance, the practitioner imitates the action of drawing a bow to either side. It is said to exercise the waist area, focusing on the kidneys and spleen.

     Regulate spleen-stomach by lifting one hand.

     This resembles a version of the first piece with the hands pressing in opposite directions, one up and one down. A smooth motion in which the hands switch positions is the main action, and it is said to especially stimulate the stomach.
4. Remedy the 5 symptoms and 7 disorders by looking backward.

     This is a stretch of the neck to the left and the right in an alternating fashion.
5. Turn the head and swing the tail to eliminate heart fire.

     This is said to regulate the function of the heart and lungs. Its primary aim is to remove excess fire from the heart. In performing this piece, the practitioner squats in a low horse stance, places the hands-on thighs with the elbows facing out, and twists to glance backward on each side.
6. Two hands grab the feet to strengthen kidneys and waist.

     This involves a stretch upwards followed by a forward bend and a holding of the toes.
7. Clench fists and look angry to increase qi and strength.

     This resembles the second piece and is largely a punching movement either to the sides or forward while in horse stance. As the most external of the pieces, this is aimed at increasing general vitality and muscular strength.
8. Jolt the back 7 times and hundred illnesses will disappear.

     This is a push upward from the toes with a small rocking motion on landing. The gentle shaking vibrations of this piece is said to "smooth out" the qi after practice of the preceding seven pieces or, in some systems, this is more specifically to follow swaying the head and shaking the tail.

4.5   Tai Chi

4.5.1   General Introduction of Tai Chi

Tai Chi means "Grand Ultimateness," and in Chinese culture, it represents an expansive philosophical and theoretical notion which describes the natural world (i.e., the universe) in the spontaneous state of dynamic balance between mutually interactive phenomena including the balance of light and dark, movement and stillness, waves, and particles. Tai Chi, the exercise, was named after this concept and was originally developed both as a martial art (Tai Chi) and as a form of meditative movement. The practice of Tai Chi as meditative movement is expected to elicit functional balance internally for healing, stress neutralization, longevity, and personal tranquility.

The concept of the Tai Chi ("supreme ultimateness") appears in both Taoist and Confucian philosophy, where it represents the fusion or mother of yin and yang into a single ultimateness, represented by the Taijitu symbol.

Tai Chi has become one of the best known forms of exercise or practice for refining qi and is purported to enhance physiological and psychological functions. The traditional Tai Chi is performed as a highly choreographed, lengthy, and complex series of movements. Today, Tai Chi has spread worldwide. Most modern styles of Tai Chi trace their development to at least one of the five traditional schools: Chen, Yang, Wu (wú), Wu (wǔ), and Sun style.

4.5.2   Brief History of Tai Chi

Tai Chi is a gentle and slow boxing, with soft and coherent movements. The word "Tai Chi" is first seen in *Zhouyi* (*The Changes of Zhou*), Tai means supreme, and Chi means the initial beginning or ultimate terminus. Tai Chi is a primitive view of the world of Chinese ancient people. After the combination of boxing and Tai Chi, gradually Tai Chi emerged.

There have always been a variety of statements about the origin of Tai Chi. The origin of Tai Chi was formed in the late *Ming* and early *Qing* dynasty. There are three main aspects in the origin of Tai Chi.

1. The integrated absorption of the famous *Ming* dynasty boxing. The *Ming* dynasty martial arts were very popular, and there were many famous and new boxing, and Tai Chi is invented by integrated absorption of the famous Ming dynasty boxing.
2. Integrated with ancient skills of breathing and Dao Yin method, Tai Chi is emphasized on both mind and action, so-called one of the inner kongfu.
3. Tai Chi has adopted Chinese traditional medicine theories of main and collateral meridians and the theories of yin-yang. Tai Chi requires "mind and intention to lead breath, guide the qi to drive body movements."

4.5.3   Main Schools of Tai Chi

Chen style: The most famous forms of Tai Chi practiced today are the Chen, Yang, Wu, Wu, and Sun styles. All the five styles can be traced back to Chen style. According to historical records, Tai Chi was founded by *Chen Wangting* (1597–1664), who lived in Chen Village, in today's Henan Province in China. There are two styles, an old Posture and a New Posture. The characteristics of Chen-style Tai Chi include showing hardness and implying softness, coupling hardness with softness, coiling and twisting the movements with changeable, disappearing, and fast-slow techniques. Practices pay attention to "internal rotation on Dantian" when breathing. The postures are commonly wide and low, containing powerful movements like jumping and foot stamping.

Yang-style: Yang-style Tai Chi is one of the important schools of Tai Chi with a long history of boxing. The Yang family first became involved in the study of Tai Chi in the early nineteenth century. The founder of the Yang-style was *Yang Luchan* (1800–1873), and his grandson *Yang Chengfu* (1883–1936) created the most popular Yang-style, which spread to the present. The national sports committee has officially publicized the type of Yang-style Tai Chi or its evolution, including the 48-style, 24-style, and many other styles which are performed popularly in many occasions. The characteristics of Yang-style Tai Chi: the movements are stretching, simple, and smooth, and the speed is even and continuous. The movements are carefully conceived and practically arranged. It embodies a unique style of beauty and grandeur.

Wu-style (wú): The Wu-style Tai Chi is a traditional boxing, one of the schools of Tai Chi, mainly from the boxing development innovation of Yang's Tai Chi. Yang-style Tai Chi has big and small frames, and Wu-style is gradually revised on the basis of small type Yang-style. Wu-styles is famous for its softness. The movements are easy and continuous with small and nimble fist type. The punches are compact and uninhibited. The hand pushing is tight, delicate, and quiet.

Wu-style (wǔ): *Wu Yuxiang* (1813–1880) was the creator of Wu-style. It is a separated family style from the more popular Wu-style. *Wu Yuxiang* was a scholar from a wealthy and influential family who was a friend of Yang Luchan and financially supported him in his endeavor to study Tai Chi. Wu-style Tai Chi is a distinctive style with small, subtle movements; highly focusing on balance, sensitivity and internal qi development. The movements of hands are within the length of toes, and each hand is in charge of the half body.

Sun-style: Sun-style Tai Chi was developed by *Sun Lutang*, who is considered an expert in two other internal martial arts styles: Xingyiquan and Baguazhang before he came to study Tai Chi. Today, Sun-style ranks fourth in popularity and fifth in terms of seniority among the five family styles of Tai Chi. The characteristics: linking forward and backward stepping, extending, swift and natural movements, and direction changes with opening and closing movements.

4.5.4   The Movement Characteristics of Tai Chi

4.5.4.1   Relax Body and Tranquilize Heart

Relaxing body and tranquilizing heart are the most important characteristics of Tai Chi. In practice, muscles are in a state of relaxation, naturally stretching, not rigid. "Peaceful heart" means to eliminate all thoughts and concentrate all attentions.

4.5.4.2   Slow and Gentle Strength

Slow and gentle strength is another important characteristic of Tai Chi. A set of simplified Tai Chi, 24 movements, according to the normal speed, should be finished in 5–6 min, slow and smooth.

4.5.4.3   Coordination of Movements, Breath, and Mind

When practicing Tai Chi, try to cooperate with the breath and the mind. The coordination of movements and mind means that you must remove all the distracting thoughts when practicing, and pay attention to movements. The consciousness should lead the movements and then make the entire body follow the mind.

4.5.5   Twenty-Four Form of Tai Chi

The 24-posture simplified form of Tai Chi is a short version of Tai Chi composed of twenty-four unique movements.

4.5.5.1   Starting Posture

Sink weight to the right leg and then step out to the left to shoulder width. Gently raise both arms up, palms facing down, to about shoulder height. Lower both arms, palms down, and lower knees.

4.5.5.2   Part the Wild Horse's Mane on Both Sides

Gently rise up both arms to normal height. Circle right arm counterclockwise up to chest height, with the palm facing down. Draw left arm to waist, with the palm facing up. Imagine holding a ball between the two hands. Draw the left foot to the side of the right foot. Step diagonally with the left leg, bring left hand out, palm up, to about chest height. Left elbow is slightly bent. Right hand moves down to right hip, with the right palm down. End with chest height. Left bow stance with 60% of weight in forward left leg, left knee bent, 40% of weight in rear right leg, with leg bend. Head upright and shoulders down. Then do the "part wild horse's mane to the right." Repeat left and right movements 3 times.

4.5.5.3   White Crane Spreads its Wings

With body turning slightly to the left, draw the right foot forward a half-step. The right hand moves upward as the left hand moves downward. Draw the left foot backward as the right hand moves up and left hand moves down. Finish with the right hand above the head and palm forward, in a left toe stance with the body weight in the back right leg, and the left hand rests along left leg with palm down. Relax and exhale as the weight settles down in the back right leg.

4.5.5.4   Brush Knees and Step Forward Left and Right

Right hand moves downward while left hand moves upward. Turn torso to the right, right hand circles past abdomen and the upward to ear level with arm lightly bend and palm facing upward, while left hand moves first in an upward, and then in a down ward curve, stopping before right part of chest, palm facing downward. Turn torso to the left. Left foot takes a step forward to form a left bow stance. At the same time, right hand draws left ward past right ear and pushes forward, while left hand drops and circles around left knee to stop beside left hip, with fingertips pointing forward.

4.5.5.5   Playing the Lute

Move the right foot half a step toward the left heel. Lightly shift the body center back to sit on the right leg. Extend the left heel a little forward touching the floor in an empty stance. At the same time, rotate the waist slightly to the right, lift the left arm and hand upward to the nose level, lower the right hand to guard the inside of the left elbow. Look at the forefinger of the left hand.

4.5.5.6   Reverse Reeling Forearm Left and Right

Turn torso slightly right, two hands turn upwards, with the right hand turning over backward arc up to the side of the ear height over shoulder, left hand stops in front of the body. Turn the upper body slightly to the left; step the left foot back, foot palm gently falls, eyes focus on the left hand. Move the upper part of the body center backward, continue to turn left, right into the empty step. The right hand is pushed to the front of the body, the left hand backward and downward, to the left side of the waist, the palm upwards; the eye looks right hand. Repeat twice these two movements.

4.5.5.7 Left Grasp Sparrow's Tail

Turn the body slightly to the right and make a hold-ball gesture at the right side. Then performs the 4 movements below.

1. Ward off.

    Turn the upper body to the left, the left foot steps to the left front into the left bow stance. Hands separate, left hand bends to the front of the body, right hand downward on the left hip side, fingers forward. Look at the left forearm.
2. Rollback.

    Turn upper body lightly to the left while extending the left hand forward with palm down. Right arm external rotate, upward and forward to the inside of the left arm, palm up. The body turns to right, and sits down at the same time. Then pulls the two hands downward past the abdomen and swing them up backward to the right until the right hand comes to the height of the shoulders with its palm upward and the left hand comes before the chest with its palm facing inward and the elbow bends horizontally. At the same time shifts the center of gravity to the right foot. The eyes are looking at the right hand.
3. Press.

    The center of gravity moves forward to the left bow stance, the right hand pushes the left forearm forward to the front of the body, and the arms turn to round.
4. Push.

    Sit back and shift weight onto the right leg which is slightly bent, raising toes of the left foot. Look straight ahead. The left hand turned down, right through the left wrist extending direction, palm steering, hands about shoulder width apart, arms bend after closing, close to the front of the abdomen, palms oblique. The center of gravity moves forward to the left bow; the two hands push along the arc to the front of the body.

4.5.5.8 Right Grasp Sparrow's Tail

Sit back and turn torso to the right, shifting weight onto the right leg and turning left toes inwards. Slowly bend arms, and assume the ball-holding position in front of the left side of the body. While in the ball-holding position, the right foot is pulled toward the left without the toes touching the ground. Then repeat the movement of left grasp sparrow's tail, just reverse the direction.

4.5.5.9   Single Whip

The upper body turns left, the right foot turns inward. Carrying both hands leftward with the left hand on top until the left arm is extended sideways at shoulder level with the palm facing outward, and the right hand is in front of the left ribs with palm facing obliquely inward. Look at the left hand.

Then turns the body to right, left foot makes a T-step. As the right arm gets to the right side, the hand is shaped into a beak style (thumb touches the other fingers and all fingers point down). The left arm is drawn up to the face level, with the palm facing the face. Look at the left hand.

The upper body turns left, left foot steps to the left front into the left bow step, turning the left palm forward.

4.5.5.10   Cloud Hands

Turn upper body to the right, the left foot turns inward. The left hand turns down, moves the left hand in a curve past abdomen to the front of the right shoulder, the palm turns inward, the right hand turns beak style to palm. Then turns to the left, move body weight to left, the left hand moves to the left side slowly, right hand moves in a curve past abdomen up to the front of the left shoulder with the palm slowly turning obliquely inward. Eyes move with the left hand. Turn torso slowly to the right, the left hand turns to right shoulder, palm turns slowly backward, left leg moves to the left a step, looks at left hand. Then repeat upper movement twice.

4.5.5.11   Single Whip

Same as Sect. 4.5.5.9.

4.5.5.12   High Pat on Horse

From single whip, draw the right foot forward a half-step. The right hand changes from a beaked hand into an open hand. The right arm moves forward at about face level from right to left, and ends with palm facing out in front of the body at face level. The torso turns to the left. The right hand stops at face level, with the palm facing out and away. The left hand moves in a downward arc to the Dan Tien level, and ends with the left palm facing up. The left leg is in an empty toe stance. Look at the right hand.

4.5.5.13   Right Heel Kick

Turn torso slightly right, the left foot steps to left front. The right hand pulls back, the left hand crosses the right hand from upside. Cross two hands, with the left palm slanted upward, and the right palm slanted downward. Next movement, move body weight forward into the left bow step; the upper body slightly right, two hands separate to the side and make a curve with palms outward. Look at right hand. Then hold back hands and foot, right foot make a T-step, two hands crossed in front of chest, right hand at out, and two palms turn inside. Next movement, two palms turn outside and pull separated to the body side. Right leg and foot kick out gradually to the right front, look at the right hand.

4.5.5.14   Strike to Ears with Both Fists

From the right heel kick position, draw the right knee back into the body to waist level. Draw both hands down and bring the elbows to the sides of the body, closing the open hands into fists and holding the hands level with the knee. Step forward with the right leg. Circle the arms outward from the body and then draw both fists toward the head level of an imaginary opponent to strike the opponent's temples with both fists. Settle into a right bow stance.

4.5.5.15   Turn Body and Left Heel Kick

The same as those kick with right heel at the left side.

4.5.5.16   Left Lower Body and Stand on One Leg

Pull back the left foot and keep at thigh level. Turn the body to the right side, the right arm pull close, the right hand turn to hook shape, move the left hand in a curve to the front of the right should. Look at the hook hand. Then turn the body to the left, the right knee bend, the left leg step forward to make a left half-squat stance, the left hand move down and along the inner side of the left leg forward, look at the left hand. Move the weight to left and make a lunge stance, then stand up with the left foot, raise the right leg up. At the same time, put the left hand at the side of left hip; right elbow is over right knee. Look at right hand.

4.5.5.17   Right Lower Body and Stand on One Leg

Repeat movement of (16), just reverse right and left.

4.5.5.18 Shuttle Back and Forth

Step left foot forward and diagonally, draw right foot to left foot, step out with right foot diagonally to right. Raise right arm to block out above head, palm facing out. Left palm strike. Right leg bow stance. Bring the left leg up, and bring arms to chest. Step diagonally to the left side with left foot. Raise left arm to block out above head, palm facing out. Right palm strikes. Left leg makes a bow stance.

4.5.5.19 Needle at Sea Bottom

From the last posture of "Shuttle back and forth, " begin by stepping forward a half-step with the right leg. The right hand moves back and up to the right until it is drawn up to around face level on the right side. The left hand moves down in an arc until it comes to stop at about waist height over the left leg. Lift up the left leg and step forward a half-step into a left toe stance. Settle the body weight into the right leg. Reach down with the right hand, fingers pointing downward, until the right hand is below the waist.

4.5.5.20 Fan Through Back

Turn the body slightly to the right to straight direction, lift the right hand to the chest level, the left arm draw back with fingers near to the wrist, takes the left foot near the right foot. Sink the body weight into the left leg, and take a left bow stance, pull the left hand to the front of body. The right hand moves up and back to the left, finishing above head level, palm facing up, and fingers pointing upward. Look at the left hand.

4.5.5.21 Turn Body, Deflect, Parry, and Punch

Sit back and shift weight onto the right leg. Turn the body right, move the right hand to the body side, and left hand to the left side of head. Look at the right hand. Then shift weight to the left, the right fist move down and left to the left rib, palm face down, left hand raise up to the left side of forehead. Look straight ahead.

Turn the body to the right side, pull the right foot near the left foot, the step forward on heel. Bring right fist up and then forward and down ward for a backhand punch. Put the left hand lower to the side of the left hip with palm down. Look at the right fist.

Shift weight to the right and turn body to right, move the right fist to the side of the body, and move the left arm outward make a curve in front of the body with palm upward. Look at the left hand. Bend the left leg for a left bow stance as you strike out the fight fist forward at chest level while the left hand withdraws to the side of the right forearm. Look at the right fist.

4.5.5.22 Apparent Close-Up

From the end of deflect, parry and punch, begin by drawing the left hand under the right hand from the forearm toward the right hand. Both hands come together in front of the body. Draw both arms backward toward the body as the weight shifts backward into the right leg. As both hands reach the waist, the weight is on the back right leg and the left toe rises. Drawing the weight into the left leg and taking a left bow stance, and then begin to move forward again. Both arms push forward, palms out, elbows bent. Look straight ahead.

4.5.5.23 Cross Hands

Begin from the push position. Gradually turn the front of the body to the right. Draw the right hand in an arc out and across to the left. Draw the weight into the right leg. Open the arms wide to both sides, palms facing forward, arms about shoulder height. Step the right foot back to shoulder width stance. Draw both arms down in an arc then up to cross the hands in front of the chest, holding the right hand in front of left hand. Look straight ahead.

4.5.5.24 Closing

The crossed-arms push slowly forward and rotate inward. Turn over both hands downward, at shoulders' width. Moving arms down and put outward until they reach the waist. Bring the foot back slightly next to the right foot, same like the "Starting posture."

You have now finished a full performance of the Tai Chi 24 Form.

4.5.6 Health Benefits

Before Tai Chi was introduced to Western people, the health benefits of Tai Chi were largely explained through traditional Chinese medicine, based on a view of the body and healing mechanisms which may not always be studied or supported by modern science. Today, Tai Chi is in the process of being subjected to rigorous scientific studies in the west.

Now that the majority of health studies have displayed a tangible benefit in some areas to the practice of Tai Chi, health professionals have called for more in-depth studies to determine mitigating factors such as the most beneficial style, suggested duration of practice to show the best results, and whether tai chi is as effective as other forms of exercise.

4.6 Summary

Massage originated from TCM and characterized by its own theory. Usually massage could classify for adult and infantile massages both of them are quite different from theory to manipulation. In adult massage, spinal manipulation as a special treatment to adjust the vertebrate subluxation is popularized in modern times. Dietary therapy and qigong are subjects under the guidance of the theory of Traditional Chinese Medicine to study diet treatment of diseases. It is an important part of TCM clinical medicine. Tai Chi has become one of the best known forms of exercise or practice for refining qi and is purported to enhance physiological and psychological function. All of those methods have enriched the therapies of TCM.

Questions
1. What's the category of massage manipulation?
2. What's the different between adult massage and infantile massage?
3. What are the methods of dietary therapy?
4. How to understand the qigong and Tai Chi?

References

1. Hongzhu J. Science of Tuina. Beijing: People's Medical Publishing House; 2007.
2. Zhihong W, Tianyuan Y. Science of Tuina. Beijing: China Press of Traditional Chinese Medicine; 2012.
3. Yikai L, Wei Z. Science of Tuina. Beijing: Science Press; 2012.
4. Enqin Z. Chinese massage. Shanghai: Publishing House of Shanghai University of Traditional Chinese Medicine; 1990.
5. Dafang Y. Science of Tuina. Shanghai: Shanghai Scientific and Technical Publishing House; 1991.
6. Changguo W. Basic theory of traditional Chinese medicine. Shanghai: Publishing House of Shanghai University of Traditional Chinese Medicine; 2006.
7. Mingjun L, Jingui W. Science of pediatric Tuina. Beijing: China Press of Traditional Chinese Medicine; 2016.
8. Tianyou F. Clinical study on the treatment of soft tissue injury by Chinese integrative medicine. Beijing: China Science and Technology Press; 2002.
9. Hongfei S, Hong F. Traditional Chinese dietary therapy. Beijing: Chinese Medicine Publishing House of China; 2016.
10. Tianjun L, Wenchun Z. Qigong of traditional Chinese medicine. Beijing: Chinese Medicine Publishing House of China; 2016.
11. Bo W. The primary course of tai chi both in Chinese and English. Beijing: Beijing Normal University Press; 2014.

Chapter 5
Common Diseases

Xinjun Wang, Yang Yang, Ying Xiong, Ruiqin Cui, Rui Wang, Xiaowen Cai, and Yong Huang

5.1 Wind Stroke

Objectives

Master the knowledge about the treatment of wind stroke based on syndrome differentiation via learning the etiology, pathogenesis, diagnosis, differentiation, treatment, and prevention of wind stroke.

Guideline

This chapter introduces the etiology, pathogenesis, diagnosis, differential diagnosis, treatment (herbal medicine and acupuncture), and prevention of wind stroke.

X. Wang · Y. Xiong
Nanjing University of Chinese Medicine, Nanjing, China

Y. Yang · R. Wang
Hebei University of Chinese Medicine, Hebei, China

R. Cui
Ningxia Medical University, Yinchuan, Ningxia, China

X. Cai
Southern Medical University, Guangzhou, China

Y. Huang (✉)
School of Traditional Chinese Medicine, Southern Medical University, Guangzhou, China

© Zhengzhou University Press 2024
Y. Huang, L. Zhu (eds.), *Textbook of Traditional Chinese Medicine*,
https://doi.org/10.1007/978-981-99-5299-1_5

5.2 Introduction

The Chinese term "wind stroke," also known as stroke or apoplexy, refers to an emergency case manifested by the sudden loss of consciousness or sensation, accompanied by a deviated mouth, slurred speech, and hemiplegia. In mild cases, there is just hemiplegia, deviation of the mouth, dysphasia, or aphasia without sudden coma.

Wind stroke is characterized by symptoms occurring abruptly and pathological changes varying quickly like the wind, from which the Chinese term comes. *Internal Classic* records the symptoms of wind stroke, even without mentioning the term itself.

This disease corresponds to the Western medicine term for cerebrovascular accident (CVA), including cerebral hemorrhage, cerebral thrombosis, cerebral infarction, subarachnoid hemorrhage, cerebral vasospasm, and even viral encephalitis, a cerebral facial paralysis in Western medicine.

5.2.1 Etiology

The onset of wind stroke is attributed to overworking, emotional stress, and irregular diet based on zang-fu viscera deficiency for a long time.

5.2.1.1 Deficiency for a Long Time

Zang-fu viscera deficiency is caused by a yin deficiency constitution or being old and feeble for a long time.

5.2.1.2 Overstrain from Physical Work and Sexual Activity with Inadequate Rest

Overstrain from physical work, such as excessive lifting or sports activities and excessive exercise with inadequate rest, takes the muscles and the meridians weakened and sweat lost too much, causing deficiency of both qi and yin. Overstrain from sexual activity in humans combined with inadequate rest consumes essence too much, causing deficiency of kidney yin. The deficient qi and yin lead to the failure in restricting yang. The internal wind is caused by unrestricted yang.

5.2.1.3   Irregular Diet

Eating irregularly or eating excessive amounts of fats, sugar, dairy foods, fried foods, barbecue or alcoholic indulgence weakens the spleen and leads to phlegm. Phlegm causes internal fire, which brings phlegm into the meridians and brain.

5.2.1.4   Emotional Disorders

Emotional disorders, such as depression, anxiety, anger, and stress, transform heart and liver qi to fire, which makes qi and blood go upward into the brain.

5.2.1.5   Exogenous Pathogenic Factors

External pathogenic qi intrudes into meridians under weakened healthy qi conditions when the weather changes.

5.2.2   Pathogenesis

5.2.2.1   Pathogenic Site

The pathogenic site of wind stroke is located in the brain and heart, involving the liver, spleen, and kidney.

5.2.2.2   Pathological Nature

The pathological nature of wind stroke is a deficiency in origin and excess in symptoms. Deficiency in origin in wind stroke includes liver and kidney yin deficiency and dual deficiency of qi. Excess symptoms in wind stroke consist of pathogenic wind, pathogenic fire, phlegm, and blood stasis.

5.2.2.3   Basic Pathogenesis

The pathology of wind stroke may be summarized in yin-yang disharmony and qi and blood disorder. Pathogenic wind and fire due to deficiency of liver and kidney yin both qi and yin for a long time forces phlegm (caused by spleen yang deficiency) and blood stasis (caused by qi deficiency) to go upward together under emotional fluctuation or weather-changing conditions. Pathogenic wind, fire, phlegm, and blood stasis attacking just meridians cause deviated mouth, slurred speech, and hemiplegia. If zang-fu viscera and meridians are affected, the diseases will manifest sudden loss of consciousness and sensation in addition to those symptoms.

5.2.2.4 Pathogenesis in Different Disease Stages

During the acute stage of a wind stroke attack, pathogenic wind, fire, phlegm, and blood stasis play the stagnation leading roles. Therefore, wind stroke shows excess symptoms. Liver wind invades meridians with phlegm, blocks qi, and blood movement in tendons and muscles, and causes loss of unilateral limb activity, facial paralysis, and pararthria. If pathogenic wind and fire are so fierce as to ascend to head with the turbid damp phlegm and blood stasis, it will obstruct the clear orifices and brain vessels; make the brain bleed, even separate yin and yang, and collapse the patient.

During the restoration and sequelae stage of a wind stroke attack, disordered qi and blood, phlegm, and blood stasis staying in meridians and collaterals cause sequelae, including limb numbness, weakness and less activities, speech, and swallowing difficulties.

5.2.3 Diagnosis

- Sudden onset, dizziness, unilateral numbness and activity difficulties, deviated mouth and slurred speech, and even loss of consciousness.
- Occurring in the middle-aged and the aged who are in poor health.
- Premonitory symptoms include dizziness, headache, and unilateral limb numbness.
- Predisposing factors include emotional stress, overwork, overdrinking, and irregular diet.

5.2.4 Differentiation

5.2.4.1 Differentiation of Zang-Fu Viscera and Meridians Attacked with Wind Stroke

Zang-fu viscera being attacked with wind stroke are characterized by loss of consciousness, possible coma, hemiplegia, numbness, and aphasia. The loss of consciousness indicates an attack on the zang-fu viscera.

Meridians being attacked with wind stroke are characterized by unilateral paralysis, numbness, deviated mouth, and slurred speech. There is no loss of consciousness or coma.

5.2.4.2 Differentiation of Tense Type and Flaccid Type

There are two types of pattern in wind stroke attacking zang-fu viscera: one called tense type (excessive syndrome corresponding to hard pathogenic qi), and the other called flaccid type (deficient syndrome corresponding to yin and yang separated from each other).

1. Tense type

    The main manifestations are sudden falling down in a fit with loss of consciousness, coma, tightly clinched hands, and clenched jaws, closed fists, red face and ears, coarse breathing, rattling in the throat, profuse sputum, constipation, retention of urine, stiff deviated red tongue with thick yellow or dark grey coating, wiry slippery, and rapid pulse.

2. Flaccid type

    The main manifestations are sudden falling down with a loss of consciousness, coma, opening hands and mouth, closed eyes, weak nasal breathing, flaccid tongue, flushed face, oily sweat beads on the forehead, cold limbs, incontinence of urine and stools, and weak faint thread pulse.

5.2.4.3 Differentiation of Yang Tense Type and Yin Tense Type

Both the yang tense type and yin tense type manifest falling down in a fit and sudden loss of consciousness with closed eyes and mouth.

1. Yang tense type

    Pathogenic factors of the yang tense type are phlegm and fire. The main manifestations are red face and ears, coarse breathing, rattling in the throat, profuse sputum, constipation, retention of urine, red tongue with a yellow greasy thick coating, and wiry slippery and rapid pulse.

2. Yin tense type

    Pathogenic factors of the yin tense type are cold dampness and phlegm. The main manifestations are a white face, purple lips, cold limbs, profuse sputum, light red tongue with a white and greasy coating, and a deep slippery fainting pulse.

5.2.4.4 Differentiation of Disease Stages

- Acute stage: 2 weeks.
- Restoration stage: from 2 weeks to 6 months.
- Scquelae stage: more than 6 months.

5.2.5 Treatment

5.2.5.1 Principles of Treatment

1. The general principles of treatment for the attack on meridians and collaterals are pacifying the liver, extinguishing wind, resolving phlegm, dispelling blood stasis, and dredging meridians.
2. The general principles of treatment for an attack of tense type on zang-fu viscera are clearing away fire, extinguishing wind, clearing up phlegm, opening orifices, relaxing bowels, and discharging heat.
3. The general principles of treatment for an attack of flaccid type on zang-fu viscera are restoring yang to stop the collapse, activating the brain, and regaining consciousness.
4. The general principles of treatment for restoration and sequelae stage of wind stroke attack are reinforcing healthy qi, clearing pathogenic qi, treating symptoms and root causes, pacifying liver, extinguishing wind, nourishing liver and kidney, resolving phlegm, dispelling blood stasis, reinforcing qi, and nourishing blood.

5.2.5.2 Chinese Medicinal Treatment

Attack on Meridians and Collaterals

Wind–Phlegm Attacking Collaterals Syndrome

Characteristic symptoms: skin numbness, especially on one-side of the body, sudden deviated mouth and slurred speech, even unilateral paralysis, light red tongue with white and thin coating, and floating rapid pulse.

Key pathogenesis: wind–phlegm attacking collaterals with deficient qi and blood.

Therapeutic principle and method: dispelling wind, resolving phlegm, and dredging meridians.

Major prescription: Zhenfang Baiwanzi Tang Vaviation.

Herbs: Banxia, Tiannanxing, Baifuzi, Tianma, Quanxie, Danggui, Baishao, Jixueteng, and Xixiancao.

Explanation:

Banxia, Tiannanxing, and Baifuzi: to dispel wind and resolve phlegm.

Tianma and Quanxie: to extinguish wind and dredge collaterals.

Danggui, Baishao, Jixueteng, Xixiancao: to nourish blood and dispel wind.

Modification: For cases with slurred speech, Shichangpu added; for cases with purple tongue with blood stasis, Danshen, Taoren, Honghua, and Chishao added.

Wind and Liver Yang Harassing Upper Energizer Syndrome

Characteristic symptoms: dizziness, headache, and tinnitus as usual, sudden deviated mouth and slurred speech, even unilateral paralysis, red tongue with yellow coating, and wiry pulse.

Key pathogenesis: liver yang transforming into wind which invades into collaterals.

Therapeutic principle and method: pacifying liver and subduing yang, activating blood, and dredging meridians.

Major prescription: Tianma Gouteng Yin.

Herbs: Tianma, Gouteng, Zhenzhumu, Shijueming, Sangye, Juhua, Huangqin, Zhizi, and Niuxi.

Explanation:

Tianma and Quanxie: to extinguish wind and dredge collaterals.

Zhenzhumu and Shijueming: to settle liver and subdue yang.

Sangye and Juhua: to clear the liver and discharge heat.

Huangqin and Zhizi: to clear the liver and drain the fire.

Niuxi: to activate blood, resolve stasis, and guide blood to flow downward.

Modification: For cases with chest stuffy, nausea, and greasy coating, Dannanxing, Yujin added; for cases with severe headache, Lingyangjiao, Xiakucao added; and for cases with heavy legs, Duzhong, Sangjisheng added.

Syndrome of Stirring Wind Due to Yin Deficiency

Characteristic symptoms: dizziness, tinnitus, and soreness of the waist as usual, sudden deviated mouth, slurred speech, and trembling fingers, even unilateral paralysis, red tongue with greasy coating, and wiry thready rapid pulse.

Key pathogenesis: liver and kidney yin deficiency and wind–phlegm obstructing meridians.

Therapeutic principle and method: nourishing yin, subduing yang, extinguishing wind, and dredging meridians.

Major prescription: Zhenggan Xifeng Tang Vaviation.

Herbs: Baishao, Tiandong, Xuanshen, Gouqizi, Longgu, Muli, Guiban, Daizheshi, Niuxi, Danggui, Tianma, and Gouteng.

Explanation:

Baishao, Tiandong, Xuanshen, and Gouqizi: to nourish yin, emolliate liver, and extinguish wind.

Longgu, Muli, Guiban, and Daizheshi: to settle liver and subdue yang.

Niuxi and Danggui: to activate blood, resolve stasis, and guide blood to flow downward.

Tianma and Gouteng: to pacify the liver and extinguish wind.

Modification: For cases with too much phlegm and fire, nausea, and yellow greasy coating, Dannanxing, Zhuli, and Chuanbeimu added; for cases with vexing heat in the chest, Zhizi and Huangqin added.

Attack on Zang-Fu Viscera

Tense Type
Syndrome of Fu-Viscera Excess Caused by Phlegm–Heat

Characteristic symptoms: headache, dizziness, dysphoria, testiness, constipation, abdominal distension, sudden loss of consciousness, possibly coma, deviated mouth and slurred speech, muscle rigidity, profuse greasy sputum, dull-red tongue with yellow greasy coating, and wiry slippery pulse.

Key pathogenesis: wind–phlegm attacking upper energizer and phlegm and heat obstructing fu-viscera.

Therapeutic principle and method: relaxing bowels, discharging heat, extinguishing wind, and resolving phlegm.

Major prescription: Taohe Chengqi Tang Vaviation.

Herbs: Taoren, Dahuang, Mangxiao, Zhishi, Dannanxing, Huangqin, Gualou, Taoren, Chishao, Mudanpi, and Niuxi.

Explanation:

Taoren, Dahuang, Mangxiao, and Zhishi: to relax bowels, discharge heat, cool blood, and resolve blood stasis.

Dannanxing, Huangqin, Gualou: to clear heat and resolve phlegm.

Taoren, Chishao, Mudanpi: to cool blood and resolve blood stasis.

Niuxi: to guide blood to flow downward.

Modification: For cases with severe headache and dizziness, Gouteng, Juhua, and Zhenzhumu added; for cases with dysphoria, insomnia, dry mouth, and red tongue, Shengdihuang, Shashen, and Yejiaoteng added.

Syndrome of Orifices Closed by Phlegm–Fire

Characteristic symptoms: sudden loss of consciousness, coma, tightly clinched hands and clenched jaws, closed fists, red face and ears, coarse fetid breathing, rattling in the throat, constipation, retention of urine, red tongue with yellow greasy coating, wiry slippery, and rapid pulse.

Key pathogenesis: phlegm–fire caused by liver yang obstructing orifices.

Therapeutic principle and method: extinguishing wind, clearing hire, eliminating phlegm, and opening orifices.

Major prescription: Lingjiao Gouteng Tang Vaviation.

Herbs: Lingyangjiao or Shanyangjiao, Gouteng, Zhenzhumu, Shijueming, Dannanxing, Zhuli, Banxia, Tianzhuhuang, Huanglian, Shichangpu, and Yujin.

Explanation:

Lingyangjiao or Shanyangjiao, Gouteng, Zhenzhumu, and Shijueming: to pacify the liver and extinguish wind.

Dannanxing, Zhuli, Banxia, Tianzhuhuang, and Huanglian: to clear heat and resolve phlegm.

Shichangpu and Yujin: to resolve phlegm and open orifices.

Modification: For cases with gurgling with sputum in the throat, Zhuli taken orally; for cases with dry red tongue with yellow rough coating, Shengdihuang, Shashen, Maidong, and Shihu added.

Syndrome of Orifices Closed by Profuse Phlegm

Characteristic symptoms: sudden loss of consciousness, coma, tightly clinched hands, and clenched jaws, red face, lip with dead color, closed fists, profuse sputum, rattling in the throat, lying still, cool limbs, constipation, retention of urine, white greasy coating, and slippery deep slow pulse.

Key pathogenesis: profuse phlegm closing orifices.

Therapeutic principle and method: eliminating phlegm and opening orifices.

Major prescription: Ditan Tang Vaviation.

Herbs: Banxia, Fuling, Hua Juhong, Zhuru, Dannanxing, Shichangpu, Yujin, Tianma, Gouteng, and Jiangcan.

Explanation:

Banxia, Fuling, Hua Juhong, Zhuru: to resolve phlegm.

Dannanxing, Shichangpu, Yujin: to eliminate phlegm and open orifices.

Tianma, Gouteng, Jiangcan: to extinguish wind and resolve phlegm.

Modification: For cases with hectic cheek and faint pulse verging on expiry, Shenfu Tang taken orally.

Flaccid Type (Syndrome of Collapse of Yang and Exhaustion of Yin)

Characteristic symptoms: sudden loss of consciousness, coma, opening hands and mouth, closed eyes, weak nasal breathing, flaccid paralysis of limbs, excess sweating, incontinence of urine and stools, and weak faint thread pulse.

Key pathogenesis: pathogenic qi defeating collapsed healthy qi.

Therapeutic principle and method: restoring yang to save from collapse with replenished qi.

Major prescription: Shenfu Tang plus Shengmai San Vaviation.

Herbs: Renshen, Fuzi, Maidong, Wuweizi, Shanzhuyu.

Explanation:

Renshen and Fuzi: to replenish qi to restore yang.

Maidong, Wuweizi, and Shanzhuyu: to nourish yin and astringe yang.

Modification: For cases with excess sweat, Longgu and Muli added.

Restoration and Sequelae Stage of Wind Stroke Attack

During the acute stage of wind stroke, the best results are obtained if treatment is given within 1 month after the attack. However, if treatments are not delivered or good effects are not got, once the occurrence of hemiplegia and facial paralysis is kept for more than 6 months, the sequelae stage comes.

Wind stroke attack during the sequelae stage manifests limb numbness and loss of activities, speech, and swallowing difficulties.

The principles of treatment are reinforcing healthy qi, clearing pathogenic qi, and treating both symptoms and causes.

Wind–Phlegm and Blood Stasis Obstructing Collaterals Syndrome

Characteristic symptoms: limb numbness, hemiplegia, facial paralysis, slurred speech, purple tongue with slippery greasy coating, and wiry slippery pulse.

Key pathogenesis: wind–phlegm and blood stasis obstructing qi and blood in collaterals.

Therapeutic principle and method: dispelling wind, resolving phlegm, activating blood, and dredging meridians.

Major prescription: Jieyu Dan.

Herbs: Tianma, Dannanxing, Tianzhuhuang, Banxia, Chenpi, Dilong, Quanxie, Jiangcan, Yuanzhi, Shichangpu, Jixueteng, Xixiancao, Sangzhi, Danshen, and Honghua.

Explanation:

Tianma, Dannanxing, Tianzhuhuang, Banxia, Chenpi: to extinguish wind and resolve phlegm.

Dilong, Quanxie, and Jiangcan: to dispel wind and dredge meridians.

Yuanzhi, Shichangpu: to resolve phlegm and open orifices.

Jixueteng, Xixiancao, Sangzhi, Danshen, and Honghua: to dispel wind, activate blood, and dredge meridians.

Modification: For cases with profuse phlegmatic and heat, Gualou, Zhuru, and Chuanbeimu added; for cases with dizziness, headache, red face, red tongue, greasy coating, and wiry powerful pulse, Gouteng, Shijueming, and Xiakucao added; for cases with a dry throat and mouth, Tianhuafen and Tiandong added.

Qi Deficiency and Blood Stasis in Collateral Syndrome

Characteristic symptoms: unilateral limb paralysis, lack of strength, sallow complexion, purple tongue, and weak unsmooth pulse.

Key pathogenesis: qi deficiency, blood stasis, and obstructed collaterals.

Therapeutic principle and method: replenishing qi, nourishing blood, resolving blood stasis, and dredging collaterals.

Major prescription: Buyang Huanwu TangVaviation.

Herbs: Huangqi, Taoren, Honghua, Chishao, Danggui and Chuanxiong, Dilong and Niuxi.

Explanation:

Huangqi: to replenish qi and nourish the blood.

Taoren, Honghua, Chishao, Danggui, and Chuanxiong: to nourish the blood, resolve blood stasis, and dredge collaterals.

Dilong and Niuxi: to activate blood, resolve stasis, and guide blood to flow downward.

Modification: For cases with blood deficiency, Gouqizi and Shouwuteng added; for cases with cold limbs, Guizhi added; for cases with soreness and weakness of the waist and knees, Xuduan, Duzhong, and Sangjisheng added.

Syndrome of Liver and Kidney Deficiency

Characteristic symptoms: unilateral paralysis, stiff muscular contracture or amyotrophy limb, slurred speech with tense tongue, deep thready pulse.

Key pathogenesis: tendon and muscle malnutrition due to liver and kidney deficiency.

Therapeutic principle and method: nourishing liver and kidney.

Major prescription: Zuogui Wan plus Dihuang Yin.

Herbs: Shengdihuang, Heshouwu, Gouqizi, Shanzhuyu, Maidong, Shihu, Danggui and Jixueteng.

Explanation:

Shengdihuang, Heshouwu, Gouqizi, and Shanzhuyu: to replenish kidney essence.

Maidong and Shihu: to nourish yin and promote fluid production.

Danggui and Jixueteng: to nourish blood and collaterals.

Modification: For cases with soreness lumber and weak legs, Duzhong, Sangjisheng, and Niuxi added; for cases with kidney yang deficiency, Roucongrong, Bajitian, Fuzi, and Rougui added; and for cases with phlegm, Yuanzhi, Shichangpu, and Fuling added.

5.2.5.3 Acupuncture and Moxibustion Treatment

Attack on Meridians and Collaterals

Acupoints: Shuigou (GV 26), Jiquan (HT 1), Chize (LU 5), Neiguan (PC 6), Weizhong (BL 40), and Sanyinjiao (SP 6).

Methods: Reducing manipulation is applied to Shuigou (GV 26), till the tears of patients fall out. Apply the reducing method with lifting and thrusting to Jiquan (HT 1), Chize (LU 5), Neiguan (PC 6), Weizhong (BL 40), and Sanyinjiao (SP 6) till the patient feels numbness in the diseased limbs.

Modification: For cases with deviation of the mouth: Dicang (ST 4) and Jiache (ST 6); for cases with upper limbs hemiplegia: Jianyu (LI 15), Quchi (LI 11), Shousanli (LI 10), Hegu (LI 4) and Houxi (SI 3); for cases with lower limbs hemiplegia: Huantiao (GB 30), Yanglingquan(GB 34), Zusanli (ST 36) and Taichong (LR 3); for cases with constipation: Tianshu (ST 25), Zhigou (TE 6), and Shangjuxu (ST 37); for cases with slurred speech and stiff tongue: Lianquan (CV 23) and Tongli (HT 5).

Attack on Zang-Fu Viscera

Acupoints: Shenque (CV 8), Shuigou (GV 26), twelve Jing (well) points, and Yongquan (KI 1).

Methods: Apply indirect moxibustion with salt to Shenque (CV 8). Reducing manipulation is applied to Shuigou (GV 26), till the tears of patients fall out. Apply the bleeding method to twelve Jing (well) points. Apply the reducing method with lifting and thrusting to Yongquan (KI 1).

Modification: For cases with lockjaw: Jiache (ST 6), Xiaguan (ST 7), and Hegu (LI 4); for cases with profuse sputum: Tiantu (CV22) and Fenglong (ST 40).

Restoration and Sequelae Stage of Wind Stroke Attack

Acupoints: Baihui (GV 20), Fengfu (GV16), Pishu (BL 20), Zhongwan (CV12), Zusanli (ST 36), Fenglong (ST 40), Guanyuan (CV 4), Sanyinjiao (SP 6) and Taixi (KI 3).

Methods: Apply reducing manipulation to Baihui (GV20) and Fengfu (GV16); reinforcing manipulation is applied to Pishu (BL 20), Zhongwan (CV 12), Zusanli (ST 36), Fenglong (ST 40), Guanyuan (CV4), Sanyinjiao (SP 6), and Taixi (KI 3).

Modification: For cases with a deviation of the mouth: Dicang (ST 4) and Jiache (ST 6); for cases with constipation: Tianshu (ST 25), Zhigou (TE 6), and Shangjuxu (ST 37); and for cases with slurred speech and stiff tongue: Lianquan (CV 23), and Tongli (HT 5).

5.2.6 Prevention

Zhu Dan Xi considered that people with dizziness were about to get wind stroke. Old people with a deficiency of qi, excessive liver yang, and phlegm should be cautious about the occurrence of wind stroke, especially those people who feel dizzy and numb in their fingers.

Attention should be paid to diet and life style and overstraining should be avoided. Moxibustion on Zusanli (ST 36) and Xuanzhong (GB 39) is beneficial for high risk groups to avoid an attack of wind stroke.

5.3 Summary

Wind stroke refers to an emergency case manifested by sudden loss of consciousness and sensation, accompanied by a deviated mouth, slurred speech, and hemiplegia. In mild cases, there is just hemiplegia, deviation of mouth, dysphasia, or aphasia without sudden coma.

Treatments for wind stroke are delivered according to the differentiation of three parts: zang-fu viscera and meridians, tense type and flaccid type, and disease stages.

Acupuncture and moxibustion are effective therapies for wind stroke, especially for improving the movement of limbs, speech, and swallowing. The earlier treatment with acupuncture and moxibustion, the better the therapeutic effect will be. During the course of treatment, the patients are strongly advised to do functional physical exercise.

Questions
1. Describe the main characteristics of wind stroke.
2. What is the differentiation of wind stroke attack between zang-fu viscera and meridians?
3. Describe the treatment principles and major prescriptions for wind–phlegm attack collaterals syndrome.

References

1. Zhongyin Z. Internal medicine of traditional Chinese medicine. Beijing: China Press of Traditional Chinese Medicine; 2007. p. 304–14.
2. Yongshen X, Hua W, Baixiao Z. Acupuncture and moxibustion. Beijing: People's Medical Publishing House; 2007. p. 457–60.
3. Zhenji L. International standard Chinese-English basic nomenclature of Chinese medicine. Beijing: People's Medical Publishing House; 2008.
4. Niancong C. Traditional Chinese medicine. Beijing: Higher Education Press; 2013.
5. Maciocia G. The practice of Chinese medicine: the treatment of diseases with acupuncture and Chinese herbs. New York: Churchill Livingstone/Elsevier; 2008.
6. Jianqiao F. Science of acupuncture and moxibustion. Beijing: China Press of Traditional Chinese Medicine; 2014.
7. Xinnong C. Chinese acupuncture and moxibustion. Beijing: Foreign Languages Press; 2010.
8. Tianshuo G, Hua B, Shuqing Z. Traditional Chinese internal medicine. Beijing: China Press of Traditional Chinese Medicine; 2004.
9. Xinhua W. Textbook of traditional Chinese medicine. Beijing: Beijing Science Press; 2016.

5.4 Arthralgia

Objective
Master the knowledge about the treatment of arthralgia based on syndrome differentiation via learning the etiology, pathogenesis, diagnosis, differentiation, treatment, and prevention of arthralgia.

Guideline
This chapter introduces the etiology, pathogenesis, diagnosis, differential diagnosis, treatment (herbal medicine and acupuncture), and prevention of arthralgia.

5.5   Introduction

Arthralgia (the Chinese term "Bi syndrome") refers to pain, heavy sensation, soreness or numbness of muscles, tendons, and joints due to obstructed meridians caused by invasion of pathogenic wind, cold, damp, and heat. The disease is manifested by pain, stiffness, swelling, deformity, and limited movement of joints. In mild cases, there are just symptoms in muscles, tendons, and joints; in serious cases, symptoms in internal organs.

In the book *Internal Classic*, the Chinese term "Bi syndrome" is proposed and its symptoms, etiology, pathogenesis, and prognosis are stated. In Chapter 43 of *Plain Questions*, the invasion of pathogenic wind, cold, and dampness causes the development of arthralgia. When pathogenic wind predominates, wind arthralgia develops; when pathogenic cold predominates, cold arthralgia develops; when pathogenic dampness predominates, dampness arthralgia develops.

The severity of arthralgia is affected by exposure to climatic factors. The weather of wind and rain tends to cause the occurrence of arthralgia.

In Western medicine, arthralgia responds to rheumatic arthritis, rheumatoid arthritis, osteoarthritis, tonic rachitis, ankylosing spondylitis, fibrositis, tendinitis, bursitis, and gout.

5.5.1   Etiology

The development of arthralgia is related to physical constitution, climate, dwelling environment, and diet. The deficient healthy qi and external pathogenic factors cause arthralgia together.

5.5.1.1   Invasion of Wind–Dampness–Cold

Wind–dampness–cold, from the damp living environment, cold injury, sleeping in the open, working in the wind and rain, and working in water, invades striae, interstice, and meridians, stays in muscles, tendons, and joints, and causes wind–dampness–cold arthralgia. The excessive yang qi in the body or protracted course may give rise to heat syndrome.

5.5.1.2 Invasion of Wind–Dampness–Heat

Unlike wind–dampness–cold, pathogenic heat comes from the hot humid living or working environment. Wind–dampness–heat blocks circulation of qi and blood, obstructs meridians, and remains in muscles, tendons, and joints, and thus arthralgia develops.

5.5.1.3 Overstrain from Physical Work and Sexual Activity with Inadequate Rest

Overstrain from physical work, such as excessive lifting or sports activities and excessive exercise with inadequate rest, injures the muscles and tendons and depletes qi and blood so that human bodies are prone to invasion by external pathogenic factors. Therefore, excessive sports or work activities are likely to develop arthralgia.

Overstrain from sexual activity in humans combined with inadequate rest consumes essence too much so as to cause deficiency of qi and blood which decreases the resistance of the body, and thus inducing the development of arthralgia too.

5.5.1.4 Weak and Aged Body with Chronic Diseases

Losing nourishment of muscles and tendons due to liver and kidney deficiency in aged bodies, or weak bodies caused by chronic disease or childbirth likely leads to the invasion of pathogenic factors. Hence, the arthralgia occurs.

5.5.2 Pathogenesis

5.5.2.1 Pathogenic Site

The pathogenic site of arthralgia is located in muscles, tendons, and joints, even zang-fu viscera.

5.5.2.2 Pathological Nature

The pathological nature of arthralgia during the beginning course is excess in symptoms, which manifests obstruction of meridians due to pathogenic factors. Once the healing is delayed, qi and blood are consumed too much, which causes liver and kidney deficiency and phlegm and blood stasis. The pathological nature of arthralgia shows deficiency-excess in complexity under that condition.

5.5.2.3 Basic Pathogenesis

The pathology of arthralgia may be summarized, which is the obstruction in the circulation of qi and blood in the meridians that causes pain, soreness, and numbness in muscles, tendons, and joints. The obstruction of the meridians is caused by wind, dampness, cold, and heat attacking weak bodies due to oldness, chronic diseases, or childbirth.

5.5.3 Diagnosis

Clinic symptoms include pain, heavy sensation, soreness or numbness of muscles, tendons, and joints, and even stiffness, swelling, deformity, and limited movement of joints.

The exacerbation of arthralgia is related to fatigue, climate, seasonal variation, and dwelling environment.

Occurring in any age. Some types of arthralgia are more common in the young and middle-aged groups.

5.5.4 Differentiation

5.5.4.1 Differentiation of Predominant Pathogenic Factors in Arthralgia

1. Wind arthralgia
    Wind arthralgia is marked by predominant pathogenic wind which is characterized by constant movement and changes. Therefore, the main manifestations of wind arthralgia are wandering pain moving from joint to joint, especially the elbows, wrists, knees, and ankles, leading to limitation of movement.
2. Cold arthralgia
    Cold arthralgia is marked by the predominant pathogenic cold, which is characterized by the property of contraction. The contracted meridians with cold cause qi and blood circulation obstruction. Therefore, the main manifestations of cold arthralgia are severe stable pain in the joints with limitation of movement, alleviated by warmth and aggravated by cold, with fixed localization but no local redness and hotness.
3. Dampness arthralgia
    Dampness arthralgia is marked by predominant pathogenic dampness, which is characterized by stickiness, heaviness, and turbidity. Dampness may impede

the qi activity when it attacks the body and impairs yang qi. Therefore, the main manifestations of dampness arthralgia are numbness and heavy sensation in the limbs, fixed pain, soreness, and swelling in muscles and joints, aggravated on cloudy and rainy days.

4. Heat arthralgia

Heat arthralgia is marked by predominant pathogenic heat, which is characterized by hotness and consumption of body fluids. The main manifestations of heat arthralgia are local redness, swelling, and excruciating pain with limitation of movement involving one or several joints that feel hot when touched, accompanied by fever and thirst. This happens especially with an underlying deficiency of yin.

5.5.4.2 Differentiation of Deficiency and Excess in Arthralgia

During the acute stage of arthralgia, the excessive syndrome is composed of severe pathogenic factors, including wind, cold, dampness, and heat.

Once symptoms of arthralgia advance to the chronic stage, too much essence is consumed and liver and kidney yin become deficient. Blood stasis and phlegm due to qi and yin deficiency obstruct meridians and cause deformity of the joints. Under that condition, arthralgia falls into deficiency and excess in the complex.

5.5.5 Treatment

5.5.5.1 Principles of Treatment

The general principles of treatment for arthralgia include clearing pathogenic factors and dredging meridians because the pathogenic wind, cold, dampness, heat, phlegm, and blood stasis obstruct the meridians and collaterals.

Treatment methods which include expelling wind, dissipating cold, removing dampness, clearing heat, resolving phlegm, activating blood, and resolving stasis are chosen based on predominant pathogenic factors.

Moreover, treatment for wind may combine nourishing and activating blood; treatment for cold and warming yang may be applied at the same time; invigorating spleen and replenishing qi may be combined with treatment for dampness; tonifying liver and kidney and replenishing qi and blood are used to patients with chronic arthralgia for a long time.

5.5.5.2 Chinese Medicinal Treatment

Invasion of Wind–Dampness–Cold

Wind Arthralgia

Characteristic symptoms: wandering pain and soreness in muscles and tendons, involving several joints with limited movements, chill and fever, white and thin coating, and floating or slow pulse.

Key pathogenesis: wind guiding with cold and dampness obstructing qi and blood in meridians.

Therapeutic principle and method: expelling wind, dissipating cold, removing dampness, and dredging meridians.

Major prescription: Fangfeng Tang modification.

Herbs: Fangfeng, Mahuang, Guizhi, Gegen, Danggui, Fuling, Shengjiang, Dazao. and Gancao.

Explanation:

Fangfeng, Mahuang, Guizhi, and Gegen: to expel wind, dissipate cold, release flesh, and relieve pain.

Danggui: to nourish and activate blood.

Fuling, Shengjiang, Dazao, and Gancao: to invigorate the spleen and drain dampness, harmonize nutrient and defensive aspects.

Modification: For cases with soreness and pain in the back and lumber, Duzhong, Sangjisheng, Roucongrong, Bajitian, and Xuduan are added to tonify kidney and liver; for cases with swelling heat joints and thin yellow coating, Guizhi Shaoyao Zhimu Tang modification is preferred.

Cold Arthralgia

Characteristic symptoms: severe stable pain in the joints with limitation of movement, alleviated by warmth and aggravated by cold, with fixed localization but no local redness and hotness, pale tongue with thin white coating, and wiry tight pulse.

Key pathogenesis: cold guiding with wind and dampness obstructing qi and blood in meridians.

Therapeutic principle and method: dissipating cold, expelling wind, removing dampness, and dredging meridians.

Major prescription: Wutou Tang Vavriation.

Herbs: Zhichuanwu, Mahuang, Baishao, Gancao, Fengmi. and Huangqi.

Explanation:

Zhichuanwu and Mahuang: to warm channel, dissipate cold, and relieve pain.

Baishao, Gancao, and Fengmi: to relieve spasms and pain.

Huangqi: to replenish qi and consolidate exterior.

Modification: For cases with severe pain in joints with cold sense, Fuzi, Xixin, Guizhi, Ganjiang, and Danggui added.

Dampness Arthralgia

Characteristic symptoms: heavy sense, fixed pain, and soreness in muscles and joints with limited movements, numbness of skin, pale tongue with a greasy white coating, and soggy slow pulse.

Key pathogenesis: dampness guiding with wind and cold obstructing qi and blood in meridians.

Therapeutic principle and method: removing dampness, dissipating cold, expelling wind, and dredging meridians.

Major prescription: Yiyiren Tang modification.

Herbs: Yiyiren, Cangzhu, Gancao, Qianghuo, Duhuo, Fangfeng, Zhichuanwu, Mahuang, Guizhi, Danggui and Chuanxiong.

Explanation:

Yiyiren, Cangzhu, and Gancao: to invigorate the spleen, replenish qi, disperse wind and cold.

Qianghuo, Duhuo, and Fangfeng: to expel wind and remove dampness.

Zhichuanwu, Mahuang, and Guizhi: to warm channel, dissipate cold, and relieve pain.

Danggui and Chuanxiong: to nourish and activate blood.

Modification: For cases with severe swelling joints, Bixie and Wujiapi added; for cases with numbness of the skin, Haitongpi and Xixiancao added; for cases with edema, Fuling, Zexie, and Cheqianzi added; for cases with profuse phlegm, Dannanxing and Banxia added.

Invasion of Wind–Dampness–Heat

Characteristic symptoms: wandering, redness, swelling, and excruciating pain in one or several joints with limited movements, relieved with cool, local subcutaneous nodule or erythema, accompanied by fever, aversion to wind, sweat, thirst, and dysphoria, red tongue with yellow greasy coating, and slippery rapid pulse.

Key pathogenesis: pathogenic wind, dampness, and heat obstructing qi and blood in meridians.

Therapeutic principle and method: clearing heat, expelling wind, removing dampness, and dredging meridians.

Major prescription: Baihu Tang, Guizhi Tang plus Xuanbi Tang modification,

Herbs: Shengshigao, Zhimu, Huangbo, Lianqiao, Guizhi, Fangji, Kuxingren, Yiyiren, Huashi, Chixiaodou, and Cansha.

Explanation:

Shengshigao, Zhimu, Huangbo, Lianqiao: to clear heat and relieve dysphoria.

Guizhi: to disperse wind and release flesh.

Fangji, Kuxingren, Yiyiren, Huashi, Chixiaodou, and Cansha: to clear heat, drain dampness, diffuse impediment, and dredge collaterals.

Modification: For cases with erythema, Mudanpi, Chishao, Shengdihuang, and Zicao added; for cases with fever, aversion to wind, and throat pain, Jingjie, Bohe, Niubangzi, and Jiegeng added; for cases with thirst and dysphria, Shengdihuang, Maidong, and Xuanshen added.

Syndrome of Phlegm and Blood Stasis Obstructing Meridians

Characteristic symptoms: stabbing pain with fixed localization in the joints, swelling stiff purple joints, numbness with heavy sensation limbs, deformity joints with limited movements, local subcutaneous nodule or ecchymosis, darkish complexion, eyelid edema, deep purple tongue with white greasy coating, and wiry unsmooth pulse.

Key pathogenesis: phlegm and blood stasis obstructing meridians.

Therapeutic principle and method: revolving phlegm, activating blood, and dredging meridians.

Major prescription: Shuanghe Tang modification.

Herbs: Taoren, Honghua, Chishao, Danggui, Chuanxiong, Banxia, Fuling, Chenpi, Baijiezi. and Zhuli.

Explanation:

Taoren, Honghua, Chishao, Danggui, and Chuanxiong: to nourish the blood, resolve blood stasis, and dredge collaterals.

Banxia, Fuling, Chenpi, Baijiezi, and Zhuli: to invigorate the spleen and resolve phlegm.

Modification: For cases with subcutaneous nodules, Dannanxing and Tianzhuhuang added; for cases with swelling pain and stiff deformity joints, Ezhu, Sanqi, and Tubiechong added; for cases with severe continued pain in joints, Chuanshanjia, Baihuashe, Quanxie, Wugong, and Dilong added.

Syndrome of Liver and Kidney Deficiency

Characteristic symptoms: delayed healing of arthralgia, joints with limited movements, becoming thin muscle, soreness and weakness of waist and knees, aversion to cold limbs, impotence, and seminal emission, or steaming bone fever, dry mouth, and dysphoria, light red tongue with thin white coating, and deep thready weak pulse.

Key pathogenesis: muscles and tendons lose nourishing due to liver and kidney deficiency.

Therapeutic principle and method: tonifying and replenishing the liver and kidney, relaxing sinew, relieving pain, and activating collaterals.

Major prescription: Duhuo Jisheng Tang modification.

Herbs: Duhuo, Fangfeng, Qinjiao, Xixin, Rougui, Renshen, Fuling, Gancao, Danggui, Shengdihuang, Baishao, Duzhong, Niuxi, and Sangjisheng.

Explanation:

Duhuo, Fangfeng, Qinjiao, Xixin, and Rougui: to expel wind, remove dampness, and dissipate cold.

Renshen, Fuling, Gancao, Danggui, Shengdihuang, and Baishao: to tonify qi and blood.

Duzhong, Niuxi, and Sangjisheng: to tonify and replenish liver and kidney.

Modification: For cases with severe soreness and weakness of the waist and knees and lack of strength, Lujiaoshuang, Xuduan, and Gouji added; for cases with aversion to cold limbs, Fuzi, Ganjiang, and Bajitian added; liver and kidney yin deficiency, pain in lumber and knees, dyphoria, lower fever, or afternoon tidal fever, Guiban, Shudihuang, and Nvzhenzi added.

5.5.5.3 Acupuncture and Moxibustion Treatment

Attack on Meridians and Collaterals

Ashi points located in the diseased areas are selected for the purpose of clearing pathogenic factors. The manipulations of acupuncture and moxibustion should be chosen by symptoms and signs that include the location and the depth of pain. Shallow insertion is for the diseased skin and muscles; deep insertion is for bones and tendons. The bleeding methods can be used to clear blood stasis and dampness. To eliminate wind and cold, moxibustion can be applied.

Prescriptions:

Disease at the shoulder joint: Jianyu (LI 15), Jianliao (TE 14), Jianzhen (TE 19), Naoshu (SI 10).

Disease at the elbow joint: Quchi (LI 11), Chize (LU 5), and Tianjing (TE 10).

Disease at the wrist: Yangchi (TE 4), Yangxi (LI 5), Yanggu (SI 5), Waiguan (TE 5).

Disease at the back and lumber: back transport points with pain, points with pain on governor's vessel, Jiaji (EX-B 2), Shuigou (GV 26), Shenzhu (GV 12), and Yaoyangguan (GV 3).

Disease at the hip joint: Huantiao (GB 30), Juliao (GB 29), and Xuanzhong (GB 39).

Disease at the knee joint: Heding (EX-LE 2), Dubi (SI 35), Neixiyan (EX-LE 4), Yanglingquan (GB 34), and Yinlingquan (SP 9).

Disease at the ankle joint: Jiexi (SI 41), Shangqiu (SP 5), Qiuxu (GB 40), Kunlun (BL 60), and Taixi (KI 3).

Disease at the hands and feet: Yanggu (SI 5), Hegu (LI 4), Houxi (SI 3), Sanjian (LI 3), Baxie (EX-UE 9), Gongsun (SP 4), Shugu (BL 65), and Bafeng (EX-LE 10).

5.5.6 Prevention

Patients with arthralgia should keep warm, avoid wind, and live in a humid room. The mild exercises are beneficial to the healing. However, the sweating body after exercise should not have a shower or stay in the wind.

5.6 Summary

Arthralgia refers to pain, heavy sensation, soreness, or numbness of muscles, tendons, and joints due to obstructed meridians caused by invasion of pathogenic wind, cold, damp, and heat. The disease is manifested by stiffness, swelling, deformity, and limited movement of joints. In mild cases, there are just symptoms in muscles, tendons, and joints; in serious cases, symptoms in internal organs.

The pathology of arthralgia may be summarized, which is the obstruction in the circulation of qi and blood in the meridians that causes pain, soreness, and numbness in muscles, tendons, and joints. The obstruction of the meridians is caused by pathogenic wind, dampness, cold, and heat taking advantage of a weak body due to oldness, chronic diseases, or childbirth.

Acupuncture is effective in treating arthralgia, especially for pain. For severe cases, Chinese medicine may be combined with acupuncture to tonify the kidney and liver.

Questions
1. Describe the main characteristics of arthralgia.
2. What is the differentiation of deficiency and excess in arthralgia?
3. Describe the treatment principles and major prescriptions of acupuncture for arthralgia.

References

1. Zhongyin Z. Internal medicine of traditional Chinese medicine. Beijing: China Press of Traditional Chinese Medicine; 2007. p. 304–14.
2. Yongshen X, Hua W, Baixiao Z. Acupuncture and moxibustion. Beijing: People's Medical Publishing House; 2007. p. 457–60.
3. Zhenji L. International Standard Chinese-English basic nomenclature of Chinese medicine. Beijing: People's Medical Publishing House; 2008.
4. Niancong C. Traditional Chinese medicine. Beijing: Higher Education Press; 2013.
5. Maciocia G. The practice of Chinese medicine: the treatment of diseases with acupuncture and Chinese herbs. New York: Churchill Livingstone/Elsevier; 2008.
6. Jianqiao F. Science of acupuncture and moxibustion. Beijing: China Press of Traditional Chinese Medicine; 2014.
7. Xinnong C. Chinese acupuncture and moxibustion. Beijing: Foreign Languages Press; 2010.
8. Tianshu G, Hua B, Shuqin Z. Traditional Chinese internal medicine. Beijing: China Press of Traditional Chinese Medicine; 2004.
9. Xinhua W. Textbook of traditional Chinese medicine. Beijing: Beijing Science Press; 2016.

5.7 Headache

Objectives
Master the knowledge about the treatment of headaches based on syndrome differentiation via learning the etiology, pathogenesis, diagnosis, differentiation, treatment, and prevention of headaches.

Guideline
This chapter introduces the etiology, pathogenesis, diagnosis, differential diagnosis, treatment (herbal medicine and acupuncture), and prevention of headaches.

5.8 Introduction

Headache is a disease that shows the main clinical feature of head pain, due to external and/or internal injuries resulting in stagnation or deficiency. Headache is not only a common disease but also a common symptom, which can occur in many kinds of acute and chronic diseases. Sometimes, it is also a sign of aggravation or deterioration of some related diseases.

There are records of head illness in the Oracle in the *Shang* dynasty. It is called "brain wind" or "head wind" in the book of *Internal Classic*. In the book *Treatise on Cold Damage Diseases*, there are different treatment methods discussed in detail in the chapters about yangming diseases, shaoyang diseases, jueyin diseases, and so on. *Dong Yuan Shi Shu* (*Dongyuan Ten Books*) pointed out that both exogenous and internal injuries are the causes of headaches. According to the etiology and symptoms, headache can be recognized as dampness–heat headache, real headache, qi deficiency headache, blood deficiency headache, taiyin headache, shaoyin headache, and so on. That provides a method for medicine choice according to meridians.

Headaches can be induced by various diseases of internal medicine, neurology, surgery, psychiatry, otolaryngology, and ophthalmology in Western medicine. It involves hypertension, neurosis, intracranial diseases, infectious fever, and so on.

5.8.1 Etiology

Headache can be led by any of the six external etiological factors, impairment of the function of internal organs, and emotional strain, resulting in external pathogens, phlegm, and hyperactivity of liver yang. Or it is caused by a deficiency of qi, blood, yin, and yang, resulting in malnutrition of the brain. Trauma, chronic disease, and accumulation of stasis also induce headaches.

5.8.1.1 The Six External Etiological Factors Caused Headache

Wind pathogens may be the main factor. Wind pathogen belongs to the yang pathogen. As is known, the head will be hurt first when one is impaired by wind. It is only the wind that can reach the peak. Wind is the chief pathogen of all diseases. When a wind pathogen attacks the head, it is usually compounded with coldness, dampness, and heat. If the wind is compounded with coldness, the coldness will hurt the yang, block the qi and blood, affect the meridian circulation, and lead to pain. If the wind is compounded with dampness, the sticky qi will make the clear yang turbid, and qi and blood cannot flow smoothly, so to lead to pain. If the wind is compounded with heat, the wind-heat will flow upward to the head and make the qi and blood revert upward, so to lead to headache.

5.8.1.2 Deficiency of Qi, Blood, Yin, and Yang Impair the Function of Internal Organs

The deficiency may be caused by congenital deficiency, aged deficiency, kidney deficiency by excessive sexual life, being ill for a long time, after giving birth to a child, after losing blood, etc. The deficient qi, blood, yin, and yang cannot nourish the head and brain and result in headaches.

5.8.1.3 Emotional Strain Lead to Headache

Being in a state of nervousness and melancholy for a long time will affect liver qi. Stagnation of liver qi makes the liver meridian lose the stretching, contract together, and be painful. An irritable man is easy to be angry. The anger contributes to the production of liver-heat. Liver-heat impairs liver-yin after a long-time of damage. Liver-heat will go upward to the head and lead to headaches.

5.8.1.4 Irregular Dining Lead to Headache

Just as *Zhu Danxi* said, most of the headache is caused by phlegm. An irregular diet such as excessively having sweet food or meat, or eating too much or too little than usual, will damage the spleen. The damaged spleen cannot transfer water normally. Stagnant water becomes dampness and phlegm. They stay in the head and become pathogenic factors covering the orifices in the head. Therefore, diet is also one of the causes of headaches.

5.8.2 Pathogenesis

5.8.2.1 Pathogenic Site

The pathogenic site of headache is located in the head, related to the liver, spleen, and kidney.

5.8.2.2 Pathological Nature

The pathological nature of headache can be related to any of the six external etiological factors, impairment of the function of internal organs, caused by emotional strain, resulting in external pathogens, phlegm, and hyperactivity of the liver yang. Or it is caused by a deficiency of qi, blood, yin, and yang, resulting in malnutrition of the brain. Trauma, chronic disease, and accumulation of stasis also induce headaches. The obstruction causes pain.

5.8.2.3 Basic Pathogenesis

According to the nature of the disease's syndrome, headache can be divided into excess syndrome and deficiency syndrome. Pathogens obstruct qi's flowing in meridians and cover the clear orifices. A deficiency of essence and blood leads to brain malnutrition. Both excess and deficiency are the basic pathogen of headache.

5.8.3 Diagnosis

5.8.3.1 Main Symptoms

It is manifested as forehead pain, frontal and temporal pain, parietal pain, occipital and parietal pain, or even all head pain. It can be jumping pain, stabbing pain, distending pain, vague pain, empty pain, etc. It will occur suddenly or repeatedly. The duration of pain can vary from several minutes to hours, days, or weeks.

Headaches can be caused by external and internal injuries or have a history of repeated episodes.

5.8.3.2 About Inspection

To do routine blood tests and measure blood pressure is a regular check. Cerebrospinal fluid test, cerebral blood flow test, and EEG are sometimes necessary. Transcranial Doppler check, cranial CT, and MRI examination are required. All of these help to make clear diagnoses and exclude organic diseases.

5.8.4   Differentiation

5.8.4.1   Wind-Cold Type

Wind-cold headache is characterized by acute occurrence, severe headache, being more serious after catching a cold, feeling chilly and aversion to wind-cold, nasal congestion, watery nasal discharge, thin whitish coating of the tongue, floating pulse, or taut floating pulse.

5.8.4.2   Wind-Heat Type

Wind-heat headache is characterized by distending pain and scorching sensation in the head, acute onset, aversion to wind, stuffy nose with turbid discharge, reddened tongue with yellowish coating, and rapid pulse.

5.8.4.3   Type of Hyperactivity of the Liver Yang

Type of hyperactivity of the liver yang is characterized by distending and radiative pain of the head induced by tension, flushed face and conjunctival congestion, bitter taste, tinnitus, red tongue with thin yellow coating, and taut pulse.

5.8.4.4   Type of Accumulation and Up-Stirring of Phlegm

The type of accumulation and up-stirring of phlegm is characterized by heavy feeling in the head, vertigo, oppressed feeling in the chest, nausea, vomiting phlegm, whitish greasy coating of the tongue, and slippery pulse.

5.8.4.5   Type of Stagnation of Qi and Blood

The type of stagnation of qi and blood in the meridians is characterized by headache with punctured feeling, fixed pain, and recurrence due to trauma in the head, purple tongue, and smooth-less pulse.

5.8.4.6   Type of Deficiency of Blood

Type of deficiency of blood is characterized by headache and dizziness worsened by movement, palpitation, insomnia, pale complexion, pale tongue, and small pulse.

5.8.5 Treatment

5.8.5.1 Principles of Treatment

The general principles of treatment for headaches include strengthening health qi and eliminating pathogens. The pathogens include wind, cold, heat, hyperactivity of the liver yang, phlegm, and stagnation of liver qi. The health qi includes qi, blood, yin, and yang.

Treatment methods, which include expelling wind, dissipating cold, clearing heat, resolving phlegm, activating blood, and resolving stasis, are applied based on predominant pathogenic factors.

5.8.5.2 Chinese Medicinal Treatment

Wind-Cold Headache

Characteristic symptoms: cute occurrence, severe headache, being more serious after catching a cold, feeling chill and aversion to wind-cold, nasal congestion, watery nasal discharge, thin whitish coating of the tongue, floating pulse, or taut floating pulse.

Key pathogenesis: wind-pathogen is one of the main pathogens that hurts the head. If the wind is compounded with coldness, the coldness will hurt the yang, block the qi and blood, and contract the pulse to lead to pain.

Major prescription: Chuanxiong Chatiao powder.

Herbs: Chuanxiong, Jingjie, Fangfeng, Baizhi, Qianghuo, Gancao, Xixin, and Chaqing.

Explanation: decocted in water for oral use.

Chuanxiong, Qianghuo, Baizhi, and Xixin: to divergent cold and dredge the meridian.

Jingjie, Bohe: to evacuate the upper wind evil, and to clear the leader.

Fangfeng: dispel the wind to solve the table, and win the wet pain.

Gancao: supplementing qi and harmonizing the medicine.

Chaqing: to clear the leader and harmonize the temperature and dryness of wind medicine.

Modification: With colder symptoms, the drugs added are Zhichuanwu, Xixin, and Gaoben; with severe headache due to dampness, the drugs added are Cang'erzi, and Cangzhu.

Wind-Heat Headache

Characteristic symptoms: distending pain and scorching sensation in the head, acute onset, aversion to wind, stuffy nose with turbid discharge, reddened tongue with yellowish coating, and rapid pulse.

Key pathogenesis: when the wind is compounded with heat, wind-heat will flow upward to the head and make the qi and blood revert upward, so to lead to headache.

Major Prescription: XiongZhishigao Decoction.

Herbs: Chuanxiong, Baizhi, Shengshigao (decocted firstly), Manjingzi, Sangye, Juhua, Qianghuo, and Gaoben.

Explanation: decocted in water for oral use.

Chuanxiong, Baizhi, Shengshigao, Juhua: to dispersing wind and clearing heat.

Qianghuo, Gaoben: to dispel dampness, and cure headache.

Manjingzi, Sangye, Juhuato evacuation wind heat and a clear head.

Modification: In case of stuffy with yellow and sticky discharge, the drugs added are Xinyi, Cang'erzi, and Yuxingcao; in case of severe fever, the drug added is Shengdahuang (decocted later); in case of severe headache, the drug added is Xixin.

Type of Hyperactivity of the Liver Yang

Characteristic symptoms: distending and radiative pain of the head induced by tension, flushed face and conjunctival congestion, bitter taste, tinnitus, red tongue with thin yellow coating, and taut pulse.

Key pathogenesis: the liver loses its characteristic of harmony and accessibility, and the qi stagnates in the body. After a long period of stagnation, the gas is converted into fire; yang qi is the type of liver that disturbs the brain.

Major prescription: Tianma Gouteng Drink.

Herbs: Gouteng(decocted later), Tianma, Shijueming(decocted first), Niuxi, Huangqin, Zhizi, Duzhong, Sangjisheng, Fuchen, and Yejiaoteng(Thunb).

Explanation: decocted in water for oral use.

Gouteng, Tianma: suppressing hyperactive liver and extinguishing wind.

Shijueming: suppressing hyperactive liver and subsiding yang, clearing heat, and improving eyesight.

Niuxi: draw blood downward.

Huangqin, Zhizi: clearing heat and purging fire.

Duzhong, Sangjisheng: nourishing liver and kidney.

Fushen, Yejiaoteng: tranquilizing and sedating the mind.

Modification: in case of up-stirring of the liver and endless radiated pain, the drugs added are Quanxie, Jiangcan; in case of deficiency of liver yin and kidney yin, vertigo, and tinnitus, the drugs added are Shengdi, Shudi, Shouwu, and Gouqizi.

Type of Accumulation and Up-Stirring of Phlegm

Characteristic symptoms: heavy feeling in the head, vertigo, oppressed feeling in the chest, nausea, vomiting phlegm, whitish greasy coating of the tongue, and slippery pulse.

Key pathogenesis: the function of transport and transformation of spleen being abnormal, phlegm turbidity hinders char, and then it blinds the brain.

Major prescription: Banxia Baizhu Tianma Decoction.

Herbs: Zhibanxia, Weitianma, Baizhu, Chenpi, Fuling, and Gancao.

Explanation: decocted in water for oral use.

Zhibanxia: eliminating dampness and phlegm, stopping the inverse and anti-nausea.

Weitianma: calming liver, extinguishing wind, stopping dizziness.

Fuling, Chenpi, and Baizhu: invigorating the spleen and infiltrating the dampness, regulating qi, and resolving phlegm.

Gancao: to reconcile the medicine.

Modification: in case of stagnation of phlegm–dampness in the stomach and sticky sputum, the drugs added are Wuzhuyu, Shengjiang; in case of accumulation of phlegm forming heat, bitter taste sticky mouth and yellow greasy coating of the tongue, the drugs added are Zhuru, Chendanxing, Huangqin, and Zhishi.

Type of Stasis of Qi and Blood

Characteristic symptoms: headache with punctured feeling, fixed pain, recurrence due to trauma in the head, purple tongue, and smooth-less pulse.

Key pathogenesis: the congestion blocks the collaterals. General pain means the balance in the body is disrupted.

Major prescription: Tongqiao Huoxue Decoction.

Herbs: Chishao, Chuanxiong, Taoren, Honghua, Shexiang, Shengjiang, Congbai, and Dazao.

Explanation: decocted in water for oral use.

Chishao, Chuanxiong, Taoren, and Honghua: promoting blood circulation for removing blood stasis and obstruction in collaterals.

Shexiang: Shengjiang, Congbai: to unobstruct the meridians and collaterals.

Modification: For ease of stasis due to cold, headache, and aversion to cold, the drugs added are Xixin and Guizhi; in case of stagnation of phlegm-dampness, the drugs added are Baifuzi, Zhinanxing, Jiangcan; and in case of deficiency of qi and blood due to chronic disease, the drugs added are Huangqi, Dangshen, Gouqizi.

Type of Deficiency of Blood

Characteristic symptoms: headache and dizziness worsened by movement, palpitation, insomnia, pale complexion, pale tongue, and small pulse.

Key pathogenesis: insufficient qi and blood on the brain and meridians causes nourishment loss of the brain and headache.

Major prescription: decoction of four drugs.

Herbs: Shudi, Danggui, Chuanxiong, and Baishao.

Explanation: decocted in water for oral use.

Shudi: nourishing yin and nourishing blood.

Danggui: nourishing the liver and activating blood circulation.

Chuanxiong, Baishao: nourishing blood, invigorating the liver activating the qi, and making the qi and blood harmonious and unobstructed.

Modification: in case of palpitation and severe insomnia due to blood failure in the nourishing heart, the drugs added are Zaoren, Guiyuanrou, and Yuanzhi; in case of deficiency of qi, the drugs added are Dangshen and Huangqi.

5.8.5.3   Acupuncture and Moxibustion Treatment

Attack on Meridians and Collaterals

According to the part of the headache, we should take the meridian following acupoint selection and select ashi point as the main. Basic moxibustion and acupuncture techniques are filiform needle deficiency-excess tonifying and purging methods. Moxibustion can be added to cold syndrome. Blood stasis headache can use the method of swift pricking blood therapy in ashi point. Patients with severe headaches can use strong stimulation and a long needle in the ashi point.

Prescriptions:

Main acupoint: Baihui (GV 20), Taiyang (EX-HN 4), Fengchi (GB 20), and Hegu (LI 4).

Taiyang headache: add Tianzhu (BL 10), Houxi (SL 3), and Kunlun (BL 60).

Yangming headache: add Yintang (GV 29) and Neiting (SI 44).

Shaoyang headache: add Shuaigu (GB 8), Waiguan (TE 5), and Zulinqi (GB 41).

Jueyin headache: add Sishencong (EX-HN 1), Taichong (LR 3), and Neiguan (PC 6).

A headache caused by wind cold: add Fengmen (BL 12) and Lieque(LU 7).

A headache caused by wind heat: add Quchi (LI 11) and Dazhui (GV 14).

A headache caused by dampness: add Touwei (SI 8) and Yinlingquan (SP 9).

A headache caused by upper hyperactivity of liver yang: add Taixi (KI 3) and Taichong (LR 3).

A headache caused by phlegm turbid: add Zhongwan (GV 12) and Fenglong (SI 40).

A headache caused by blood stagnation: add Xuehai (SP 10) and Geshu (BL 17).

A headache caused by blood deficiency: add Pishu (BL 20) and Zusanli (SI 36).

5.8.6   Prevention

Patients with a headache should participate in physical exercise, enhance their physique, and keep warm, in order to resist the invasion of external evil.

Keep a good mood and avoid bad emotional stimulation. Do not eat greasy, fast spicy, or fried foods. Discontinue smoking and drinking. For severe or gradually worsening headaches or headaches accompanied by nausea and vomiting of patients, other lesions and timely examination should be considered.

5.9   Summary

Headache due to exopathy is common in the wind-heat type. Headache due to internal injury is often seen in deficiency of yin and excess of yang. For Severe headaches with persistent attacks, the possibility of intracranial tumor should be excluded.

For severe headaches, acupuncture should be applied at first. For mild headaches, the decoction of medicinal herbs should be used with some guiding herbs according to the types of the disease. For bitemporal headache the drugs added are Chuanxiong, Chaihu; for forehead ache the drug added is Baizhi; for pain in the arcus superciliaris the drug added is Manjingzi; for ache all over the head the drugs added are Qianghuo, Fangfeng; for headache with the neck the drug added is Gegen; for headache in the top the drugs added are Wuzhuyu, Gaoben; for severe headache without remission the drugs added are Quanxie, Wugong, Jiangcan in order to dispel wind and remove obstruction in the meridians.

Patients with headaches due to exopathy should avoid attacks of wind and cold. Patients with headaches due to internal injury should keep calm and serene. Avoid irritability. Give up smoking and drinking. Avoid over-intake of greasy and sweet food. Keep a proper balance between work and rest.

Questions
1. Describe the main characteristics of headache.
2. What is the TCM classification of headache? How to treat?
3. Describe the treatment principles and major prescriptions of acupuncture for headache?

Reference
1. Fanrong L, Jiping Z. Acupuncture and moxibustion. Beijing: People's Medical Publishing House; 2014. p. 259–61.

5.10   Insomnia

Objectives
Master the knowledge about the treatment of insomnia based on syndrome differentiation via learning the etiology, pathogenesis, diagnosis, differentiation, treatment, and prevention of insomnia.

Guideline
This chapter introduces the etiology, pathogenesis, diagnosis, differential diagnosis, treatment (herbal medicine and acupuncture), and prevention of insomnia.

5.11   Introduction

Insomnia refers to difficulty in falling asleep, frequent waking from sleep, and dyssomnia by night. It is manifested by dizziness, headache, palpitation, and amnesia. In Western medicine, it is found in neurosis, anemia, and chronic asthenic diseases.

In the book of *Internal Classic,* it was called "cannot sleep," resulting from disorders in the viscera, and yang qi cannot enter the yin. The book *Plain Questions* records "inverse regulating the stomach and treating insomnia." *Zhang Zhongjing* of the *Han* dynasty in *Treatise on Cold Damage Diseases* and *Synopsis of Golden Chamber* divided the etiology of insomnia into two types: exogenous and internal injuries, and put forward the "dysphoria and consumptive disease leading to insomnia," which still has application value.

Insomnia can be the main clinical manifestation of various diseases like neurosis, menopausal syndrome, chronic indigestion, anemia, and atherosclerosis. These diseases can refer to this section of dialectical treatment.

5.11.1   Etiology

5.11.1.1   Improper Diet

Overeating causes food retention and stagnant, which results in spleen and stomach damage, and then brews phlegm, which disturbances the spleen and stomach and causes insomnia. In addition, tea, coffee, and wine are also the factors that cause insomnia.

5.11.1.2   Emotional Disorders

Emotion failures can lead to the dysfunction of zang-fu viscera. For example, rage injures the liver and causes stagnation of liver qi. Pathogenic fire derived from the stagnation of liver qi disturbs the mind, causing lassitude of spirit and insomnia. Joy of laughing, mental excitement, and uneasiness can also cause insomnia.

5.11.1.3   Work and Rest Disorders

Excessive fatigue will hurt the spleen and excessive idleness will weaken the spleen qi. Lack of blood and qi cannot nourish the heart and result in loss of mind and insomnia.

5.11.1.4   Deficiency After the Illness

Non-urgency illness causes deficiency including less heart blood and limitation of movement of heart qi, leading to insomnia. Some elderly patients are physically weak, so the deficiency of yin and yang causes insomnia.

5.11.2   Pathogenesis

5.11.2.1   Pathogenic Site

Insomnia is often caused by a deficiency of the heart and is closely related to the liver, spleen, and kidney.

5.11.2.2   Pathological Nature

There is a difference between deficiency and excess. In clinical practice, the type of deficiency of both the heart and spleen, the type of hyperactivity of fire due to yin deficiency, and the type of accumulation of phlegm in the interior are often found.

5.11.2.3   Basic Pathogenesis

The basic pathogenesis is the deficiency of the heart, gallbladder, spleen, and kidney yin. It leads to pathogenic fire derived from the stagnation of liver qi, phlegm-heat attacking internally, deficiency of both heart and spleen and impaired nourishment of heart and mind. Long-term illness can present intermingled deficiency and excess.

5.11.3 *Diagnosis*

5.11.3.1 Main Symptoms

It is difficult to fall asleep and easy to wake up at night for more than 3 weeks, often accompanied by headache, dizziness, palpitation, amnesia, lassitude, dreams, and other symptoms. This disease often has improper diet, emotional disorders, fatigue, excessive anxiety, disease, and weakness a history.

5.11.3.2 About Inspection

Clinically detectable polysomnography:

1. The duration of the average sleep latency is prolonged (longer than 30 min);
2. The actual sleep time is reduced (less than 6. 5 h per night);
3. The arousal time increased(more than 30 min per night).

5.11.4 *Differentiation*

5.11.4.1 Liver Fire Disturbing Heart

Insomnia and dreaming a lot, irritability, dizziness with red swollen eyes, tinnitus, dry and bitter taste in the mouth, no desire to eat, dark urine, red tongue, string, and rapid pulse.

5.11.4.2 Phlegm–Heat Disturbing Heart

Upset wakefulness, chest tightness, fullness, belching, nausea, accompanied by pain, head, dizziness, the yellow coating on the tongue, slippery, and rapid pulse.

5.11.4.3 Heart–Spleen Deficiency

It is not easy to sleep or wake up, accompanied by palpitations, forgetfulness, lassitude, eating less, dizziness, abdominal distension, diarrhea, pale tongue, thin, and weak pulse.

5.11.4.4 Disharmony Between Heart and Kidney

Upset wakefulness, sleep difficulties, palpitation and dreaminess, red tongue, little coating, and thready pulse.

5.11.4.5 Heart and Gallbladder Deficiency

Virtual trouble insomnia, getting frightened easily, timidness, palpitation, shortness of breath and sweating, fatigue, pale tongue, and thready pulse.

5.11.5 Treatment

5.11.5.1 The Principle of Treatment

The principle of adjusting the yin and yang of viscera should be made in the treatment of deficiency and diarrhea. Treat excess with reinforcement and deficiency with expelling. Tranquillization is necessary on this basis, such as nourishing blood, calming the spirit, and clearing the heart.

5.11.5.2 Chinese Medicinal Treatment

Liver Fire Disturbing Heart

Typical symptoms: wakefulness and excessive dreams, irritability accompanied by dizziness and distention in the head, red tongue with thin fur, and wiry rapid pulse.
   Key pathogenesis: the liver is depressed and the heart is disturbed.
   Major prescription: Longdan Xiegan Decoction.
   Herbs: Longdancao, Huangqin, Zhizi, Zexie, Cheqianzi, Danggui, Shengdi, Chaihu, Gancao, Shenglonggu, Shengmuli, and Cishi.
   Explanation: Decocted in water for oral use.
   Longdancao, Huangqin, and Zhizi: clearing liver fire. Zexie, Cheqianzi: to clear damp and hot.
   Danggui, Shengdi: nourish yin and yang.
   Chaihu: to unblock qi of liver and gallbladder.
   Shenglonggu, Shengmuli, and Cishi: heart fire, calming the nerves.
   Gancao: supplementing qi and harmonizing the medicine.
   Modification: in case of chest distress, Xiangfu, Yujin Foshou added; in case of dizziness and a headache with constipation, Danggui Longhui Wan used.

Phlegm–Heat Disturbing Heart

Typical symptoms: upset insomnia, chest tightness, fullness, tongue red, yellow greasy moss, and pulse slide.

Key pathogenesis: eating some high-fat food causes phlegm accumulation in the chest, and the phlegm becomes phlegm-fire to affect the consciousness of the heart.

Major prescription: Huanglian Wendan Soup.

Herbs: Banxia, Chenpi, Fuling, Zhishi, Huanglian, Zhuru, Longchi, Zhenzhumu, and Cishi.

Explanation: Decocted in water for oral use.

Banxia, Chenpi, Fuling, and Zhishi: to fortify the spleen, dry dampness, dissolve phlegm, and remove accumulation.

Huanglian and Zhuru: to clear heat, dissolve phlegm, and harmonize the stomach.

Longchi, Zhenzhumu, and Cishi: tranquilize the heart and calm the mind.

Modification: in case of insomnia with a choking sensation in the chest, abdominal fullness and distention, ungratifying defecation, greasy fur, and slippery pulse, Banxia Shumi Tang is to be added; if the stomach is not comfortable and ache in the belly, Shenqu, Jiaoshanzha, Laifuzi to be added to promote the digestion.

Heart-Spleen Deficiency

Typical symptoms: difficulty sleeping, excessive dreams, forgetfulness, pale tongue, thin and weak pulse.

Key pathogenesis: lack of blood in the spleen and heart results in failure of nourishment of the heart.

Major prescription: Guipi Decoction.

Herbs: Renshen, Baizhu, Gancao, Danggui, Huangqi, Yuanzhi, Suanzaoren, Fushen, Longyanrou and Muxiang.

Explanation: Decocted in water for oral use.

Renshen, Baizhu, Danggui, and Huangqi: to boost the qi and fortify the spleen.

Yuanzhi, Suanzaoren, Fushen, and Longyanrou: nourish the heart and calm the mind.

Muxiang: to move qi and relieve the pain.

Gancao: harmonize nutrient and defensive aspects.

Modification: if the blood of the heart is not enough, Shudi, Shaoyao, and Ejiao are added; if insomnia is serious, Yejiaoteng, Hehuanpi, and Baiziren are added or adding Shenglonggu, Shengmuli to tranquilize and allay excitement. If accompanied by food indigestion, a greasy coating on the tongue, we raise Cangzhu, Banxia, Chenpi, Fuling, and Houpo to invigorate the spleen and dry the qi and phlegm. If one can not sleep well after giving birth to a baby, or if old people wake up too early, the treatment is the same as that of deficiency of qi and blood

Disharmony Between Heart and Kidney

Typical symptoms: insomnia, palpitation, dreaminess, accompanied by soreness and weakness of the waist and knees, red tongue, little coating, and thready pulse.

Key pathogenesis: deficient kidney water deficiency fails to nourish the heart and excessive heart fire fails to move down to the kidney.

Major prescription: Liuwei Dihuang Wan combined with Jiaotai Wan.

Herbs: shudi, Shanzhuyu, Shanyao, Fuling, Zexie, Danpi, Huanglian, and Rougui.

Explanation: Decocted in water for oral use.

Shudi, Shanzhuyu, and Shanyao: nourishing liver and kidney, replenishing vital essence, and nourishing the bone marrow.

Fuling, Zexie, and Danpi: invigorating the spleen to transform dampness and clearing ministerial fire.

Huanglian, Rougui: conducting the fire back to its origin.

Modification: For the shortness of heart yin, we can use Tianwang Buxin Dan to nourish yin and produce blood, tonifying the heart and calming the nerves; if insomnia stays all night, Zhusha, Cishi, Longgu, and Longchi are added to tranquilize and allay excitement.

Heart and Gallbladder Deficiency

Typical symptoms: insomnia, getting frightened easily, shortness of breath and spontaneous sweating, pale tongue, and thin pulse string.

Key pathogenesis: Heart-gallbladder vacuity timidity, failure of nourishment of the heart, and uneasiness.

Major prescription: AnShengdingzhi Pills and Suanzaoren decoction.

Herbs: Renshen, Fuling, Gancao, Fushen, Yuanzhi, Longchi, Shichangpu, Chuanxiong, Suanzaoren, and Zhimu.

Explanation: Decocted in water for oral use.

Renshen, Fuling, and Gancao: replenishing qi of heart and gallbladder.

Fushen, Yuanzhi, Longchi, and Shichangpu: reducing phlegm, calming one's mind, tranquilizing, and allaying excitement.

Chuanxiong, Suanzaoren: regulating blood and nourishing heart.

Zhimu: Clearing heat and relieving fidgetness.

Modification: for shortness of blood of heart and liver, palpitation with fear, reusing Renshen, adding Baishao, Danggui, and Huangqi to nourish the blood of the liver; if heaving deep sighs and eating less food, adding Chaihu, Chenpi, and Shaoyao, and Baizhu to clear the liver and tonify spleen; if one feels more palpitation and restlessness with fear, adding Shenglonggu, Shengmuli, and Zhusha to tranquilize and allay excitement.

5.11.5.3 Acupuncture and Moxibustion Treatment

According to the part of the insomnia, we should take meridian-following acupoint selection and select ashi point as the main. Basic moxibustion and acupuncture techniques are very effective in the treatment of insomnia.

Prescriptions:

Main acupoints: Shenmen (HT 7), Sanyinjiao (SP 5), Baihui (GV 20), Shenmai (BL 62), and Anmian.

Liver fire disturbing heart: add Xingjian (LR 2).

Phlegm heat disturbing syndrome: add Fenglong (ST 40), Zhongwan (CV 12), and Neiting (ST 44).

Heart-spleen deficiency: add Xinshu (BL 15), Pishu (BL 20), and Zusanli (ST 36).

Disharmony between heart and kidney: add Taixi (KI 13).

Heart and gallbladder deficiency: add Xinshu (BL 15) and Danshu (BL 19).

5.11.6 Prevention

Pay attention to the cultivation of the mind. Pay attention to sleep hygiene. Establish a regular system of interests. Light diet do not overeat and do not take thick tea or coffee.

5.12 Summary

Insomnia is related to emotional factors, improper diet, overwork disorders, illness, and other factors caused by viscera functional disorders, blood loss, and imbalance between yin and yang. The main disease is heart disease and it involves disorders of the liver, gallbladder, spleen, stomach, kidney, and so on. Liver fire, phlegm heat, and uneasiness cause excess syndrome while deficiency of both heart and spleen, deficiency of both heart and gallbladder, and disharmony between heart and kidney cause deficiency syndrome.

Treatment of insomnia should include three key points: first, pay attention to adjusting the balance of yin and yang, qi and blood; second, emphasize the tranquilizing on the basis of syndrome differentiation and treatment; and third, pay attention to the effect of psychotherapy.

Questions
1. Describe the main characteristics of insomnia.
2. How kinds of differentiations does it include?
3. Describe the treatment principles of insomnia.

Reference
1. Chunsheng J, Yong H. Acupuncture and moxibustion. Beijing: Science Press; 2016.

5.13   Cough

Objectives
Master the knowledge about the treatment of cough based on syndrome differentiation via learning the etiology, pathogenesis, diagnosis, differentiation, treatment, and prevention of cough.

Guideline
This chapter introduces the etiology, pathogenesis, diagnosis, differential diagnosis, treatment (herbal medicine, acupuncture, and Tuina), and prevention of cough.

5.14   Introduction

Cough is a common problem that occurs in the lung system. In Chinese, we call it Kesou. "Ke" refers to coughing with sound but without sputum production, while "Sou" to the presence of sputum without coughing sound. Clinically, the symptoms of "Ke" and "Sou" are combined together.

TCM treatment of cough here may be applicable to some respiratory diseases in Western medicine in which cough is a major symptom, such as upper respiratory infection, acute and chronic laryngopharyngitis or bronchitis, pneumonia, cough variant asthma, and bronchiectasis.

5.14.1   Etiology and Pathogenesis

Cough is usually caused by the failure of the lung qi in dispersion and descent and adverse ascent, which results from the attack of six external pathogenic factors or zang-fu viscera dysfunctions.

5.14.1.1   Six External Pathogenic Factors Attacking the Lung

When the weather changes suddenly or abnormally, the lung is attacked externally from the mouth, nose, body hair, and skin, by pathogenic wind, cold, summer heat, dampness, dryness, or fire. The lung qi fails in dispersion and descent, which leads to the adverse ascent and causes cough.

5.14.1.2 Deficiency of the Lung

Prolonged diseases in the lung may consume the lung qi and lung yin, which affects the lung's function in governing qi and thus causes cough.

5.14.1.3 Dysfunction of Other Zang-Fu Viscera

Zang-fu viscera' dysfunction may block the ascent and descent of qi flow and impair the lung's function in governing qi, which also causes cough. The phlegm–dampness due to spleen deficiency, fire transformed from liver qi stagnation, or kidney qi deficiency may affect the lungs and induce cough.

The following factors like improper diet, excessive drinking or smoking, or excessive intake of spicy and greasy food may cause the spleen dysfunction of transportation and transformation. Then phlegm–dampness occurs in the body, which affects the lungs and causes cough. As the saying goes: "The spleen is the origin of phlegm production and the lung is the place where phlegm stays."

Stress, anger, and other emotional upset cause liver qi stagnation, which may transform into liver fire over time. Liver fire flame upwards through the liver channel, which may cause adverse ascent of lung qi and cause cough.

The kidney is the root of qi and takes in qi. Therefore, deficient kidney qi or yin-yang deficiency may result in kidney failure in the intake of qi and cause the adverse ascent of lung qi, which is followed by cough.

5.14.2 Diagnosis and Differential Diagnosis

Cough can be diagnosed by cough with or without sputum. Cough is generally divided into cough due to external attack and cough due to internal injury. The former is characterized by a sudden onset, a short duration, and the symptoms of the exterior syndrome, while the latter is characterized by recurrent attack, a prolonged duration, and the symptoms of other zang-fu viscera' dysfunction.

5.14.3 Differentiation

Cough is mainly caused by the lungs and is closely related to the liver, spleen, and kidney. As the saying goes, "dysfunction of all of five zang viscera and six fu viscera can cause cough besides the lung." Cough due to external attack usually manifests excess syndrome and cough due to internal injury manifests deficiency in root but excess in symptoms such as phlegm–dampness, phlegm–heat, and liver fire.

5.14.3.1 Cough Due to External Attack

1. Wind-cold attacking the lung
   Cough with heavy sound, clear thin white sputum, itchy throat, fast breathing, stuffy nose with clear discharge, headache, limbs soreness, aversion to cold, fever, no sweating, a thin white tongue coating, and a superficial tense pulse.
2. Wind-heat attacking the lung
   Cough with difficult expectoration, fast breathing, dry sore throat, sticky thick yellow sputum, stuffy nose with yellow discharge, thirst, headache, fever, and a red tongue with thin yellow coating, a superficial rapid or slippery pulse.
3. Wind-dryness attacking the lung
   Frequent cough with scanty sticky sputum or with no sputum or with blood-streaked sputum, itchy or dry sore throat, dry lips and nose, stuffy nose, head-ache, aversion to wind or cold, fever, a dry red tongue with thin white or yellow coating, and a superficial rapid pulse.

5.14.3.2 Cough Due to Internal Injury

1. Phlegm–dampness accumulating in the lung
   Cough with a heavy sound, profuse sticky white sputum, easy expectoration, chest tightness, cough relieved after expectoration, lassitude, abdominal disten-sion and fullness, nausea or vomiting, loose stools, greasy white tongue coating, and a soft moderate pulse.
2. Phlegm–heat accumulating in the lung
   Cough with profuse sticky thick yellow sputum or with foul-smelling or bloody sputum, fast breathing or even wheezing sound in the throat, distension and fullness or even pain in the chest, and hypochondriac region, red face, mild fever, dry mouth with a desire to drink water, a red tongue with thin greasy yel-low coating, and a slippery rapid pulse.
3. Liver fire affecting the lung
   Paroxysmal cough with scanty sticky sputum, difficult expectoration, flushed face, distending pain in the chest and hypochondriac region, dry throat, bitter taste in the mouth, the symptoms variable with emotional fluctuation, a dry red tongue with thin yellow coating, and a wiry rapid pulse.
4. Lung yin consumption
   Abrupt short cough with scanty sticky white sputum or with blood-streaked sputum or without sputum, tidal fever, flushed cheeks in the afternoon, night sweating, dry mouth and throat, a red tongue with scanty coating, and a rapid thready pulse.

5.14.4 Treatment

5.14.4.1 Chinese Medicinal Treatment

Cough Due to External Attack

To disperse the lung and eliminate external pathogenic factors.

Wind-Cold Attacking the Lung

Treatment principle: to eliminate wind, dissipate cold, disperse the lung, and stop coughing.

Chinese medicinal treatment:

Major Prescription: Sanao Tang plus Zhisou San.

Herbs: Mahuang, Xingren, Zhigancao, Shengjiang, Jingjie, Jiegeng, Baiqian, Chenpi, Baibu and Ziyuan.

Explanation: Sanao Tang is applied to disperse the lungs and dissipate the cold. Zhisou San is applied to slightly disperse the lung, regulate the lung qi, and stop the cough.

Mahuang: to relieve the exterior and dissipate cold.

Xingren: to descend the lung qi and stop coughing.

Zhigancao: to harmonize the actions of other herbs.

Ziyuan and Baibu: to resolve phlegm and stop coughing.

Jiegeng and Baiqian: to disperse the lung qi and resolve phlegm.

Jinjie: to eliminate wind and relieve the exterior.

Chenpi: to regulate qi and resolve phlegm.

Modification: For cases with an itchy throat, add Niubangzi and Chanyi; for cases with a severe stuffy nose, add Cangerzi and Xinyihua; for cases with chest tightness with a greasy tongue coating, add Fuling, Banxia, and Houpu.

Wind-Heat Attacking the Lung

Treatment principle: to eliminate wind, clear heat and stop coughing.

Chinese medicinal treatment:

Major prescription: Sangjuyin.

Herbs: Sangye, Juhua, Lianqiao, Bohe, Jiegeng, Xingren, Lugen, and Gancao.

Explanation: Sangye: to eliminate wind and clear heat.

Juhua, Xingren, and Jiegen: to disperse wind-heat and descend the lung qi.

Lianqiao, Bohe, and Lugen: to relieve the exterior, clear heat, and generate fluid.

Gancao: to coordinate the other herbs and soothe sore throat.

Modification: For cases with severe productive cough, add Chuanbeimu, Qianhu, and Pipaye; for cases with fever, add Zhimu, Huangqin, Yuxingcao, and Jinyinhua; for cases with a sore throat and hoarse voice, add Niubangzi, Shegan, and Shandougen; and for cases with thirst, add Tianhuafen and Zhimu.

Wind-Dryness Attacking the Lung

Treatment principle: to eliminate wind, moisten dryness, and stop coughing.

Chinese medicinal treatment:

Major Prescription: Sangxing Tang.

Herbs: Sangye, Douchi, Xingren, Xiangbeimu, Shashen, Lipi, and Zhizi.

Explanation: Sangye and Xingren: to clear heat, disperse, and moisten the lung.

Douchi, Xiangbeimu, and Shashen: to clear heat, moisten the throat, and relieve cough.

Zhizi and Lipi: to clear the lung-heat, moisten the throat, and relieve cough.

Modification: For cases with blood-streaked sputum, add Shengdihuang and Baimaogen; for cases with fluid damage, add Maidong, Shihu, and Yuzhu; for cases with lung-heat, add Shengshigao and Zhimu.

Cough Due to Internal Injury

To eliminate pathogenic factors and supplement anti-pathogenic qi.

Phlegm–Dampness Accumulating in the Lung

Treatment principle: to dry dampness, resolve phlegm, regulate qi, and stop coughing.

Chinese medicinal treatment:

Major Prescription: Ercheng Tang and Sanzi Yangqin Tang.

Herbs: Jiangbanxia, Chenpi, Fuling, Juhong and Zhigancao, Suzi, Baijiezi, and Laifuzi.

Explanation: Erchen Tang is applied to resolve phlegm–dampness and Sanzi Yangqin Tang to warm the lung, resolve phlegm, descend the lung qi, and promote digestion.

Jiangbanxia: to dry dampness and resolve phlegm.

Chenpi: to regulate qi and resolve phlegm and dampness combined with Banxia.

Fuling: to strengthen the spleen to resolve phlegm.

Zhigancao: to coordinate other herbs and harmonize the middle Jiao.

Modification: For cases with poor appetite due to spleen deficiency, add Dangshen, Baizhu, and Fuling; for cases with difficult expectoration, add Gualouren, Zhebeimu, and Haifushi; for cases with cold–phlegm with symptoms such as sticky foamy white sputum, aversion to cold and cold sensation in the back, add Xixin and Ganjiang.

Phlegm–Heat Accumulating in the Lung

Treatment principle: to clear heat, disperse the lung qi, resolve phlegm, and stop coughing.

Chinese medicinal treatment:

Major Prescription: Qingjin Huatan Tang.

Herbs: Huangqin, Zhizi, Jiegeng, Maidong, Sangbaipi, Beimu, Zhimu, Gualouren, Juhong, Fuling, and Gancao.

Explanation: Sangbaipi, Huangqin, Zhizi, and Zhimu: to clear the lung-heat,

Beimu, Gualouren, and Jiegeng: to clear heat and resolve phlegm.

Fuling, Juhong, and Gancao: to regulate qi and resolve phlegm.

Modification: For cases with thick yellow sputum or with foul-smelling sputum, add Yuxingcao, Yiyiren, and Dongguaren; for cases with profuse sputum, chest fullness, and constipation, add Tinglizi and Dahuang; for cases with phlegm–heat impairing the lung fluid with symptoms, add Xianlugen, Tianhuafen, and Beisharen; and for cases with fever and restlessness, add Zhimu and Shengshigao.

Liver Fire Affecting the Lung

Treatment principle: to soothe the liver, clear the lung, resolve phlegm, and stop coughing.

Chinese medicinal treatment:

Major Prescription: Xiebai San and Daibe San.

Herbs: Sangbaipi, Diguapi, Jingmi, Zhigancao, Qingdai and Haigeqiao.

Explanation: Xiebai San is applied to clear the lung heat, relieve dyspnea and cough while Daige San is to clear the liver fire, facilitate lung's function, and relieve restlessness.

Sangbaipi: to clear the lung-heat.

Diguapi: to reduce hidden fire in the lungs and nourish the lung yin.

Jingmi and Zhigancao: to nourish the stomach and harmonize the middle Jiao.

Qingdai: to clear toxic-heat in the liver channel.

Haigeqiao: to resolve phlegm and relieve cough.

Modification: For cases with pronounced liver fire, add Danpi and Zhizi; for cases with adverse ascent of the lung qi and chest oppression, add Tinglizi, Zhike, and Gualou; for cases with chest fullness and hypochondriac pain, add Yujin and Sigualuo; for cases with sticky sputum, add Dannanxing, Haifush,i and Zhebeimu; and for cases with fire injuring fluid, add Xianlugen, Maidong, and Beisharen.

Lung Yin Consumption

Treatment principle: to nourish yin, clear heat, moisten the lung, and stop coughing.

Chinese medicinal treatment:

Major Prescription: Shashen Maidong Tang.

Herbs: Shashen, Maidong, Yuzhu, Dong Sangye, Tianhuafen, Shengbiandou, and Gancao.

Explanation: Shashen, Maidong, Yuzhu, and Tianhuafen: to nourish yin and moisten the lung.

Dong Sangye: to clear the lung-heat and descend the lung qi.

Shengbiandou and Gancao: to coordinate and harmonize the middle Jiao.

Modification: For cases with prolonged fever and cough due to dryness-heat in the lung, add Sangbaipi and Diguapi; for cases with blood-streaked sputum, add Zhizi, Danpi, and Baimaogen; for cases with night sweating, add Shengmuli, Fuxiaomai, and Nuodaogen; and for cases with cough with yellow sputum, add Huangqin, Haigefen, and Zhimu.

5.14.4.2 Acupuncture and Moxibustion Treatment

Cough Due to External Attack

Main acupoints: Lieque (LU 7), Hegu (LI 4), Feishu (BL 13), and Taiyuan (LU 9).

Modification: In cases with a wind-cold attack, add Fengmen (BL 12), in cases with a wind-heat attack, add Dazhui (GV 14) and Quchi (LI 11); in cases with a sore throat, add Shaoshang (LI 11) with pricking for bloodletting.

Methods: The reducing method is applied to the above points. Moxibustion can also be combined in a wind-cold attack.

Cough Due to Internal Injury

Main acupoints: Feishu (BL 13), Taiyuan (LU 9), and Sanyinjiao (SP 6).

Modification: In cases with phlegm–dampness in the lung, add Fenglong (SI 40), Zusanli (SI 36), and Pishu (BL 20); in cases with liver fire affecting the lung, add Xinjian (LR 2); in cases with lung yin consumption, add Gaohuang (BL 43); in cases with phlegm–heat accumulating the lung, add Chize (LU 5).

Methods: reinforcing manipulation is applied to Pishu (BL 20) and Zusanli (SI 36). The reducing method is applied to the rest points.

5.14.4.3 Tuina

Principal acupoints and locations: Tiantu (CV 22), Danzhong (CV 17), Zhongfu (LU 1), Yunmen (LU 2), Shenzhu (GV 12), Dazhu (BL 11), Fengmen (BL 12), Feishu (BL 13), Dingchuan (EX-B 1), Fengchi (GB 20), Fengfu (GV 16), Jianjing (GB 21), hypochondriac region, chest, and upper back.

Manipulations: one-finger pushing, kneading, pushing, rolling, grasping, wiping, and scrubbing manipulations.

Basic procedure: patient takes a supine position; apply one-finger pushing or kneading manipulation on the route from Tiantu (CV 22) to Danzhong (CV 17) 5–10 times; apply pressing–kneading manipulation on Zhongfu (LU 1) and Yunmen (LU 2) for 1 min each point; apply separate-pushing manipulation on the chest to the hypochondriac region for 5–10 times; apply pressing–kneading manipulation on Chize (LU 5), Taiyuan (LU 9), Yuji (LU 10), and Lieque (LU 7) for 1 min each point; apply grasping–kneading manipulation on Hegu (LI 4) for 1 min.

A patient takes a prone position; apply rolling manipulation on the upper back along the urinary bladder channel 3–5 times; apply pressing–kneading manipulation on Dazhu (BL 11), Dingchuan (EX-B 1), Shenzhu (GV 12), Fengmen (BL 12), and Feishu (BL 13) for 1 min each point; apply grasping manipulation on Jianjing (GB 21).

Modification: In cases with wind-cold attacking the lung, add applying scrubbing manipulation on the upper back along the urinary bladder channel till a hot sensation appears; in cases with wind-heat attacking the lung, add applying pressing–kneading Quchi (LI 11) and patting on the upper back till hot sensation appears; in cases with phlegm–dampness accumulating the lung, add pressing–kneading Fenglong (SI 40) and Zusanli (SI 36), wiping on the chest till hot sensation appears; in cases with phlegm–heat or liver fire, add pressing–kneading Taichong (LR 3), palm-twisting hypochondrium.

5.14.5 Prevention

Patients with a cough should keep a warm, light diet and avoid sweet, salty, greasy, and spicy food. Try to expectorate sputum with the assist of tapping the back or sputum aspirator. Give up cigarette smoking or alcohol drinking, do more outdoor exercises, and keep good ventilation in the room.

5.15 Summary

Pathogenesis	Syndromes	Treatment principles	Prescriptions
External attack	Wind–cold attacking the lung	Eliminate wind, dissipate cold, disperse the lungs, and stop cough	Sanao Tang and Zhisou San
	Wind–heat attacking the lung	Eliminate wind, clear heat, and stop cough	Sangju Yin
	Wind–dryness attacking the lung	Eliminate wind, moisten dryness, and stop cough	Sangxing Tang
Internal injury	Phlegm–dampness accumulating in the lung	Dry dampness, resolve phlegm, regulate qi, and stop cough	Ercheng Tang and Sanzi Yangqin Tang
	Phlegm–heat accumulating in the lung	Clear heat, disperse the lung qi, resolve phlegm, and stop cough	Qingjin Huatan Tang
	Liver fire affecting the lung	Soothe the liver, clear the lungs, resolve phlegm, and stop cough	Xiebai San and Daige San
	Lung yin consumption	Nourish yin, clear heat, moisten the lungs, and stop cough	Shashen Maidong Yin

Questions
1. Describe the key diagnostic points of cough due to external attack and internal injury.
2. Describe the clinical manifestations, treatment principle, and major prescription of cough due to the liver fire affecting the lung.
3. Describe the treatment principles and major prescriptions for cough due to different external pathogenic factors.

References
1. Du Y, Dong Q. Therapeutic of acupuncture and moxibustion. Beijing: People's Medical Publishing House; 2016.
2. Peng B. Traditional Chinese internal medicine. Beijing: People's Medical Publishing House; 2007.
3. Shen X. Acupuncture and moxibustion. Beijing: People's Medical Publishing House; 2007.
4. Xie J, Li M, Han C. Chinese internal medicine. Beijing: People's Medical Publishing House; 2011.
5. Yan J. Tuina Science. Beijing: China Press of Traditional Chinese Medicine; 2006.

5.16 Asthma

Objectives
Master the knowledge about the treatment of asthma based on syndrome differentiation via learning the etiology, pathogenesis, diagnosis, differentiation, treatment, and prevention of asthma.

Guideline
This chapter introduces the etiology, pathogenesis, diagnosis, differential diagnosis, treatment (herbal medicine and acupuncture), and prevention of asthma.

5.17 Introduction

Asthma is a paroxysmal respiratory disease that occurs when lung qi fails to disperse and descend in the latent phlegm body. It is a joint name for wheezing syndrome and dyspnea syndrome, which is characterized by recurrent attacks of dyspnea with bronchial wheezing. "Wheezing" refers to polypnea with phlegm rale in the throat. "Dyspnea" means hasty panting, with the mouth open and shoulders raised, and inability to lie flat.

According to the *Internal Classic*, which records "The lung may thus be damaged and wheezing will ensue." In the treatise on the differentiation of yin and yang chapter, the clinical feature of wheezing is similar to asthma, ALthough there is no exact name. In the *Han* dynasty, by stating "for coughing with qi ascent and a frog-like rale in the throat, Shegan Mahuang Tang is indicated." *Zhang Zhongjing* presented the typical symptoms and treatment when an asthmatic attack happened. In the *Yuan* dynasty, *Zhu Danxi* created the phrases of asthma disease and pointed out the therapeutic principles. During the *Ming* dynasty, *Yu Tuan* made an explicit differentiation between "wheezing" and "dyspnea." He suggested that wheezing could be confirmed with sound, and panting with breath.

In Western medicine, the relevant disease includes bronchial asthma, asthmatic bronchitis, allergic asthma, and cardiac asthma.

5.17.1   Etiology

5.17.1.1   Exogenous Pathogenic Factors

Due to the attack of wind–cold, wind–heat, or inhalation of extrinsic factors such as smoke, pollen, animals' fur, and irritant gas, the lung qi may fail to disperse and descend, which causes the disturbance of water metabolism and the stagnation of phlegm–wetness. Thus, asthma happens.

5.17.1.2   Irregular Diet

Over-consumption of raw and cold, spicy, sweet, and fatty food affects the transportation and transformation of the spleen and the digestive function of the stomach, leading to phlegm–turbidity or phlegm–heat, and the excessive phlegm could directly flame up along the meridian of the lung and block the airway to be asthma.

5.17.1.3   Deficiency Status

The deficiency of the lung, spleen, or kidney due to constitutional or post illness may damage body resistance and affect water metabolism. This may cause susceptibility to allergic factors, such as infant asthma owing to the congenital kidney qi deficiency, and the retention of phlegm-fluid. Also, lung yin deficiency could cause a deficient fire which may evaporate body fluids to the phlegm-turbidity stagnation in the lung, subsequently resulting in asthma.

5.17.2 Pathogenesis

5.17.2.1 Pathogenic Site

Asthma is mainly located in the lungs and is closely associated with the spleen and kidney. Besides, because the conditions between each organ are closely related, the heart and liver may also be involved.

Phlegm–dampness, the predominant factor during asthma, may be produced by the dysfunction of the spleen due to the improper diet. Phlegm could affect water metabolism by blocking the normal flow of qi. As the lung dominates qi and is the container of phlegm, and the kidney is responsible for deep breath and is the root of phlegm, the main pathogenic site contains the lung, spleen, and kidney.

By means of association with the circulation of fluid and qi, the liver should also be involved. In one term, the liver qi stagnation could hinder the fluid movement, in the other, such status always transforms into fire conditions and evaporates body fluids. Both of them will lead to phlegm.

Since blood circulation is closely connected with the heart and lungs, severe deficiency of the lung may damage heart function. Thus, it leads to the deadly wheeling collapse.

5.17.2.2 Pathological Nature

Asthma should be divided into acute and relieving stages, which means asthenia in origin and sthenia in superficiality. The sthenia in symptom appears in the acute stage while the asthenia in viscera happens in the relieving stage. The sthenia in symptom exhibits different characteristics for various exogenous pathogenic factors: wind, cold, heat, etc. Besides, the asthenia in zang-fu viscera should distinguish both the main sites and the natures of yin, yang, or qi.

5.17.2.3 Basic Pathogenesis

The fundamental cause of asthma lies in phlegm-qi binding and obstructing the airway due to the exogenous pathogen induced by the latent phlegm in the body.

5.17.2.4 Pathogenesis in Different Disease Stages

In the attack stage, the main pathogenesis is phlegm blocking the airway causing the failure of the lung to disperse and descend, which triggers wheezing and panting. The common factors include external pathogens, emotional stress, irregular diet, fatigue, etc. The main factor should be the sudden climate change. Due to the differentiation between constitution and causes, the sthenia in symptoms differs in four conditions: cold, heat, deficiency, and excess. The categories include:

Cold asthma is due to exposure to external colds or lack of vital energy.
Pyretic asthma is due to external heat or the constitutional yang excess.
Frigiopyretic asthma is due to the external cold and the internal pyretic.
Anemophlegmatic asthma is due to the latent phlegm in the lung and the external wind attack.

Deficient asthma is due to recurrent episodes of asthma, manifesting in insufficient symptoms. The lung, spleen, and kidney could be sick concurrently, owing to the interrelationships between visceral organs.

In the status asthmatics attacking, the deficiency in the root cause and excessiveness in the manifestation could emerge at the same time, which is characterized by persistent dyspnea. If the lung-energy cannot assist the blood circulation and the fire in the vital gate is too weak to support the heart yang, the collapse due to dyspnea will happen.

In the remission stage, the deficiency of qi is the predominant factor to the insufficient symptoms. However, the character is a combination of deficiency and excess. For example, the excess syndrome could transform into the deficient syndrome when yin, yang, or qi is damaged by the pathogenic products. Besides, because yin, yang, and qi are fundamental materials in metabolism, their deficiency creates pathogenic products, which could increase the deficiency symptoms and thus cause the boundless cycle between deficiency and excess.

5.17.3 Diagnosis

5.17.3.1 Disease Diagnosis

Because of factors such as sudden change, unsuitable foods, and emotional disorder, it typically has recurrent wheezing, dyspnea, inability to lie flat, even pale complexion, cyanotic lips, and nails that could last for minutes or hours. Previous symptoms include rhinocnesmus, sneezing, cough, and chest distress.

If the wheezing or panting cannot be relieved constantly, it should be treated as the status asthmaticus.

The patient's behavior is usually normal except for a bit of fatigue, a poor appetite, or abundant phlegm.

A history of other allergic diseases (eczema or allergic rhinitis) or asthma is in first-degree relatives.

The blood tests, the lung function, and the X-ray could be auxiliary examinations.

5.17.3.2   Differential Diagnosis

Asthma should be distinguished from dyspnea and pleural fluid retention.

1. The difference between asthma and dyspnea
     Asthma is the combination name of wheezing and dyspnea, which is charac-
terized by paroxysmal whistling sounds in the throat and the breathless while
dyspnea involves panting rapidly, not necessarily accompanied by the wheezing sounds.
2. The difference between asthma and pleural fluid retention
     Pleural fluid retention is characterized by coughing, panting, chest fullness,
or pain after a persistent and forceful coughing, not involving wheezing sounds
such as asthma.

5.17.4   Differentiation

5.17.4.1   Major Points

Before the treatment, it is necessary to distinguish a deficiency syndrome from an
excess syndrome.
     During asthma attacks, cold, pyretic, frigiopyretic, and anemophlegmatic asthma
are included as excessive patterns.
     During remissions, the deficiency of the lung, spleen, and kidney is often
included.

5.17.4.2   Cold Asthma

Clinical manifestations:
     Patients may have wheezing dyspnea, tachypnea, shortness of breath, a sense of
fullness and tightness in the chest, mild cough with dilute, whitish, and frothy sputum, which is difficult to spit out, no thirst or thirst with a preference for hot drinks,
pale or bluish complexion, cold limbs, and coldness intolerance. The typical symptoms could be triggered by cold weather or getting cold.
     Tongue: pale tongue with a whitish and slippery coating.
     Pulse: wiry tense pulse or floating tense pulse.
     Analysis of clinical manifestations:
     Wheezing dyspnea and tachypnea may be induced by the latent-cold phlegm in
the lung and the narrow airway due to the obstruction of the phlegm-qi conjugate.
     Cold and phlegm may block the lung and cause an inability of lung qi to disperse,
which causes the sensation of fullness or tightness in the chest and mild cough.
     Lack of heat pathogen or pathogenic products, patients neither bring out thirst
nor prefer hot water.

Because the esoteric cold could trigger the intense fluid retention, asthma will attack during the cold weather.

As internal yin excess overwhelms yang qi, the bluish complexion, cold limbs, and cold intolerance will come together. The features of the tongue and pulse are typical signs of cold excess.

5.17.4.3 Pyretic Asthma

Clinical manifestations:

The symptoms include ecphysesis with roar like wheezing, breathing with a gruff voice, fullness in chest and hypochondrium, frequent cough with yellow and thick sputum, which is difficult to spit out, a bitter taste in the mouth, feeling of thirst and preferring to drink water, sweating red face, or general fever. Some cases are triggered in the summer.

Tongue: red tongue with a thin and yellowish greasy coating.

Pulse: slippery rapid pulse or taut slippery pulse.

Analysis of clinical manifestations:

Heat and phlegm may block the airway and cause the inability of lung qi to disperse and descend, which causes the ecphysesis with roar like wheezing, breath with a gruff voice, fullness in the chest, and hypochondrium and frequent cough.

The combining heat-phlegm evaporates the latent phlegm and causes the yellow and thick sputum which is difficult to spit out. It also evaporates the body fluid and causes a bitter taste in the mouth and thirst the desire to drink water.

Excess of inner heat causes sweating, a red face, or general fever.

The features of the tongue and pulse are typical signs of heat excess.

5.17.4.4 Frigiopyretic Asthma

Clinical manifestations:

Patients may undergo wheezing dyspnea, tachypnea, shortness of breath, a febrile sensation and fullness in the chest, dysphoria, chills, fever, and body ache, absence of sweat, cough with yellow and thick or yellow and white sputum, which is difficult to spit out, thirst with desire to drink water, and feces lack of fluid.

Tongue: red tip and margin of the tongue with white bias in the yellow and greasy coating.

Pulse: wiry tense pulse.

Analysis of Clinical manifestations:

The airway may be blocked or narrow due to the heat–phlegm binding, thus causing the inability of lung qi to disperse and descend, which results in wheezing dyspnea, tachypnea, shortness of breath, febrile sensation, and fullness in the chest subsequently.

External colds attack the Taiyang channel and stay in the skin impairing the circulation of defense qi and then causing chills, absence of sweat, fever, and body aches.

The combining heat–phlegm evaporates the body fluid and then causes thirst and a desire to drink water.

The features of the tongue and pulse are typical signs of cold external and heat–phlegm internal excess.

5.17.4.5 Anemophlegmatic Asthma

Clinical manifestations:

The symptoms include excessive sputum in the throat with a voice similar to sawing wood or whistle, panting and tachypnea, a sense of fullness in the chest, orthopnea and inability to lie flat, frothy sputum or sticky sputum which is hard to spit out, acute break with the sense organs itch, and sneeze in the beginning.

Tongue: thick and turbid coating with normal tongue.

Pulse: floating and forceful pulse.

Analysis of clinical manifestations: wind could trigger the latent-phlegm in the body, which may affect the function of lung qi and hinder the airway simultaneously. As a result, patients may get a fullness sensation in the chest, wheezing sounds in the throat, typical sputum, panting, and hard to lie flat.

5.17.4.6 Deficient Asthma

Clinical manifestations:

Patients may have frequent and chronic relapse, wheezing in the throat, low voice, breathlessness, which becomes more serious after exercise, and weakness of the lung qi. With the deficiency of yang, dilute and pale sputum, no thirst, wind intolerance, pale or even dark-purple complexion and lips, white coating tongue, and small deep pulse would be exhibited.

As for insufficiency of yang: stick sputum or lack of sputum, flushed cheeks, fever, red tongue with little coating, and small or deep and thready pulse.

Analysis of clinical manifestations:

The basic pathogenesis is due to the frequent and chronic relapse, the phlegm and qi binding together, then causing the blockage of lung qi and also damage the organs such as the lung and kidney, and finally creating the dysfunction of lung's director of qi and kidney's storage.

5.17.4.7 Status Asthma

Clinical manifestations:

Patients may present severe dyspnea with an open mouth, raised shoulders and inability to lie flat, wheezing sound in the throat, restlessness, unconsciousness, cyanotic complexion, peripheral coldness, and bead-like sweats.

Tongue: bluish tongue with greasy or floating coating.

Pulse: small and rapid pulse, large and forceless pulse, or fainting pulse.

Analysis of clinical manifestations:

The excessive phlegm could not only block the dispersing and descending function of lung qi, which causes severe dyspnea with an open mouth, raised shoulders, and inability to lie flat and wheezing sound in the throat, but also blocks upper orifices, which causes unconsciousness.

Due to the blockage of phlegm, the energy cannot be transported all over, and cyanotic complexion and peripheral coldness happen then.

The features of the tongue and pulse are typical signs of deficiency.

5.17.4.8 The Deficiency of Lung and Spleen

Clinical manifestations:

The symptoms include no strength to talk, shortness of breath, slight wheezing occasionally, a lot of clear and white sputum, spontaneous sweating, aversion to wind, frequent common cold in changing seasons, sleep, poor appetite, and easy diarrhea.

Tongue: pale tongue with thin or white-slippery coating.

Pulse: weak and soft pulse.

Analysis of clinical manifestations:

Spleen qi deficiency may cause shortness of breath, sleepiness, and little strength to talk.

Spleen fails to transport and transform leading to poor appetite and easy to have diarrhea.

Weakness of defense qi leads to an aversion to wind, frequent common cold in season-changing times, and spontaneous sweating.

Lung fails to handle qi and the dysfunction of lung qi to transform fluid leads to phlegm-fluid stagnation in the lung, causing shortness of breath, lots of clear and white sputum, and slight wheezing occasionally.

5.17.4.9 The Deficiency of Lung and Kidney

Clinical manifestations:

The symptoms include shortness of breath, dyspnea that is triggered by physical exercises, difficulty in inhalation, cough with spicy sputum, tinnitus and rotating dizziness, aching and weakness of the waist and knees, fluster, and intolerance of work. With the kidney yang deficiency, cold limbs with coldness intolerance and pale complexion will occur. With the lack of kidney yin, symptoms include the feverish sensation of five-palm, hot flush, red cheeks, night sweating, and dry mouth.

Tongue: red tongue with lack of liquid and thin coating or pale and plump tongue with white coating.

Pulse: small and rapid pulse or deep thready pulse.

Analysis of clinical manifestations:

Lung fails to handle qi and the dysfunction of lung qi to transform fluid leads to phlegm-fluid stagnation in the lung, causing shortness of breath and cough with spicy sputum.

The kidney fails to receive qi, leading to shortness of breath, dyspnea, and difficulty in inhalation that is triggered by physical exercises.

Essential deficiency of qi causes tinnitus and rotating dizziness, aching, and weakness of the waist and knee.

The deficiency of kidney yang may cause internal cold with symptoms such as cold limbs coldness intolerance and pale complexion.

The deficiency of kidney yin may cause internal deficient heat leading to the feverish sensation of five-palm, hot flush, red cheeks, night sweating, and dry mouth.

5.17.5   Treatment Principles

General principles during episodes are dispelling phlegm, directing qi, and relieving asthma. Specifically, warming the lung, eliminating cold, resolving phlegm, regulating the lung qi downward for cold asthma and dissipating heat, dispersing the lung, resolving phlegm, and directing qi downward for pyretic asthma.

General principles during remission states are supplying qi, tonifying yang, nourishing yin and strengthening the lung, spleen, or kidney for deficient patterns.

5.17.5.1   Chinese Medicinal Treatment

Cold Asthma

Treatment Principle: Disseminate the lung, eliminate cold, reduce phlegm and relieve asthma.

Prescription: She Gan Mahuang Tang or Xiaoqinglong Tang modification.

Herbs:Monarch: Zhimahuang, Shegan, Ziwan, Zhibanxia, Ganjiang, Xixin, Kuandonghua, Wuweizi, Dazao, and Gancao.

Administration: Take the herbals decoction for oral use, twice a day.

Explanation:

Zhimahuang and Shegan: to ventilate lungs, relieve dyspnea, resolve phlegm, and benefit throat.

Ganjiang, Xixin, and Zhibanxia: to warm lungs, reduce fluid retention, and bring adverse qi downward.

Ziwan and Kuandonghua: to resolve phlegm to stop cough.

Wuweizi: to astringe lung qi.

Dazao and Gancao: to coordinate the drug actions and harmonize the middle energizer.

Modification: For cases with chills, fever, and body aches, add Guizhi and Ganjiang to reduce wind and ventilate the cold; for cases with excessive phlegm with an inability to lie flat, add Tinglizi to purge the lung and direct qi downward. It is also necessary to add Xinren, Suzi, Baiqian, and Jupi to resolve phlegm and associate the circulation of qi; for cases with severe cough with breathless and profuse sweat, Baishao should be added to astringe lung qi.

Pyretic Asthma

Treatment Principle: Regulate the lung and clear away heat, resolve phlegm, relieve asthma, and send the adverse qi down.

Prescription: Dingchuan Tang or Yuebijia Banxia Tang.

Herbs:Zhimahuang, Baiguo, Xingren, Zhibanxia, Zi Suzi, Kuandonghua, Sangbaipi, Huangqin, and Gancao.

Administration: take the herbals decoction for oral use, twice a day.

Explanation:

Zhimahuang: to ventilate the lung and relieve dyspnea.

Huangqin and Sangbaipi: to clear heat and regulate the function of lung qi.

Xingren, Banxia, Kuandonghua, and Zisuzi: to resolve phlegm and bring adverse qi downward.

Baiguo: to astringe lung qi and restrain the excessive disperse from Mahuang.

Gancao: to coordinate the drug actions.

Modification: for cases with exterior cold binding with internal intense lung-heat, the drug added is Shengshigao, Gypsum Fibrosum (initial usage) to clear the internal heat; for cases of inability to lie flat, Tinglizi and Guangdilong are added to clear lung and stop panting; for cases with excessive lung heat and spit yellow and thick sputum, add Haigeqiao, Shegan, Zhimu and Yuxingcao to remove heat-phlegm; for cases with constipation, add Dahuang, Gualou, Mangxiao and Zhishi to remove heat by catharsis; for cases with prolonged heat which impairs body fluids and cause the rapid breathing, coughing with a little thick phlegm mixed with blood, dry and sore throat, red and dry tongue and thready rapid pulse, Maimendong Tang or other drugs such as Shashen, Zhimu, Tianhuafen should be used to nourish yin and clear inner heat.

Frigiopyretic Asthma

Treatment Principle: Relieve superficial pathogenic factors: dissipating cold, clearing away heat, and eliminating sputum.

Prescription: Xiaoqinglong plus Shigao Tang or Houpo Hahuang Tang modification.

Herbs: Mahuang, Shigao, Houpo, Xingren, Shengjiang, Banxia, Dazao, and Gancao.

Administration: take the herbals decoction for oral use, twice a day.

Explanation:

Mahuang: to ventilate lung.

Shigao: to relieve lung-heat, the combination of both two could disseminate exterior cold and remove the interior heat.

Houpo and Xingren: to relieve asthma and stop cough.

Shengjiang and Banxia: to resolve phlegm and bring adverse qi downward.

Dazao and Gancao: to coordinate the drug action.

Modification: for cases with severe outside cold, add Guizhi and Xixin; for cases with excessive phlegm with panting, add Tinglizi, Suzi, and Shegan to resolve phlegm and relieve asthma; for cases with yellow and thick sputum which is difficult to spit out, Huangqin, Qianhu, and Gualoupi should be added to remove the phlegm–heat.

Anemophlegmatic Asthma

Treatment principle: Eliminate wind, resolve phlegm, and direct lung qi downward.

Prescription: Sanzi Yangqin Tang plus Erchen Tang modification.

Herbs: Suzi, Baijiezi, Laifuzi, Jiangbanxia, Chenpi, Xingren, Jiangcan, Houpo, Fuling, and Mahuang.

Explanation:

Suzi: to direct lung qi downward and stop asthma.

Baijiezi: to ventilate lung qi and resolve phlegm.

Laifuzi: to assist Suzi and Laifuzi to direct lung qi and reduce phlegm.

Mahuang: to ventilate the lung and relieve dyspnea.

Xingren and Jiangcan: to eliminate wind and resolve phlegm.

Houpo, Banxia, and Chenpi: to resolve phlegm and bring adverse qi downward.

Fuling: to invigorate the spleen to dissolve phlegm.

Modification: for cases with severe panting with an inability to lie flat, add Tinglizi and Zaojiaoci or Kunxian Dan; for cases with the attack triggered by the exotic wind evil, add Suye, Fangfeng, Caoercao, Chanyi, and Dilong.

Deficient Asthma

Treatment principle: Invigorate the lung, strengthen the kidney, resolve phlegm, and bring adverse qi downward.

Prescription: Pingchuan Guben Tang modification.

Herbs: Dangshen, Huangqi, Chenxiang, Suzi, Qidai, Hutaorou, Banxia, Kuandong, Jupi, Dongchongxiacao, and Wuweizi.

Administration: take the herbals decoction for oral use, twice a day.

Explanation:

Dangshen and Huangqi: to reinforce the lung.

Hutaorou, Chenxiang, Qidai, Dongchongxiacao, and Wuweizi: to strengthen the kidney and keep the inspired air going downward.

Suzi, Banxia, Kuandong, and Jupi: to keep the inspired air going downward and dispel phlegm.

Modification: for cases with deficiency of kidney yang, add Fuzi, Lujiaopian, Buguzhi and Zhongrushi; for cases with lack of yin, add Shashen, Maidong, Shengdi and Dang Gui; for cases with excessive panting after moving and direct the qi to be downward, add Zishiyin, Ci; for cases with dark purple lips and the obstruction of phlegm, add Taoren and Sumu.

Status Asthmatics

Treatment principle: Tonify yang and prevent collapse.
    Prescription: Huiyang Jiuji Tang and Shengmai Yin modification.
    Herbs: the ingredients of Huiyang Jiuji Tang: Fuzi, Ganjiang, Rougui, Shengshaishen, Baizhu, Fuling, Ganpi, Zhigancao, Wuweizi, Banxia, and Shexiang.
    The ingredients of Shengmai Yin: Renshen, Maidong, Wuweizi.
    Explanation:
    Huiyang Jiuji Tang: to recuperate depleted yang and rescue the patient from collapse, and supplement qi to activate pulse, to cure syndrome of dominance of internal cold and exhaustion of yang qi.
    Shengmai Yin: to strengthen qi and nourish yin, to cure weakness of qi and yin.
    Modification: for cases with severe panting, restlessness, bead-like sweat with cold limbs, thick-purple tongue, and thin pulse, take Heixi Dan immediately; for cases with serious weakness of yang, breathlessness, and sweat with cold limbs, add Rougui and Ganjiang; for cases with rapidly panting, restlessness, bead-like sweat and dry mouth with red tongue, add Shengdi and Yuzhu to nourish yin.

The Deficiency of Lung and Spleen

Treatment principle: Tonify the lung, invigorate the spleen, and strengthen the sickness of qi.
    Prescription: Liujunzi Tang modification.
    Herbs:Renshen, Baizhu, Fulin, Banxia, Chenpi, Gancao.
    Administration: take the herbals decoction for oral use, twice a day.
    Explanation:
    Dangshen, Baizhu, Fulin, and Zhigancao: to invigorate the spleen and replenish qi.
    Chenpi and Banxia: to direct qi and dispel phlegm.
    The indication of Liujunzi Tang is spleen qi deficiency with phlegm, marked by shortness of breath, cough with white and clear sputum or vomiting, and poor appetite.
    Modification: for cases with a lack of qi and serious spontaneous sweat, add Huangqi and Fuxiaomai; for cases with a lack of resistance to external evils, add Yupinfeng San for usual use; for cases with a lack of spleen yang with cold limbs, add Guizhi and Ganjiang to warm yang and resolve fluid retention.

The Deficiency of Lung and Kidney

Treatment principle: Tonify the lung and strengthen the kidney.

Prescription: Shengmai Dihuang Tang and Jinshui Liujun Jian modification.

Herbs: Shudihuang, Shanzhuyu, Hutaorou, Renshen, Maidong, Wuweizi, Fulin, Gancao, Banxia, and Chenpi.

Explanation:

Shudihuang, Shanzhuyu, and Hutaorou: to strengthen the kidney and assistant qi to be received.

Renshen, Maidong, and Wuweizi: to nourish the kidney yin.

Baizhu, Fulin, and Zhigancao: to invigorate the spleen and replenish qi.

Chenpi and Banxia: to direct qi and dispel phlegm.

Modification: For cases with tonifying the kidney yang, combine with Buguzhi, Lujiaopian, Zhifuzi, and Rougui; for cases with lack of lung ying and qi, add Huangqi, Shashen, Baihe; for insufficient kidney yin, combine with Shengdihuang, Dongchongxiacao, also the Heche Dazao Wan could be used to nourish yin; for cases with failing to receive qi, add Dongchongxiacao, Zishiying or Shenge San. In addition, the powder of Ziheche could be used normally.

5.17.5.2 Acupuncture and Moxibustion Treatment

Main acupoints: Feishu (BL 13), Zhongfu (LU 1), Taiyuan (LU 9), Dingchuan (EX-B 1), and Danzhong (CV 17).

Methods: a reduced manipulation should be given to the above points. The needles are retained for 15–30 min. Give the treatment qd.

Modification: For cases with difficult breathing: Tiantu (CV 22); excess syndrome: Chize (LU 5) and Yuji (LU 10); and deficiency syndrome: Gaohuang (BL 43) and Shenshu (BL 23).

5.17.6 Prevention

Patients with asthma should keep warm and avoid being triggered by the sudden change in climate. Take measures to prevent the common cold or flu. Try appropriate exercise according to your physical condition. Give up smoking. Be away from inhaling dust or other irritative gas. Avoid excessive intake of cold, greasy, sour, salty, sweet, and marine food. Keep off overwork and maintain a peaceful mind. Take patented Chinese medicine such as Yupingfeng San or Shenqi Wan to strengthen body resistance.

5.18 Summary

Asthma is a paroxysmal respiratory disease, which is characterized by wheezing syndrome, dyspnea syndrome, and fullness, tightness, or pain in the chest.

The episode of asthma is due to the failure of lung qi in dispersing and descending, which caused the disturbance of water metabolism and the stagnation of phlegm–wetness.

The general treatment during episodes is dispelling phlegm, directing qi, and relieving asthma, while during in remission states are supplement qi, tonify yang, nourish yin, and also strengthen the lung, spleen, or kidney for deficient patterns.

During the onset of asthma, the treatment of acupuncture can be used prior to the prescription of medicinal herbs. During the remission stage, decoction, moxibustion, acupuncture, and other external therapies can be used to tonify the inside resistance in order to reduce the relapse of asthma.

Questions
1. Describe the concept of asthma.
2. Describe the etiology and pathogenesis of asthma.
3. Describe the difference between asthma and dyspnea.
4. Describe the general treatment principles of asthma.

References
1. Xinnong C. Chinese acupuncture and moxibustion. Beijing: Foreign Languages Press; 2010.
2. Chunsheng J, Yong H. Acupuncture and moxibustion. Beijing: People's Medical Publishing House; 2013.
3. Peng B. Traditional Chinese internal medicine. Beijing: People's Medical Publishing House; 2007.
4. Xie J, Li M, Han C. Chinese internal medicine. Beijing: People's Medical Publishing House; 2011.

5.19 Dysmenorrhea

Objectives
Master the knowledge about the treatment of dysmenorrhea based on syndrome differentiation via learning the etiology, pathogenesis, diagnosis, differentiation, treatment, and prevention of cough.

Guideline
This chapter introduces the etiology, pathogenesis, diagnosis, differential diagnosis, treatment (herbal medicine, acupuncture, and tuina), and prevention of dysmenorrhea.

5.20   Introduction

Dysmenorrhea, also known as painful periods, or menstrual cramps, is characterized by periodic lower abdominal pain or other discomforts before, during, or after
menstruation. The pain may be even beyond tolerance and cause pale complexion,
nausea, vomiting, cold sweating, and cold limbs. Clinically, dysmenorrhea can be
divided into primary one and secondary one based on the absence or presence of
organic problems. Primary dysmenorrhea usually occurs after menarche, while secondary dysmenorrhea occurs after menarche. Dysmenorrhea often occurs among
unmarried young women, among whom primary one is more common.

In Western medicine, the higher levels of prostaglandins and other inflammatory
mediators cause the uterus to contract, which is believed to be a major factor in the
occurrence of primary dysmenorrhea. Other developmental problems, such as uterine hypoplasia, cervical stenosis, or uterine over-flexion, may cause unsmooth menstrual flow and then cause painful periods.

Dysmenorrhea is closely related to the chong vessel, the conception vessel, and
the uterus. Emotional upset, irregular life style, or attack by six external pathogenic
factors are the common causes of dysmenorrhea.

5.20.1   Etiology

5.20.1.1   Qi Stagnation and Blood Stasis

Emotional upset or external pathogenic factors may cause the disturbance of qi flow
and thus blood stasis in the uterus, which causes painful menstruation.

5.20.1.2   Congealed Cold and Dampness

If being attacked by cold, such as being caught in rain, contracting pathogenic cold,
taking in cold drinks, and sitting or lying on the cold or damp ground, the uterus
may be affected by accumulation of cold and dampness, which leads to the unsmooth
flow of qi and blood.

5.20.1.3   Deficiency of Qi and Blood

Congenital deficiency of qi and blood or consumption of qi and blood due to severe
or prolonged diseases can lead to weak blood circulation, which causes pain due to
malnutrition.

5.20.1.4   Deficiency of the Kidney and Liver

Insufficiency of congenital essence, excessive sexual activity, or prolonged diseases may injury the liver and kidney, which causes yin-blood deficiency, and thus malnutrition of the uterus occurs.

5.20.1.5   Down-Pouring Dampness–Heat

Dampness–heat attacks the body and affects thoroughfare and conception vessels or uterus, which leads to the stagnation of qi and blood, and thus pain occurs.

5.20.2   Diagnosis and Differential Diagnosis

Periodic lower abdominal pain or painful lumbosacral region during, before, or after menstruation.

Common among young unmarried women.

Gynecological examination and ultrasound B can be applied to differentiate the primary dysmenorrhea from the secondary one.

Dysmenorrhea should be distinguished from the acute abdominal pain caused by extra-uterine pregnancy or torsion of ovarian cyst and also from the lower abdominal pain caused by acute pelvic inflammation, acute cystitis, urinary lithiasis, appendicitis, colitis or acute gastroenteritis, etc.

5.20.3   Differentiation

5.20.3.1   Qi Stagnation and Blood Stasis

Distending or bearing-down pain in the abdomen during menstruation or 1 or 2 days before, an abundant amount of or scanty menses or inhibited dripping menses, or dark purple menses with clots or even with big pieces, pain is aggravated by pressing and relieved with clot discharge, distending pain in the breasts and hypochondriac region, dark purple tongue with petechiae on the edges, and a deep wiry pulse.

5.20.3.2   Congealed Cold–Dampness

Cold pain in the lower abdomen that occurs before or during menstruation, pain may be aggravated by pressing and relieved by warming, scanty dark purple menses with clots, aversion to cold, loose stools, a light purple tongue with a moist or slimy white coating, and a wiry deep pulse.

5.20.3.3 Deficiency of Qi and Blood

Persistent dull pain during or after menstruation, pain may be relieved by pressing, bearing-down sensation, an abundant amount of menses without any clot or scanty menses, pale complexion, dizziness and palpitation, fatigue, a pale tongue with teeth-marked edges, a thin coating, and a fine pulse.

5.20.3.4 Deficiency of the Kidney and Liver

Dull pain or cold and bearing-down sensation in the lower abdomen with soreness and distension in the lumbar region 1 or 2 days after menstruation, thin scanty menses dark or light in color, tinnitus, dizziness, blurred vision, or tidal fever, malar flushing, a pale tongue with a thin white or yellow tongue coating, a deep thready pulse.

5.20.3.5 Down-Pouring Dampness–Heat

Pain or burning sensation in the lower abdomen during menstruation, aggravated by pressing, distending pain in the lumbar region, or frequent pain in the lateral lower abdomen, which is worsened at the beginning days of menstruation, frequently slight fever, thick darkish red menses with clots, thick yellowish vaginal discharge, scanty dark urine, a red tongue with a slimy yellow coating, a wiry fast, or soggy fast pulse.

5.20.4 Treatment

5.20.4.1 Chinese Medicinal Treatment

Qi Stagnation and Blood Stasis

Treatment principle: to sooth the liver, regulate qi, remove blood stasis, and relieve pain.

Major Prescription: Gexia Zhuyu Tang.

Herbs: Danggui, Chuanxiong, Chishao, Taoren, Zhiqiao, Yuanhu, Wulingzhi, Mudanpi, Wuyao, Xiangfu, and Gancao.

Explanation:

Zhiqiao, Wuyao, and Xiangfu: to regulate qi and harmonize the liver.

Danggui: to nourish and harmonize blood.

Chuanxiong, Chishao, Taoren, and Mudanpi: to activate blood circulation and resolve blood stasis.

Yuanhu and Wulingzhi: to resolve blood stasis and relieve pain.

Gancao: to relieve pain and harmonize other herbs.

Modification: for cases with the stomach being attacked by the liver qi, add Wuzhuyu and Banxia; for cases with bearing-down and distending sensation in the lower abdomen, add Chaihu and Shengma.

Congealed Cold and Dampness

Treatment principle: to warm the meridians to dispel cold, eliminate dampness to remove stasis, and relieve pain.

Major prescription: Shaofu Zhuyu Tang and Fuling.

Herbs: Xiaohuixiang, Ganjiang, Yuanhu, Moyao, Danggui, Chuanxiong, Rougui, Chishao, Puhuang, and wulingzhi.

Explanation:

Rougui, Xiaohuixiang, and Ganjiang: to warm the meridians, dispel cold, and eliminate dampness.

Danggui, Chuanxiong, and Chishao: nourish blood, activate blood circulation, and resolve blood stasis.

Yuanhu, wulingzhi, Puhuang, and Moyao: to resolve blood stasis and relieve pain.

Cangzhu: to dry dampness and resolve the turbidity.

Fuling: to strengthen the spleen and eliminate dampness by diuresis.

Modification: for cases with pronounced cold pain, add Danggui Jianzhong Tang plus Aiye and Wuzhuyu.

Deficiency of Qi and Blood

Treatment principle: to strengthen the spleen qi and nourish the blood to relieve pain.

Major Prescription: modified Sheng Yu Tang.

Herbs: Rensheng, Huangqi, Danggui, Chuanxiong, Shudihuang, Baishao, Xiangfu, and Yuanhu.

Explanation:

Rensheng and Huangqi: to replenish qi.

Danggui, Chuanxiong, Shudihuang, and Baishao: to nourish and harmonize blood.

Xiangfu and Yuanhu: to regulate qi and relieve pain.

Modification: for cases with soreness in the lumbar region, add Tusizi and Duzhong.

Depletion of the Liver and Kidney

Treatment principle: to nourish the blood, harmonize the liver, tonify the kidney, and supplement the essence.

Major Prescription: Tiaogan Tang.

Herbs: Danggui, Baishao, Bajitian, Ejiao, Shanyao and Shanyurou.

Explanation:

Danggui and Baishao: to nourish blood and harmonize the liver.

Shanyurou: to nourish the liver and kidney and supplement the essence-qi.

Bajitian: to warm and tonify the kidney yang.

Ejiao: to nourish blood and yin.

Shanyao: to strengthen the spleen and replenish qi.

Modification: for cases with scanty menses, add Lujiaojiao.

Down-Pouring Dampness–Heat

Treatment principle: to clear heat, remove dampness, resolve blood stasis, and relieve pain.

Major prescription: modified Qingre Tiaoxue Tang and Yiyiren.

Herbs: Mudanpi, Huanglian, Shengdihuang, Danggui, Baishao, Chuanxiong, Honghua, Taoren, Yuanhu, Ezhu, Xiangfu, Hongteng, and Yiyiren.

Explanation:

Mudanpi: to clear heat, cool blood, and resolve blood stasis.

Shengdihuang: to clear heat and cool blood.

Huanglian: to clear toxic heat.

Danggui and Baishao: to nourish blood and harmonize the liver.

Chuanxiong, Honghua, Taoren, and Ezhu: to activate blood circulation and resolve blood stasis.

Xiangfu and Yuanhu: to regulate qi and relieve pain.

Hongteng and Yiyiren: to remove dampness and resolve blood stasis.

5.20.4.2 Acupuncture and Moxibustion

Main acupoints: Guanyuan (CV 4), Zigong (EX-CA 1), Shiqizhui (EX-B 8), Sanyinjiao (SP 6), and Hegu (LI 4).

Methods: Reducing manipulation on Hegu (LI 4) and Sanyinjiao (SP 6). Reducing manipulation on the rest points for excess syndrome and reinforcing manipulation for deficiency syndrome.

Modification: in cases with cold congealing and blood stasis, add Shenque (CV 8) and Guilai (SI 29); in cases with qi stagnation and blood stasis, add Taichong (LR 3) and Xuehai (SP 10); in cases with kidney qi deficiency, add Shenshu (BL 23) and Taixi (KI 3); in cases with qi-blood deficiency, add Qihai (CV 6) and Zusanli (SI 36).

5.20.4.3 Tuina

Principal acupoints and locations: Qihai (CV 6), Guanyuan (CV 4), Baliao (BL 31–34), Zhangmen (LR 13), Ganshu (BL 18), Geshu (BL 17), Pishu (BL 20), Weishu (BL 21), Shenshu (BL 23), Baliao (BL 31–34), Xuehai (SP 10), Sanyinjiao (SP 6), Zusanli (SI 36), Taixi (KI 3), and Yongquan (KI 1), back and lumbar area.

Manipulation: one-finger pushing, rubbing, kneading, pressing, grasping, and scrubbing manipulations.

Basic procedure: The patient takes a supine position; apply rubbing manipulation clockwise on the lower abdomen; apply one-finger pushing or pressing–kneading manipulation on Qihai (CV 6) and Guanyuan (CV 4) for 3–5 min at each point.

A patient takes a prone position; apply rolling manipulation on bilateral lumbar areas along the urinary bladder channel; apply pressing–kneading manipulations on Shenshu (BL 23) and Baliao (BL 31–34) for 2–3 min at each point; apply scrubbing manipulation on the lumbosacral area and Baliao (BL 31–34) until it is warm enough in the local area.

Modification: in cases with qi stagnation and blood stasis, apply pressing and kneading manipulations on Zhangmen (LR 13), Ganshu (BL 18), Geshu (BL 17), grasp Xuehai (SP 10), and Sanyinjiao (SP6) until there is local distending feeling; in cases with cold–dampness coagulation, apply scrubbing manipulation first along governor vessel, and then, transversely over lumbosacral region until it is warm enough in the local area and apply pressing–kneading manipulation on Xuehai (SP 10) and Sanyinjiao (SP 6); in cases with qi and blood deficiency, apply scrubbing manipulation along governor vessel, and then transversely over both sides of the back until it is warm enough in the local area, apply rubbing manipulation clockwise on the lower abdomen, applying pressing–kneading manipulations on Zhongwan (CV12), apply pressing–kneading manipulations on Pishu (BL 20), Weishu (BL 21), and Zusanli (SI 36); in cases with liver-kidney depletion, apply scrubbing manipulation first along governor vessel, and then transversely over lumbar area until it is warm enough in the local area; apply pressing–kneading manipulations on Taixi (KI 3) and Yongquan (KI 1), Ganshu (BL 18), and Shenshu (BL 23).

5.20.5 Prevention

Patients with dysmenorrhea should keep warm during menstruation. Pay attention to menstrual hygiene. Have a proper rest and avoid overstrain. Avoid irritability and depression. Avoid cold drinks and strenuous exercises before and during menstruation.

5.21 Summary

Pathogenesis	Syndromes	Treatment principles	Prescriptions
Emotional upset, external pathogenic factors, or congenital weakness	Qi stagnation and blood stasis	Sooth the liver, regulate qi, remove blood stasis, and relieve pain	Gexia Zhuyu Tang
	Congealed cold–dampness	Warm the meridians to dispel clod, eliminate dampness to remove stasis, and relieve pain	Shaofu Zhuyu Tang
Disturbance of qi flow and blood stasis in the uterus	Deficiency of qi and blood	Strengthen the spleen qi and nourish blood to relieve pain	Shengyu Tang
	Deficiency of the kidney and liver	To nourish the blood, harmonize the liver, tonify the kidney, and supplement the essence	Tiaogan Tang
	Down-pouring dampness–heat	Clear heat, remove dampness, resolve blood stasis, and relieve pain	Qingre Tiaoxue Tang

Questions

1. What kind of condition can be called dysmenorrhea?
2. Describe the key points of diagnosis in different syndromes of dysmenorrhea.

References

1. Du Y, Dong Q. Therapeutic of acupuncture and moxibustion. Beijing: People's Medical Publishing House; 2016.
2. Tan Y. Gynecology of traditional Chinese medicine. Beijing: People's Medical Publishing House; 2007.
3. Shen X. Acupuncture and moxibustion. Beijing: People's Medical Publishing House; 2007.
4. Xie J, Li M, Han C. Chinese internal medicine. Beijing: People's Medical Publishing House; 2011.
5. Yan J. Tuina Science. Beijing: China Press of Traditional Chinese Medicine; 2006.
6. Jamieson DJ, Steege JF. The prevalence of dysmenorrhea, dyspareunia, pelvic pain, and irritable bowel syndrome in primary care practices. Obstet Gynecol. 1996;87(1):55–8.
7. Proctor M, Farquhar C. Diagnosis and management of dysmenorrhea. BMJ. 2006;332(7550):1134–8.
8. Nasir L, Bope ET. Management of pelvic pain from dysmenorrhea or endometriosis. J Am Board Fam Pract. 2004;17(suppl):S43–7.

5.22 Stomachache

Objectives
Master the knowledge about the treatment of stomachache based on syndrome differentiation via learning the etiology, pathogenesis, diagnosis, differentiation, treatment, and prevention of stomachache.

Guideline
This chapter introduces the etiology, pathogenesis, diagnosis, differential diagnosis, treatment (herbal medicine and acupuncture), and prevention of stomachache.

5.23 Introduction

Stomachache may be a paroxysmal, intermittent, or seasonal disease that occurs when stomach qi fails to descend, qi stagnation and blood disorder, food retention, or stomach qi blockage. The symptom manifested as pain in the stomach and upper abdomen.

Early in *Internal Classic*, there was a record of the stomachache when it was still confused with real heart pain. Until the *Song Jin Yuan* dynasty, "stomach pain" was first put forward as an independent disease. The name "stomach pain" was first recorded in *Yi Xue Qi Yuan* (*Medicine Origin*). Then *Lan Shi Mi Cang* (*Secret Book of Orchid Chamber*), for the first time, individually separated "stomach pain" as a disease and elaborated its etiology and pathogenesis, principle, and treatment. Since then, "stomach pain" has been treated as an independent disease. In addition, the etiology and pathogenesis, principle, and treatment of stomach pain were relatively systematically understood. *Treatise on the Pathogenesis and Manifestations of All Diseases* considered that the etiology of stomach pain resulted from internal cause (damage by the excess of seven emotions), external cause (invasion of six climatic exopathogens), and non-endo-non-exogenous cause (diet, overstrain, and contacts with foreign substances), and the principle of treatment was to relieve pain by eliminating pathogens and helped the pattern differentiation to be much clear.

In Western medicine, the relevant disease includes acute and chronic gastritis, peptic ulcer, gastroptosis or prolapsed gastric mucosa, gastroneurosis, functional dyspepsia, gastric cancer, and esophagitis.

5.23.1 Etiology

5.23.1.1 Exogenous Pathogenic Factors

Due to the attack of cold, heat, or pathogenic damp, especially, cold evil could obstruct the circulation of stomach qi, which causes the dysfunction of stomach qi, leading to pain.

5.23.1.2 Irregular Diet

On the one hand, surfeit harms the spleen and stomach, leading to stomach distension and pain, or even abdominal pain and diarrhea. On the other hand, overconsumption of fatty, spicy, or sweet food or alcohol will produce inner-heat and impair the descending of stomach qi, subsequently causing gastric pain.

5.23.1.3 Emotional Maladjusted

Emotional disorders such as excessive anger, upset, or stress may damage the liver and lead to the stagnation of liver qi, which not only hinders the movement of stomach qi but also restrain the spleen and stomach, resulting in stomachache.

5.23.1.4 Deficiency Status of the Spleen and Stomach

The spleen and stomach are the main organs for digestion. The improper diet or other factors that damage the two organs led to the deficiency of the spleen and stomach. Lack of spleen yang may produce an internal deficient cold and neglect the duty to warm the stomach system, which may cause the pain in stomach. Lack of stomach yin may cause malnourishment of the stomach and subsequent pain in the stomach.

5.23.1.5 Medicine Injury

Over ingestion of cold-natured or hot-natured medications may hurt the stomach qi or stomach yin, which leads to the obstruction of digestion, then, caused the stomachache.

5.23.2 Pathogenesis

5.23.2.1 Pathogenic Site

Stomachache is mainly located in the stomach, majorly relates to the liver and spleen and involves the gallbladder and kidney.

According to the five elements theory, the liver, known as the resolute viscus, should be ascribed to the character of wood, and the stomach, known as the sea of grains and water, should be ascribed to the character of the earth. Because of the liver controlling dispersion, the pathogenic products that affect the circulation of qi may cause the stagnation of liver qi. As same as the restriction among wood and earth, the stagnation of liver qi may affect the stomach and lead to stomach pain subsequently. In addition, the stagnation of liver qi may transform into inner fire and damage stomach yin, which causes malnourishment of the stomach.

Lack of spleen yang may produce an internal deficient cold and neglect the duty to warm the stomach system, which may cause the pain in stomach.

The kidney is the gate of the stomach. The warm energy from the kidney yang is essential to the transportation and transformation of the spleen and stomach. Lack of kidney yang may cause deficient cold in the spleen, leading to stomach pain.

5.23.2.2 Pathological Nature

Stomach pain should be divided into cold or heat, excess or deficiency, and qi level or blood level patterns. Above all, it should be ascribed to excess patterns and deficiency patterns.

Excess patterns include cold attacking the stomach, food retention, coordination between the liver and stomach, stasis of blood, and dampness–heat stagnation of the liver and stomach.

Deficiency patterns include deficiency of spleen qi and stomach qi, deficiency cold of spleen and stomach, and deficiency of stomach yin.

Between excess syndrome and deficiency syndrome, there is complication and transformation.

5.23.2.3 Basic Pathogenesis

The fundamental of stomachache lies in the disorder of qi and blood, imbalance of cold and heat, and accumulation of pathological products, such as dampness and stasis, which are consequences of improper diet, emotional disturbance, invasion by six exogenous pathogens, or weakness of habitus, resulting in qi disorder, and ascending and descending disorder of spleen and stomach, then the chronic gastritis relative symptoms such as gastric distention and stomach pain are generated. It is usually manifested as asthenia in origin and sthenia in superficiality and deficiency complicated with excess. Asthenia in origin majorly performs as deficiency of spleen qi and stomach yin, while sthenia performs as qi stagnation, damps heat, and blood stasis. The qi disorder of the spleen and stomach is the most direct pathogenic factor.

5.23.3 Diagnosis

5.23.3.1 Disease Diagnosis

Because of external factors, such as colds, overeating unsuitable foods, emotional disorders, and hurt with medicines with the typical stomachache symptom or other manifestations of pain, with the associated symptoms such as poor palpitation, nausea, vomiting, acid regurgitation, and belching with a foul breath.

Middle-aged youth patients are in the majority and the disease may frequently recur in an acute or chronic way.

The normal blood tests, bilirubin, diastase tests, ultrasound, and CT scan as well as the X-ray could be the assistants.

5.23.3.2 Differential Diagnosis

Before the proper treatment, it is necessary to distinguish stomachache from cardiac pain, hypochondriac pain, intestinal abscesses, and abdominal pain.

1. The difference between stomachache and angina pectoris
   The site of the pain for angina pectoris is in the chest while stomachache is in the central of the upper abdomen. The symptoms are different in cardiac pain with severe, persistent stabbing pain, a sense of death, breathless, white complexion with cold limbs, and dark purple lips.
2. The difference between stomachache and hypochondriac pain
   The main difference between the two diseases is the site of the pain, in which the hypochondriac pain is left or right flank, and stomachache is central of the upper abdomen.
3. The difference between stomachache and intestinal abscesses
   The pain site in intestinal abscesses is an epigastric region or the right lower abdomen with the sudden pain in the epigastric region first and then rapidly transferring to the right lower abdomen.
4. The difference between stomachache and abdominal pain
   The site of the pain for abdominal pain is between the stomach and the pubis with the symptoms including distending and dull pain or sever pain with diarrhea or constipation.

5.23.4 Differentiation

5.23.4.1 Major Points

First, to identify the excess from deficiency: the excess patterns manifest in sudden attack, short duration, and severe pain with tenderness and forceful pulse while the deficient patterns show a chronic episode, long duration, mild pain with preference for pressure, and weak pulse.

Second, to identify the cold from heat: the cold patterns manifest in the wiry or tight pulse and the pain, which could be triggered by cold and removed by warmth while the heat patterns show a sudden, burning pain which could be triggered by the warmth and alleviated by cold, along with a yellow tongue or tongue coating and wiry-rapid or slippery-rapid pulse.

Third, to identify the conditions between qi level and blood level: the patterns stay in qi level include qi stagnation with the distending pain associated with emotional fluctuation, qi deficiency with dull pain, decreased food ingestion, abdominal distension after eating food and weak pulse while the blood level only includes the blood stasis with the symptoms, such as stabbing pain with a fixed position, purple tongue, and choppy pulse.

5.23.4.2   Accumulation of Exotic Cold

Clinical manifestations:

Patients may present with sudden abrupt stomachache, which could be increased by cold and decreased by warmth, no thirst, or preference for hot water.

Tongue: thin and white.

Pulse: wiry and tense.

Analysis of clinical manifestations:

Cold attacking in the stomach may influence the movement of qi causing the warm and nourishing functions beyond the ability of qi, leading to sudden stomachache.

Because the heat could warm the body and cold could worsen the stagnation of qi, the pain could be increased by cold and decreased by warmth.

Since cold belongs to the yin pathogen and cannot damage the fluid in the body, patients may present with no thirst or preference for hot water.

Both the tongue and pulse indicate cold too.

5.23.4.3   Food Retention

Clinical manifestations:

The symptoms include: stomach pain, fullness in the gastric, belching, acid regurgitation, vomiting undigested food, and feeling relief after vomiting.

Tongue: thick and greasy coating.

Pulse: slippery.

Analysis of clinical manifestations:

Food retention may block the flow of stomach qi, causing stomachache with fullness in the gastric, belching, acid regurgitation, vomiting, and feeling relief after vomiting.

The dysfunction of the spleen and stomach may cause an inability to digest food.

5.23.4.4   Inharmonious Between Liver and Stomach

Clinical manifestations:

Distention and ache in the gastral cavity or scurrying hypochondrium pain, frequent eructation, and exacerbation when emotional discomfort.

Tongue: pink or red tongue with thin white or thin and yellowish coating.
Pulse: stringy pulse.

5.23.4.5 Heat Stagnation of Liver and Stomach

Clinical manifestations:

Urgent burning pain in the gastral cavity, dysphoria, gastric discomfort, acid regurgitation, dry mouth, bitter taste in the mouth, dry, and unsmooth defecation.

Tongue: red tongue with yellow coating.
Pulse: stringy and rapid pulse.

5.23.4.6 Blood Stasis

Clinical manifestations:

Stomachache with a fixed stabbing pain in the epigastrium, tenderness, pain triggered by eating food, hematemesis, and black stools.

Tongue: purplish tongue.
Pulse: choppy pulse.

5.23.4.7 Deficiency of Stomach Yin

Clinical manifestations:

Burning pain in the gastral cavity, hunger but no appetite, dry mouth, dry and unsmooth defecation, red and dry tongue with scanty fur or without fur or with fissure, thin and rapid pulse or stringy and thin pulse.

Critical pathogenesis:

Deficiency of stomach yin, deficient fire flaring stomach.

5.23.4.8 Deficient Cold of Spleen and Stomach

Clinical manifestations:

Dull ache in the gastral cavity, relief with warmness and pressure, relief after diet, cold of limbs, vomiting watery fluid, diarrhea with undigested food, plump and teeth-printed tongue with white and slippery fur, deep and thin pulse, or deep and moderate pulse.

Critical pathogenesis:

The deficient cold of the spleen and stomach, asthenia spleno-gastric yang, loss of warming of the stomach, and stagnation of qi movement.

5.23.5   *Treatment*

General principles direct the movement of qi and harmonize the stomach.

For excess patterns, the principle is to remove the pathogenic factors. Distinguishing the different types from cold accumulation, qi stagnation, blood stasis, and stomach heat prior to the proper treatment, such as warming the stomach, smoothing the liver, moving the blood, and clearing heat is necessary.

For deficient patterns, the main point is to identify the insufficiency in yin or yang, in order to nourish yin or strengthen yang.

5.23.5.1   Chinese Medicinal Treatment

Accumulation of Exotic Cold

Treatment principle: Dissipate cold and relieve pain.
  Prescription: Xiangsu San plus Liangfu Wan modification.
  Herbs: Gaoliangjiang, Cuxiangfu, Zisuye, Zisugen, Ganpi, Zhigancao.
  Administration: take the herbals decoction for oral use, twice a day.
  Explanation: Liangfu Wan, Gaoliangjiang, Cuxiangfu: to warm the stomach and regulate the flow of qi.
  Xiangsu San, Xiangfu, Zisuye, Ganpi, Zhigancao: to dispel cold to relieve the exterior syndrome, regulate qi and the function of the stomach.
  Modification: in case of severe cold, combine with Wuzhuyu and Chenpi to reduce the effect of cold and associate the circulation of qi; in case of food intention, combine with Zhishi, Shenqu, Banxia, and Jiaoshanzha to promote digestion.

Food Intention

Treatment principle: assist digestion and relieve pain.
  Prescription: Baohe Wan modification.
  Herbs: Shanzha, Banxia, Fuling, Shenqu, Chenpi, Lianqiao, and Laifuzi.
  Explanation:
  Shanzha: to digest fatty food.
  Shenqu: to pormote digestion.
  Laifuzi: to assist stomach qi downward.
  Banxia, Chenpi, and Fuling: to regulate qi and resolve dampness.
  Modification: in case of severe pain or distention, add Zhishi, Sharen, and Binglang to promote digestion and assist the movement of qi; in case of severe blockage inside the stomach, combine with Zhishi Daozhi Wan or Xiaochengqi Tang; in case of severe, acute stomachache with tenderness, constipation and yellow, dry tongue coating, and forceful pulse.

Inharmonious Between Liver and Stomach

Treatment principle: Dispersing stagnated liver qi for regulating stomach qi.
　　Prescription: Chaihu Shugan San.
　　Herbs: Chaihu, Baishao, Zhiqiao, Xiangfu, Chuanxiong, Chenpi, and Gancao.
　　Administration: decoct with water one dose per day, take 2 or 3 times per dose.
　　Explanation:
　　Chaihu and Xiangfu: to smooth the liver, direct qi, and reduce pain.
　　Zhiqiao: to regulate qi and coordinate the stomach.
　　Chuanxiong: to assist the movement of qi and blood.
　　Baishao and Gancao: to harmonize the stomach and reduce the pain.
　　Modification: for fullness in the chest, belching and retching, combine with Chenxiang, Xuanfuhua, and Sugeng to direct the qi downward; for the transformation trend into the fire of stagnation qi, add Huangqin.

Heat Stagnation of the Liver and Stomach

Treatment principle: Dispersing stagnated liver qi and purging heat to regulate stomach.
　　Prescription: Danzhi Xiaoyan San or Qingzhong Tang modification.
　　Herbs: Danggui, Baishao, Baizhu, Chaihu, Fuling, Danpi, and Zhizi.
　　Administration: decoct with water one dose per day, take 2 or 3 times per dose.
　　Explanation:
　　Baishao and Chaihu: to soothe the liver.
　　Danpi and Zhizi: to remove heat and soothe the liver.
　　Modification: for the disorder of qi and pain or distention in the chest and hypochondrium, combine with Yujin and Foshou; for fullness in the abdomen and constipation, combine with Shengdahuang and Binglang; for facilitating the effect of the above formula, add Zuoji Wan to drain the liver fire; for the severe retention of dampness, add Huoxiang, Baidoukou, and Houpo.

Blood Stasis

Treatment principle: Remove blood stasis to reduce the pain.
　　Prescription: Shixiao San plus Danshen Yin Modification.
　　Herbs: Puhuang, Wulinzhi, Danshen, Tanxiang, Sharen.
　　Explanation:
　　Wulinzhi and Danshen: to move the blood to resolve stasis.
　　Puhuang and Tanxiang: to promote the movement of qi and blood.
　　Sharen: to harmonize the stomach and resolve dampness.

Deficiency of Stomach Yin

Treatment Principle: Nourishing yin to strengthen the stomach.
    Prescription: Yiguan Jian plus Shaoyao Gancao Tang.
    Explanation:
    Yiguan Jian.
    Ingredients: Beisharen, Maidong, Danggui, Shengdihuang, Gouqizi, Chuanlianzi.
    Administration: Decoct with water one dose per day, take 2 or 3 times per dose.
    Action: to nourish yin and soothe the liver.
    Indication: hypochondriac and thoracic pain due to deficiency of yin of the liver
and kidney, and stagnancy of the liver qi, the formula is often used for chronic hepatitis, chronic cholecystitis, gastritis, and gastro-duodenal ulcer.
    Shaoyao Gancao Tang.
    Herbs: Baishao, Zhigancao.
    Indication: spasms of the muscles and abdominal pain.

Deficient Cold of Spleen and Stomach

Treatment Principle: Warming middle energizer and invigorating spleen.
    Prescription: Huangqi Jianzhong Decoction.
    Herbs: Huangqi, Baishao, Guizhi, Gancao, Shengjiang, Dazao, and Yitang.
    Administration: Decoct with water; decoct Huangqi, Bai Shao, Guizhi, Gan Cao,
Sheng Jiang, and Da Zao together, add Yi Tang after filtering the residue; one dose
per day, take 2 or 3 times per dose.
    Explanation:
    Huangqi Jianzhong Decoction.
    Action: to warm the middle energizer, restore qi, and regulate the internal organs
to relieve acute symptoms. Indications: abdominal pain, spontaneous sweating, dyspnea due to deficiency, and cold in the spleen and stomach; the formula is now often
used for gastro-duodenal ulcer, neurosis, and aplastic anemia, with above-mentioned
symptoms.

5.23.5.2 Acupuncture and Moxibustion Treatment

Main acupoints: Zusanli (ST 36), Zhongwan (CV 12), Guanyuan (CV 4), and
Tianshu (ST 25).
    Methods: apply reducing manipulations and combing with moxibustion.
    Modification: in cases with pathogenic cold attacking stomach: Shenque (CV 8);
food retention: Xiawan (CV 10), and Liangmen (ST 21); inharmonious between
liver and stomach: Qimen (LR 14), Taichong (LR 3); blood stasis: Geshu (BL 17),
Ashi points; deficient cold of spleen and stomach: Pishu(BL 20) and Shenque (CV 8).

5.23.6 *Prevention*

Patients with stomach pain need to develop good diet habits and avoid overfeeding with spicy, hot, and greasy food. They need to keep their mind at ease, avoid stimulation by unhealthy emotions, and consult a psychologist. Enhancing psychological counseling for stomach pain patients has certain help to alleviate disease onset, attenuate symptoms, and improve life quality. In addition, this kind of patient should avoid long-term overwork and pay attention to life regulations, especially in winter and spring. Regular physical training is recommended.

5.24 **Summary**

Pathogenesis	Syndromes	Treatment principles	Prescriptions
Exogenous pathogenic factors Irregular diet Emotional maladjusted Deficiency status of the spleen and stomach Medicine injury	Accumulation of exotic cold	Dissipate cold and relieve pain	Xiangsusan plus Liangfuwan modification
	Food intention	Assist digestion and relieve pain	Baohe Wan modification
	Inharmonious between the liver and stomach	Dispersing stagnated liver qi for regulating stomach qi	Chaihu Shugan San
	Heat stagnation of the liver and stomach	Dispersing stagnated liver qi and purging heat to regulate stomach	Danzhi Xiaoyan San or Qingzhong Tang modification
	Blood stasis	Remove blood stasis to reduce the pain.	Shixiao San plus Danshen Yin modification
	Deficiency of stomach yin	Nourishing yin to strengthen wei	Yiguan Jian plus Shaoyao Gancao Tang
	Deficient cold of spleen and stomach	Warming middle energizer and invigorating spleen	Huangqi Jianzhong decoction

Questions
1. Describe the main characteristics of stomachache.
2. What is the differentiation of stomachache between the accumulation of exotic cold and deficient cold of the spleen and stomach?
3. Describe the treatment principles and major prescriptions of inharmonious between liver and stomach syndrome.

References
1. Jianqiao F. Science of acupuncture and moxibustion. Beijing: China Press of Traditional Chinese Medicine; 2014.

2. Peng B. Traditional Chinese internal medicine. Beijing: People's Medical Publishing House; 2007.
3. Shen X. Acupuncture and moxibustion. Beijing: People's Medical Publishing House; 2007.
4. Xie J, Li M, Han C. Chinese internal medicine. Beijing: People's Medical Publishing House; 2011.

5.25   Diarrhea

Objectives
Master the etiology and pathogenesis of diarrhea under the guidance of TCM theory.

Master the law of syndrome differentiation and treatment of diarrhea under the guidance of TCM theory.

Guideline
This chapter introduces the etiology, pathogenesis, diagnosis, differential diagnosis, treatment (herbal medicine, acupuncture, and moxibustion), and prevention of diarrhea.

5.26   Introduction

Diarrhea is a disease referring to frequent defecation with a bellyache, loose stool, and even water stool at times occurring in all seasons but mostly in the summer and autumn.

In traditional Chinese medicine, diarrhea is included in the categories of diarrhea, dysentery, abdominal pain, and so forth. The etiology and pathogenesis were detailedly discussed in *Internal Classic*, which laid the foundation for the diagnosis and treatment of diarrhea.

In Western medicine, the relevant disease includes acute and chronic enteritis, gastrointestinal dysfunction, diarrhea-predominant irritable bowel syndrome, and intestinal tuberculosis.

5.26.1   Etiology and Pathogenesis

It usually results from the influence of cold, heat and dampness attack, improper diet, emotional upsets, and a part of which caused weak physique when it takes longer than usual, which leads to functional disorders of the spleen and stomach, accompanied by the dysfunction of the small intestine to digest food and the dysfunction of the large intestine in transportation. In this case, the clear and excreting turbid mix together and transport to the intestines. The main pathogenic factor is dampness and invasion of external pathogenic factors which cause the dysfunction of the spleen with the involvement in the spleen, stomach, and intestines with relation to the kidney and liver.

5.26.2 Diagnosis

With the pain and hyperactive bowel sounds in the abdomen, diarrhea is mainly marked by mucus, blood, and pus present in the stools. By the repeated attacks of damage, long-term diarrhea can cause emaciation and malnutrition. In microscopic stool examination, a small amount of leucocytes can be found. Congestion and edema of the intestine mucosa plica and mucous secretion can be seen under colonoscopy. Derangement of the intestinal plica mucosa is examined under X-ray with barium contrast of the colon.

5.26.3 Differentiation

5.26.3.1 Major Points

Excess and deficiency syndromes are usually set apart in this disease. Cold, heat, and dampness attacks, improper diet damaging the middle energizer, and emotional upsets causing the stagnant liver qi to invade the spleen are presented in excess syndromes; A prolonged illness, weak constitution, or an old age will result in deficiency syndromes, including splenic dysfunction of transportation and transformation, and declination of kidney yang, qi, and yin, which cause the inability to control the defecation.

5.26.3.2 Damp Cold Attacking the Middle Energizer

Clinical Manifestations:
   Abdominal pain, loose, watery, or even pus and blood stools, gasteremphraxis, borborygmus, anorexia, shiver, fever, weakness, and muscular soreness.
   Tongue: thin, white, and greasy tongue coating.
   Pulse: soft-superficial and soft pulse.
   Analysis of clinical manifestations:
   Loose and watery stools are the result of indigestion of water and food as well as a mixture of clear and turbid caused by dysfunction of the spleen in transportation. Gasteremphraxis, anorexia, and shivering are caused by cold–dampness disturbing the spleen. Cold–dampness also hampers intestine qi movement, which leads to abdominal pain and borborygmus. If combined with a wind-cold attacking exterior,

patients can have syndromes like aversion to cold, fever, muscular soreness, and soft-superficial and soft pulse. Thin, white, and greasy tongue coating are indications of damp cold attacking the middle energizer.

5.26.3.3 Damp Heat Attacking the Middle Energizer

Clinical manifestations:

Abdominal pain, urgent watery and yellowish-brown stools with extremely foul smell, difficulty defecation, burning pain in anus, fever, thirst, and scanty deep yellow urine.

Tongue: yellow and greasy tongue coating.

Pulse: soft-superficial and rapid pulse or smooth and rapid pulse.

Analysis of clinical manifestations:

Urgent watery and yellowish-brown stools with an extremely foul smell are because of heat in the intestine. Difficult defecation is caused by dampness-heat. When dampness-heat flows downward, it leads to burning pain in the anus and scanty deep yellow urine. Fever, thirst, yellow and greasy tongue coating, as well as soft-superficial and rapid pulse or smooth and rapid pulse are all indications of damp heat attacking the middle energizer.

5.26.3.4 Food Retention

Clinical manifestations:

Fullness in the epigastrium and abdomen, foul belching, poor appetite, diarrhea with a foul smell like rotten eggs and abdominal pain alleviated after bowel movements.

Tongue: dirty, thick, and greasy tongue coating.

Pulse: smooth pulse.

Analysis of clinical manifestations:

Fullness in the epigastrium and abdomen is caused by improper diet, food retention, and dysfunction of the spleen in transportation. Foul belching is the result of indigestion. Food indigested flowing downward leads to diarrhea with a foul smell like rotten eggs. Abdominal pain alleviates after bowel movements because of exerting indigestion. Dirty, thick, and greasy tongue coating and smooth pulse are indications of food retention.

5.26.3.5 Liver Qi Attacking the Spleen

Clinical manifestations:

This syndrome includes distending pain, borborygmus, abdominal pain before diarrhea, and the pain relieved after diarrhea, which is caused by anger, anxiety, depression, or stress, and the symptoms are belching, stiffness in the chest and anorexia.

Tongue: light red tongue.

Pulse: wiry pulse.

Analysis of clinical manifestations:

Distending pain and borborygmus are caused by a disorder of qi movement when patients feel anger, anxiety, depression, or stress. These symptoms alleviate diarrhea. Diarrhea is a result of dysfunction of the spleen in transportation. Combined with dysfunction of the liver in controlling conveyance and dispersion, patients can have belching, stiffness in the chest, and anorexia. Light red tongue and wiry pulse are indications of hyperactivity of liver qi.

5.26.3.6 Deficiency of the Spleen and Stomach

Clinical manifestations:

Usually, the patient with this type of diarrhea has distention and stuffiness in the chest and hypochondrium. Loose stools or diarrhea with undigested food, after intaking greasy food bowl movement increases, poor appetite, abdominal flatulence, sallow complexion, and tiredness.

Tongue: pale tongue with white coating.

Pulse: thread and weak pulse.

Analysis of clinical manifestations:

Loose stools or diarrhea with undigested food are due to deficiency of spleen and stomach deficiency, which cannot digest water and food or separate clear and turbid. Deficiency of the spleen yang and dysfunction of the spleen in governing movement and transformation leads to poor appetite, abdominal flatulence, and increased bowel movement after taking greasy food. Because of long-time diarrhea and deficiency of the spleen and stomach, the source of qi and blood lacks and patients can present with sallow complexion and tiredness. A pale tongue with a white coating and thread and weak pulse are indications of deficiency of the spleen and stomach.

5.26.3.7 Declination of Kidney Yang

Clinical manifestations:

Abdominal pain and borborygmus followed by diarrhea, pain relieved after diarrhea, cold body and limbs, and soreness of the waist and knees.

Tongue: pale tongue.

Pulse: deep and thread pulse.

Analysis of clinical manifestations:

Kidney yang is too weak to war.m spleen and stomach, leading to failure of the spleen in governing movement and transformation. Because yang qi has not been aroused before dawn and the cold is stronger, patients can have abdominal pain and borborygmus followed by diarrhea, which is also called "morning diarrhea." Pain will be relieved after diarrhea. Cold body and limbs, soreness of the waist and knees, pale tongue as well as deep and thread pulse are all indications of declination of kidney yang.

5.26.3.8 Deficiency of Both Qi and Yin

Clinical manifestations:

Long-term diarrhea with pus and bloody stools, dull pain in the abdomen, low fever in the afternoon, dizziness, insomnia, night sweating, restlessness, irritability, and emaciation.

Tongue: red tongue with less coating.

Pulse: thread and rapid pulse.

Analysis of clinical manifestations:

This type of diarrhea is usually based on the type of damp heat attacking the middle energizer. Because long-term diarrhea, qi, yin, and fluid are wasted, leading to dull pain in the abdomen and emaciation. Lack of qi and yin causes low fever in the afternoon, dizziness, insomnia, night sweating, restlessness, and irritability. Red tongue with less coating as well as thread and rapid pulse are indications of deficiency of both qi and yin.

5.26.4 Treatment

5.26.4.1 Treatment Principles

To clarify the pathogenic factor, the primary treatment is to dispel dampness, strengthen the spleen, adjust the middle energizer, straighten out liver qi, and warm kidney yang. Astringents are commonly used in long-term diarrhea also.

5.26.4.2 Chinese Medicinal Treatment

Damp Cold Attacking the Middle Energizer

Treatment Principle: to remove dampness, expel cold and heat with aromatic herbs.

Prescription: Huoxiang Zhengqi San.

Herbs: Huoxiang, Banxiaqu, Chenpi, Baizhu, Fuling, Houpo, Zisuye, Dafupi, Jiegeng, and Baizhi.

Administration: Take the herbals decoction for oral use, twice a day.

Explanation: Huoxiang: to warm cold and resolve dampness. Banxiaqu, Chenpi, Baizhu, and Fuling: invigorate the spleen and resolve phlegm.

Houpo: to invigorate the spleen and dry the qi and phlegm. Zisuye and Baizhi: to dispel cold to relieve the exterior syndrome. Dafupi: to refresh the spleen and resolve dampness.

Jiegeng: to disperse the lung qi and resolve phlegm.

Modification: If dampness is severely causing abdominal fullness, borborygmus, dripping, and lassitude, with white and greasy tongue coating, Weiling Tang should be used to invigorate the spleen to promote dieresis. Meanwhile, add Jingjie and Fangfeng; Baikouren (to be decocted later); Sharen (to be decocted later) and Paojiang.

Damp Heat Attacking the Middle Energizer

Treatment Principle: clearing heat away to disperse dampness and promote diuresis.
Prescription: Gegen Qinlian Tang.
Herbs: Gegen, Huangqin, Huanglian, Gancao.
Administration: Take the herbals decoction for oral use, twice a day.
Explanation: Gegen: to clear heat and release flesh.
Huangqin and Huanglian: to clear heat and resolve phlegm.
Gancao: to harmonize nutrient and defensive aspects.
Modification: In the case of an attack of summer heat dampness, which is fever, headache, thirst, scanty deep yellow urine, and soft-rapid pulse, Xinjia Xiangru Yin and Liuyi San should be used to clear summer heat dampness. For severe dampness with fullness in the abdomen, add Shichangpu and Fuling.

Food Retention

Treatment Principle: promoting digestion to benefit the spleen and relieve stagnation.
Prescription: Baohe Wan.
Herbs: Shanzha, Shenqu, Banxia, Fuling, Chenpi, and Laifuzi.
Administration: Take the herbals decoction for oral use, twice a day.
Explanation: Shanzha: to digest fatty food.
Shenqu: to pormote digestion.
Laifuzi: to assist stomach qi to downward.
Banxia, Chenpi, and Fuling: to regulate qi and resolve dampness.

Liver Qi Attacking the Spleen

Treatment Principle: to depress the wood (liver) and strengthen the earth (spleen), regulate the middle energizer, and relieve diarrhea.
Prescription: Tongxieyao Fang.
Herbs: Baizhu, Baishao, Chenpi, Fangfeng.
Administration: Take the herbals decoction for oral use, twice a day.

Explanation: Baizhu: to invigorate the spleen.

Baishao: to emolliate the liver and nourish the blood.

Chenpi: to invigorate the spleen and regulate qi.

Fangfeng: to ascend clear and relieve diarrhea.

Modification: For spleen deficiency with lassitude and loose stools, add Fuling and Shanyao; for recurrent diarrhea, add Mugua and Hezi.

Deficiency of the Spleen and Stomach

Treatment Principle: to invigorate the spleen and tonify qi, promote transportation, and relieve diarrhea.

Prescription: Shenling Baizhu San.

Herbs: Renshen, Baizhu, Fuling, Shanyao, Lanzirou, Biandou, Yiyiren, Suosharen, Jiegeng, Zhigancao.

Administration: Take the herbals decoction for oral use, twice a day.

Explanation: Renshen, Baizhu, Fuling, and Zhigancao: to nourish spleen qi.

Shanyao, Lanzirou, Biandou, Yiyiren, Suosharen, and Jiegeng: to nourish the spleen, eliminate dampness, and relieve diarrhea.

Modificaion: For declination of spleen yang with cold pain in the abdomen and cold limbs, add Shu Fuzi and Ganjiang: for long-term diarrhea, add Yingsuke and Hezi; for indigestion, add Maiya and Jianqu.

Declination of Kidney Yang

Treatment Principle: warm the kidney, strengthen the spleen, induce astringency, and relieve diarrhea.

Prescription: Sishen Wan.

Herbs: Buguzhi, Roudoukou, Wuzhuyu, Wuweizi, Shengjiang, Dazao.

Administration: Take the herbals decoction for oral use, twice a day.

Explanation: Buguzhi: to warm yang and nourish kidneys. Roudoukou and Wuzhuyu: to warm the interior and disperse cold.Wuweizi: to relieve diarrhea with astringents, Shengjiang: warming stomach for dispelling cold, Dazao: nourishing spleen and stomach.

Modification: For long-term diarrhea, and Yuyuliang, Yingsukeand Hezi.

Administration and dosage: twice daily.

Deficiency of Both Qi and Yin

Treatment Principle: to nourish yin, clear away heat, replenish qi, and relieve diarrhea.

Chinese medicinal treatment.

Prescription: Shengmai San and Liujunzi Tang Modification.

Herbs: Renshen, Maidong, Baizhu, Wuweizi, Fuling, Chenpi, Banxia, and Zhigancao.

Administration: Take the herbals decoction for oral use, twice a day.

Explanation: Renshen: to replenish qi to restore yang. Maidong and Wuweizi: to nourish yin and astringe yang. Dangshen, Baizhu, Fulin, and Zhigancao: to invigorate the spleen and replenish qi. Chenpi and Banxia: to direct qi and dispel phlegm.

Modification: For feverish sensation in the chest, palms, and soles, add Qinghao and Yinchaihu; for restlessness and insomnia, add Chaosuanzaoren, Huanglian, and Danshen; for dizziness, add Tianma and Zhenzhumu; for severe diarrhea, add Chishizhi and Yuyuliang; for red and white mucus in the stools, add Baihuasheshecao and Machixian.

5.26.4.3 Acupuncture and Moxibustion Treatment

Main acupoints: Tianshu (ST 25), Shangjuxu (ST 34), Shenque (CV 8), Dachangshu (BL 25), and Sanyinjiao (SP 6).

Methods: Apply indirect moxibustion with Shengjiang to Shenque (CV 8). Needle at Tianshu (ST 25), Sanyinjiao (SP 6), and Shangjuxu (ST 34) with reducing technique. The acupoints above are respectively needled perpendicularly at a depth of 1–2 cun, bringing about the local soreness and distention sensation. The needles are retained for 20–40 min.

Modification: in cases with cold–dampness: Yinlingquan (SP9) and Pishu (BL 20); food retention: Xiawan (CV 10), and Liangmen (ST 21); liver qi attacking the spleen: Qimen (LR 14) and Taichong (LR 3); deficiency of the spleen and stomach: Pishu(BL 20) and Zusanli (ST 36); declination of kidney yang: Shenshu (BL 23) and Mingmen (GV 4).

5.26.5 Prevention

During the treatment, patients with diarrhea should pay attention to dietary hygiene and develop a light diet. They should avoid raw, cold, spicy, or greasy food.

5.27 Summary

Diarrhea is a disease referring to frequent defecation with a bellyache, loose stool, and even water stool at times occurring in four seasons but mostly in summer and autumn.

Treatments for diarrhea are delivered according to the differentiation of five parts: external pathogenic factors, zang-fu viscera, improper diet, emotional upsets, and decline of kidney yang.

Acupuncture and moxibustion are effective therapies for diarrhea, especially for the deficiencies of spleen and kidney yang.

Questions
1. Describe the main characteristics of diarrhea.
2. What is the differentiation of diarrhea between zang-fu viscera and emotional upsets?
3. Describe the treatment principles and major prescriptions of different syndromes.

References
1. Gao T, Bai H, Zheng S. Traditional Chinese internal medicine. Beijing: China Press of Traditional Chinese Medicine; 2004.
2. Zuo Y. Internal medicine of traditional Chinese medicine. Shanghai: Shanghai Pujiaing Education Press; 2002.

5.28 Edema

Objectives
Master the etiology and pathogenesis of edema under the guidance of TCM theory.

Master the law of syndrome differentiation and treatment of edema under the guidance of TCM theory.

Guideline
This chapter introduces the etiology, pathogenesis, diagnosis, differential diagnosis, treatment (herbal medicine, acupuncture, and moxibustion), and prevention of edema.

5.29 Introduction

Edema is marked by abnormal fluid retention in the body, which affects the head, face, eyelids, limbs, abdomen and back, and even the whole body.

Edema, called "water" in the book of Internal Classic, could be divided into three syndromes: the Chinese terms "Fengshui," "Shishui," and "Yongshui." The treatment principles of edema were put forward in *Plain Questions*, "to dislodge blood stasis, open pores, and empty bladder." In the *Song* dynasty, edema was divided into "Yinshui" and "Yangshui" in Chinese terms.

In Western medicine, the relevant disease includes acute and chronic glomerulonephritis, nephrotic syndrome, and secondary glomerulonephropathy.

5.29.1 Etiology

Edema is a morbid condition caused by invasion of pathogenic wind, damp toxin, water-dampness, dampness-heat, and improper diet, which result in dysfunction of the lung to regulate the water passage, the spleen to govern the transport and transform body fluids, the kidney to regulate water metabolism, and qi transformation in the urinary bladder to control urination, thus giving rise to abnormal fluid retention in the body and further involving the muscles and skin.

5.29.2 Pathogenesis

Invasion of pathogenic wind, noxious dampness, water and dampness, improper diet, prolonged illness, stress, and anxiety are considered as the main reasons for edema. It usually occurs when the function of qi activity is declined. In the aspect of purtenance, the transportation and transformation of body fluids are related to the lungs, spleen, and kidneys, but kidneys are more significant to edema. Besides, if there exists blood stasis and the functioning of the triple energizers is impaired, edema will be obstinate and need prolonged treatment. Edema may be seen in acute and chronic glomerulonephritis, nephritic syndrome, congestive heart failure, endocrine disturbance, and dystrophy in Western medicine.

5.29.3 Diagnosis

Edema usually begins from the eyelids or lower limbs and then spreads to four limbs and the entire body. In mild cases, there may be light swelling around the eyelids or in the tibia while in severe cases, generalized swelling, abdominal fullness and enlargement, and asthmatic breathing with an inability to lie supine may be present. In even more severe cases, retention of urine, nausea, vomiting, foul breath, nasal bleeding, atrophy of the gum, or even headache, convulsion, coma, and delirium may occur.

The patient may have a history of tonsillitis, palpitation, septicemia or purpura, or invalidism.

Urine routine examination, 24-h quantitative determination of urinary protein, blood routine examination, determination of blood sedimentation rate, plasma albumin, creatinine, urea nitrogen in blood and humoral immunity, as well as electrocardiography, cardiac functional test and B-type ultrasonic examination for the kidneys are the necessary means in the diagnosis of edema.

5.29.4 Differentiation

5.29.4.1 Major Points

In making the diagnosis of edema, it is essential to clarify whether the complaint is edema of the yang type or edema of the yin type. Usually, the yang-type edema is characterized by a short duration, rapid development, and more pronounced edema on the head and face with the skin shiny and thin. However, the yin-type edema is marked by a longer duration, a gradual development, more pronounced pitted edema of lower limbs, and sallow and grayish skin.

5.29.4.2 Invasion by Wind and Overflow of Water

Clinical Manifestations:

Acute onset, edema starting from the eyelids, followed by four limbs and the whole body, aversion to cold, fever, soreness of the limbs and joints, dysuria, etc.

Tongue: thin white tongue coating.

Pulse: superficial, smooth, or superficial, tense pulse.

Analysis of clinical manifestations:

Edema and dysuria are caused by wind attacking the exterior. Wind evil, mobile, and changeable, usually attacks the yang portion of the body, so edema often starts from the eyelids, followed by four limbs and the whole body. Pathogenic qi stuck on the exterior blocks the movement of wei qi, so patients can have an aversion to cold, fever, and soreness of the limbs and joints. In the case of predominant wind heat, there may also be swelling and pain in the throat, red tongue, and superficial, smooth, and rapid pulse. In cases with predominant wind cold, aversion to cold, cough, and dyspnea.

5.29.4.3 Retention of Noxious Dampness

Clinical manifestations:

Edema of the eyelids followed by generalized edema, dysuria, pyogenic infection, or even ulceration of the skin, and fever with aversion to wind.

Tongue: red tongue with thin yellow coating.

Pulse: superficial, rapid, or smooth, rapid pulse.

Analysis of clinical manifestations:

Being the primary pathogen, wind evil is often combined with other diseases, so edema often starts from the eyelids, followed by four limbs and the whole body, and patients can have a fever with aversion to wind. Noxious dampness flows into the lung and spleen, damaging the function of the lung in governing the regulation of water passages and the spleen in governing water and dampness, which leads to dysuria, pyogenic infection, or even ulceration of the skin. Red tongue with a thin yellow coating as well as superficial, rapid, or smooth, rapid pulse are indications of retention of noxious dampness.

5.29.4.4 Rententin of Water and Dampness

Clinical manifestations:

Pitted edema of the whole body, scanty urine, heaviness of the body, feeling of oppression in the chest, poor appetite, and nausea.

Tongue: greasy white tongue coating.

Pulse: deep, even-soft pulse.

Analysis of clinical manifestations:

Water and dampness stagnate on the skin and the interior, damaging the function of sanjiao and bladder in transformation, which causes pitted edema of the whole body and scanty urine. The pathogen also disturbs the spleen yang and spleen qi, resulting in the heaviness of the body, a feeling of oppression in the chest, poor appetite, and nausea. Greasy white tongue coating and deep, even-soft pulse are indications of retention of water and dampness.

5.29.4.5 Excess of Dampness–Heat

Clinical manifestations:

General edema with the skin shiny and taut, fullness in the chest and abdomen, restless fever, thirst, scanty deep yellow urine, or dry stools.

Tongue: red tongue with a yellow greasy coating.

Pulse: deep, rapid, or soft-superficial, rapid pulse.

Analysis of clinical manifestations:

General edema with the skin shiny and taut is due to long-term dampness-water turning into heat or dampness-heat stagnation on skin or in meridians. Fullness in the chest and abdomen may be caused by dampness-heat stagnation in sanjiao which disturbs the movement of qi. If heat predominates, fluid could be wasted and patients may have restless fever, thirst, scanty deep yellow urine, or dry stools. Red tongue with yellow greasy coating as well as deep, rapid or soft-superficial, rapid pulse are indications of excess dampness–heat.

5.29.4.6 Deficiency of Spleen Yang

Clinical Manifestations:

General pitted edema which is more pronounced below the loins, abdominal flatulence, impaired appetite, loose stools, lusterless complexion, lassitude, cold limbs, and a small amount of urine.

Tongue: pale tongue with greasy white coating or smooth white coating.

Pulse: deep, even-soft, or deep, weak pulse.

Analysis of clinical manifestations:

General pitted edema which is more pronounced below the loins, abdominal flatulence, impaired appetite, and loose stools may be caused by dysfunction of the spleen in governing water due to deficiency of spleen yang. Lusterless complexion, lassitude, and cold limbs are results of lack of qi and blood generated by the spleen due to deficiency of spleen yang, too. Spleen yang cannot transform to spleen qi, so patients have little urine. A pale tongue with a greasy white coating or smooth white coating as well as a deep, even-soft, or deep, weak pulse are indications of deficiency of spleen yang.

5.29.4.7 Deficiency of Kidney Yang

Clinical manifestations:

General pitted edema which is more pronounced below the loins, palpitation, short breath, soreness and heaviness in the loins, decreased quantity of urine, cold limbs, aversion to cold, lassitude, and pale or grayish dim complexion.

Tongue: pale and swollen tongue with white tongue coating.

Pulse: deep and thread or deep, slow, and forceless pulse.

Analysis of clinical manifestations:

A deficiency of kidney yang leads to a deficiency of kidney qi, so water and dampness flow downward and edema is generally pitted and more pronounced below the loins. Water pathogen insults the heart, so patients may have palpitation and shortness of breath. Waist, the house of the kidney, could feel soreness and heaviness because of deficiency of kidney yang. The kidney and bladder share the relationship of exterior and interior, so a deficiency of kidney yang may cause dysfunction of the bladder in qi transformation and decreased quantity of urine. Lack of kidney yang can also cause cold limbs, aversion to coldness, lassitude, and pale or grayish dim complexion. A pale and swollen tongue with white tongue coating as well as deep and thread or deep, slow, and forceless pulse are indications of deficiency of kidney yang.

5.29.5 Treatment Principles

The treatment for the yang-type should aim at eliminating pathogenic factors, with such methods as diaphoresis and diuresis. When necessary, purgation should be used. For the yin-type, it is advisable to support healthy qi to eliminate pathogenic factors, for instance, to promote diuresis by invigorating the spleen and warming the kidneys. If edema is persistent, promoting diuresis by activating blood circulation and dissipating blood stasis is recommended as the accessory treatment.

5.29.5.1 Chinese Medicinal Treatment

Invasion by Wind and Overflow of Water

Treatment Principle: eliminating wind, dispersing lung qi, and circulating water to relieve edema.

Prescription: Yuebi Jiazhu Tang.

Herbs: Mahuang, Shigao (to be decocted first), Xingren, Baizhu, Fuling, and Zexie.

Administration: Take the herbals decoction for oral use, twice a day.

Explanation:

Mahuang, Shigao, Xingren, Fuling, and Zexie: to induce sweating to release the exterior.

Baizhu: to clear damp and promot diuresis.

Modification: For the predominance of wind heat, add Lianqiao, Jiegeng, Banlangen, and Xianmaogen; for the predominance of wind cold, remove Shigao and add Zisuye, Guizhi, and Fangfeng; for severe cough and dyspnea, add Qianhu and Ziyuan; and for sweating with an aversion to wind and defensive qi, add Fangji and Huangqi.

Retention of Noxious Dampness

Treatment Principle: to disperse lung qi, remove toxic substances, and promote diuresis to relieve edema.

Prescription: Modified Mahuang Lianqiao Chixiaodou Tang and Wuwei Xiaodu Yin.

Herbs: Mahuang, Xingren, Sangbaipi, Chixiaodou, Jinyinhua, Lianqiao, Yejuhua, Pugongying, Zihuadiding, and Zibeitiankui.

Administration: Take the herbals decoction for oral use, twice a day.

Explanation:

Mahuang and Xingren: to release the exterior with acrid-warm.

Sangbaipi, Chixiaodou, Lianqiao, Jinyinhua, Yejuhua, Pugongying, Zihuadidingand Zibeitiankui: to clear away heat and toxic material.

Modification: For predominant dampness with skin ulceration, add Kushen and Tufuling; for predominant wind with itching, add Baixianpi and Difuzi; for blood heat with red and swollen skin, add Mudanpi; and for constipation, add Shengdahuang (to be decorated later) and Mangxiao (to be infused separately).

Retention of Water and Dampness

Treatment Principle: to invigorate the spleen, eliminate dampness, activate yang, and promote diuresis.

Prescription: Modified Wupi Yin and Weiling Tang.

Herbs: Cangzhu, Houpo, Chenpi, Guizhi, Fuling, Zexie, Shengjiangpi, and Dafupi.

Administration: Take the herbals decoction for oral use, twice a day.

Explanation:

Cangzhu, Houpo, Chenpi, and Shengjiangpi: to clear dampness and harmonize the stomach.

Fuling, Zexie, Dafupi, and Guizhi: to induce diuresis to alleviate edema.

Modification: For severe edema with asthma, add Mahuang and Xingren.

Excess of Dampness–Heat

Treatment Principle: to clear away heat, promote dieresis, and regulate qi circulation.
 Prescription: Shuzao Yinzi modification.
 Herbs: Mutong, Zexie, Fulingpi, Chixiaodou, Huangbai, Zhuling, Shanglu, Binglang, Cangzhu, and Shengyiren.
 Administration: Take the herbals decoction for oral use, twice a day.
 Explanation:
 Mutong, Zexie, Fulingpi, Zhuling, Shanglu, Binglang and Chixiaodou: to induce diuresis to alleviate edema.
 Huangbai, Cangzhu, and Shengyiren: to dry dampness and strengthen the spleen.
 Modification: For abdominal flatulence and constipation, add Shengdahuang and Tinglizi; for retention of damp heat in the urinary bladder damaging the blood vessels, manifested as painful urination and hematuria, add Daji, Xiaoji, and Baimaogen; for severe edema accompanied by chest oppression, asthmatic breathing, inability to lie supine, and wiry, forceful pulse, add Tinglizi, Xingren, and Fangji; and for long-standing retention of damp heat transforming into dryness which further damages yin, manifested as dry mouth and throat, and dry stools, add Zhuling, Huashi, Maimendong, and Ejiao.

Deficiency of Spleen Yang

Treatment Principle: to warm and invigorate spleen yang so as to promote diuresis.
 Chinese medicinal treatment:
 Prescription: Modified Shipi Yin.
 Herbs: Ganjiang, Caoguo, Baizhu, Fuling, Jiaomu, Houpo, Muxiang, and Dafupi.
 Administration: Take the herbals decoction for oral use, twice a day.
 Explanation:
 Zhifuzi and Ganjiang: to warm nourishing spleen and kidney.
 Baizhu and Fuling: to dry dampness and strengthen the spleen.
 Caoguo, Jiaomu, Houpo, Muxiang, and Dafupi: to refresh the spleen and resolve dampness.
 Modification: For short breath and weak voice, add Danshen and Huangqi; for a small amount of urine, add Guizhi and Zexie.

Deficiency of Kidney Yang

Treatment Principle: to warm the kidney, assist yang, and activate qi to promote dieresis.

Prescription: Modified Jisheng Shenqi Wan and Zhenwu Tang.

Herbs: Zhifuzi, Rougui, Bajitian, Yinyanghuo, Baizhu, Fuling, Zexie, Cheqianzi, Niuxi, and Shanyao.

Administration: Take the herbals decoction for oral use, twice a day.

Explanation:

Zhifuzi, Rougui, Bajitian, and Yinyanghuo: to warm yang for resolving fluid retention.

Baizhu, Fuling and Zexie: to clear damp and promote diuresis.

Cheqianzi: to clear away heat and promote diuresis.

Niuxi: to nourish yin and nourish kidney.

Shanyao: to invigorate the liver and benefit the spleen.

Modification: If there is palpitation, cyanotic lips, feeble pulse, or slow-irregular and intermittent pulse, increase Zhifuzi and add Guizhi, Zhigancao, and Danshen. If there is asthmatic breathing, sweating, and superficial, feeble, and rapid pulse, add Hongshen (to be decocted separately), Gejiefen (to be infused separately), Wuweizi, Shanzhuyu, Muli (to be decocted first), and Longgu (to be decocted first). If the deficiency of kidney yang is persistent, it impairs yin, giving rise to deficiency of kidney yin. In this case, there appear such manifestations as recurrence of edema, lassitude, soreness in the loins, nocturnal emission, dry mouth and throat, feverish sensation in the palms, soles, and chest, red tongue and thready, and rapid pulse. The treatment should aim at nourishing kidney yin and promoting diaresis concurrently. The alternative prescription is Shanyao, Shanzhuyu, Gouqizi, Mudanpi, Zexie, and Fuling.

5.29.5.2 Acupuncture and Moxibustion

Main acupoints: Sanjiaoshu (BL 22), Shuifen (CV 9), Weiyang (BL 39), Shuidao (ST 28), and Yinlingquan (SP 9).

Methods: The acupuncture manipulation is the same as type one. Yingshui adds moxibustion.

Modification: Yangshui: Feishu (BL 13) and Lieque (LU 7); Yinshui: Sanyinjiao (SP 6) and Guanyuan (CV 4).

5.29.6 Prevention

Patients with edema should develop a regular life style and try to avoid getting cold or tired. During treatment, sexual activity should be abstinent.

5.30   Summary

Edema refers to abnormal fluid retention of the head, face, eyelids, limbs, abdomen and back, and even the whole body. It is a morbid condition caused by invasion of pathogenic factors, improper diet, or overstrain, which results in failure of the lungs, spleen, kidneys, and qi.

Treatments for edema are delivered according to the differentiation of three parts: zang-fu viscera and meridians, yin type and yang type, and disease stages.

Acupuncture and moxibustion are effective therapies for edema, especially for edema in the lower limbs.

Questions
1. Describe the main characteristics of edema.
2. What is the differentiation of edema between zang-fu viscera and meridians?
3. Describe the treatment principles and major prescriptions of different syndromes.

Reference
1. Tianshu G, Hua B, Shuqin Z. Traditional Chinese internal medicine. Beijing: China Press of Traditional Chinese Medicine; 2004.

Appendixes

Brief Introduction to Classics

Basic Classics

(Huangdi's) Internal Classic
Written in the *Spring and Autumn* states by numerous experts, it is China's earliest comprehensive traditional medical work including two parts, *Plain Questions*and *Miraculous Pivot*.

Classic of Difficult Issues

Written in the *Western Han* dynasty by *Qin Yueren* (*Bian Que*), it is also known as *Classic on 81 Medical Problems*, which includes a total of eighty-one difficult issues and covers the basic theory of Chinese traditional medicine through questions and answers.

Treatise on Cold Damage Diseases

Written in the *Eastern Han* dynasty by *Zhang Zhongjing*, it is a monograph on the treatment of exogenous disease.

Synopsis of Golden Chamber

Written in the *Eastern Han* dynasty by *Zhang Zhongjing*, it is the earliest extant monograph on diagnosing and treating diseases.

© Zhengzhou University Press 2024
Y. Huang, L. Zhu (eds.), *Textbook of Traditional Chinese Medicine*,
https://doi.org/10.1007/978-981-99-5299-1

Treatise on the Pathogenesis and Manifestations of All Diseases

Written in the *Sui* dynasty by *Cao Yuanfang*, it is a monograph on the origins and manifestations of diseases.

Chinese Medicinal Classics

Shennong's Classic of Materia Medica

Written in the *EasternHan* dynasty by numerous experts, it is the earliest extant monograph on science of Chinese Materia Medica.

Variorum of the Classic of Materia Medica

Written in the *Liang* dynasty by *Tao Hongjing*, it is written on the basis of *Shennong's Classic of Materia Medica*, adding 365 kinds of medicine.

Newly Revised Materia Medica

Written in the *Tang* dynasty by *Li Ji*, *Su Jing* and other 23 people following the Emperor's order, it is China's first pharmacopoeia promulgated by the government.

Classified Emergency Materia Medica

Written in the *Northern Song* dynasty by *Tang Shenwei*, it is a brilliant monograph on collective Materia Medica.

Compendium of Materia Medica

Written in the *Ming* dynasty by *Li Shizhen*, it includes 1892 kinds of medicine.

Prescription Classics Lei's Treatise on Processing of Drugs

Written in the *Northern* and *Southern* dynasties by *Lei Xiao*, it is China's earliest science of Chinese medicine processing.

Prescriptions for Fifty-Two Diseases

Written in the *Warrior States* period, it is China's earliest extant medical classics.

Handbook of Prescriptions for Emergencies

Written in the *Eastern Jin* dynasty by *Ge Hong*, it is China's first monograph on the clinical emergency treatment.

Essential Prescriptions Worth a Thousand Gold for Emergencies

Written in the *Tang* dynasty by *Sun Simiao*, it is the first medical encyclopedia in China.

Supplement to the Essential Prescriptions Worth a Thousand Gold

Arcane Essentials from the Imperial Library

Written in the *Tang* dynasty by *Wang Tao*, it is a compilation on medical works in the *Tang* dynasty.

Prescriptions from the Great Peace Imperial Grace Pharmacy

Written in the *Song* dynasty by Taiping People's Welfare Bureau, it is the first official medicine standard.

Effective Formulas Handed Down for Generations

Written in the *Yuan* dynasty by *Wei Yilin*, it contains a total of more than 3300 prescriptions, including internal medicine, surgery, gynecology, pediatrics, orthopedics, otolaryngology and other diseases in TCM.

Diagnostic Classics

Pulse Classic

Written in the *Jin* dynasty by *Wang Shuhe*, it is a brilliant monograph on sphygmology before the *Han* dynasty.

Essentials for Diagnosticians

Written in the *Yuan* dynasty by *Hua Shou*, the book was written by combining pulse theory before *Yuan* dynasty and private insight.

Binhu's Sphygmology

Written in the *Ming* dynasty by *Li Shizhen*, this book discusses 27 kinds of pulse conditions.

Pulse Diagnosticians

Written in *Ming* dynasty by *Li Zhongzi*, it is a work on the basic theory and clinical application of the pulse.

Obey the Rules of Inspection

Written in the *Qing* dynasty by *Wang Hong*, it is an all-around monograph on inspection.

Internal Medicine Classics

Confucian's Duties to Their Parents

Written in the *Jin* dynasty by *Zhang Congzheng*, it charts *Zhang Congzheng*'s academic thinking and clinical experience.

The Origin of Medicine

Written by in the *Jin* dynasty *Zhang Yuansu*, it expounds zang-fu viscrea, meridians, pathogeny and the law of the treatment.

Treatise on the Spleen and Stomach

Written in the *Jin* dynasty by *Li Dongyuan*, it is his representative work of his theory on spleen- stomach.

Treatise on Inquiring the Properties of Things

Written in the *Yuan* dynasty by *Zhu Zhenheng*, it is a collection of medical journals by Zhu and puts forward the famous academic viewpoints such as the theory of ministerial fire, the theory of yang in excess and yin in asthenia and so on.

Complete Works of Jingyue

Written in the *Ming* dynasty by *Zhang Jiebin*, it is a famous book, combining ancient medical experts' and his own experience.

Systematized Identification of Warm Diseases

Written in the *Qing* dynasty by *Wu Tang* in 1798, it is a work on warm diseases.

Treatise on Warm-Heat Diseases

Transcribed in the *Qing* dynasty from *Ye Gui*'s dictation, it is a foundational work on warm diseases.

Classified Patterns Clear- Cut Treatments

Written in the *Qing* dynasty by *Lin Peiqin*, it is a work on practice in internal medicine.

Correction of Errors in Medical Classics

Written in the Qing dynasty by *Wang Qingren*, it corrects some thinking of the ancients on anatomy and physiology.

Secret Formulary Bestowed by Immortals for Treating Injuries and Mending Fractures

Written in the *Tang* dynasty by *Lin Daoren*, it is a monograph on orthopedics and traumatology during the early period in China.

Orthodox Manual of External Medicine

Written in the *Ming* dynasty by *Chen Shigong*, it is a monograph on orthopedics and traumatology.

Essence on the Silvery Sea

Written in the *Ming* dynasty, it is a monograph on ophthalmology.

Longmu's Secret Treatiseon Ophthalmology

Written in the *Song* and *Yuan* dynasty, it concludes the general theory of ophthalmology and the treatment and prescription of 72 kinds of eye diseases.

Gynaecology and Pediatrics Classics

Tested Treasures in Obstetrics

Written in the *Tang* dynasty by *Zan Yin*, it is the earliest extant monograph on obstetrics and covers the treatment of various diseases for women during the period from pregnancy to puerperium.

Compendium of Effective Prescriptions for Women

Written in the Song dynasty by *Chen Ziming*, it is the first all-round monograph on gynecology and obstetrics.

Fu Qingzhu's Obstetrics and Gynecology

Written in the *Qing* dynasty by *Fu Shan*, it is a famous work on gynecology.

Synopsis of Treating Women's Diseases

Written in the *Ming* dynasty by *Wu Zhiwang*, it is a monograph on gynecology.

Standards of Syndrome Identification and Treatment

Written in the *Ming* dynasty by *Wang Kentang*, it is a monograph on gynecology.

Key to Therapeutics of Children's Diseases

Written in the *Song* dynasty by *Qian Yi*, it is a monograph on pediatrics.

Acupuncture Classics

Huangdi's Bright Hall Moxibustion Classic

Written in the *Tang* dynasty, it covers the acupuncture methods of the general points for adults and children.

Systematic Classic of Acupuncture and Moxibustion

Written in the *Western Jin* dynasty by *Huangfu Mi*, it sums up science of acupuncture and moxibustion again after *Internal Classic*.

Treatise on the Eight Extra Meridians

Written in the *Ming* dynasty by *Li Shizhen*, it is a monograph on eight extra meridians.

Elucidation of the Fourteen Meridians

Written in the *Yuan* dynasty by *Hua Shou*, it is a monograph on meridians.

Complete Compendium of Acupuncture and Moxibustion

Written in the *Ming* dynasty by *Yang Jizhou*, it compiles the ancients' academic viewpoints and experience on acupuncture and moxibustion.

Prescriptions

Pingyin	English	Chinese
Exterior-releasing prescription		
Mahuang Tang	Ephedra decoction	麻黄汤
Guizhi Tang	Cinnamon twig decoction	桂枝汤
Xiaoqinglong Tang	Small blue dragon decoction	小青龙汤
Yinqiao San	Lonicera and forsythia powder	银翘散
Heat-cleaning prescription		
Baihu Tang	White tiger decoction	白虎汤
Qingying Tang	Decoction for cleaning heat in nutrient aspect	清营汤
Huanglian Jiedu Tang	Decoction of coptis for detoxification	黄连解毒汤
Purgative prescription		
Dachengqi Tang	Major purgative decoction	大承气汤
Wenpi Tang	Warming spleen decoction	温脾汤
Jichuan Jian	Blood replenishing decoction	济川煎
Wind-dispelling prescription		
Chuanxiong Chatiao San	Ligusticum powder	川芎茶调散
Duhuo Jisheng Tang	Pubescent Angelica and Taxillus decoction	独活寄生汤
Tianma Gouteng Yin	Gastrodia and Uncaria decoction	天麻勾藤饮
Dampness-draining prescription		
Huoxiang Zhengqi San	Patchouli Qi-restoring powder	霍香正气散
Yinchenhao Tang	Oriental wormwood decoction	茵陈蒿汤
Wuling San	Five Poria powder	五苓散
Digestant prescription		
Baohe Wan	Harmony-preserving pill	保和丸
Phlegm-dispelling and cough-suppressing prescription		
Erchen Tang	Two old ingredients decoction	二陈汤
Qingqi Huatan Wan	Clear heat and dispel phlegm pill	清气化痰丸
Suzi Jiangqi Tang	Perilla fruit decoction for directing Qi downward	苏子降气汤
Warm-interior prescription		
Lizhong Wan	Middle-regulating pill	理中丸
Sini Tang	Resuscitation decoction	四逆汤
Qi-regulating prescription		
Yueju Wan	Relieving stagnation pill	越鞠丸

Pingyin	English	Chinese
Chaihu Shugan San	Bupleurum soothing liver powder	柴胡疏肝散
Banxia Houpo Tang	Pinellia and Magnolia decoction	半夏厚朴汤
Blood-regulating prescription		
Xuanfu Zhuyu Tang	Expelling chest stasis decoction	血府逐瘀汤
Buyang Huanwu Tang	Tonifying Yang and Returning five decoction	补阳还五汤
Tranquilizing prescription		
Suanzaoren Tang	Wild jujube seed decoction	酸枣仁汤
Tonifying and replenishing prescription		
Sijunzi Tang	Four gentlemen decoction	四君子汤
Buzhongyiqi Tang	Tonify and replenish middle Qi decoction	补中益气汤
Siwu Tang	Four Ingreddients decoction	四物汤
Guipi Tang	Fortifying spleen decoction	归脾汤
Liuwei Dihuang Wan	Six Ingreddients with Rehmanniae pill	六味地黄丸
Shenqi Wan	Kidney Qi pill	肾气丸
Astringent prescription		
Muli San	Oyster Shell powder	牡蛎散
Harmonizing prescription		
Xiaochaihu Tang	Minor bupleurum decoction	小柴胡汤
Xiaoyao San	Ease powder	逍遥散
Banxia Xiexin Tang	Pinellia heart-draining decoction	半夏泻心汤
Resuscitative prescription		
Angong Niuhuang Wan	Peaceful palace bezoar pill	安宫牛黄丸

Manipulations

English	Chinese Pinyin
Rubbing manipulation	Mo fa
Five mimic-animal exercise	Wu Qin Xi
Tendons along twelve meridians	Jing jin theory
Muscle and bones theory	Jin gu theory

English	Chinese Pinyin
Shaolin internal cultivation exercise	Shaolin Neigong
Sinew-transforming exercise	Yi Jin Jing
Massage practice	Massage gong fa
Qi-concentrated single-finger pushing manipulation	Yi zhi chan tui fa
Rolling manipulation	Gun fa
Kneading manipulation	Rou fa
Palm-base kneading manipulation	Zhang gen rou fa
Major thenar kneading manipulation	Da yu ji rou fa
Finger kneading manipulation	Zhi rou fa
Forearm kneading manipulation	Qian bi rou fa
Circular rubbing manipulations	Mo fa
Palm circular rubbing manipulation	Zhang mo fa
Finger circular rubbing manipulation	Zhi mo fa
Pushing manipulation	Tui fa
Separating pushing manipulation	Fen Tui
Scrubbing manipulation	Ca fa
Pressing manipulation	An fa
Grasping manipulation	Na fa
Patting manipulation	Pai fa
Knocking manipulation	Ji fa
Shaking manipulation	Dou fa
Twisting manipulation with both palms	Cuo fa
Vibrating manipulation	Zhen fa
Rotating manipulation	Yao fa
Pulling-stretching manipulation	Ba shen fa
Grasping-kneading manipulation	Na rou fa
Thumb-pushing and circular-rubbing manipulation	Tui mo fa
Sweeping manipulation	Sao san fa

Pediatric Tuina

English	Chinese Pinyin
Pinching of the two sides of spine	Nie ji fa
Pressing, rubbing, pinching, circularly pushing, kneading, pushing, nipping and pounding	An, Mo, Qia, Yun, Rou, Tui, Nie, and Dao
Gate of sky	Tianmen
Cervical column	Tianzhu
Four transverse creases	Sihengwen
Small palmar transverse crease	Zhangxiaohengwen
Small transverse crease	Xiaohengwen
Major thenar	Banmen
Small center of sky	Xiaotianxin

English	Chinese Pinyin
Triple pass	Sanguan
The river in sky	Tianheshui
The ulnar side of palmar transverse striation at wrist	Yinchi
Six fu viscera	Liufu
Double gate	Ershanmen
Climbing upon the horse	Shangma
Lower abdomen	Dantian
Side of abdomen	Dujiao
Seven lunbosacral vertebrae	Qijiegu
Coccyx	Guiwei
Oblique pulling of the cervical vertebra	Jing zhui xie ban fa
Positioning rotating-pulling of the cervical vertebra	Jing zhui ding wei xuan zhuan ban fa
Positioning rotating-pulling of the thoracic-vertebrae	Xiong zhui xuan zhuan ding wei ban fa
Antagonistic reduction of thoracic vertebrae	Xiong zhui dui Kang fu wei fa
Positioning rotating-pulling of the lumbar vertebrae in sitting position	Yao zhui zuo wei ding wei xuan zhuan ban fa
Oblique pulling of the lumbar vertebrae	Yao zhui xie ban fa
Backward stretching and pulling of the lumbar vertebrae	Yao zhui hou shen ban fa
Six healing sounds	Liu Zi Jue
Eight-sectioned exercise	Ba Duan Jin
'Way' or 'path'	Tao
Muscle and tendon changing qigong	Yi Jin Jing
Inner kongfu	Neigong quan

Taichi 24 Actions

English	Chinese pinyin
Starting posture	Qi shi
Part the wild horse's mane on both sides	Zuoyou yema fenzong
White crane spreads its wings	Bai he Liang chi
Brush knees and step forward left and right	Zuo you lou xi ao bu
Playing the lute	Shou hui pi pa
Reverse reeling forearm left and right	Zuo you daojuan gong
Left grasp sparrow's tail	Zuo lan que wei
Ward off	Peng
Rollback	Lv
Press	Ji
Push	An
Right grasp sparrow's tail	You lan que wei

English	Chinese pinyin
Single whip	Dan bian
Cloud hands	Yun shou
High pat on horse	Gao tan ma
Right heel kick	You deng jiao
Strike to ears with both fists	Shuang feng guan er
Turn body and left heel kick	Zhuan shen zuo deng jiao
Left lower body and stand on one leg	Zuo xia shi du li
Right lower body and stand on one leg	You xia shi du li
Shuttle back and forth	Zuo you chuan suo
Needle at sea bottom	Hai di zhen
Fan through back	Shan tong bi
Turn body, deflect, parry, and punch	Zhuan shen ban lan chui
Apparent close-up	Ru feng si bi
Cross hands	Shi zi shou
Closing	Shou shi

Printed in the United States
by Baker & Taylor Publisher Services